SPEECH & AUDIOLOGY DEPARTMENT
CHARLOTTE INSTITUTE OF REHABILITATION
1100 BLYTHE BOULEVARD
CHARLOTTE, NC 28203

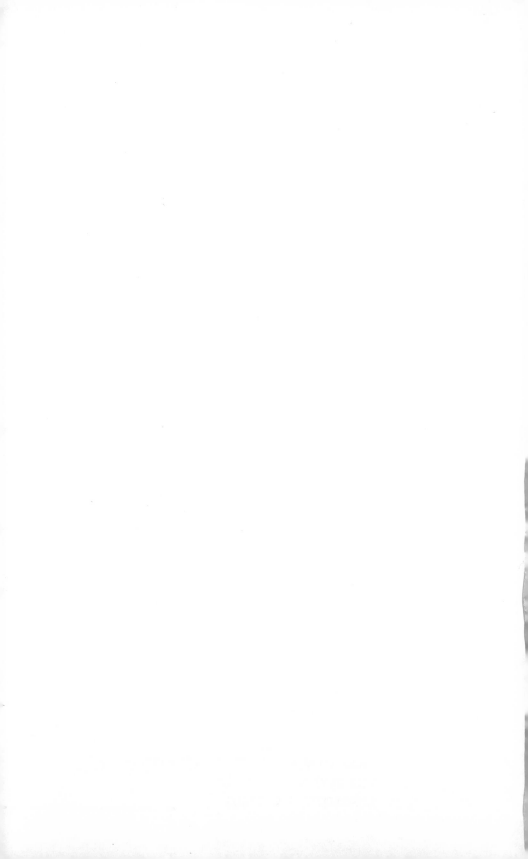

Handbook
of
Neurological
Speech and
Language
Disorders

NEUROLOGICAL DISEASE AND THERAPY

Series Editor

WILLIAM C. KOLLER

Department of Neurology
University of Kansas Medical Center
Kansas City, Kansas

Handbook of Neurological Speech and Language Disorders

edited by
Howard S. Kirshner

Vanderbilt University School of Medicine
Nashville, Tennessee

Marcel Dekker, Inc.   New York • Basel • Hong Kong

Library of Congress Cataloging-in-Publication Data

Handbook of neurological speech and language disorders / edited by
  Howard S. Kirshner.
      p.   cm. — (Neurological disease and therapy ; 33)
    Includes bibliographical references and index.
    ISBN 0-8247-9282-3 (alk. paper)
    1. Language disorders.   2. Speech disorders.   I. Kirshner, Howard
  S. II. Series: Neurological disease and therapy ; v. 33.
    [DNLM: 1. Aphasia—diagnosis. 2. Aphasia—therapy. 3. Language
  Disorders.   W1 NE33LD v. 33 1995 / WL 340.5 H236 1995]
  RC423.H3263   1995
  616.85'52—dc20
  DNLM/DLC
  for Library of Congress   94-33915
                                                                       CIP

The publisher offers discounts on this book when ordered in bulk quantities.
For more information, write to Special Sales/Professional Marketing at the
address below.

This book is printed on acid-free paper.

Marcel Dekker, Inc.
270 Madison Avenue, New York, New York   10016

Current printing (last digit):
10   9   8   7   6   5   4   3   2   1

PRINTED IN THE UNITED STATES OF AMERICA

Series Introduction

The *Handbook of Neurological Speech and Language Disorders* addresses an important area of neurological science and clinical medicine. The first section of the book deals with aphasia, lower motor neuron speech disorders, and apraxia of speech. The topic of vocalization is addressed, as well as basic scanning procedures, including PET. Various types of aphasic syndromes, including conduction and naming, are discussed in detail. Disorders of writing, speaking, and alexias are addressed in separate chapters. Aphasia in special circumstances, such as in the old, in the young, and related to closed head trauma, is discussed in separate chapters that will be of particular interest to the clinician. Testing used in aphasic patients is discussed as well as therapeutic approaches to the patient with aphasia.

This book is in keeping with this series of handbooks in providing in-depth, basic and clinical knowledge. The clinician will find this book exceedingly helpful when evaluating patients with language and speech disorders in the clinic.

William C. Koller

Preface

As the 21st century approaches, an update on neurological speech and language disorders seems especially timely. The subject has always had obvious importance, dealing with the relationships of language symbols to thought, to the workings of the brain, and to the practical ability of human beings to communicate with one another. Language was the first "higher" function to be correlated with brain pathology, and the study of language has led the way in mind/brain and brain/behavior correlations. Disorders of speech and language create medical, psychological, and social disruptions that challenge the expertise of numerous specialists, including neurologists, neurosurgeons, psychologists, speech–language pathologists, physical and occupational therapists, social workers, and nurses. Linguists and cognitive psychologists, among others, have studied aphasic patients to discover what the loss of language function can teach us about the organization of language in the brain. All these professional groups have contributed to our understanding of speech and language disorders and our ability to help patients.

In keeping with the congressional designation of the 1990s as the "Decade of the Brain," several converging areas of research promise a new era of progress in speech and language disorders. While 19th- and early 20th-century physicians studied language by describing single cases and correlating them with autopsy findings, new neurodiagnostic technologies now make possible the delineation of lesions causing aphasia in "real time," in the living patient.

Computerized tomographic (CT) scanning, introduced in the United States in 1973, allows the immediate mapping of brain lesions causing aphasia. Magnetic resonance imaging (MRI) provides even more precise localization, without need for X-ray exposure or administration of iodinated contrast agents. Positron emission tomography (PET) allows visualization of the functional activity of brain regions, according to blood flow or metabolism, in both normal subjects and patients with language disorders, both at rest and during language tasks. Electrophysiological techniques such as brain stimulation with subdural electrodes permit mapping of cortical neurons involved in speech and language. These neuroscientific and technological advances permit the topographical analysis of language-related structures at a level of precision only dreamed of previously.

As the anatomical techniques for mapping brain lesions have advanced, so have the behavioral techniques for studying abnormal language. Speech-language pathologists have developed standardized batteries that allow quantitative measurement of language performance and of improvement over time. Neurolinguists have devised language tasks that specify precise breakdowns in language function. Cognitive neuropsychologists have applied these findings to create models of normal language, with specification of the steps that are deranged in language disorders. Studies are now emerging that combine brain imaging or physiological techniques with sophisticated behavioral testing, promising a better understanding of the organization of speech and language in both normal persons and patients with brain disorders. This new information is beginning to be used to design individualized therapy programs for the restoration of language skills. Even drug therapy with dopaminergic and other agents is being applied to patients with language disorders.

This volume updates the field of speech and language disorders, with emphasis on new knowledge from these neuroanatomical, brain imaging, and behavioral techniques. The traditional motor speech disorders and the aphasias, alexias, and agraphias are reviewed, along with the topics of aphasia in children, aphasia in head injury, language disorders of aging and dementia, and right-hemisphere involvement in language. Chapter 5 reviews the localization of lesions by CT scan, prediction of prognosis for recovery from the anatomy of the lesion, and the selection of therapy techniques individualized to the patient's lesion anatomy and language test results. Chapters on PET and on EEG/brain electrical stimulation summarize the application of these techniques to speech and language functions. Aphasia therapy, pharmacotherapy of aphasia, psychiatric aspects of aphasia, and related disorders such as apraxia and agnosia are considered in the final chapters. The result is a marriage of contributions to language science from the diverse areas of clinical studies, neuroscience, brain imaging, and linguistics.

The book is designed to provide useful information for neurologists, neurosurgeons, medical students, cognitive neuropsychologists, neurolinguists, and rehabilitation personnel including speech–language pathologists, physical and occupational therapists, and nurses — indeed, all the professionals who work with patients with speech and language disorders. We hope that this volume will aid not only in the understanding of communication disorders, but in the essential communication among members of different professional specialties, who must understand one another's language if patients are to be well served.

I would like to thank my colleagues from several disciplines and numerous institutions who contributed to this book; my clinical mentors in neurology, especially the late Dr. Norman Geschwind, Dr. C. Miller Fisher, and Dr. J. P. Mohr; and my current co-workers at Vanderbilt University and the Vanderbilt Stallworth Rehabilitation Hospital. I particularly want to mention Dr. R. Terry Wertz, a colleague at Vanderbilt, who has honed my ideas on motor speech disorders and speech apraxia. Most of all, I thank the patients, who have taught me what I know about language disorders. Finally, I thank my wife, Carol, and children, Josh and Jodie, who put up with my involvement in yet another project that kept me away from family life. The book owes its existence to all these individuals.

Howard S. Kirshner

Contents

Contributors

Bassel Abou-Khalil, M.D.   Department of Neurology, Vanderbilt University School of Medicine, Nashville, Tennessee

Martin L. Albert, M.D., Ph.D.   Department of Neurology, Boston University School of Medicine, Boston, Massachusetts, and Medical Research Service, Department of Veterans Affairs, Washington, D.C.

Alfredo Ardila, M.D.   Colombian Institute of Neuropsychology, Bogotá, Colombia

Kathryn A. Bayles, Ph.D.   Department of Speech and Hearing Sciences, National Center for Neurogenic Communication Disorders, University of Arizona, Tucson, Arizona

Pelagie M. Beeson, Ph.D.   Department of Speech and Hearing Sciences, National Center for Neurogenic Communication Disorders, University of Arizona, Tucson, Arizona

D. Frank Benson, M.D.   Department of Neurology, UCLA School of Medicine, Los Angeles, California

Hiram Brownell, Ph.D.   Department of Psychology, Boston College, Chestnut Hill, and Department of Veterans Affairs Medical Center and Department of Neurology, Boston University School of Medicine, Boston, Massachusetts

xi

Sandra Bond Chapman, Ph.D.   Department of Human Development, Callier Center for Communication Disorders, University of Texas at Dallas, Dallas, Texas

Ann H. Craig, M.D.   Department of Neurology, UCLA School of Medicine, Los Angeles, California

Kathleen A. Culhane, M.D.   Department of Psychology, University of Houston, Houston, Texas

Jeffrey L. Cummings, M.D.   Departments of Neurology and Psychiatry, UCLA School of Medicine, and Psychiatry Service, West Los Angeles Veterans Affairs Medical Center, Los Angeles, California

Howard Gardner, Ph.D.   Department of Human Development and Psychology, Harvard Graduate School of Education, Cambridge, Massachusetts

Victor W. Henderson, M.D.   Departments of Neurology and Psychology, Andrus Gerontology Center, and the Program in Neural, Informational, and Behavioral Sciences, University of Southern California, and the Los Angeles County/University of Southern California Medical Center, Los Angeles, California

Audrey L. Holland, Ph.D.   Department of Speech and Hearing Sciences, National Center for Neurogenic Communication Disorders, University of Arizona, Tucson, Arizona

Howard S. Kirshner, M.D.   Department of Neurology, Vanderbilt University School of Medicine, and Vanderbilt Stallworth Rehabilitation Hospital, Nashville, Tennessee

Harvey S. Levin, Ph.D.   Division of Neurosurgery, University of Maryland Medical System, Baltimore, Maryland

Marjorie Perlman Lorch, Ph.D.   Department of Applied Linguistics, Birkbeck College, University of London, and National Hospital for Neurology and Neurosurgery, London, England

Russell J. Love, Ph.D.   Division of Hearing and Speech Sciences, Vanderbilt University School of Medicine, Nashville, Tennessee

Gail Martino   Department of Psychology, Boston College, Chestnut Hill, Massachusetts

Patrick McNamara, Ph.D.   Department of Psychology, State University of New York at Buffalo, Buffalo, New York

E. Jeffrey Metter, M.D.   Longitudinal Studies Branch, Gerontology Research Center, National Institute on Aging, National Institutes of Health, Baltimore, Maryland

Masaru Mimura, M.D. Department of Neurology, Boston University School of Medicine and Boston Veterans Affairs Medical Center, Boston, Massachusetts

Margaret A. Naeser, Ph.D. Department of Neurology, Boston University Aphasia Research Center, Boston University School of Medicine and Veterans Affairs Medical Center, Boston, Massachusetts

Carole L. Palumbo Department of Neurology, Boston University Aphasia Research Center, Boston University School of Medicine and Veterans Affairs Medical Center, Boston, Massachusetts

Penny Prather, Ph.D. Department of Vetrans Affairs Medical Center and Department of Neurology, Boston University School of Medicine, Boston, Massachusetts, and Center for Complex Systems, Brandeis University, Waltham, Massachusetts

Wanda G. Webb, Ph.D. Division of Hearing and Speech Sciences, Vanderbilt University School of Medicine, Nashville, Tennessee

Bryan T. Woods, M.D. Departments of Medicine and Psychiatry, Texas A&M University School of Medicine, Temple, Texas

1

Introduction to Aphasia

Howard S. Kirshner

Vanderbilt University School of Medicine, Nashville, Tennessee

INTRODUCTION

Aphasia involves the loss of symbolic communication, the attribute that has set man the farthest apart from lower animals. Patients who have been rendered deficient in verbal communication suffer a disability that strikes at the heart of the human condition. The skills of physicians and a team of other health care professionals are required to understand the experiences of these patients and help them adapt to their impairments.

Aphasiology began with physicians describing their patients with language disorders, and aphasic patients have provided the main source of information on the organization of language in the brain. In modern times the field of aphasiology has involved the study of human language by a multitude of disciplines, including neurology, psychology, linguistics, speech/language pathology, and even computer science and philosophy. The contributions of these disciplines have rendered the field terminologically complex and confusing. While the theoretical aspects of aphasiology are of great interest to any study of aphasia, an increasing body of practical knowledge of language disorders has developed, knowledge that students of asphasia must understand to be of service to patients with these disorders. This practical information regarding language disorders is the major emphasis of this book.

Neurological speech and language disorders are impairments of verbal communication brought about by dysfunction of the nervous system. We attempt to distinguish disorders of speech articulation, or dysarthrias; disorders of voice, or dysphonias; and disorders of language, or aphasias. The dysarthrias and dysphonias are discussed in Chapter 2, while the bulk of this chapter and most of the other chapters of the book are dedicated to aphasia. Somewhat intermediate between the dysarthrias and aphasias is the syndrome called *apraxia of speech*, in which utterance of syllables is deranged in a nonstereotyped way, but central language processes are largely intact. Apraxia of speech is discussed in Chapter 3.

DEFINITION

Aphasia has been defined as an acquired disorder of previously intact language ability secondary to brain disease (1). Language is a system of symbols used to convey thoughts — internal, nonverbal images and representations — from one individual to another. Language also consists of a set of rules by which these symbols are combined and expressed. The words in the definition of aphasia are carefully chosen to emphasize the acquired nature of the disorder, the involvement of language and not only speech, and the relationship to brain disease. First, we must distinguish acquired language disorders, or aphasias, from developmental disorders of language, often termed *dysphasias*. Childhood aphasia, by this definition, refers only to language disorders in children that are acquired as a result of brain injury or disease. In England, the term dysphasia is often used to mean a partial, as opposed to total, loss of language function. Second, the definition of aphasia requires that language functions, and not just motor speech expression, are disturbed, thus excluding the dysarthrias, dysphonias, and apraxia of speech. Language is distinguished not only from speech, but also from thought. While philosophers have debated whether thought can exist without symbolic language, patients with severe aphasia are clearly capable of nonverbal thought. This is just one of the areas in which the study of aphasia contributes to our understanding of mind–brain relationships. Disturbed thought, moreover, can be conveyed in perfectly normal language, as is often seen in the psychotic thought disorder of schizophrenia and other psychoses (2–4). Since these disorders involve thought rather than language, they should not be called aphasias. Finally, the definition of aphasia requires that the derangement of language must result from brain disease. Again excluded are disorders of language content resulting from functional or psychiatric disorders such as the tangential associations and "clang" associations of bipolar affective disease or the "word salad" speech of schizophrenia.

Aphasia usually results from focal damage to the language centers of the brain, but language disorders are also seen in diffuse brain diseases, such as encephalopathies, or acute confusional states, and dementias. While language dysfunction is not prominently mentioned as an aspect of dementia, Alois Alzheimer, in the 1907 case report (5) of the dementing disease that now bears his name, clearly described aphasic disturbances. While some would prefer that the term be used solely for syndromes due to focal brain disease (1), syndromes of language disorder in diffuse diseases of the central nervous system share most of the characteristics of language dysfunction secondary to focal lesions of the brain, and for the purposes of this volume they qualify as aphasias.

HISTORY

Historically, speech and language were the first of the "higher cortical functions" to be localized to a specific region of the brain. While earlier descriptions have been discovered (6,7), Broca's 1861 report (8) of two patients with nonfluent aphasia secondary to left frontal lesions was the starting point of the modern field of aphasiology. The subsequent decades of the nineteenth century saw a steady increase in knowledge, accruing largely from physicians' clinical descriptions of patients, often correlated with findings in the brain at autopsy. The major clinical syndromes of aphasia were described and classified according to studies of this type, mostly before 1900. Many of these classical descriptions of aphasic syndromes are discussed in the context of the specific language disorders in Chapters 4, 6, 7, 10, and 11. The rate of progress of our understanding of aphasia, dependent on the physician's outliving his patient and studying the brain at autopsy, was exceedingly slow.

During the early years of the twentieth century, neurological interest in the higher cortical functions waned, in favor of the "harder" deficits of motor and sensory dysfunction. Psychologists such as Lashley promulgated the idea that the higher functions of the cerebrum were not well localized to specific regions of the brain, but rather that widespread areas were functionally equipotential. Philosophical objections to the study of higher functions as physical attributes of disease of focal brain regions also impeded progress in aphasia.

CONTEMPORARY TRENDS

Aphasiology has had a profound reawakening in the latter part of the Twentieth Century. First, a few clinicians, most notably Norman Geschwind, rekindled an interest in behavioral deficits resulting from brain injury, expanding on the classical descriptions. Second, the technology for brain imaging underwent a revolution, beginning with computerized axial tomography (CT scanning) in the 1970s, magnetic resonance imaging (MRI) in the 1980s,

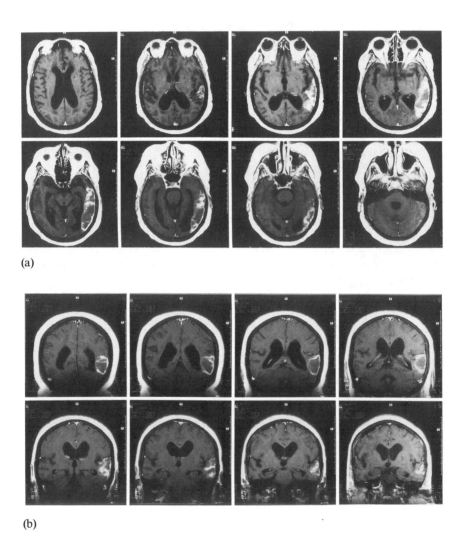

(a)

(b)

Figure 1   MRI scans in (a) axial and (b) coronal planes. A large left temporal lesion is seen in an elderly patient with generalized brain atrophy. The coronal section is useful in confirming that the infarct lies below the sylvian fissure.

and most recently the isotope imaging modalities of single photon emission computed tomography (SPECT) and positron emission tomography (PET). CT and MRI allow the anatomical definition of the brain lesion in the living patient, while SPECT and PET provide imaging of tissue metabolism or blood flow, reflecting changes in the function of brain tissue, either at rest or during actual cognitive activities.

Figure 1 shows an MRI of the brain in a patient with Wernicke's aphasia; Figure 2 shows a PET slice showing decreased metabolic activity in the same area. These modalities are discussed in much greater detail in subsequent chapters of this book; Chapter 5 summarizes the use of CT scanning in aphasia research, and Chapter 8 reviews SPECT and PET applications to aphasia.

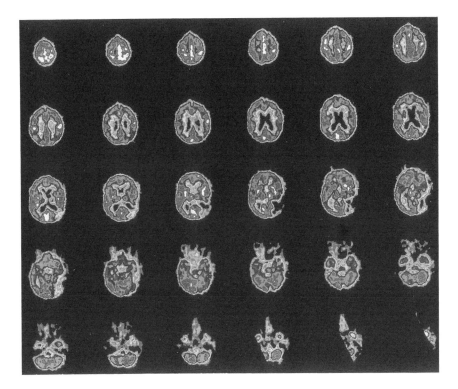

Figure 2 PET image of the same patient as in Figure 1. The patient was unable to give a history, and the family described an apparently gradual onset of aphasia, leading to suspicion of a brain tumor. The PET image shows a metabolically inactive area corresponding to the MRI lesion of Figure 1, consistent with a large infarction, or stroke.

In addition to these advances in medical technology, the study of aphasia has also advanced because of greater specification of the behaviors themselves. Whereas the nineteenth-century neurologist described aphasic disorders at the bedside, the contemporary aphasiologist can apply the testing methods of several other disciplines, including speech–language pathology, neuropsychology and cognitive neuropsychology, and neurolinguistics. The field of speech–language pathology has developed to provide both standardized testing and therapy for patients with acquired language disorders. Linguistic analysis of both normal and aphasic language has contributed detailed study of abnormal language phenomena. Cognitive psychologists have broken down psychological and cognitive functions into component parts called "modules" and have then constructed models of normal and abnormal language production and comprehension. Results of language testing in individual patients are then used to refine the models themselves, and occasionally to break down functions into even smaller modules (9,10). The greater precision of behavioral testing of patients has permitted more reliable classification of aphasic patients, as well as more specific behavioral measures to correlate with brain imaging procedures such as PET. As is seen in Chapters 5 and 18, this information is also leading to advances in aphasia therapy.

Most studies of aphasia have continued to involve patients with aphasia secondary to focal lesions of the brain. Strokes are the most common focal lesions studied, since they have the advantage of being restricted to one area of the brain, with other areas left intact. Stroke thus represents an "experiment of nature," in which the effects of ablation of one area of the brain can be studied. The consistency of vascular territories also makes strokes relatively stereotyped in different patients. Approximately 500,000 persons suffer strokes annually in the United States, and of these 20%, or 100,000, are rendered aphasic (11,12). Patients with focal lesions secondary to head injuries, brain tumors, and encephalitis also develop aphasia. Traumatic brain injury is the most common etiology of aphasia in the United States, if the cognitive disruptions that affect the organization of discourse are included (13). Disorders such as brain tumors and head injuries are less represented than strokes in research studies of aphasia, largely because these disorders tend to be less localized, with greater edema and "remote" pressure effects to tissue not directly involved in the lesion.

Newer technologies of brain imaging have not only provided more precise lesion localization but have also permitted new models for aphasia research. PET studies in normal volunteers have allowed mapping of the activation of the language cortex during functional language tasks (14). These studies have indicated that more extensive areas of the brain are activated during language tasks than previously believed. When a subject hears a word, for example, the areas of the brain activated include both primary temporal auditory cortices, inferior anterior cinglate cortex, the left temporoparietal cortex, and the anterior superior temporal cortex. The last two of these areas do not become active when subjects listen to non-word auditory sounds (15). This anatomical evidence that multiple brain regions simultaneously increase their metabolism has rendered outdated the concept of simple, localized "centers" for language function, and we must now speak of systems or "networks" of interconnected areas simultaneously functioning during language tasks. PET techniques have also been utilized to study the areas of abnormal brain metabolism in traditional aphasia syndromes (16,17), and to delineate subcortical structures involved in aphasia (18). Mechanisms of recovery can potentially be studied by similar activation techniques in patients with aphasia, to see how new brain areas become recruited into language tasks with recovery from aphasia. These studies are technically difficult, but one pioneering series has found PET with language activation to account for much of the variability in recovery among patients with aphasia (19).

Studies of language have also been undertaken in patients undergoing electrical stimulation and neurosurgical resections for intractable epilepsy. These procedures have allowed mapping of the language cortex in patients who do not have destructive brain lesions; most are young and healthy except for their epilepsy. The results of electrical-stimulation mapping, like those of PET scanning, have forced some modification of our concepts of the language areas of the brain. Electrophysiological studies indicate those areas that disrupt language functions when electrically stimulated. They define only those areas of the brain that are essential for language function, whereas PET indicates all areas activated during a language task (20). In contrast to the large areas designated as Broca's and Wernicke's areas from CT or PET studies of patients with stroke, electrophysiological studies have shown that the brain regions in which stimulation disrupts production or comprehension of language are restricted to approximately 1–2 square centimeters each (21). There is also much more variability from subject to subject than predicted from studies of stroke. For example, in tests of object naming, 21% of subjects showed no interference with stimulation of the traditional Broca's area, and 15% had none with stimulation anywhere in the left frontal lobe. Sixty-five percent had disruption of naming with stimulation of the posterior superior temporal gyrus, but in many subjects this involved only a small portion of the traditional Wernicke's area. Naming was sensitive to stimulation of the middle temporal gyrus or inferior parietal lobule in some patients (21,22). In addition, new areas not previously associated with language function have been discovered, such as the inferior temporal language area found by Luders and colleagues (23,24) to have a function in receptive language. Chapter 9 reviews knowledge about language function derived from epilepsy and electrical stimulation.

LANGUAGE TERMINOLOGY

Just as many disciplines have contributed to the study of aphasia, many different terminologies have been applied. Descriptive terms and eponymic syndromes are the legacy of classical neurology, including the classifications of aphasia discussed in Chapter 4. Linguists have borrowed terms from the study of normal language and development, while cognitive neuropsychologists have adopted terms from normal cognitive psychology and computer science. A brief, introductory discussion of aphasia terminology is presented here, to facilitate understanding of the information presented from these various disciplines throughout this book.

Spoken language is broken up into *phonemes*, which are the smallest units of speech that can alter the meaning of a word. *Phonology* refers to the encoding and decoding of phonemes, both as individual sounds and as combinations. Printed letters that correspond to phonemes are called *graphemes*, while the term *orthographic* refers to the visual pattern of a group of printed letters. Words, or *lexical units*, are the subunits of phrases and sentences, while the *lexicon* is the dictionary of words stored in the brain. Lexical units are patterned according to a grammatical plan referred to as *syntax*. This organization changes not only the order of words, but also the structure of some words, such as singular and pleural endings; past, present, and future tenses; and, in some languages, the masculine and feminine genders. These different word forms, which change according to the context of the word in a phrase, are called *morphemes*, and their study is called *morphology*. *Semantics* refers to the meaning carried by individual words or phrases. The flow of speech, including emotional tone and placement of emphasis within phrases, is called *prosody*. The production of longer, meaningful spoken or written language expressions is referred to as *discourse*.

While aphasia denotes the loss of any language function after brain injury, *alexia* specifically refers to acquired disorders of reading, and *agraphia* signifies the loss of writing ability. Errors of speech are called *paraphasic errors* or *paraphasias*. These are divided into *literal* or *phonemic* errors, which involve substitutions of similar sounding phonemes, and *verbal* or *semantic* errors, in which an incorrect word is substituted. Nonexistent word utterances are called *neologisms*, and speech made up of such words is called *jargon*. Errors in reading aloud are called *paralexias*, while errors in writing are referred to as *paragraphias*.

BRAIN ANATOMY

Just as a knowledge of language terms is necessary for reading the literature of aphasia, at least an elementary knowledge of brain anatomy is likewise needed. Relevant brain anatomy for language functions is reviewed in many chapters of this book, but a very simple introduction is provided here. Figure 3 is a diagram of the cortical gyri, as seen from the lateral surface of the brain. Gyri of the brain have names and are also referred to by Brodmann numbers, derived by differences in cellular architecture of the cortex.

Language begins with perception of language stimuli, generally through heard words. The anatomy of the auditory pathway starts in the ear, progresses through the eighth cranial nerve and a series of relay nuclei in the brainstem and the medial geniculate body of the thalamus, culminating in the auditory cortices in both temporal lobes. The primary auditory cortices — Brodmann areas 41 and 42, also called Heschl's gyri — are located on the superior surface of the superior temporal gyri, buried within the sylvian fissure. By traditional theory, sounds are decoded into words in the posterior portion of the superior temporal gyrus of the dominant hemisphere; this area for understanding speech is referred to as Wernicke's area, or Brodmann area 22. If language is read from visual stimuli, the input is the visual system, which begins with the eye, proceeds through the optic nerves, optic tracts, lateral geniculate body of the thalamus, and thence via the optic radia-

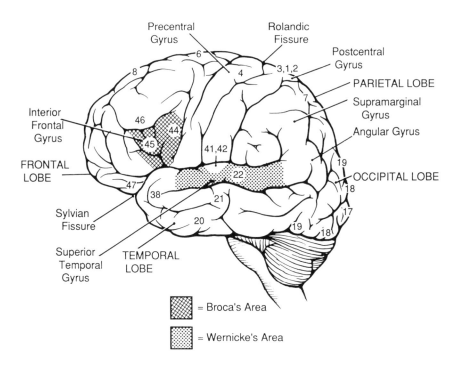

Figure 3 Diagram of the lateral surface of the left cerebral hemisphere. The names of gyri and corresponding Brodmann numbers are indicated, as described in the text.

tions to the primary visual cortex in the medial occipital pole. The primary visual area is called the striate cortex, or Brodmann area 17. Information from the visual cortex and visual association areas is somehow translated into language in posterior areas of the left hemisphere, although the right hemisphere may also have some elementary capacities in word recognition. The left angular gyrus (Brodmann area 39), the gyrus that overlies the superior temporal sulcus and makes up part of the inferior parietal lobule, is thought to have a special involvement in associating information from different sensory modalities such as vision and hearing. If a patient is asked to repeat a spoken word, the information must be transmitted from the left-hemisphere Wernicke's area to the left frontal areas involved in speech. The arcuate fasciculus, a bundle of white matter connecting the temporal and frontal cortices, may be involved in this transfer.

Expressive speech is known to involve the inferior frontal gyrus; traditionally, the posterior parts of this gyrus, or parts of the pars opercularis and pars triangularis, Brodmann areas 44 and 45, are referred to as Broca's area. This area is in close proximity to the primary motor cortex for the face, lips, and tongue, located in the inferior portion of the precentral gyrus, area 4. Presumably, the motor programs for production of specific speech sounds lie in this primary motor cortex, and the Broca's area contains programming instructions for production of strings of phonemes, or words and phrases. Writing is directed by similar language cortices but also involves the parts of the motor cortex that control the contralateral hand. However, evidence for a primary writing area, formerly referred to as Exner's area and localized to the left superior frontal region, has not been supported either by stroke cases or by electrical-stimulation studies. Stimulation of Broca's area interferes with writing, while excitation of other frontal regions does not produce agraphia without disturbing speech (25).

In addition to this cortical circuitry, speech involves the basal ganglia, which help control motor behavior in general, and the cerebellum, a coordination center of the brain. The thalamus, a sensory relay nucleus located above the brainstem in the diencephalon, contains both motor relay nuclei involved in speech and sensory projections to Wernicke's area and other cortical regions relevant to language. The subcortical contribution to language expression, as well as greater detail on cortical anatomy, are discussed in Chapters 4 and 5.

HANDEDNESS AND CEREBRAL DOMINANCE

Since the time of Broca, aphasiologists have known that most right-handed people have at least relative language dominance in the left hemisphere. Over 90% of normal people are right-handed, and 99% of lesions causing aphasia in right-handed people involve the left cerebral hemisphere (26). Among left-handers, a majority have relative left-hemisphere language dominance, but this dominance may be less complete than in right-handers. Thus, left-handed persons who suffer a stroke may develop aphasia regardless of the side of the brain affected, but recovery is sometimes better than in right-handers (27). Basso and colleagues (28) found that most cases of non-right-handed and right-handed patients with aphasia have similar syndromes and recovery, except for a few atypical cases in whom a specific language center seems to be in the other hemisphere.

The basis of language dominance is generally thought to be grounded in brain anatomy, and not dependent on education or literacy. Damasio and colleagues (29) studied 38 illiterate patients with acquired brain lesions and found that the association of left-hemisphere lesions with aphasia was as strong as in educated patients. Geschwind and Levitsky (30) first showed that there is a normal asymmetry in the superior temporal plane (planum temporale), the left-hemisphere area being larger than the right in 65 of 100 brains, while the right-hemisphere temporal plane was larger in only 11 brains. The sylvian fissure, which separates the frontal and temporal lobes in the vicinity of the left-hemisphere speech areas, appears longer and lower in the left hemisphere, and shorter but higher on the right (31).

Witelson and Pallie (32) found similar asymmetries in neonatal brains, again indicating that hemispheric asymmetry is a "hard-wired" aspect of brain inheritance, and not a hypertrophy of the language area with use or linguistic experience. Several investigators (31,33,34) have found similar asymmetries in CT scans, especially a difference in the length of the occipital lobes, measured on a CT scan slice at the level of the bodies of the lateral ventricles (31). This occipital-length asymmetry on CT scan was shown to correlate well with planum temporale measurements taken of the same 15 brains postmortem, although none of the other measured CT scan asymmetries had such a correlation. Eidelberg and Galaburda (35) have found in microscopic studies of the cerebral cortex that the cytoarchitechtonic area making up most of the angular gyrus is also larger in the left hemisphere of brains in which the left planum temporale is larger than the right. These brain asymmetries, so closely involved with the language areas, are commonly assumed to relate to language dominance, although the correlation has not been rigorously proved. Studies of the relationship of brain asymmetries to handedness have been conflicting; Le May and Kido (33) found that the typical asymmetries are much more common in right-handed than left-handed people, but Chui and Damasio (34) found no association between CT scan asymmetries and handedness. Further studies are needed to correlate brain asymmetries and cerebral dominance for language.

Attempts have also been made to predict the language dominance in left-handed people based on handwriting posture: some write with the left hand held straight and the hand below the line of writing ("straight-hand posture"), while others write with the hand hooked and held alongside the ling of writing ("inverted-hand posture"). Levy and Reid (36) postulated that left-handed patients with straight-hand posture have contralateral (right) hemisphere language dominance, while those with inverted-hand posture have ipsilateral (left) language dominance. Volpe, Sidtis, and Gazzaniga (37) failed to confirm this association with Wada tests and dichotic listening studies.

Currently, the standard test for determination of hemisphere dominance for language is the Wada test, which involves the infusion of sodium amobarbital into the carotid artery during a cerebral arteriogram (38). Naming or other language tasks are administered during the infusion, and interruption of language ability indicates language specialization in the hemisphere ipsilateral to the infusion. The predictive value of the Wada test has been reliable enough to serve as the standard preoperative test for epilepsy surgery. (The Wada test is discussed further in Chapter 9.) We have recently studied patients who had MRI scans and Wada tests as part of evaluation for epilepsy surgery; while the occipital asymmetry did tend to correlate with the hemisphere of language dominance, the measurement could not be used for prediction of dominance in an individual case (39).

Other methods of testing language dominance include neuropsychological tests such as dichotic listening and activation tests with PET. Dichotic listening tests indicate a hemisphere preference in listening to competing auditory stimuli in both ears (40). This method also correlates with dominance, but the results are less clear-cut than those of the Wada test. Most recently, PET scanning has been used to map the activation of the language areas during language tasks in patients who are candidates for epilepsy surgery. This method appears to have promise but is not as well documented as the Wada test. PET studies of language activation are discussed in Chapter 8.

BEDSIDE SPEECH/LANGUAGE ASSESSMENT

The bedside aphasia test is a part of the neurological examination that can be accomplished in a few minutes with most patients. The examination is used to test the function of separate aspects of the speech/language system, such that a language disorder can be characterized. The pattern of abnormalities allows both an aphasia classification and a preliminary localization of the responsible brain lesion.

The bedside language examination is nonstandardized and qualitative, and therefore does not provide sufficient documentation for planning of speech therapy or for research into language disorders. Standardized bedside examinations such as Folstein's Mini Mental State Examination (41) contain only one example of each language function and are even less adequate for detailed exploration of a patient's language disorder; in addition, the scoring system does not distinguish between focal and diffuse brain disease (42,43). Other, more detailed versions of bedside mental status examinations have been provided by Strub and Black (44), Kirshner (45), and Weintraub and Mesulam (46). The examination shown in Table 1 is based on one developed at the Boston Veterans Administration Hospital by Geschwind, Goodglass, and others (1).

Speech pathologists and neuropsychologists use standardized language test batteries, which can be considered extensions of the bedside examination. These provide detailed, quantitative, and standardized measures. Two of the most popular test batteries—the Boston Diagnostic Aphasia Examination (47) and its modification, the Western Aphasia Battery (48)—use

Table 1   The Bedside Language Examination

   I. Spontaneous speech
      A. Articulation
      B. Fluency
      C. Circumlocutions, paraphasic errors
      D. Automatic utterances
  II. Naming
      A. Confrontation naming
          1. Objects
          2. Object parts
          3. Body parts
          4. Colors
      B. Series naming
 III. Auditory comprehension
      A. Commands
      B. Yes/no questions
      C. Complex grammatical constructions
 IV. Repetition
      A. Polysyllabic words
      B. Complex grammatical phrases
  V. Reading
      A. Reading aloud
      B. Reading for meaning
 VI. Writing
      A. Copying
      B. Writing from dictation
      C. Spontaneous writing

Source: Adapted from Ref. 1.

the same classification system as the bedside examination summarized here. Others, such as the Porch Index of Speech Ability (PICA) (49), measure specific functions at a simple level and quantitate a patient's performance as compared to that of other aphasics, making the test useful in following the patient's progress during speech therapy. (An overview of available aphasia test batteries and their use is provided in Chapter 17.) Finally, aphasia research has also utilized specific language tests designed by linguists, cognitive neuropsychologists, and others. Such tests are referred to throughout this volume.

The bedside aphasia examination consists of six items: spontaneous speech, naming, auditory comprehension, repetition, reading, and writing. While the details of the testing may vary from examination to examination, all six items should be tested explicitly.

Spontaneous Speech

Spontaneous speech is characterized by several variables reflecting both speech articulation and language content. The parameters of articulation, as summarized by Alexander and Benson (1), include: loudness or volume, rate of utterance and initiation of speech, precision of articulation, melodic intonation or prosody, and speed of initiation. Abnormalities of these aspects of speech expression are seen both in motor speech disorders and in aphasias. Reduced speech volume is seen in disorders involving muscle weakness secondary to dysfunction of the peripheral nerves, neuromuscular junction, or muscle, in extrapyramidal syndromes such as Parkinson's disease, and even in pulmonary diseases with shortness of breath. Abnormal vocal quality, such as hoarseness, is called *dysphonia*. Slowed speech is seen in some aphasias, while increased rate is characteristic of Parkinson's disease and related diseases. Imprecise articulation is seen in the dysarthrias (see Chapter 2). In the aphasias and speech apraxias (see Chapter 3), articulation errors are also seen but tend to be inconsistent from attempt to attempt, whereas in the dysarthrias the errors occur consistently with specific consonants or consonant-vowel combinations.

Prosody refers to the melodic pattern of speech expression. Articulation difficulties—as in the dysarthrias—impair prosody, as do aphasic disturbances, with pauses and hesitations. *Prosody* has also been used to refer to the emotional tone of speech and intended emotional effects on the listener, including sarcasm, irony, and humor; these latter aspects of speech prosody involve the right cerebral hemisphere (see Chapter 12).

The language content of the speech output is also characterized according to fluency, presence of pauses or word-finding difficulty, circumlocutions or use of several words where one would do, grammatical disturbances, and paraphasic errors, or substitutions. Fluency is perhaps the most important single quality in speech: does the speech issue forth in an effortless manner, or is it halting, effortful, and reduced in quantity and rate? Fluent speech should contain phrases of several words, strung together with some grammatical relationship, and articulated without hesitancy. Nonfluent speech is often dysarthric, but aphasia and dysarthria can occur independently. Word-finding difficulty in spontaneous speech corresponds to anomia, when naming is deliberately tested. Patients may learn to give a description, or circumlocution, such as "the thing you write with" for "pen." Grammatical disturbances, or errors of syntax, are divided into *agrammatism* and *paragrammatism.* Agrammatism refers to the omission of grammatical words, especially prepositions, so that the speech sounds telegraphic (see Chapter 4, Broca's aphasia), while paragrammatism refers to grammatical errors, often made as part of a fluent speech pattern. Paraphasic errors, neologisms, and jargon productions are noted in spontaneous speech. An example of a literal paraphasia is "skoon" for spoon, while a verbal paraphasia might be "fork" for spoon.

As part of the testing of speech, automatic utterances are also tested. Alexander and Benson (1) refer to this function as *recitation* and list it as a separate part of the bedside examination. Automatic utterances include counting to 10 and reciting the days of the week or the months of the year. Some aphasics produce automatic speech more successfully than they fulfill other language tasks. In addition, the examiner has a body of speech expression to analyze, in which the target of the patient's attempted speech is clear.

This description of spontaneous speech may sound complex, but it can usually be simplified to a description of articulatory or prosodic disturbances and a description of fluency. The principal questions being asked are: (1) is there dysphonia or dysarthria present?, (2) is aphasia present?, and (3) is the aphasia fluent or nonfluent?

Naming

Naming is customarily tested by asking the subject to name objects pointed to by the examiner. Objects, colors, and body parts should all be tested. Parts of objects, such as a watchband or the clip of a pen, are especially difficult for aphasic patients. Some examiners also test series naming, such as the maximum number of animals or words beginning with a specific letter that the patient can name in 60 seconds. These tests of naming speed are especially affected by frontal lobe lesions and dementing diseases.

Auditory Comprehension

Auditory comprehension is customarily tested by commands comprising one, two, or three steps. For example, the command "close your eyes" is a one-step command, while "take your left thumb and touch your nose" is a two-step command. Following commands, of course, requires that the subject hear the command, understand its language content, and have the motor ability to execute it. The examiner must therefore ensure that the patient is not deaf, understands English, and is not paralyzed in the limb required to perform the command. A more complicated issue is *apraxia*, the inability to carry out a motor command despite intact comprehension and intact motor ability; this subject is discussed in Chapter 21.

As a practical matter, if a patient fails to carry out even one-step commands, comprehension should be tested by a means that does not require a motor response. The examiner may ask yes/no questions or offer commands that require only a pointing response. More detailed tests of auditory comprehension may also be constructed in which grammatical relationships within a sentence must be understood. For example, the patient listens to the sentence "Tom lent Betty's book to Bill" and then is asked who received the book. Such tests detect subtle deficits of comprehension of syntax, as are seen in Broca's aphasia (Chapter 4).

Repetition

Repetition is tested for both words and sentences. Patients with dysarthria and apraxia of speech have difficulty with polysyllabic words such as "Methodist Episcopal"; repetition of the same multisyllabic word five times also brings out the variable errors characteristic of apraxia of speech. Nonsense polysyllables such as "pa-da-ca" are also useful, since transitions from one consonant to another are particularly vulnerable to both dysarthria and speech apraxia (see Chapters 2 and 3). Aphasics, on the other hand, tend to have more difficulty with grammatically complex or unfamiliar phrases, particularly those with prepositions. The phrase "no ifs, ands, or buts about it" is especially difficult for aphasic patients. The Boston Diagnostic Aphasia Examination (47) contains a number of other unfamiliar or "low-probability" phrases, such as "pry the tin lid off" and "the spy fled to Greece."

Reading

Reading is tested for both reading aloud and reading for comprehension. An easy way to test reading comprehension is to present cards with one-, two-, and three-step printed commands. Direct comparison can then be made between auditory and reading comprehension. Reading of paragraphs should be tested in patients with milder deficits.

Writing

Writing is tested for copying, writing from dictation, and spontaneous writing. Many patients with aphasia have an associated right hemiparesis, or right-sided paralysis. These patients may refuse to attempt to write with the left, nondominant hand. Normal subjects can write, albeit awkwardly, with the left hand, and aphasic patients should be encouraged to try. Usually their inability to write is language-based and not simply secondary to right-sided weakness. Experimental studies have also shown that some hemiparetic subjects can write better with the paretic right arm when a special splint resembling a skate is used (50,51) (see Chapter 11). Writing shares with speech the expression of language; as in speech, there can be word or sound substitutions, called *paragraphias* in written productions. In addition to the variables seen in speech, however, written language output involves spelling, which provides further insight into disturbed language. Very mild aphasic deficits, for example, may be detected more readily in written than in spoken expression (52).

In general, writing is more affected than speech in aphasias. The exceptions involve severe aphasias in which the patient is nearly mute but can write a few words, and the syndrome of aphemia (see Chapter 4). Some would interpret the superiority of writing over speech as evidence of an apraxia of speech (Chapter 3).

Application of Bedside Testing in Aphasia Diagnosis

The profile of these six language elements is used to classify the aphasic deficit, as described in Chapter 4. The neurologist also applies knowledge of the rest of the neurological examination, particularly the presence or absence of a right visual field defect, right hemiparesis, right hemisensory loss, and related behavioral deficits, such as memory loss, apraxia, and agnosia (see Chapter 21). These examination findings indicate the localization of the brain lesion and thus contribute to medical diagnosis. Lesion localization is confirmed by brain imaging studies. The etiology of the aphasia, or disease diagnosis, is ascertained by the history of how the deficit evolved, as well as by the appearance of the lesion on brain imaging studies. For example, an embolic stroke produces sudden aphasia, while a brain tumor produces the more gradual onset of progressive language difficulty.

The first and most important task of the bedside aphasia test is to determine whether the patient is aphasic. Motor speech disorders are characterized by the sound characteristics of the spontaneous speech, naming, and repetition subtests of the bedside examination. The language functions assessed by naming, repetition, comprehension of auditory and visual material, and writing should be normal in patients with dysarthria but no aphasia. In general, if the patient's speech can be typed or transcribed into print and then read aloud with a normal-sounding pattern, the patient is not aphasic.

The mute patient is a special source of confusion, since the absence of any speech output prevents the analysis of language needed to diagnose an aphasic disturbance. If the patient can comprehend spoken and printed language and write normally, aphasia is almost certainly not present. If the patient is alert and appears to be trying to speak, he may or may not be aphasic. Failure to comprehend commands makes it more likely that the patient is aphasic. Other signs of left-hemisphere injury, such as right hemiparesis or a right-visual-field deficit, also increase the likelihood of aphasia. Patients who are mute and do not appear to make any effort to speak might be aphasic but might also have other abnormalities such as akinetic mutism related to frontal-lobe disease, psychiatric disorders such as catatonia, or simple uncooperativeness. Patients who are mute because of a severe aphasia are usually active in other ways, such as grunting or gesturing (53); their lack of behavior applies only to language, not to other activities.

CONCLUSION

Aphasia comprises a series of language disorders caused by acquired disease of the brain. As in other areas of brain function, the nature and location of the brain disorder can be ascertained by careful observation of the patient's behavior at the bedside. In contemporary practice, these bedside observations are complemented both by more detailed behavioral testing by speech-language pathologists and neuropsychologists and by sophisticated brain imaging techniques. The result has been a burgeoning of new information on language and the brain. As can be seen in the rest of this volume, the new information is of both practical value in patient care and theoretical value in extending our understanding of brain function.

REFERENCES

1. Alexander MP, Benson DF. The aphasias and related disturbances. In: Joynt RJ, ed. Clinical neurology. 1. Philadelphia: JB Lippincott 1992:1–58.
2. Critchley M. The neurology of psychotic speech. Br J Psychiatry 1964;110:353–364.
3. Gerson SN, Benson DF, Frazier SH. Diagnosis: schizophrenia versus posterior aphasia. Am J Psychiatry 1977;134:966–969.
4. DiSimon FG, Darley FL, Aronson AE. Patterns of dysfunction in schizophrenic patients on an aphasia test battery. J Speech Hear Disord 1977;62:498–513.
5. Alzheimer A. A unique illness involving the cerebral cortex. In: Rottenberg DA, Hochberg FH, eds. Neurological classics in modern translation. New York: Hafner 1977:41–43 (originally 1907).
6. Benton AL, Joynt RJ. Early descriptions of aphasia. Arch Neurol 1960;3:205–222.
7. Boller F. Comprehension disorders in aphasia: A historical review. Brain Lang 1978;5:149–165.

8. Broca P. Remarques sur le siège de la faculté du langage articulé suiviés d'une observation d'aphemie. Bulletin de la Societe d'Anatomie 1861;6:330–364.
9. Margolin DI. Cognitive neuropsychology. Resolving enigmas about Wernicke's aphasia and other higher cortical disorders. Arch Neurol 1991;48:751–765.
10. Moscovitch M, Umilta C. Modularity and neuropsychology: modules and central processes in attention and memory. In: Schwartz MF, ed. Modular deficits in Alzheimer-type dementia. Cambridge, MA: MIT Press, 1990:1–59.
11. American Heart Association. 1992 heart and stroke facts, quoted in Medical news and perspectives. JAMA 1992;267:335–336.
12. Brust JCM, Shafer SQ, Richter RW, Bruun B. Aphasia in acute stroke. Stroke 1976;7:167–174.
13. Kurtzke JF. The current neurologic burden of illness and injury in the United States. Neurology 1982;32:1207–1214.
14. Posner MI, Petersen SE, Fox PT, Raichle ME. Localization of cognitive operations in the human brain. Science 1988;240:1627–1631.
15. Petersen SE, Fox PT, Posner MI, Mintun M, Raichle ME. Positron emission tomographic studies of the cortical anatomy of single-word processing. Nature 1988;331:585–589.
16. Metter EJ, Wasterlain CG, Kuhl DE, Hanson SR, Phelps ME. [18]FDG positron emission computed tomography in a study of aphasia. Ann Neurol 1981;10: 173–183.
17. Metter EJ, Kempler D, Jackson C, Hanson WR, Mazziotta JC, Phelps ME. Cerebral glucose metabolism in Wernicke's, Broca's, and conduction aphasia. Arch Neurol 1989;46:27–34.
18. Metter EJ, Riege WH, Hanson WR, Jackson CA, Kempler D, van Lancker D. Subcortical structures in aphasia. An analysis based on (F-18)-fluorodeoxyglucose, positron emission tomography, and computed tomography. Arch Neurol 1988;45:1229–1234.
19. Heiss W-D, Kessler J, Karbe H, Fink GR, Pawlik G. Cerebral glucose metabolism as a predictor of recovery from aphasia in ischemic stroke. Arch Neurol 1993;50:958–964.
20. Ojemann G, Ojemann J, Lettich E, Berger M. Cortical language localization in left, dominant hemisphere. An electrical stimulation mapping investigation in 117 patients. J Neurosurg 1989;71:316–326.
21. Ojemann GA, Fried I, Lettich E. Electrocorticographic (ECoG) correlates of language. I. Desynchronization in temporal language cortex during object naming. Electroencephalog Clin Neurophysiol 1989;73:453–463.
22. Ojemann GA. Cortical organization of language. J Neurosci 1991;11:2281–2287.
23. Luders H, Lesser J, Hahn J, Dinner DS, Morris H, Resor S, Harrison M. Basal temporal language area demonstrated by electrical stimulation. Neurology 1986; 36:505–510.
24. Luders H, Lesser RP, Hahn J, Dinner DS, Morris HH, Wyllie E, Godoy J. Basal temporal language area. Brain 1991;114:743–754.
25. Lesser RP, Luders H, Dinner DS, Hahn J, Cohen L. The location of speech and writing functions in the frontal language area. Results of extraoperative cortical stimulation. Brain 1984;107:275–291.

26. Subirana A. Handedness and cerebral dominance. In: Vinken PJ, Bruyn GW, eds. Handbook of clinical neurology. Vol 4. Amsterdam: North Holland, 1969: 248–272.
27. Satz P. A test of some models of hemispheric speech organization in the left- and right-handed. Science 1979;203:1131–1133.
28. Basso A, Farabola M, Pia Grassi M, Laiacona M, Zanobio ME. Aphasia in left-handers. Comparison of aphasia profiles and language recovery in non-right-handed and matched right-handed patients. Brain Lang 1990;38:233–252.
29. Damasio AR, Castro-Caldas A, Grosso JT, Ferro JM. Brain specialization for language does not depend on literacy. Arch Neurol 1976;33:300–301.
30. Gaschwind N, Levitsky W. Human brain: left-right asymmetries in temporal speech region. Science 1968;161:186–187.
31. Pieniadz JM, Naeser MA. Computed tomographic scan cerebral asymmetries and morphologic brain asymmetries. Correlation in the same cases post-mortem. Arch Neurol 1984;41:403–409.
32. Witelson SF, Pallie W. Left hemispheric specialization for language in the new-born: Neuroanatomical evidence of asymmetry. Brain 1973;96:641–647.
33. Le May M, Kido DK. Asymmetries of the cerebral hemispheres on computed tomograms. J Comp Assist Tomog 1978;2:471–476.
34. Chui HC, Damasio AR. Human cerebral asymmetries evaluated by computed tomography. J Neurol Neurosurg Psychiatry 1980;43:873–878.
35. Eidelberg D, Galaburda A. Symmetry and asymmetry in the human posterior thalamus. I. Cytoarchitectonic analysis in normal persons. Arch Neurol 1982; 39:325–332.
36. Levy J, Reid M. Variations in writing posture and cerebral organization. Science 1976;184:337–339.
37. Volpe BT, Sidtis JJ, Gazzaniga MS. Can left-handed writing posture predict cerebral language laterality? Arch Neurol 1981;38:637–638.
38. Wada J, Rasmussen T. Intra-carotid injection of sodium amytal for the lateral-ization of cerebral speech dominance. J Neurosurg 1960;17:266–282.
39. Charles PD, Abou-Khalil R, Abou-Khalil B, Wertz RT, Ashmead DH, Welch L, Kirshner HS. MRI asymmetries and language dominance. Neurology. In press.
40. Kimura D. Functional asymmetry of the brain in dichotic listening. Cortex 1967; 3:163–178.
41. Folstein MF, Folstein SE, McHugh PR. "Mini mental state." A practical method for grading the cognitive state of patients for the clinician. J Psychiatr Res 1975; 12:189–198.
42. Dick JPR, Guiloff RJ, Stewart A, Blackstock J, Bielawska C, Paul EA, Mars-den CD. Mini-mental state examination in neurological patients. J Neurol Neuro-surg Psychiatry 1984;47:496–499.
43. Nelson A, Fogel BS, Faust D. Bedside cognitive screening instruments. A criti-cal assessment. Nerv Ment Dis 1986;174:73–83.
44. Strub RL, Black FW. Language. In: Strub RL, Black FW, eds. The mental status examination in neurology. Philadelphia: FA Davis, 1977:39–61.

45. Kirshner HS. Bedside mental status examination. In: Kirshner HS, ed. Behavioral neurology: A practical approach. New York: Churchill-Livingstone, 1986: 3-13.
46. Weintraub S, Mesulam M-M. Mental state assessment of young and elderly adults in behavioral neurology. In: Mesulam M-M, ed. Principles of behavioral neurology. Philadelphia: FA Davis, 1985:71-124.
47. Goodglass H, Kaplan E. The assessment of aphasia and related disorders. 2nd ed. Philadelphia: Lea & Febiger, 1982.
48. Kertesz A. Aphasia and associated disorders: Taxonomy, localization and recovery. New York: Grune & Stratton, 1979.
49. Porch BE. The Porch index of communicative ability: Administration, scoring and interpretation. Palo Alto, CA: Consulting Psychologists, 1971.
50. Brown JW, Leader BJ, Blum CS. Hemiplegic writing in severe aphasia. Brain Lang 1983;19:204-215.
51. Whurr M, Lorch M. The use of a prosthesis to facilitate writing in aphasia and right hemiplegia. Aphasiology 1991;5:411-418.
52. Critchley M. The detection of minimal dysphasia. In: The divine banquet of the brain and other essays. New York: Raven Press, 1979:63-71.
53. Geschwind N. Non-aphasic disorders of speech. Int J Neurol 1964;4:207-214.

2

Motor Speech Disorders

Russell J. Love

Vanderbilt University School of Medicine, Nashville, Tennessee

DEFINITIONS

The term *motor speech disorder* traditionally refers to speech impairment, as opposed to language impairment, caused by lesion or dysfunction of the motor control centers of the peripheral or central nervous systems or a combination of both systems. The primary neurological sign of this disorder is an inability to regulate normally the movements of the speech mechanism. Historically, two broad classes of speech disorder have been subsumed under the rubric of motor speech disorders: (1) *dysarthria* and (2) *apraxia of speech.* These two concepts were introduced early in the history of clinical neurological medicine and are associated with Jean Charcot (1) and Hugo Liepmann (2).

Dysarthria currently refers to a group of speech disorders characterized by disturbances in the dimensions of strength, speed, tone, steadiness, accuracy, and range of movement in the muscles of the speech mechanism. When the disturbances in any or all of the motor dimensions of speech are severe enough to preclude articulate speech, the term *anarthria* has been used. Present-day speech–language pathologists, however, tend to employ the following less precise terms when referring to any person who does not communicate through oral language or is a completely unintelligible speaker on a motor basis: *nonspeaking, nonoral, nonverbal,* or *nonvocal.* Anarthria may still be the better term.

When there are disturbances in any motor dimension of speech production, the *basic speech processes* (respiration, phonation, resonance, articulation, prosody) may become deviant. These basic processes of speech production are supported by four major interrelated muscular systems: the respiratory, laryngeal, palatopharyngeal, and articulatory systems. The muscles of the four speech-production systems are innervated by what have been called the *cranial nerves for speech*: trigeminal (V), facial (VII), glossopharyngeal (IX), vagus (X), spinal accessory (XI), and hypoglossal (XII).

Several vocal disturbances traditionally labeled *dysphonia* (difficulty in producing voice) might be more appropriately designated as dysarthrias because of mounting evidence of neurological etiology. For instance, the dysphonia that accompanies a unilateral vocal-fold paralysis is caused by a compromised vagus nerve and is clearly a type of dysarthria. Similarly, the condition known as spasmodic dysphonia has always had a controversial etiology, but growing evidence places it in a neurological context (see below).

Stuttering is generally defined as dysfluency of speech. It has been considered an adult motor speech disorder by many neurologists and some speech-language pathologists if associated with evidence of cerebral dysfunction (3). Currently, many neurologists recognize a disorder known as *cortical* or *neurogenic stuttering*, which occurs in adults after brain injury. A recent term, suggested by speech–language pathologists who believe in cortical stuttering, is the phrase *acquired neurogenic dysfluency* (4) (see below).

Apraxia of speech has been defined in various ways, but speech–language pathologists usually view it as an impaired ability to execute voluntarily the appropriate movements for articulation of speech in the absence of paralysis, weakness, or incoordination of the speech musculature (5). Apraxia of speech is often considered a disorder of motor programming of articulatory postures and movements, while dysarthria is a disorder of impaired muscle control of motor execution of speech (see Chapter 3 for discussion of various definitions of speech apraxia).

Speech–language pathologists also recognize a nonspeech ideomotor disorder of the oral muscles called *oral apraxia*. It is defined as an inability to perform nonspeech movements with the muscles of the pharynx, larynx, tongue, cheeks, and lips, although automatic and sometimes imitative movements of the same muscles may be preserved. The muscles do not display signs of paralysis, weakness, or the incoordination of either a basal ganglia disorder or a cerebellar disorder. Oral apraxia is usually called *buccofacial apraxia* by neurologists. Speech apraxias and oral apraxias are generally conceived to be the result of a higher-level motor programming disturbance of the oral musculature as opposed to disturbances of motor power and coordination mediated at lower levels of the motor system. Speech apraxia and oral apraxia may appear independently or may coexist in the same individual (6–8). Speech apraxia in children is controversial, and well-documented cases are uncommon (9).

THE MAYO CLINIC STUDIES OF DYSARTHRIA

Over the past century, a small but steady stream of publications, primarily from neurologists, has been devoted to dysarthria. Historically notable is the extensive coverage of the topic by the British neurologist W. R. Gowers in his widely used 1888 textbook, *A Manual of Diseases of the Nervous System* (10). He differentiated a cerebral and bulbar group of dysarthrias. In 1943, Froeschels (11) presented a neuroanatomical classification of the dysarthrias by site of lesion. He included pyramidal, extrapyramidal, palladum-projectional, cerebellar, and peripheral dysarthria.

In 1948, Brain (12) presented a similar classification, as did Luchsinger and Arnold (13) in 1949; the latter suggested that audible symptoms varied with the site of lesion. In 1950, Peacher (14) presented a complex neuroanatomical classification system with five levels of CNS dysarthria and four levels of PNS dysarthria. Grewel (15), in 1957, presented a classification of 14 major types and several subtypes. His was a mixed classification in that it was based on neuroanatomical site, etiology, and disease entities. However, Grewel stressed the value of dysarthric signs in neurological diagnosis, pointing out that motor speech signs might suggest a diagnosis even before a standard neurological examination provided evidence of a neurological disorder.

It was not until 1969 that two speech–language pathologists (Darley and Aronson) and a neurologist (Brown) from the Mayo Clinic reported a comprehensive empirical study of 212 dysarthric speakers, with unequivocal neurological diagnoses that documented the deviant perceptual speech and vocal signs that were associated with sites of lesion of given diseases (16,17). Six groups of dysarthria, each with different patterns of abnormal speech signs, were identified: flaccid, spastic, ataxic, hypokinetic, hyperkinetic, and mixed, as in amyotrophic lateral sclerosis (spastic-flaccid), Wilson's disease (spastic-hypokinetic-ataxic), and multiple sclerosis (spastic-ataxic). The classification system, appropriate for any dysarthria, was based on sites of lesion in the traditional clinical divisions of the motor system that neurologists routinely employ.

Flaccid dysarthria results from a lower motor neuron lesion at specific points of the motor unit: anterior horn cell, nerve, neuromuscular junction, or muscle. Spastic dysarthria is associated with bilateral upper motor neuron lesions, while ataxic dysarthria arises from cerebellar or cerebellar pathway lesions. Hypo- and hyperkinetic dysarthrias are found with extrapyramidal lesions, and mixed dysarthrias are present when there are lesions in multiple

Table 1 Speech Signs in the Adult Dysarthrias

Flaccid dysarthria		*Ataxic dysarthria* (continued)	
Rank		Rank	
1	Hypernasality	6	Prolonged phonemes
2	Imprecise consonants	7	Prolonged intervals
3	Continuous breathiness	8	Monopitch
4	Monopitch	9	Monoloudness
		10	Slow rate
5	Nasal emission		
6	Audible inspiration	*Hypokinetic dysarthria* (*Parkinsonism*)	
7	Harsh voice	Rank	
8	Short phrases		
9	Monoloudness	1	Monopitch
		2	Reduced stress
Spastic dysarthria		3	Monoloudness
Rank		4	Imprecise consonants
		5	Inappropriate silences
1	Imprecise consonants	6	Short rushes
2	Monopitch	7	Harsh voice
3	Reduced stress	8	Continuous breathiness
4	Harsh voice		
5	Monoloudness	9	Pitch level disturbances
6	Low pitch	10	Variable rate
7	Slow rate		
8	Hypernasality	*Quick hyperkinetic dysarthria* (*chorea*)	
9	Strained-strangled quality	Rank	
10	Short phrases		
		1	Imprecise consonants
11	Distorted vowels	2	Prolonged intervals
12	Pitch breaks	3	Variable rate
13	Continuous breathiness	4	Monopitch
14	Excess and equal stress	5	Harsh voice
		6	Inappropriate silences
Ataxic dysarthria		7	Distorted vowels
Rank		8	Excessive loudness variation
1	Imprecise consonants	9	Prolonged phonemes
2	Excess and equal stress	10	Monoloudness
3	Irregular articulatory breakdown	11	Short phrases
4	Distorted vowels	12.5	Irregular articulatory breakdown
5	Harsh voice	12.5	Excess and equal stress
		14.5	Hypernasality
		14.5	Reduced stress
		16	Strained-strangled quality

Table 1   (Continued)

Slow Hyperkinetic dysarthria (*dystonia*)		*Mixed spastic-flaccid dysarthria* (*amyotrophic lateral sclerosis*)	
Rank		Rank	
1	Imprecise consonants	1	Imprecise consonants
2	Distorted vowels	2	Hypernasality
3	Harsh voice	3	Harsh voice
4	Irregular articulatory breakdown	4	Slow rate
5.5	Strained-strangled quality	5	Monopitch
5.5	Monopitch	6	Short phrases
7	Monoloudness	7	Distorted vowels
-----	-----	8	Low pitch
8.5	Inappropriate silences	9	Monoloudness
8.5	Short phrases	10	Excess and equal stress
10	Prolonged intervals	11	Prolonged intervals
11	Prolonged phonemes	-----	-----
12	Excess loudness variation	12	Reduced stress
13	Reduced stress	13	Prolonged phonemes
14	Voice stoppages	14	Strained-strangled quality
15	Rate	15	Breathiness
		16	Audible inspiration
		17	Inappropriate silences
		18	Nasal emission

All speech signs above dashed line have mean scale value of 2.00 or more.
Source: Adapted from Ref. 18.

motor systems. The empirically derived deviant speech signs of seven dysarthrias reported in the 1975 summary (18) of the work are listed in Table 1. The speech signs determined by ear are ranked in mean order by their degree of deviancy and/or saliency in each of the dysarthrias.

Recognition of the various types of dysarthria at bedside is clinically useful for both the neurologist and the speech–language pathologist. Using the data of Table 1 and other research, several speech pathologists have provided short lists of the most distinctive speech signs of the dysarthrias described in the Mayo Clinic studies. This short-list information can be used in establishing an early clinical impression of the type of dysarthria that a given patient presents. This bedside diagnosis can be confirmed later with a more complete perceptual and instrumental analysis by the speech–language pathologist. The most distinctive speech signs of nine well-known dysarthrias are:

1. *Flaccid dysarthria*: marked hypernasality, often with nasal air emission; breathiness; imprecise consonants
2. *Spastic dysarthria*: harsh strained-strangled voice, hypernasality, slow rate, very imprecise consonants, low pitch
3. *Ataxic dysarthria*: imprecise consonants, excess and equal stress, irregular articulatory breakdown
4. *Hypokinetic dysarthria (Parkinsonism)*: monopitch, monoloudness, reduced stress, imprecise consonants, inappropriate silences, variable rate, short rushes of speech
5. *Quick hyperkinetic dysarthria (chorea)*: imprecise consonants, prolonged intervals, variable rate, monopitch, harsh voice, inappropriate silences, distorted vowels, excess loudness variation
6. *Slow hyperkinetic dysarthria (dystonia)*: imprecise consonants, harsh strained-strangled voice, irregular articulatory breakdown, monopitch, monoloudness
7. *Spastic-flaccid dysarthria (amyotrophic lateral sclerosis)*: imprecise consonants, hypernasality, harsh voice, slow rate, monopitch, short phrases, distorted vowels, low pitch, monoloudness, excess and equal stress, prolonged intervals, bizarre quality
8. *Variable spastic-ataxic dysarthria (multiple sclerosis)*: variable slow rate, harsh voice, irregular articulatory breakdown; half of cases are dysarthric
9. *Spastic-ataxic-hypokinetic dysarthria (Wilson's disease)*: reduced stress, monopitch, monoloudness, imprecise consonants, slow rate, excess and equal stress, low pitch, irregular articulatory breakdown

The unique array and severity of deviations in a given dysarthric speaker suggested a set of seven clusters of speech signs. (For instance, hypernasality, nasal emission, imprecise consonants, and short phrases comprise a *resonatory incompetence cluster*.) Identification of the various clusters in a given dysarthria imply certain underlying physiological dysfunctions. In the case of resonatory incompetence one might predict a deficit in muscle contraction as well as velopharyngeal inadequacy. (See Table 2 for the clusters found in the Mayo Clinic studies.) Information from cluster analysis can be used for therapeutic intervention. Resonatory incompetence, for instance, might indicate the need for a speech prosthesis, such as a palatal lift, to aid velopharyngeal closure and reduce hypernasality and imprecise articulation.

The impact of the Mayo Clinic studies on the field of neurological speech-language pathology cannot be overestimated. On a clinical level, the studies allowed the well-trained listener to recognize a given dysarthria, separate it from other neurogenic communication disorders involving language disturbance, differentiate it from speech apraxia or other types of dysarthria, and record the unique pattern of speech deviations of the individual case.

Table 2 The Clusters Characterizing Each of the Dysarthrias Studied in the Mayo Clinic Research

Pseudobulbar palsy: spastic dysarthria
  Prosodic excess
  Prosodic insufficiency
  Articulatory-resonatory imcompetence
  Phonatory stenosis
Bulbar palsy: flaccid dysarthria
  Phonatory incompetence
  Resonatory incompetence
  Phonatory-prosodic insufficiency
Amyotrophic lateral sclerosis: mixed spastic-flaccid dysarthria
  Prosodic excess
  Prosodic insufficiency
  Articulatory-resonatory incompetence
  Phonatory stenosis
  Phonatory incompetence
  Resonatory incompetence
Cerebellar lesions: ataxic dysarthria
  Articulatory inaccuracy
  Prosodic excess
  Phonatory-prosodic insufficiency
Parkinsonism: hypokinetic dysarthria
  Prosodic excess
  Prosodic insufficiency
  Phonatory stenosis
Dystonia: slow hyperkinetic dysarthria
  Articulatory inaccuracy
  Prosodic insufficiency
  Phonatory stenosis
Chorea: quick hyperkinetic dysarthria
  Articulatory inaccuracy
  Prosodic excess
  Prosodic insufficiency
  Articulatory-resonatory incompetence
  Phonatory stenosis
  Resonatory incompetence

Source: Adapted from Ref. 67.

The Mayo Clinic studies not only enhanced clinical practice in speech pathology but also introduced a modern, comprehensive, scientific concept of dysarthria to neurology and speech pathology. In the decades since the initial research, there has been an explosion of interest in the motor speech disorders in speech science. The Mayo Clinic research has no doubt had less

Table 3 Studies of Dysarthria Employing the Mayo Clinic Perceptual Analysis Procedures

Multiple sclerosis — Darley, Brown, and Goldstein, 1972 (19)
Wilson's disease — Berry, Aronson, Darley, and Goldstein, 1974 (20)
Motor neuron disease — Carrow, Rivera, Mauldin, and Shamblin, 1974 (21)
Shy-Drager syndrome — Linebaugh, 1979 (22)
Friedreich's ataxia — Joanette and Dudley, 1980 (23)
Athetoid and spastic cerebral palsy — Workinger and Kent, 1991 (24)
Reye's syndrome — Stuart, Beukelman, Kenyon, Healy, and Bernthal, 1991 (25)
Progressive supranuclear palsy — Metter and Hanson, 1991 (26)

impact on neurologists than on speech pathologists, probably because physicians have neurodiagnostic instruments (CT, MRI, PET, and SPECT) that are more objective than the well-trained ear to establish a reliable neurological diagnosis. The Mayo Clinic approach has stimulated research studies on the acoustic perceptual approach to dysarthria diagnosis useful to both the neurologist and the speech pathologist. These are listed in Table 3.

DIFFERENTIAL DIAGNOSIS

An examiner inexperienced in the diagnosis of motor speech disorders may find the task complex and difficult, since these disorders must be carefully differentiated from several other neurological conditions that cause speech or language problems.

Motor Speech Disorders vs. Language Disorders

The three language disturbances most likely to be confused with motor speech disorder are aphasia, confused language, and demented language (27).

Aphasia is commonly defined as a deficit in the comprehension and/or expression of language involving one or more of the primary modalities of language function (listening, reading, speaking, writing, or gesturing). Putative sites of lesions for loss of specific language functions are discussed in Chapter 4. Dysarthric or dyspraxic speech, or a combination of the two, may coexist with aphasia if lesions appear in motor areas or pathways in addition to language areas or pathways. Aphasia test batteries are discussed in Chapter 17.

Demented language is found in individuals who present generalized intellectual impairment marked by progressive deterioration of memory, reasoning, judgment, orientation in time and space, personality, and language. Although controversial (28), distinctions have been made between cortical and subcortical dementias and their corresponding language and speech symptoms (29). In cortical dementias, such as Alzheimer's disease, speech is usually fluent and is characterized by normal syntax and phonology until the later stages of the disease. Motor speech disorder, particularly dysarthria, does not characterize the cortical dementias. In contrast, the subcortical dementias — such as Parkinson's disease, Huntington's disease, Wilson's disease, and progressive supranuclear palsy — are characterized by well-documented and distinct patterns of dysarthria in addition to progressive cortical language deterioration. Speech–language pathologists in the past have often relied on the Boston Diagnostic Examination of Aphasia (BDEA) (30) and a companion test, the Boston Naming Test (31), to assess dementias. A newer test, the Arizona Battery for Communication Disorders of Dementia (ABCD) (32) is specifically designed to assess the language of dementia (see Chapter 13). A profile for the bilaterally brain-damaged with dementia can be found on the well-known language battery, the Porch Index of Communicative Ability (PICA) (33).

Confused language arises in acute confusional states, which are caused by such conditions as traumatic brain injury, metabolic imbalance, adverse drug reactions, and withdrawal from drugs or alcohol. Patients with acute confusion display inattention and irrelevancies in their language. At times they demonstrate fluctuating levels of consciousness. Generally, expressive vocabulary and syntax are intact. Striking deviant features of the language behavior are confabulation and irrelevant response. These two language symptoms are also seen in the dementias. Speech articulation errors and vocal deviations of a dysarthria rarely coexist with confused language.

Dysarthria vs. Apraxia of Speech

Finally, a differential diagnosis of dysarthric subtypes versus apraxia of speech must be made. It is not always a simple matter to make a clear-cut distinction between them by ear alone. In fact, recent evidence suggests that the issues of diagnosis are more controversial than originally thought. Early work by Johns and Darley (34) reported that the articulatory errors of both dysarthric and apraxic speakers were similar when tested with a perceptual articulation battery. Dysarthrics produced more substitutions and distortions of speech sounds, while apraxics uttered more repetitions and additive sound substitutions. Overall, the speech errors of the apraxics were more inconsistent than those of the dysarthrics.

Recent research, however, has suggested that the two groups may be more similar in some ways. Ataxic dysarthrics and apraxics produce similar syllabic stress errors and have similar difficulties with speech initiation and open-juncture and long-stop closure (35). Abnormal force and position control of the articulators have been reported in both ataxics and apraxics (36).

Likewise, increased speech movement durations have been documented for both ataxic and apraxic speakers (37).

Questions have also been raised about the differences in the perceived speech errors in dysarthrics and apraxic speakers. Studies of apraxic individuals (35) suggest that distortions in pure apraxic speakers may actually be the most predominant error. Based on the above, Rosenbek and McNeil (38) advise that major speech differences between the two groups must not be assumed until more data are available.

Questions also remain about the validity and reliability of the differential diagnosis of the subtypes of dysarthria. The popular Mayo Clinic approach of perceptual analysis of the varied articulatory and vocal patterns in the dysarthrias has been criticized because of the subjective nature of the listening task upon which the technique rests (39). Well-trained and highly experienced listeners are quite reliable in making neurological speech diagnosis by ear. However, the reliability of perceptual diagnosis of dysarthria has not been reported for listeners not as expert as those in the original Mayo Clinic studies. Moreover, speech signs change over time with the evolution of a disease. Speech signs typical of a fullblown disease state may not be typical at its early onset. The occasional unreliability of perceptual judgments by ear sometimes demands additional confirmation for a correct diagnosis of dysarthria. It has been my practice in training students to teach them to recognize and elicit a series of confirming motor signs that are typically associated with dysfunction of the various motor subsystems (spasticity of upper motor neuron disorder, flaccidity of lower motor neuron disorder, involuntary movements of basal ganglia disorder, and incoordination of cerebellar disorder).

Diagnosis of dysarthria can also be made without major attention to deviant perceptual speech signs. The Frenchay Dysarthria Assessment (40) is an evaluation form that allows rating of reflex behavior and the function of lip, jaw, palatal, laryngeal, and tongue musculature as well as levels of intelligibility of speech in dysarthric patients. The results of the ratings of individual patients provide a profile of the oral performance of patients. Profiles of patients with similar dysarthrias tend to cluster together; the Frenchay Assessment scale identifies five dysarthrias: spastic, flaccid, extrapyramidal, cerebellar, and mixed. This assessment scale can help confirm or disprove diagnoses made by the Mayo Clinic procedures alone.

Another scale used widely by speech–language pathologists, called Assessment of Intelligibility of Dysarthric Speech (AIDS) (41), has proven very useful in the assessment of the dysarthric patient. Since intelligibility levels are probably the most widely used index of speech function for both layperson and professional, such a measure is very significant. The test assesses both single-word and sentence intelligibility as well as rate. These measures can be used for predicting a speaker's intelligibility in a variety of daily life situations.

Another aspect of the diagnosis of dysarthric speakers is the assessment of the speech musculature and its contribution to articulatory and vocal deviations in speech. Neurologists routinely assess the function of the cranial motor nerves (V, VII, IX–X, XI, XII) to discover gross signs of neurological dysfunction that aid in localization and lateralization of lesions causing dysarthria. Speech-language pathologists take a quite different view toward examination of the cranial motor nerves for speech; they attempt to determine if and how neurological dysfunction in these nerves affects the speech processes of phonation, resonance, articulation, and prosody. A complete discussion of the clinical motor speech examination may be found in Darley, Aronson, and Brown's *Motor Speech Disorders* (Ref. 18, pp. 69–88).

Speech scientists have argued that the instrumental assessment of speech physiology provides more accurate and comprehensive information in neurological cases than do clinical speech tests. Netsell, Lotz, and Barlow (42) have described a sophisticated instrumentation model for assessment of the dysarthric speaker. However, such a well-equipped speech laboratory is not available to many speech pathologists in the field, nor is it necessary for examination of every case. A survey of 66 Veterans Administration clinics (43) indicates that speech pathologists tend to rely first on readily available perceptual and nonspeech (oromotor maneuvers) measures and secondarily on instrumental results. Lack of evidence for justification of instrumental measures plus lack of knowledge of current technology probably account for these results. In any event, it appears that a combination of perceptual measures, nonspeech maneuvers, and instrumental measures provides the most reliable and valid assessment of dysarthria.

CURRENT ISSUES IN DYSARTHRIA

Two speech and voice disorders, spasmodic dysphonia and acquired neurological dysfluency, have been controversial for decades because of debate as to whether they are primarily psychogenic or neurogenic. Recent evidence suggests that they are best classified under the rubric of motor speech disorders.

Spasmodic Dysphonia

This voice disorder is extremely serious, often disrupting occupational pursuits and family ties as well as leading to social withdrawal, depression, and occasional considerations of suicide. It is frequently designated as a family of disorders resulting from several etiologies rather than a single cause. Vocal symptoms vary, but prominent is voice stoppage, in the context of strained-strangled laryngeal phonation and/or breathy or aspirate perturbations. Patients generally exhibit more normal voice quality for nonspeech behaviors such as yawning and laughing. Singing and phonating of the pitch range are also often free of vocal symptoms. Likewise, the superlaryngeal process of articulation is relatively unimpaired.

Aronson and Lagerlund (44) hold that spasmodic dysphonia is psychogenic in some patients and is fairly responsive to voice therapy and psychotherapy, but in the majority the dysphonia is neurogenic and resistant to all therapies except weakening of one or both of the vocal folds by resection of the recurrent laryngeal nerve or injection of botulism toxin. Aronson (45) asserts that two syndromes are responsible for the majority of neurogenic spasmodic dysphonic cases: (1) organic (essential) voice tremor and (2) focal dystonia or dyskinesia. A high incidence of spasmodic dysphonia has been reported among movement-disordered extrapyramidal syndromes (46). In cervical-cranial dystonia, blepharospasm as well as spasms of the lower face and/or oromandibular muscles (Meige syndrome) frequently occur. Other forms of cranial dystonia are lingual and pharyngeal dystonia. A similar pathophysiology is thought to underlie these various forms of focal cranial dystonia, but as yet the specific etiology remains essentially unknown.

Although neuromotor signs in spasmodic dysphonia have been associated with movement disorders of extrapyramidal origin, lesions at various other sites in the nervous system have also been suggested (47). The evidence is inconclusive concerning the brain mechanism involved in the disorder, but the consensus is that the majority of cases should be considered motor speech disorders (48).

Acquired Neurogenic Dysfluency (Neurological Stuttering)

This disorder is fraught with more controversy than spasmodic dysphonia. It is generally defined as dysfluent behavior that arises or disappears in adults after brain injury. It may also refer to dysfluent behavior that occurs in an adult neurologic disorder such as multiple sclerosis (49). It is generally agreed that developmental stuttering may differ from the acquired neurogenic dysfluency of adulthood. In fact, some writers (50) would reserve the term "stuttering" for the speech behavior of the developmental disorder.

Developmental stuttering is usually defined as an involuntary, repetitive prolongation or cessation of speech sounds. The disorder is considered a well-defined and researched dysfluency disorder whose etiologies remain unknown. It affects approximately 1% of the prepubertal school population, with boys more frequently affected than girls. It is reported that nearly four of five children recover by 16 years of age (51).

Acquired neurogenic dysfluency frequently follows bilateral or left-sided lesions associated with aphasia. However, acquired neurogenic dysfluency may also occur without aphasia, suggesting that language mechanisms need not be involved. It is rare to have acquired neurogenic dysfluency in right-handed adults with right-sided lesions. Acute onset of acquired dysfluency is most common in stroke and head trauma.

Acquired dysfluency may also be marked by a gradual onset and slow progression. This is seen in degenerative diseases such as Parkinsonism, supranuclear palsy, dialysis dementia, and Alzheimer's disease (52).

The disorder appears to be a distinct clinical entity, although stuttered or dysfluent speech is sometimes considered a component of aphasia, apraxia of speech, dysarthria, and palilalia. Several theories have been evoked to explain acquired dysfluency. A well-known theory, particularly appealing to neurologists, is the old Orton-Travis theory (53,54), which popularized the concept that stutterers had incomplete cerebral dominance resulting in interhemispheric competition that in some way produced a fluency disorder. Other theories are that the dysfluency is a problem of impaired word or phoneme retrieval or that it may be a form of speech apraxia (55). Deal and Cannito (50), after a comprehensive review of the topic, suggest that the core of the problem is disordered motor control of the speech musculature and therefore a motor speech disorder.

MANAGEMENT

The prognosis for increased intelligibility in the moderately severe to mild dysarthric speaker or the establishment of communication through communication-aid technology for the totally anarthric speaker has vastly improved since the Mayo Clinic studies of 25 years ago. An early and seminal report on modern dysarthric rehabilitation by Netsell and Daniel (56) illustrates concepts in current dysarthria management. This report documents how a traumatically brain-injured 20-year-old man with flaccid dysarthria was shifted from an initial 5–10% level of speech intelligibility to a 90–95% level in a mere 6 weeks of therapy. Therapy consisted of a speech symptom–reduction approach utilizing systematic analysis of the nature and severity of the motor involvement in the four muscular subsystems supporting normal speech production. Adroit selection and sequencing of treatment procedures resulted in improvement in a timely and effective manner.

The symptoms of reduced loudness and hypernasality were attacked initially in the first 4 weeks of management. To maintain and increase subglottal air pressure for improved loudness, the patient worked with a water manometer with a continuous air leak monitoring his ability to produce subglottal air pressure. In eight 20-minute sessions the patient achieved sufficient air-pressure levels for increased loudness.

To improve velopharyngeal closure, attempts were first made to train the patient to use a strain-gauge transducer attached to the velum. Visual signaling of the positioning of the height of the velum was transmitted to an oscilloscope so that the patient could monitor progress through visual biofeedback. The flaccid paralysis of the velum was resistant to this exercise. This prompted the construction and fitting of a palatal lift prosthesis (57), which improved velopharyngeal function, reduced the threat of hypernasality to intelligibility, and increased the intraoral breath pressure for clearer speech articulation. During the next 2 weeks, laryngeal therapy was aimed at reducing breathiness from flaccid vocal folds. Recording of oral and nasal airflow during phonation employed a facial mask, a pneumotachometer, and a pressure transducer. This instrumentation allowed monitoring of laryngeal performance. Glottal airflow was normalized, breathiness was reduced, and loudness was increased even further.

In the last 2 weeks before discharge, therapy for the orofacial articulatory system was instituted. Lip weakness was monitored by auditory signals corresponding to changes in the voltage of a surface EMG lead as the lips were pressed together for 10-second intervals. In the final three sessions before discharge, the patient doubled his EMG levels, indicating increased lip strength. A bite-block (58) held between the molars reduced jaw forces from contributing to lip closure. Finally, resistance exercises to increase the strength of tongue movements aided articulation performance.

This case is reported in some detail to illustrate how careful sequencing of intervention procedures combined with appropriate prosthetic devices, biofeedback equipment, and the technology of the present-day speech-science laboratory is far superior to dysarthria management of the past, which chiefly employed oral exercises and articulation drills. Current clinical laboratories employ fiberoptics (59), video fluoroscopy (60), nasoendoscopy (61), instrumental visualization of fundamental frequency (Visipitch) (62), vocal-intensity measures (subglottal air pressure) (63), lung-volume assessment (Respitrace) (64), nasality evaluation (Nasometer) (65), and high speech computer data acquisition for the study of dysarthric speech physiology (66).

Yorkston, Buekelman, and Bell (67) have contributed a masterful textbook on the treatment of dysarthria, stressing intelligibility measures, control of speaking rate, linguistic stress training, and selection of augmentative communication devices. Dworkin's textbook (68) emphasizes speech exercises and drills for the dysarthric speaker. Love (9) has extended the principles of speech subsystem management and symptom reduction to childhood dysarthrics.

Neurologists (69,70) have recently called for comanagement of neurogenic communication disorders by both the physician and the speech–language pathologist. Lozona (70) has defined the individual roles of both professions, and Rosenfield (71) has provided lucid information on pharmacological approaches to treatment of motor speech disorders. Communication-aid technology—including devices from simple word and picture boards through personal computers modified for access even in severe disability, to computers that produce digitized and synthetic speech—ensure that any anarthric or severe dysarthric will have access to a viable means of communication (72).

The outlook for functional communication even in severe dysarthria and anarthria is improving. The armamentarium of management techniques and technologies has been broadened considerably, and the prognosis for compensated intelligibility or communication-aid use is the likelihood for most patients.

REFERENCES

1. Charcot JM. Lectures on the diseases of the nervous system. Vol 1. London: New Sydenham Society, 1877.
2. Liepmann H. Drei aufsatze dem apraxiege beit. Vol 1. Berlin: Krager, 1908.
3. Helm NA, Butler RB, Benson DF. Acquired stuttering. Arch Neurol 1978;28: 1159–1165.
4. Deal J, Cannito MP. Acquired neurogenic dysfluency. In: Vogel D, Cannito MP, eds. Treating disordered speech motor control. Austin, TX: PRO-ED, 1991:217–239.
5. Love RJ, Webb WG. Neurology for the speech–language pathologist. 2nd ed. Boston: Butterworth-Heinemann, 1992:209.
6. Hier DB, Goreliek PD, Shindler AG. Topics in behavioral neurology and neuropsychology. Boston: Butterworths, 1987:72–73.
7. Wertz RT, LaPointe LL, Rosenbek JC. Apraxia of speech in adults. Orlando, FL: Grune & Stratton, 1984:40–46.
8. DeRenzi E, Piezuro A, Vignolo LA. Oral apraxia and aphasia. Cortex 1966; 2:50–73.
9. Love RJ. Childhood motor speech disability. New York: Macmillan, 1992.
10. Gowers WR. A manual of diseases of the nervous system. Philadelphia: Blakiston, 1888.
11. Froeschels E. A contribution to the pathology and therapy of dysarthria due to certain cerebral lesions. J Speech Discord 1943;8:301–321.
12. Brain WR. Diseases of the nervous system. 3rd ed. London: Oxford University Press, 1948.
13. Luchsinger R, Arnold GE. Lehrbuch der stimm- und sprachheilkinde. Vienna: Springer-Verlag, 1949.
14. Peacher WG. The etiology and differential diagnosis of dysarthria. J Speech Hear Disord 1950;1:252–265.
15. Grewel F. Classification of dysarthrias. Acta Psychiat Neurol Scand 1957;32: 325–337.
16. Darley FL, Aronson AE, Brown JR. Clusters of deviant speech dimensions in the dysarthrias. J Speech Hear Res 1969;12:462–469.
17. Darley FL, Aronson AE, Brown JR. Differential diagnostic patterns of dysarthria. J Speech Hear Res 1969;12:246–269.
18. Darley FL, Aronson AE, Brown JR. Motor speech disorders. Philadelphia: Saunders, 1975.
19. Darley FL, Brown JR, Goldstein NP. Dysarthria in multiple sclerosis. J Speech Hear Res 1972;15:229–245.
20. Berry WR, Darley FL, Aronson AE, Goldstein NP. Dysarthria in Wilson's disease. J Speech Hear Res 1974;17:169–183.
21. Carrow E, Rivera V, Mauldin M, Shamblin L. Deviant speech characteristics in motor neuron disease. Arch Otolaryngol 1974;100:212–218.
22. Linebaugh C. The dysarthrias of Shy-Drager syndrome. J Speech Hear Disord 1979;44:55–60.
23. Joanette Y, Dudley JG. Dysarthria symptomatology of Friedreich's ataxia. Brain Lang 1980;10:39–50.

24. Workinger MS, Kent RD. Perceptual analysis of the dysarthrias in athetoid and spastic cerebral palsy. In: Moore CA, Yorkston KM, Beukelman DR, eds. Dysarthria and apraxia of speech. Baltimore: Paul H Brookes, 1991:109–126.

25. Stuart SL, Beukelman DR, Kenyon KK, Healy EC, Bernthal JE. Dysarthria following Reye's syndrome: A case report. In: Moore CA, Yorkston KM, Beukelman DR, eds. Dysarthria and apraxia of speech. Baltimore: Paul H Brookes, 1991:97–107.

26. Metter EJ, Hanson WR. Dysarthria in progressive supranuclear palsy. In: Moore CA, Yorkston KM, Beukelman DR, eds. Dysarthria and apraxia of speech. Baltimore: Paul H Brookes, 1991:127–136.

27. Halperin H, Darley FL, Brown JR. Differential language and neurological characteristics in cerebral involvement. J Speech Hear Disord 1973;38:162–173.

28. Whitehouse PJ Jr. The concept of cortical and subcortical dementia: Another look. Ann Neurol 1986;19:1–6.

29. Cummings JL, Benson DF. Subcortical dementia: Review of an emerging concept. Arch Neurol 1984;41:874–879.

30. Goodglass H, Kaplan E. The Boston diagnostic aphasia examination. Philadelphia: Lea & Febiger, 1983.

31. Goodglass H, Kaplan E. The Boston naming test. Philadelphia: Lea & Febiger, 1983.

32. Bayles KA, Tomoeda CA. Arizona battery for communication disorders of dementia. Tucson, AZ: Canyonland Publishing, 1991.

33. Porch BE. Porch index of communicative ability. Pal Alto, CA: Consulting Psychologists Press, 1981.

34. Johns DF, Darley FL. Phonemic variability in apraxia of speech. J Speech Hear Res 1970;13:556–583.

35. Odell KH, McNeil MR, Rosenbek JC, Hunter L. Perceptual characteristics of consonant production by apraxic speakers. J Speech Hear Disord 1990;55:345–359.

36. McNeil MR, Weismer G, Adams S, Mulligan M. Oral structure nonspeech motor control in normal, dysarthric, aphasic and apraxic speakers: Isometric force and static fine position control. J Speech Hear Res 1990;33:255–268.

37. McNeil MR, Caliguri M, Rosenbek JC. A comparison of labio-mandibular kinematic durations, displacements, velocities and dysmetrias in apraxic and normal adults. In: Prescott TE, ed. Clinical aphasiology. Vol 18. Boston: College-Hill Press, 1989:173–179.

38. Rosenbek JC, McNeil MR. A discussion of classification in motor speech disorders: Dysarthria and apraxia of speech. In: Moore CA, Yorkston KM, Beukelman DR, eds. Dysarthria and apraxia of speech. Baltimore: Paul H Brookes, 1991:289–295.

39. Wertz RT, Rosenbek JC. Where the ear fits: A perceptual evaluation of motor speech disorders. Semin Speech Lang 1992;13:39–54.

40. Enderby PM. Frenchay dysarthria assessment. San Diego: College-Hill Press, 1983.

41. Yorkston K, Beukelman DR. Assessment of intelligibility of dysarthric speech. Tigard, OR: CC Publications, 1981.

42. Netsell R, Lotz WK, Barlow SM. A speech physiology examination for individuals with dysarthria. In: Yorkston KM, Beukelman DR, eds. Recent advances in clinical dysarthria. Boston: College-Hill Press, 1989:3–37.

43. Gerratt BR, Till JA, Rosenbek JC, Wertz RT, Boysen AE. Use and perceived value of perceptual and instrumental measures in dysarthria management. In: Moore CA, Yorkston KM, Beukelman DR, eds. Dysarthria and apraxia of speech. Baltimore: Paul H Brookes, 1991:77–93.

44. Aronson AE, Lagerlund TD. Letter to the editor: Neuroimaging studies do not prove the existence of brain abnormalities in spastic (spasmodic) dysphonia. J Speech Hear Res 1991;34:801–811.

45. Aronson AE. Clinical voice disorders. 3rd ed. New York: Thieme, 1990.

46. Hartman DE, Abbs JH. Dysarthrias of movement disorders. In: Jankovic J, Tolsa E, eds. Advances in neurology. Vol 49. Facial dyskinesias. New York: Raven Press, 1988:298–306.

47. Finitzo T, Freeman F. Spastic dysphonia, whether and where: Results of seven years of research. J Speech Hear Res 1989;32:541–555.

48. Cannito MP. Neurobiological interpretation of spastic dysphonia. In: Vogel D, Cannito MP, eds. Treating disordered speech motor control. Austin, TX: PRO-ED, 1991:275–317.

49. Miller AE. Cessation of stuttering with progressive multiple sclerosis. Neurology 1985;35:1341–1343.

50. Deal J, Cannito MP. Acquired neurologic dysfluency. In: Vogel D, Cannito MP, eds. Treating disordered speech motor control. Austin, TX: PRO-ED, 1991:217–239.

51. Andrews G, Craig A, Feyer AM, Hoddinott S, Howie P, Neilson A. Stuttering: A review of research findings and theories circa 1982. J Speech Hear Disord 1983;48:226–246.

52. Fleet WS, Heilman KM. Acquired stuttering from a right hemisphere lesion in a right hander. Neurology 1985;35:1343–1346.

53. Orton ST. A physiological theory of reading disability and stuttering in children. N Engl J Med 1928;199:1045–1052.

54. Travis LE. Speech pathology. New York: Appleton Century, 1931.

55. Rosenbek J. Apraxia of speech—Relationship to stuttering. J Fluency Disord 1980;5:233–253.

56. Netsell R, Daniel B. Dysarthria in adults: Physiologic approach to rehabilitation. Arch Phys Med Rehabil 1979;60:502–508.

57. LaVelle WE, Hardy JC. Palatal lift prosthesis for the treatment of palatopharyngeal incompetence. J Prosthet Dent 1979;42:308–315.

58. Netsell R. Construction and use of a bite-block for use in evaluation and treatment of speech disorders. J Speech Hear Disord 1985;50:103–106.

59. D'Antonio L, Lotz W, Chait D, Netsell R. Fiberoptic recordings of velopharyngeal and laryngeal function during normal speech. J Am Speech Hear Assoc 1984;26:130A.

60. McWilliams BJ, Morris HL, Shelton RL. Instrumentation for assessing the velopharyngeal mechanism. In: McWilliams BJ, Morris HL, Shelton RL, eds. Cleft palate speech. 2nd ed. Philadelphia: BC Decker, 1990:163–196.

61. D'Antonio L, Chait D, Lotz W, Netsell R. Pediatric videonasoendoscopy in speech and voice evaluation. Otolaryng Head Neck Surg 1986;94:578–583.
62. Visipitch. Kay Elemetrics Corp., Pine Brook, NJ 07058-9798.
63. Netsell R, Hixon T. A non-invasive method for clinically estimating subglottal air pressure. J Speech Hear Disord 1978;43:326–330.
64. Respitrace. Ambulatory Monitoring Inc., Ardsley, NY 10502.
65. Nasometer. Kay Elemetrics Corp., Pine Brook, NJ 07058-9798.
66. Barlow SM, Netsell R. Clinical neurophysiology for individuals with dysarthria. In: Yorkston KM, Beukelman DR, eds. Recent advances in clinical dysarthria. Boston: College-Hill Press, 1989:53–82.
67. Yorkston KM, Beukelman DR, Bell KR. Clinical management of dysarthric speakers. Boston: College-Hill Press, 1988.
68. Dworkin J. Motor speech disorders: A treatment guide. St. Louis: Mosby-Year Book, 1991.
69. Kirshner HS. Foreword: Speech pathology and neurology: Intersecting specialities. In: Love RJ, Webb WG, eds. Neurology for the speech–language pathologist. Boston: Butterworth-Heinemann, 1992:ix–x.
70. Lozona R. Comanagement of disturbed speech motor control: The role of the neurologist and the speech pathologist. In: Vogel D, Cannito MP, eds. Treating disordered speech motor control. Austin, TX: PRO-ED, 1991:17–41.
71. Rosenfield DB. Pharmacologic approaches to speech motor disorders. In: Vogel D, Cannito MP, eds. Treating disordered speech motor control. Austin, TX: PRO-ED, 1991:111–152.
72. Beukelman DR, Yorkston KM, Dowden PA. Communication augmentation: A casebook of clinical management. Boston: College-Hill Press, 1985.

3

Apraxia of Speech

Howard S. Kirshner

Vanderbilt University School of Medicine, Nashville, Tennessee

INTRODUCTION

Speech apraxia, or apraxia of speech, is a disorder intermediate between the motor speech disorders, or dysarthrias, and the aphasias. The diagnosis is controversial, recognized by some but not all specialists in aphasia, and generally used by speech–language pathologists but rarely by neurologists and other physicians. Descriptions of speech apraxia, however, have involved a consistent pattern of articulatory disturbances that should be diagnosable at the bedside and amenable to scientific study. Recent experimental studies have shown specific breakdowns of speech expression. Since the treatment of patients with disorders of communication requires that members of the treatment team understand each other's language, it is important that physicians and speech pathologists agree on the clinical phenomena of speech apraxia and its relationship to other speech and language disorders. This chapter reviews the clinical findings of speech apraxia, summarizes some of the data from recent experimental studies that yield insight into the mechanisms of the disorder, and discusses the relationship of speech apraxia to the dysarthrias, the aphasias, and the apraxias.

Deal and Darley (1) defined speech apraxia as

articulatory disorder resulting from impairment, as a result of brain damage, of the capacity to program the positioning of speech musculature and the sequencing of muscle movements for the volitional production of phonemes. The speech musculature does not show significant weakness, slowness or incoordination when used for reflex and automatic acts.

This definition specifies that speech apraxia involves an abnormal articulation and sequencing of phonemes and implies that the disorder is not one of weakness or ataxia of the articulatory muscles, but rather an apraxia. Apraxia is discussed later in this chapter and also in Chapter 21. The definition also implies that there is no disturbance of central language functions, or aphasia.

While *apraxia of speech* generally refers to syndromes acquired in adult life, a developmental apraxia of speech has been recognized in children (2,3). This chapter considers only acquired speech apraxia.

CLINICAL DESCRIPTIONS

Johns and Darley (4) described apraxia of speech as involving phonemic errors, characterized by substitutions, additions, and repetitions, with marked disturbance of the prosody or cadence of speech. Substitution errors are more common than the distorted phonemes typically seen in dysarthria. Most importantly, the speech errors are inconsistent from one trial to the next, while those of dysarthria are more constant, regardless of context (5).

The key elements of speech apraxia, as defined by Darley and colleagues (1,4), are listed in Table 1. First, a triad of essential components must be fulfilled: articulatory substitution errors, often involving consonants; difficulty with initiation of articulation of the required word or phrase, giving the speech pattern a hesitant, groping quality; and variability in error pattern, such that the errors of articulation are not consistent from one trial to the next. Normal articulation may be seen at times, especially in automatic phrases. A number of minor criteria or characteristics are also usually seen in apraxic utterances: greater difficulty with initial consonants than with later consonants within a word; increasing difficulty with increasing word length or numbers of syllables; marked disturbance of prosody, with an effortful, slow delivery characterized by starts, stops, and repetitions; greater difficulty with imitation of speech than with oral reading; a spontaneous tendency to repeat incorrect utterances several times, often with eventual production of the correct articulation; and a discrepancy between intact speech perception and impaired speech production (1,4).

For a neurologist, the critical feature that distinguishes speech apraxia from aphasia is the preservation of speech comprehension, reading, and writing. The sparing of these functions indicates a disorder of articulation, not of language.

Table 1   Clinical Characteristics of Speech Apraxia

A. Major criteria
  1. Articulatory substitution errors — especially involving consonants
  2. Difficulty with initiation of articulation — starts, stops, repetitions
  3. Variability in error pattern — inconsistency from trial to trial, normal articulation at times
B. Minor criteria
  1. Greater difficulty with initial consonants than with later consonants
  2. Increasing difficulty with longer words or phrases
  3. Marked disturbance of prosody
  4. Greater difficulty with repetition than with oral reading
  5. Spontaneous repetitions
  6. Discrepancy between intact speech perception and disturbed speech production

Source: Adapted from Refs. 1 and 4.

HISTORY

The phenomena of speech apraxia have been described under many different names, all sharing the central features just discussed and the correlation with predominantly left-frontal lesions. While descriptions of abnormal speech secondary to brain injury appeared even in ancient times, the modern study of speech disorders began with Paul Broca in 1861. Broca (6) described altered articulation with preserved comprehension in his patient LeBorgne, or "Tan," yet he noted that LeBorgne could move his tongue in all directions on command. By modern terminology, Broca's patient manifested nonfluent aphasia without oral apraxia. Broca chose the term *aphemia* for this speech/language pattern, but Trousseau's 1864 (7) term *aphasia* was adopted instead. Pierre Marie (8) doubted the existence of a language disorder from left-frontal lesions, declaring that the associated speech disorder was a simple *anarthria*. Weisenburg and McBride's 1935 reference on language disorders (9) referred to nonfluent aphasia from frontal lesions as *Predominantly expressive aphasia*, which became the most commonly used designation; Goldstein (10) and Russell and Espir (11) adopted the similar term *motor aphasia*. As is discussed in Chapter 4, the terms *expressive* or *motor* aphasia have misled many students of aphasia, since they do not make any reference to comprehension, and virtually all aphasias impair language expression in one way or another. Nathan (12) was the first modern author to apply the term *apraxia* to speech disorders, in his description of *apraxic dysarthria*. Macdonald Critchley (13) used the term *cortical dysarthria*, while Denny-

Brown (14) preferred the term *apraxia of verbal expression.* These and other authors led to the coinage of the term *verbal apraxia* by Darley and colleagues at the Mayo Clinic, later modified to *apraxia of speech.*

Disturbed articulation of phonemes lies at the root of all these descriptive terms. The field of aphasiology, unfortunately, has been encumbered by continued use of these terms, made more confusing by differing definitions and interpretations. This terminological morass, along with differences in theoretical interpretation of the phenomena, has interfered with communication among professionals working with speech- and language-impaired patients. It is ironic that the study of language disorders has been the scene of so much difficulty with linguistic terms.

TESTING

Apraxia of speech is ascertained by the bedside language examination described in Chapter 1, with additional criteria for motor speech disorders in Chapter 2. Wertz (personal communication) suggests, in addition to the usual spontaneous speech sample and oral reading sample, the use of specialized repetition tasks, including: repetition of polysyllabic, multiconsonant utterances such as "pa-da-ca," repeated trials with the same polysyllabic word such as "artillery" or "impossibility," and repetition of words of increasing length such as "jab, jabber, jabbering." Patients with speech apraxia have particular difficulty with these tasks, producing variable errors from trial to trial on the polysyllabic word test and showing increasing difficulty with increasing numbers of syllables. For example, a speech-apraxic patient repeated artillery as "artilerp, artifferet, artriffert, artillery, artiperil."

EXPERIMENTAL STUDIES

Modern studies, using sophisticated testing methodologies, have contributed a body of factual knowledge to our understanding of the phenomena of apraxia of speech. Blumstein (15) has reviewed experimental analyses of phoneme errors in aphasia. In general, phonetic errors made by patients with anterior aphasias are close approximations of the correct sound. If consonant utterances are analyzed according to the three features of place of articulation, voicing, and manner of articulation (e.g., stop consonant versus fricative), errors in consonant production tend to differ by only one feature from the correct sound. For example, "p" may be substituted for "b," but not for "d." The "p" and "b" share the same place of articulation (labial) and differ only in voicing, while "d" differs in both place and voicing from "p." Similar errors apply to the timing of voicing and to the opening of the velum to produce a nasal sound, as in the difference between "b" and "m"; these share place of articulation and voicing but differ in velum opening, such that "m" has a nasal quality. By this analysis, phonetic errors are inconsistent, as emphasized by Deal and Darley (1), but they are not random. Vowel-sound errors, while less evident than those of consonants, also appear to vary by single-feature changes.

According to Blumstein's analysis, posterior aphasics make substitutions of words or phonemes but few phonetic errors, while anterior aphasics make many phonetic errors, as well as some phonemic errors (phonetic substitutions differ by only one consonant or vowel sound, while phonemic substitutions involve choice of an inappropriate phoneme, the smallest part of a word that determines meaning). In fact, many of the phoneme substitutions referred to by Deal and Darley (1) as the predominant type of error in speech apraxia may actually be simple phonetic errors.

Blumstein (15) concluded from these phonetic analyses that articulations are particularly likely to show errors when they require rapid sequencing or timing of two independent articulators. These independent articulators may be separate consonants, the sequence between a consonant sound and voicing, or that between a consonant sound and the opening of the velum. In general terms, speech apraxia is a deficit of the timing and integration of articulatory movements (15).

Kent and Rosenbek (16) reported a detailed acoustic analysis of apraxic speech. The slow speaking rate of patients with apraxia of speech was caused by slowness of transitions between articulations, steady states, and pauses. Articulatory movements themselves were slow and inaccurate, particularly for consonants, and there was associated mistiming of voicing with articulation. Difficulty with initiation of speech resulted in false starts and restarts. In general, errors occur in the sequencing of complex speech sounds.

Modern instrumental methods have further contributed to the analysis of articulation in speech apraxia, as reviewed by Miller (17). Fromm et al. (18) applied techniques of electromyography, force transducers on the lips and mandible, and a laryngeal accelerometer for voice-onset time. Patients with speech apraxia showed disturbed temporal sequencing of muscle contractions for articulation; for example, agonist and antagonist muscles contracted simultaneously. Itoh and Sasanuma (19) found similar incoordination or mistiming between movements of the tongue and velum. Hardcastle, Morgan Barry, and Clark (20), in electropalatographic studies of lingual-palatal approximation, reported poor timing, excessive force, and overshooting or undershooting of the target. Ryalls (21) reported timing and sequencing errors in the articulation of vowels. Miller (17) concluded that the deficit is not one of phoneme selection, but rather of "disintegration or dyssynchronization of the relative movement onsets and terminations of the articulators entrained, or coupled, to produce a sound."

Apraxia of speech, according to these instrumental acoustic and phonetic studies, appears to involve a specific disorder of articulation, characterized by difficulty with sequencing of timed articulations, such as transitions between consonants and the sequential timing of consonant articulation and voice onset or of consonant articulation and opening of the velum. These misarticulations have an inconsistent but nonrandom pattern. Any theory of apraxia of speech must account for these phenomena.

APRAXIA OF SPEECH AND DYSARTHRIA

The relationship of speech apraxia to dysarthria is relatively straightforward. As summarized in Chapter 2, dysarthria refers to a consistent pattern of misarticulation. In apraxia of speech, the same phonemes may be articulated correctly in one context, particularly in automatic sequences, and incorrectly in another, and the specific substitutions may vary from error to error. Dysarthria is a loss of the ability to articulate specific sounds, while speech apraxia is a disorder of the sequencing of speech sounds, each of which can be articulated correctly as individual utterances.

APRAXIA OF SPEECH AND APHASIA

The relationship of speech apraxia to the aphasias is more complex. Darley and colleagues have long held that Broca's aphasia does not represent a true aphasia, but rather an apraxic misrendering of phonemic expression (22). This position is reminiscent of Pierre Marie's 1906 contention (8) that left-frontal-lobe lesions produce only anarthria. As will be discussed in Chapter 4, modern descriptions of Broca's aphasia (23–25) include not only disturbed phoneme articulation, but also a grammatical language disturbance, consisting of "telegraphic" or agrammatic speech, anomia, impaired comprehension of syntax, alexia (26), and inability to write with the nonparalyzed left arm. Shewan (27) demonstrated that Broca's aphasics have difficulty with comprehension as well as expression of phoneme sequences. The agrammatism of expressive speech also corresponds to similar difficulty in the comprehension of complex syntax (28,29). Broca's aphasia is thus an aphasia, and not an isolated apraxia of speech. In Broca's and other aphasias, however, speech apraxia may contribute to the articulatory disorder. Apraxia of speech is especially likely to be a contributing factor to aphasia in patients who write better than they speak (30).

Broca's aphasia is only one of several syndromes of speech and language abnormality associated with left-frontal lesions (31). As discussed in Chapter 4, Mohr and colleagues (23) have established that the full syndrome of Broca's aphasia is a lasting deficit that usually evolves from global aphasia over a period of weeks to months. The responsible lesions are typically much larger than the traditional Broca's area in the left inferior frontal gyrus, involving extensive areas of the left frontal and parietal lobes, subcortical white matter, the insula, and parts of the basal ganglia, especially the anterior limb of the internal capsule and putamen (23,31). More restricted lesions involving Broca's area and the lower motor cortex of the face area produce an early Broca's aphasia, which tends to resolve nearly completely over a period of weeks. This syndrome has been called *little Broca aphasia* (23) or *Broca's area aphasia* (31). The presence of a grammatical disturbance is less evident in these cases, but literal or phonemic paraphasias and disturbed grammatical comprehension are usually present early in recovery. These patients, too, have a language disorder, and not simply a motor speech impairment.

More problematic is the syndrome referred to as *aphemia* by contemporary authors (31,32). These patients are often mute acutely, then speak hesitantly, with dysarthria and some agrammatism. Evidence of a language disturbance in naming, comprehension, or writing tends to disappear rapidly, but the motor speech disorder may persist. The lesions involve the lower motor cortex for the face in the precentral gyrus, with variable extension into the inferior frontal convolution and subjacent white matter (32). The lesions are smaller than those of the Broca's area aphasia. Alexander, Stuss, and Benson (31), in their review of frontal lesions and language, equated aphemia with apraxia of speech. The principal features of the two disorders are certainly similar, especially the nonfluent speech output in the setting of preserved comprehension, reading, and writing. Both aphemia and pure or isolated apraxia of speech are rare compared to Broca's aphasia and Broca's area aphasia, which share the articulatory or speech output disorder but have aphasic deficits as well.

Other left frontal and deep, basal ganglia syndromes are less closely related to apraxia of speech. Lesions purely involving the subcortical structures, especially the head of the caudate nucleus, anterior limb of the internal capsule, and anterior putamen (33,34), produce dysarthria and slow, nonfluent speech, but little grammatical disturbance. Transcortical motor aphasia is a syndrome in which spontaneous speech is nonfluent or mute, but repetition and comprehension are normal. The lesions lie in the frontal lobe anterior to Broca's area, in the medial frontal lobe in the region of the supplementary motor cortex, or in the deep frontal white matter, all areas supplied by the anterior cerebral artery (35–38). These patients have hesitant speech but lack a prominent articulatory disorder, of either the speech-apraxic or the dysarthric type, unless the lesion also involves the white matter underlying Broca's area and the lower motor cortex (31). Finally, disorders of discourse, without articulatory or language deficits, are seen with left prefrontal lesions, well anterior to the traditional Broca's area (31). These discourse disorders are more closely related to frontal-lobe syndromes of disinhibited behavior than to the aphasias.

In summary, apraxia of speech is closely related to nonfluent aphasia. The phenomena of apraxia of speech are present in the three syndromes of Broca's aphasia, Broca's area aphasia, and aphemia. In the first two, the phenomena exist as part of a larger deficit, involving a language disorder, or aphasia. The third syndrome, aphemia, may simply represent another term for pure apraxia of speech. Both syndromes are uncommon, and it is difficult from the limited case descriptions to distinguish them. For these reasons, many neurologists have not adopted the term *apraxia of speech* at all, and even some speech–language pathologists have preferred to consider apraxia of speech simply a part of aphasia (39).

APRAXIA OF SPEECH AND LIMB APRAXIA

The relationship of speech apraxia to limb apraxia is even more problematic than that of speech apraxia to aphasia. The complex subject of limb apraxias is reviewed in Chapter 21 and elsewhere (40,41). Geschwind (41) defined apraxias as "disorders of learned movement which cannot be accounted for either by weakness, incoordination, or sensory loss, or by incomprehension of or inattention to commands." The patient cannot carry out a motor act on command, despite evidence of understanding of the command and ability to perform the same motor act in a different context. The resemblance of this definition of apraxia to the Deal and Darley (1) definition of verbal apraxia cited earlier is obvious. Liepmann (42) originally described three types of limb apraxia: ideomotor, ideational, and limb-kinetic. We shall consider the relationship of apraxia of speech to each of these classical apraxia syndromes. The term *apraxia* has also been applied to a number of other neurological syndromes, enumerated in Chapter 21, that have little relevance either to Liepmann's models of apraxia or to the phenomena of apraxia of speech. These other apraxias will not be discussed here.

Ideomotor apraxia is a failure to translate the idea of a movement into its execution. The patient with ideomotor apraxia fails to carry out a motor command, such as "show me how to use a comb," producing either a very crude movement or running the fingers through the hair ("use of the body part as object"). The patient understands the command, as indicated either by a verbal description of the movement or by choice of the correct action from multiple pantomimes. The patient usually performs only modestly better in imitating the examiner's movement than in responding to a verbal command. Finally, the patient must also be able to carry out the movement in another context, for example by use of an actual object, such as a comb. Since the patient performs normally with the actual object, ideomotor apraxia is evident only in an artificial test situation, as in these pantomimes, and not in manipulation of real objects in the environment.

Oral apraxia, as stated earlier, is an inability to perform nonverbal, oral movements on command, despite the occurrence of the same movements spontaneously. The patient may fail to carry out a command to lick the lips or cough, yet have no trouble licking ice cream from his lips or coughing spontaneously. Imitative movements of the facial, oral, lingual, and pharyngeal muscles may also be impaired. Oral apraxia is simply ideomotor apraxia involving the oral-facial-lingual muscles. Like apraxia of speech, oral apraxia can be found in many patients with nonfluent aphasia (43,44). Lesions in patients with oral apraxia tend to involve the frontal and central opercula, insula, and superior temporal gyrus (44). Oral apraxia and apraxia of speech, however, do not always occur together. Broca (6), as stated earlier, noted articulatory disturbance without oral apraxia in his original patient. LaPointe and Wertz (45) found oral apraxia in only 50% of patients with apraxia of speech. Oral apraxia is thus not identical with and cannot explain apraxia of speech.

The relationship of apraxia of speech to ideomotor apraxia of the limbs is also problematic. As stated earlier, ideomotor limb apraxia is seen only in artificial pantomimes, and not in manipulation of actual objects in the environment. Since apraxia of speech occurs in spontaneous speech, and not only on command, and since the movements of speech always involve the actual structures of the vocal tract, there cannot be a complete analogy between apraxia of speech and ideomotor apraxia of the limbs. The two disorders also have important differences in terms of theoretical models of brain functioning. Ideomotor apraxia has been interpreted by Liepmann (42) and Geschwind (41) as a disconnection between the brain centers for understanding a motor command and those that program the movement (see Chapter 21). As discussed by Buckingham (46), apraxia of speech is usually considered to result from direct damage to the centers for encoding motor speech, rather than from a disconnection between centers of understanding and motor function. In more specific neuroanatomical terms, speech apraxia involves damage to the secondary motor cortex, which controls the speech musculature, while dysarthria results from damage to the primary motor cortex or its axons (47). For both descriptive and theoretical reasons, apraxia of speech is not an example of ideomotor apraxia.

While ideomotor apraxia does not explain the phenomena of speech apraxia, ideomotor apraxia of the limbs does have a strong correlation with aphasia. DeRenzi, Motti, and Nichelli (48), in a study of imitation of gestures, found ideomotor apraxia in most aphasics, whether the aphasia was of a Broca's, Wernicke's, or conduction type. These authors, as well as Kertesz, Ferro, and Shewan (49), however, found poor correlations between the degree of deficit in language and that of praxis, and occasional cases in which the two were dissociated. Assuming that the left hemisphere is dominant for skilled motor acts as well as language (41), the anatomical proximity of structures responsible for these two functions may explain their frequent co-occurrence. This shared neuroanatomy is more likely the basis of the correlation of apraxia and aphasia than a theoretical linking of the two deficits on the basis of symbolic expression of learned motor and language concepts (49).

The second type of apraxia, ideational apraxia, is less well understood than ideomotor apraxia. The term has been used by different authors to describe different phenomena. Some authors (50,51) have used the term to refer to loss of ability to carry out a series action, such as filling and lighting a pipe or brewing and pouring a cup of coffee. DeRenzi and Lucchelli (52), on the other hand, defined ideational apraxia as an inability to use an actual object. These authors found that failure to use single objects correlated well with inability to perform a series action involving real objects, but not with ideomotor apraxia. By either definition, ideational apraxia is a genuine problem in the real world, in that patients mishandle actual objects. The lesions of ideational apraxia can be diffuse, as in dementing diseases, or localized to the posterior left hemisphere (52).

Heilman (53) proposed another definition of ideational apraxia: failure to perform a movement on command in the setting of preserved ability to imitate the movement and describe it verbally. More recently, Heilman and colleagues (54) have used DeRenzi's definition of ideational apraxia as an inability to use an actual object in a case report of a 67-year-old left-handed man with a right-hemisphere stroke. His initial aphasia improved to the point that he could name objects and point to objects named by the examiner. By contrast, he could not use objects appropriately or describe their use, even though he could name them. Many patients with severe aphasia misuse objects; a patient with global aphasia, for example, might take a toothbrush prepared with toothpaste and rub it into his hair. In most cases, this ideational apraxia is accompanied by severe aphasia and is difficult to distinguish from comprehension loss, confusion, or agnosia. The patient in the above report, however, could name the objects, indicating a selective loss of knowledge or memory of the use of objects or tools.

Ideational apraxia, defined as an inability to use an actual object, deviates from Geschwind's definition of apraxia, in that the patient cannot be said to have full understanding of the movement. Any attempt to relate ideational apraxia to apraxia of speech is also problematic, since the speech musculature is not analogous to an object or tool.

Liepmann's third category of apraxia is limb-kinetic apraxia, a loss of motor engrams for skilled movement of a single limb. Geschwind (41) rejected limb-kinetic apraxia as a true apraxia, in that it cannot be separated from mild pyramidal tract involvement or primary motor impairment. Neurologists frequently see stroke patients whose hemiparesis recovers to the point that gross strength is intact but fine movements remain clumsy. This deficit is somewhat reminiscent of apraxia of speech, in which the strength of individual muscle groups making up the speech apparatus is intact but there are difficulties with the timing of articulation. According to Buckingham (46), Liepmann himself referred to articulatory disturbances as a limb-kinetic apraxia applied to the speech apparatus. Even Broca (6) was aware that the simple oral movements that are preserved in some aphasics cannot compare to the much finer coordination and timing of movement required for speech. As in limb-kinetic apraxia, the operative deficit may be a primary motor deficit of mild degree. Limb-kinetic apraxia is thus the closest of the traditional apraxias to apraxia of speech. The question remains, however, whether either apraxia of speech or limb-kinetic apraxia is a true apraxia.

SUMMARY AND CONCLUSIONS

Apraxia of speech is a disorder intermediate between dysarthria and aphasia. It may exist as an isolated deficit or as a contributing factor to the speech and language disturbance of syndromes such as Broca's aphasia. While theoretical explanations of speech apraxia differ, the phenomena involved in speech apraxia have been clearly described and analyzed. Recent experimental studies have provided greater specificity to the errors of apraxia of speech and have confirmed the existence of a disorder of the temporal sequencing of articulation of consonants and vowels, of consonants and voice onset, and of consonants and the opening of the velum. These descriptive features must be taken into account in any theoretical explanation of the syndrome.

Apraxia of speech differs from dysarthria in the inconsistency of the errors and in the occasional production of normal articulation, especially in automatic sequences. Apraxia of speech cannot be separated so easily from nonfluent aphasia. Most patients with the features of speech apraxia also have aphasia, as judged by agrammatism, anomia, reduced comprehension of syntax, alexia, and agraphia. Those few patients who have an articulatory disturbance but no discernible language deficit have been diagnosed as having either aphemia or isolated apraxia of speech (31). These two syndromes, aphemia and pure speech apraxia, are both rare and limited in description. Whether they are separate or identical syndromes is thus uncertain at present.

Apraxia of speech and apraxia of the limbs are separate phenomena. The traditional syndromes of ideomotor and ideational apraxia do not account for speech apraxia. Oral apraxia, an ideomotor apraxia involving the face, lips, tongue, and pharynx, may occur with or without apraxia of speech and cannot serve as an explanation for it. Limb-kinetic apraxia shares with speech apraxia the presence of a disturbance of fine movements without gross weakness. Neither syndrome, however, has been clearly demonstrated to be a true apraxia rather than a mild form of elementary motor deficit.

The term *apraxia of speech* describes a syndrome of abnormal speech articulation, of increasingly precise and mechanistic description, but it has not gained acceptance by neurologists and has impeded communication between physicians and speech–language pathologists. Until a better term is adopted, however, speech and language researchers of all disciplines should seek to understand and promulgate the increasingly sophisticated knowledge of the mechanisms of speech apraxia, for the benefit of patients with speech and language impairments.

REFERENCES

1. Deal JL, Darley FL. The influence of linguistic and situational variables on phonemic accuracy in apraxia of speech. J Speech Hearing Res 1972;15:639–653.
2. Yoss KA, Darley FL. Developmental apraxia of speech in children with defective articulation. J Speech Hearing Res 1974;17:399–416.
3. Love RJ, Fitzgerald M. Is the diagnosis of developmental apraxia of speech valid? Australian J Human Comm Dis 1984;12:71–82.
4. Johns DF, Darley FL. Phonemic variability in apraxia of speech. J Speech Hearing Res 1970;13:556–583.
5. LaPointe LL. Neurologic abnormalities affecting speech. In: Tower DB, ed. The nervous system. Vol 3. Human communication and its disorders. New York: Raven Press, 1975:493–499.
6. Broca P. Remarques sur le siège de la faculté du langage articulé, suivies d'une observation d'aphemie (perte de la parole). Bull Soc Anat Paris, 2nd series, 1861:6:332–333 and 343–357. Translated in: Rottenberg DA, Hochberg FH, eds. Neurological classics in modern translation. New York: Hafner Press, 1975: 136–149.
7. Trousseau A. Clinique Médicale de l'Hôtel-Dieu de Paris. 2nd ed. Paris: JB Ballière, 1864.
8. Marie P. La troisième circonvolution frontale gauche ne joue aucun rôle spécial dans la fonction du langage. Sem Med 1906;26:565–571.
9. Weisenburg T, McBride K. Aphasia: A clinical and psychological study. New York: Commonwealth Fund, 1935. Reprinted in 1964, New York: Hafner Press.
10. Goldstein K. Language and language disturbance. New York: Grune & Stratton, 1948.
11. Russell WR, Espir MLE. Traumatic aphasia. London: Oxford University Press, 1961.
12. Nathan PW. Facial apraxia and apraxic dysarthria. Brain 1947;70:449–478.
13. Critchley M. Articulatory defects in aphasia. J Laryngol Otol 1952;66:1–17.

14. Denny-Brown D. Physiological aspects of disturbances of speech. Australian J Exp Biol Med Sci 1965;43:455–474.
15. Blumstein S. Phonological aspects of aphasia. In: Sarno MT, ed. Acquired aphasia. 2nd ed. San Diego: Academic Press, 1991:151–180.
16. Kent RD, Rosenbek JC. Acoustic patterns of apraxia in speech. J Speech Hearing Res 1984;26:231–249.
17. Miller N. Apraxia of speech. In: Code C, ed. The characteristics of aphasia. London: Taylor & Francis, 1991:131–154.
18. Fromm D, Abbs J, McNeil M, Rosenbek J. Simultaneous perceptual-physiological method for studying apraxia of speech. In: Brookshire RH, ed. Clinical aphasiology conference proceedings. Minneapolis: BRK, 1982:251–262.
19. Itoh M, Sasanuma S. Articulatory movements in apraxia of speech. In: Rosenbek JC, McNeil MR, Aronson AE, eds. Apraxia of speech: Physiology, acoustics, linguistics, and management. San Diego: College-Hill Press, 1984:135–166.
20. Hardcastle W, Morgan Barry RA, Clark C. Articulatory and voicing characteristics of adult dysarthric and verbal dyspraxic speakers: an instrumental study. Br J Dis Commun 1985;20:249–270.
21. Ryalls J, Vowel production in aphasia: towards an account of the consonant-vowel dissociation. In: Ryalls J, ed. Phonetic approaches to speech production in aphasia and related disorders. An Diego: College-Hill Press, 1987:23–43.
22. Rosenbek JC, Kent RD, LaPointe LL. Apraxia of speech: an overview and some perspectives. In: Rosenbek JC, McNeil MR, Aronson AE, eds. Apraxia of speech: physiology, acoustics, linguistics, management. San Diego: College-Hill Press, 1984:1–72.
23. Mohr JP, Pessin MS, Finkelstein S, Funkenstein HH, Duncan GW, Davis KR. Broca aphasia: pathologic and clinical. Neurology 1978;28:311–324.
24. Caramazza A, Berndt RS, Basili AG, Koller JJ. Syntactic processing deficits in aphasia. Cortex 1981;17:333–348.
25. Tramo JJ, Baynes K, Volpe BT. Impaired syntactic comprehension and production in Broca's aphasia: CT lesion localization and recovery patterns. Neurology 1988;38:95–98.
26. Benson DF. The third alexia. Arch Neurol 1977;34:327–331.
27. Shewan CM. Phonological processing in Broca's aphasia. Brain Lang 1980;10:72–88.
28. Goodglass H, Blumstein SE, Gleason JB, Hyde MR, Green E, Statlender S. The effect of syntactic encoding on sentence comprehension in aphasia. Brain Lang 1979;7:201–209.
29. Heilman KM, Scholes RJ. The nature of comprehension errors in Broca's, conduction, and Wernicke's aphasics. Cortex 1976;12:258–265.
30. Kirshner HS. Apraxia of speech: A linguistic enigma: A neurologist's perspective. Sem Speech Lang 1992;13:14–24.
31. Alexander MP, Benson DF, Stuss DT. Frontal lobes and language. Brain Lang 1989;37:656–691.
32. Schiff HB, Alexander MP, Naeser MA, Galaburda AM. Aphemia. Clinical-anatomic correlations. Arch Neurol 1983;40:720–727.

33. Naeser MA, Alexander MP, Helm-Estabrooks N, Levine HL, Laughlin SA, Geschwind N. Aphasia with predominantly subcortical lesion sites: Description of three capsular/putaminal aphasia syndromes. Arch Neurol 1982;39:2-14.

34. Damasio AR, Damasio H, Rizzo M, Varney N, Gersh F. Aphasia with non-hemorrhagic lesions in the basal ganglia and internal capsule. Arch Neurol 1982; 39:15-20.

35. Rubens AB. Aphasia with infarction in the territory of the anterior cerebral artery. Cortex 1975;11:239-250.

36. Masdeu JC, Schoene WC, Funkenstein H. Aphasia following infarction of the left supplementary motor area. Neurology 1978;28:1220-1223.

37. Alexander MP, Schmitt MA. The aphasia syndrome of stroke in the left anterior cerebral artery territory. Arch Neurol 1980;37:97-100.

38. Freedman M, Alexander MP, Naeser MA. Anatomic basis of transcortical motor aphasia. Neurology 1984;34:409-417.

39. Martin AD. Some objections to the term *apraxia of speech*. J Speech Hearing Dis 1974;39:53-64.

40. Kirshner HS. The apraxias. In: Bradley WG, Daroff RB, Fenichel GM, Marsden CD, eds. Neurology in clinical practice. Vol 1. Boston: Butterworth-Heinemann, 1991:117-122.

41. Geschwind N. The apraxias: neural mechanisms of disorders of learned movement. Amer Sci 1975; 63:188-195.

42. Liepmann H. The syndrome of apraxia (motor asymboly) based on a case of unilateral apraxia. Monatschrift fur Psychiatrie und Neurologie 1900;8:15-44. Translated in: Rottenberg DA, Hochberg FH, eds. Neurological classics in modern translation. New York: Hafner Press, 1977:155-183.

43. Mateer C, Kimura D. Impairment of nonverbal oral movements in aphasia. Brain Lang 1977;4:262-276.

44. Tognola G, Vignolo LA. Brain lesions associated with oral apraxia in stroke patients: a clinico-neuroradiological investigation with the CT scan. Neuropsychologia 1980;18:257-272.

45. LaPointe LL, Wertz RT. Oral-movement abilities and articulatory characteristics of brain-injured adults. Percept Motor Skills 1974;39:39-46.

46. Buckingham H. Explanations for the concept of apraxia of speech. In: Sarno MT, ed. Acquired aphasia. 2nd ed. San Diego: Academic Press, 1991:151-180.

47. Keller E. The cortical representation of motor processes of speech. In: Keller E, Gopnik M, eds. Motor and sensory processes of language. Hillsdale: Lawrence Erlbaum, 1987:125-162.

48. DeRenzi E, Motti F, Nichelli P. Imitating gestures. A quantitative approach to ideomotor apraxia. Arch Neurol 1980;37:6-10.

49. Kertesz A, Ferro JM, Shewan CM. Apraxia and aphasia: the functional-anatomical basis for their dissociation. Neurology 1984;34:40-47.

50. Pick A. Studien uber motorische apraxia und ihr nahestehende erscheinungen; ihre bedeutung in der symptomatologie psychopathischer symptomen-komplexe. Leipzig: Deuticke, 1905.

51. Poeck K. Ideational apraxia. J Neurol 1983;230:1-5.
52. DeRenzi E, Lucchelli F. Ideational apraxia. Brain 1988;111:1173-1185.
53. Heilman KM. Ideational apraxia—a re-definition. Brain 1973;96:861-864.
54. Ochipa C, Rothi LJG, Heilman KM. Ideational apraxia: a deficit in tool selection and use. Ann Neurol 1989;25:190-193.

4

Classical Aphasia Syndromes

Howard S. Kirshner

Vanderbilt University School of Medicine, Nashville, Tennessee

INTRODUCTION

Since Broca's 1861 study (1), aphasiologists have applied widely varying classification schemes, based on contrasting theories of aphasia. These classifications have employed different terminologies, which have discouraged students and given the impression that aphasia is an arcane subject, more a topic of philosophical debate than of practical usefulness in patient care. The phenomena of aphasia, although cloaked in different terms, have remained the same. This chapter describes the typical features of each aphasia syndrome, the associated neurological signs, and the neuroanatomical data from brain imaging studies. The classification of Benson and Geschwind (2), recently modified by Alexander and Benson (3), is generally favored by neurologists because it is based on a bedside language examination like that of Chapter 1, it follows logically from neuroanatomical lesion localizations, and it correlates with standardized testing by the Boston Diagnostic Aphasia Examination (BDAE) (3) or its modified form, the Western Aphasia Battery (WAB) (4). A physician can diagnose an aphasia syndrome at the bedside, confirm it by standardized aphasia tests administered by a speech–language pathologist, and correlate it with localization information from brain imaging studies.

In contrast to the routine clinical use of bedside examinations and standardized aphasia batteries, research studies of aphasia often utilize single or small series of subjects, evaluated with individualized methodologies designed to test a specific language hypothesis or create a theoretical model of language function. The categories of language dysfunction in such studies do not always break down according to classical aphasia syndromes. Even in these studies, however, the classical syndromes serve as a starting point for new neurolinguistic models.

The traditional aphasia classification system divides aphasias into eight syndromes: Broca's, global, Wernicke's, conduction, anomic, transcortical motor, transcortical sensory, and mixed transcortical aphasia, also called the *syndrome of the isolation of the speech area*. This chapter considers these eight classical syndromes, as well as several other language disorders. Two additional minor syndromes, aphemia and pure word deafness, involve selective deficits of expressive speech and auditory comprehension, respectively. A new category of aphasia classification involves atypical language syndromes associated with subcortical lesions, such as those involving the dominant thalamus or basal ganglia. These *subcortical aphasias* are defined more by the anatomy of the responsible lesion than by the characteristics of the language symptoms. Those language disorders that predominantly affect reading and writing — the alexias and agraphias — are discussed in Chapters 10 and 11. Other topics discussed are aphasia in left-handers, rare aphasia syndromes encountered with right-hemisphere lesions in right-handed people (*crossed aphasia in dextrals*), and aphasia in speakers of more than one language (*aphasia in polyglots*).

One problem with commonly used aphasia terminology is the tendency to use a dichotomous classification, such as *motor* versus *sensory* aphasia, *expressive* versus *receptive* aphasia, *fluent* versus *nonfluent* aphasia, or *anterior* versus *posterior* aphasia. Of these dichotomies, the motor/sensory and expressive/receptive terminologies are the most widely used, and also the most potentially misleading. Virtually all aphasias affect both expression and comprehension. It is common, for example, for a patient with fluent, paraphasic speech to be labeled an expressive aphasic, even though language comprehension is also grossly disturbed. The fluent/nonfluent dichotomy is less misleading, since it simply describes the patient's running speech; we prefer this dichotomy if one must be used, though some cases fall between the two ends of the spectrum of fluency. Nonfluent aphasias include aphemia, Broca's aphasia, global aphasia, transcortical motor aphasia, and mixed transcortical aphasia, while fluent aphasias include Wernicke's, conduction, pure word deafness, and transcortical sensory aphasia. The anterior/posterior dichotomy refers to brain anatomy rather than to aphasia characteristics, but in general the split among syndromes is similar to the fluent/nonfluent categorization.

A final point about aphasia classification is that even the experts often disagree on labels for a specific patient. Given the frequent disagreements about aphasia classification by bedside examination, it is best for all students of aphasia, regardless of experience, to describe the patient's deficits first and classify the patient second.

BROCA'S APHASIA

In 1861 (1), the French physician Paul Broca described two patients with nonfluent speech and preserved comprehension, under the term *aphemia*. While the name has not survived, the syndrome and its eponym have continued to dominate the field of language disorders. Spontaneous speech production in Broca's aphasia is reduced, varying from complete mutism to single word utterances, to full sentences spoken in a halting, effortful manner, with an economy of words. The expressive deficit in Broca's aphasia usually involves a phoneme-articulation difficulty, with elements of dysarthria and apraxia of speech, as discussed in Chapters 2 and 3. In addition to the articulatory disorder, however, Broca's aphasia involves a grammatical language disturbance. The speech pattern of a Broca's aphasic is "telegraphic," resembling the style of a telegram that contains the major, meaning-carrying nouns and verbs of a sentence but omits nonessential prepositions and articles. Neurolinguists refer to this pattern as *agrammatism*, since it lacks grammatical constructions. An example of a telegraphic sentence of a Broca's aphasic would be, "Call wife," meaning "I need to call my wife."

The naming of a Broca's aphasic is usually deficient, although many patients give the impression of having some idea of the correct word; in one study, Broca's aphasics were more accurate in designating the first phoneme or number of syllables of the correct word than other aphasics (6). This knowledge of the correct word has been called the "tip of the tongue" phenomenon. Auditory comprehension is relatively preserved in Broca's aphasia, such that the patient appears to understand simple conversation. Detailed testing, however, usually demonstrates some comprehension deficit, especially for complex grammatical phrases, the same types of construction that cause difficulty in expression. For example, Goodglass et al. (7) reported that embedded phrases in sentences caused more deterioration of comprehension of single sentences in Broca's than in other aphasics. Heilman and Scholes (8) likewise showed that syntactic errors predominated in the comprehension deficit of Broca's aphasics. Repetition is impaired, usually to a degree similar to that of spontaneous speech.

Reading in patients with Broca's aphasia often seems more impaired than auditory comprehension. Benson (9) has referred to this phenomenon as the "third alexia," distinguishing the alexia of patients with Broca's aphasia from the two classical syndromes of alexia with and without agraphia, to be discussed in Chapter 10. Finally, writing in Broca's aphasia is complicated by the presence of right hemiparesis in most patients. As stated earlier, these patients often resist testing of writing with the left hand. When forced to attempt writing, however, their writing is usually not only awkward, but also abnormal in language content. Many patients cannot write even words of a few letters.

Patients with Broca's aphasia usually have associated right hemiparesis, often involving the face and arm more than the leg. Some patients have sensory deficits on the right as well, but the visual fields are usually intact. Broca's aphasics typically seem cognitively intact; they appear to understand normal conversation. Some have an associated ideomotor apraxia, or inability to follow motor commands (see Chapter 21). Since the right limbs are usually paretic, this apraxia may be evident only in skilled motor use of the left limbs on command. Ideomotor apraxia may create the false impression of a comprehension deficit, if comprehension is tested only by response to commands. For this reason, patients who fail to follow spoken commands should be given additional comprehension tests involving yes/no questions or commands that require only a pointing response.

Broca's aphasics are typically aware of their language deficits and are frustrated by them. Depression is a common concomitant of Broca's aphasia (10). The subject of emotional states related to aphasia is discussed by Dr. Cummings in Chapter 20.

Most patients with lasting Broca's aphasia have large lesions in the left frontal area. The original patients described by Broca had large areas of softening of the brain, visible from the cortical surface, in the left frontoparietal region. Broca judged that the most crucial area was the posterior portion of the inferior frontal gyrus, or pars triangularis and pars opercularis,

Table 1 Broca's Aphasia

1. Spontaneous speech	Nonfluent, agrammatic, often dysarthric
2. Naming	Impaired ("Tip-of-the-tongue")
3. Comprehension	Intact (difficulty with complex syntax)
4. Repetition	Impaired
5. Reading	Impaired ("third alexia")
6. Writing	Impaired (dysmorphic but also linguistically impaired)
7. Associated signs	Right hemiparesis
	Right hemisensory loss
	± Apraxia of left limbs
8. Lesion location	Left inferior frontal, subcortical white matter

now often referred to as "Broca's area," or Brodmann areas 44 and 45 (see Figure 1 in Chapter 1). Broca's area lies just anterior to the face area of the primary motor cortex (Brodmann area 4, precentral gyrus). Its blood supply is from branches of the superior division of the left middle cerebral artery. Mohr and colleagues (11) pointed out that patients who manifest Broca's aphasia immediately after a stroke usually recover nearly normal language function within several weeks. These patients tend to have smaller lesions, located in the vicinity of the traditional Broca's area. This syndrome has been called "Baby Broca syndrome" or "Broca's area aphasia," in distinction to the classical syndrome of Broca's aphasia.

Recent studies of CT scans in patients with nonfluent aphasia have further refined the correlation of Broca's aphasia with specific lesion sites. Alexander, Naeser, and Palumbo (12) found in nine cases that lesions restricted to the lower motor cortex of the precentral gyrus produced a motor speech disorder consisting of dysarthria and mild expressive disturbance, while those of the more anterior frontal operculum (Brodmann areas 44 and 45) produced mainly an initiation difficulty without true language difficulty; this syndrome is equivalent to transcortical motor aphasia (13), discussed later. Finally, lesions combining these two lesion sites, plus additional damage to the subcortical white matter and periventricular white matter, produced deficits of Broca's aphasia, including both literal and verbal paraphasias, anomia, shortened phrase length, and agrammatism. The authors postulated that these additional aphasic disturbances resulted not from the local damage to frontal structures, but from interruption of pathways from the posterior language areas and from the limbic system. Naeser and colleagues (14) have also shown that damage to two areas is necessary and sufficient to produce lasting loss of functional expressive speech: 1) the most medial, rostral subcallosal fasciculus (a deep white-matter area located deep to Broca's area, in the lateral angle of the frontal horn) and 2) the portion of the periventricular white matter adjacent to the body of the left lateral ventricle, deep to the motor and sensory cortex for the mouth and face. Illustrative lesions and more detailed consideration of the neuroanatomy of Broca's aphasia are presented in Chapter 5.

Knopman and colleagues (15) reported findings of recovery of language from an extensively studied group of 54 patients with left-hemisphere strokes. In this study, persistent nonfluency of speech after 6 months of recovery was seen only in patients with large perirolandic lesions involving the frontoparietal cortex and subcortical white matter. Patients with more restricted lesions near Broca's area had only transitory nonfluency, as did patients with deep lesions of the anterior insula, putamen, and globus pallidus. Lesion volume was usually more than 25 cc in patients with persistent nonfluency, while patients with smaller lesions almost invariably recovered fluency.

APHEMIA

The term *aphemia*, which Broca originally chose for the syndrome now called Broca's aphasia, has in modern parlance become restricted to a transitory syndrome of muteness or nonfluent speech with initiation difficulty and dysarthria. After the muteness resolves, the patient remains hesitant in speech, with abnormal prosody and sometimes phonemic substitutions. Repetition is impaired in a way similar to spontaneous speech. Both auditory and reading comprehension are preserved, and even writing is normal. Most patients have a right facial weakness, but the right upper limb may be strong enough to produce normal writing. As discussed in Chapter 3, the deficit profile of aphemia is more akin to a motor speech disorder than to a true language disorder, or aphasia, and it may be synonymous with the syndrome of apraxia of speech (14). Schiff and coworkers (16) found lesions involving the lower motor cortex for the face in the precentral gyrus, with extension in some cases into the inferior frontal convolution and subjacent white matter. Alexander, Naeser, and Palumbo (12) reported this syndrome with lesions restricted to the lower motor cortex of the left precentral gyrus.

WERNICKE'S APHASIA

In 1874, the German physician Wernicke (17) published a monograph in which he defined a syndrome of aphasia quite distinct from that of Broca's aphasia. Wernicke described patients who had fluent speech output but made both literal and verbal paraphasic errors. Wernicke's aphasics have poor auditory comprehension, sometimes to the point of total inability to understand spoken language. Their repetition is also disturbed. Attempts at naming often result in bizarre paraphasic substitutions. Unlike the Broca's aphasic who struggles with the initial syllable of the correct name, the Wernicke's aphasic may effortlessly produce a string of incorrect responses, without apparent awareness of error. Reading in Wernicke's aphasia is usually disturbed in a manner similar to auditory comprehension, but occasional patients show a dissociation between these two modalities of comprehension (18–21). These "modality-selective" deficit patterns are important to detect, since intact reading allows communication with the patient who cannot be reached by spoken language. Most patients with Wernicke's aphasia have no hemiparesis and write effortlessly. The language content of their written productions, however, is abnormal, often more so than their speech. Mild Wernicke's aphasics may speak intelligibly, although with word substitutions, but writing will show obvious errors of spelling that make the presence of a language disorder obvious.

Associated neurological deficits are often lacking in patients with Wernicke's aphasia. Most patients have no hemiparesis or sensory loss, and they

Table 2 Wernicke's Aphasia

1. Spontaneous speech	Fluent, paraphasic errors ± logorrhea
2. Naming	Impaired (bizarre, paraphasic misnamings)
3. Comprehension	Impaired
4. Repetition	Impaired
5. Reading	Impaired for comprehension, reading aloud
6. Writing	Well-formed, paragraphic
7. Associated signs	± Right hemianopsia; motor, sensory signs usually absent
8. Lesion location	Left superior temporal gyrus ± inferior parietal

may be fully ambulatory. Deficits of vision in the right homonymous field may be present. The lack of obvious physical deficits sometimes leads to misdiagnosis of a psychiatric condition or acute confusional state. Psychiatric disorders rarely produce paraphasic speech, and the abrupt onset of a fluent aphasia should always be assumed to be related to a focal brain lesion until proved otherwise. Encephalopathies, or acute confusional states, are more difficult to distinguish from Wernicke's aphasia, but even these patients tend not to have the severe abnormalities of language expression and comprehension seen in Wernicke's aphasia.

Unlike Broca's aphasics, Wernicke's aphasics are often unaware of their deficits. They may become angry when their paraphasic speech is not understood. In the chronic phase, they may become paranoid, thinking others are talking about them in some incomprehensible tongue (22). Psychiatric aspects of Wernicke's aphasia are discussed in Chapter 20.

The lesions of Wernicke's aphasia generally involve the left superior temporal region (23). Some patients also have damage in the inferior parietal lobule, including the supramarginal and angular gyri, Brodmann areas 39 and 40. Naeser and associates (24) have shown that damage to Wernicke's area itself (area 22) correlates most closely with loss of comprehension of single words; only patients with major damage to this cortical area suffer sustained loss of comprehension at the single-word level (see Chapter 5 for illustrative material from Naeser's work). The crucial importance of the anatomical Wernicke's area for decoding of spoken words has also been confirmed in the series of Kirshner and colleagues (20). Selnes and coworkers (25), on the other hand, found that damage to Wernicke's area alone did not preclude the recovery of single-word comprehension in a mixed group of aphasics; only patients with much larger areas of left-hemisphere damage had persistent loss of understanding of single words.

Recently, Kertesz and colleagues (26) found that poor recovery in Wernicke's aphasia was most highly correlated with damage to Wernicke's area, but there were also strong correlations with damage to the angular and supramarginal gyri; persistent, severe Wernicke's aphasia was usually associated with large lesions comprising all three areas. Electrical-stimulation studies involving Wernicke's area have produced consistent and reversible interference with auditory comprehension, further confirming the importance of the left superior temporal region for decoding of auditory language (27).

Patients with lesions of the inferior parietal lobule may present with an initial picture of Wernicke's aphasia, but auditory comprehension often recovers well. Kirshner and colleagues (19,20) have reported that some patients with lesions of the inferior parietal lobule have more severe involvement of reading than of auditory comprehension, while some patients with strictly temporal lobe lesions have more severe involvement of auditory comprehension than of reading (18,20).

The Comprehension Disorder of Wernicke's Aphasia

Considerable research has examined the deficit of auditory comprehension that is so striking in Wernicke's aphasia. Comprehension errors might arise from three linguistic sources: (1) inability to perceive or discriminate phonemes, (2) inability to decode syntactic relationships within a sentence, and (3) inability to understand the semantic meanings of words. Several investigators have studied the ability of patients with Wernicke's aphasia to perceive phonemes. Luria and Hutton (28) believed that deficits in phoneme perception lay at the heart of the comprehension deficit of Wernicke's aphasia. Blumstein, Baker, and Goodglass (29) examined the discrimination of closely related phonemes such as "pear" and "bear"; subjects with Wernicke's aphasia showed deficits even on this simple phonological task. The phonemic discrimination deficit, however, did not correlate with the level of language comprehension; patients with mixed or global aphasia had poorer phoneme discrimination but better comprehension than Wernicke's aphasics. Subjects also performed better if the phonemes to be discriminated were real words rather than nonsense syllables, indicating that the task may involve semantic coding in addition to simple phoneme perception. Similarly, Gainotti and colleagues (30), in an experiment requiring aphasic patients to match spoken words to pictures, found that Wernicke's aphasics made fewer phonemic errors and more semantic errors than Broca's aphasics.

Baker, Blumstein, and Goodglass (31) reported that Wernicke's aphasics had more difficulty in discriminating phonemes when they differed by only one feature (place of articulation or voicing, discussed in Chapter 3) than when they differed by two or more features. Broca's aphasics showed a similar but less severe phoneme-discrimination deficit. In addition, the Wernicke's aphasics had much greater difficulty than Broca's aphasics when a semantic aspect was added to the test. In a test requiring the patients to match a spoken phoneme to a drawing, Wernicke's aphasics made many more total errors and a greater percentage of semantic errors, as compared with Broca's aphasics. The comprehension deficit in Wernicke's aphasia thus appears to involve not simply the appreciation of the phonemic aspects of spoken language, but the relationship of perceived phonemes to the meanings of words.

Other investigators have questioned whether the comprehension deficit of Wernicke's aphasics relates to a reduced speed of auditory sequencing of perceived phonemes. Tallal and Newcombe (32) tested patients with left-and right-hemisphere lesions with a nonverbal tone sequence and a speech-sound test. Patients with left-hemisphere lesions and aphasia showed selective impairments on both the nonverbal and verbal tests, and this deficit of auditory processing of rapid acoustic events correlated with the degree of comprehension disburtance. As Blumstein (33) has pointed out, however, patients with temporal lobectomy show similar disorders of temporal-order judgments for acoustic events, without any associated disorder of language comprehension (34). In addition, deliberate efforts to increase the duration of transitions between sounds do not abolish the comprehension disorder (35), although slower speech rates (36,37) or pauses between major syntactic elements of a sentence (38) do improve language comprehension in aphasic patients.

In summary, elementary auditory aspects of speech perception, such as the differentiation of phonemes or the sequencing of rapid acoustic stimuli, are impaired in Wernicke's aphasia but do not appear to play a major role in the comprehension disturbance of these patients. More complex linguistic aspects of comprehension, especially semantics, are more important determinants of comprehension in Wernicke's aphasia.

The second linguistic aspect of comprehension, syntax, has not been found to be greatly deficient in Wernicke's aphasics. At the sentence level, Wernicke's aphasics make fewer syntactically based but more semantic errors than Broca's aphasics; Wernicke's aphasics more often fail to grasp the major nouns and verbs of a sentence.

In addition to the linguistic factors in comprehension, normal conversation contains extralinguistic cues, such as tone of voice, facial expression, emotion, context, and mode of presentation (e.g., spoken versus taped). Boller and colleagues (39) investigated two paralinguistic factors—emotional content and mode of presentation—in six global and two Wernicke's aphasics, all of whom had severe comprehension disturbance. The aphasic patients performed consistently better with emotional than with neutral sentences, and with those spoken by a live examiner as compared with tape recordings. It thus appears that extralinguistic factors improve an aphasic patient's ability to perform phonemic, syntactic, and semantic tasks. These extralinguistic factors have been utilized to improve communication in speech therapy (see Chapter 18). They are also the very factors found deficient in the comprehension of nonaphasic patients with right-hemisphere lesions (see Chapter 12).

The Reading Disorder of Wernicke's Aphasia

Another recent field of research in aphasia has been the creation of cognitive models of the linguistic mechanisms that go awry. One of the best examples of such a model is the reading disorder of Wernicke's aphasia. According to Wernicke's original concept, the superior temporal area was a center for stored sound images, by which spoken sounds were decoded into words. Failure of speech-sound perception produced both a loss of language comprehension and an inability to transmit the perceived sounds to Broca's area for repetition. The abnormality of spontaneous speech in Wernicke's aphasia presumably resulted from the loss of self-monitoring of use of words. Reading, by this model, required translation of printed words into the sound images of words stored in Wernicke's area, before any meaning could be derived from printed language. A lesion of Wernicke's area would thus disrupt not only auditory comprehension, but also reading.

This simple model of reading does not account for the phenomena of Wernicke's aphasia. While most Wernicke's aphasics are impaired to a more or less equal degree in reading and auditory comprehension, interesting dissociations do occur. Wernicke himself mentioned in his original monograph (17) that some highly educated individuals might have the ability to derive meaning directly from printed words. Modern case descriptions have documented patients with Wernicke's aphasia who have shown spared reading comprehension (18,40,41), ability to read aloud (42), preservation of both reading aloud and for comprehension (21,43), and spared written naming and spelling (44). These variations in the deficit profile of Wernicke's aphasia require a more complex model of reading (45), in which printed words can be processed without access to auditory language. Modern models of reading are discussed in Chapter 10.

PURE WORD DEAFNESS

Pure word deafness is a syndrome in which auditory comprehension is impaired in isolation. The patient with pure word deafness has normal speech, naming, reading, and writing; only auditory comprehension and repetition are defective (46). The deficit is classically described in patients with bilateral temporal lesions. Elementary hearing is intact in this syndrome; meaningful nonverbal sounds such as animal cries can be appreciated normally (47). In this pure form, pure word deafness is not truly an aphasia, but rather a selective auditory deficit.

Studies of patients with pure word deafness have differed as to the degree of primary auditory disorder and the degree of language deficit. In some cases of bilateral temporal lobe damage, pure word deafness has evolved from an initial deficit of cortical deafness, in which both auditory nonverbal stimuli and auditory language stimuli were affected (48). Tanaka and colleagues (49), for example, reported a patient in whom temporal sequencing was defective in the auditory, tactile, and visual modalities, but only in the auditory modality was a clinical deficit apparent. This patient was entirely unable to appreciate rhythm, despite only mild pure tone hearing loss. The authors postulated that the defect in sequencing or timing of stimuli is more critical to auditory comprehension than to perception in other sensory modalities. On the other hand, Kanshepolsky, Kelly, and Waggener (50) described a similar case of bilateral temporal infarctions in which temporal ordering tests were normal, pure tone acuity was only mildly affected, but loudness discrimination and auditory threshold-duration parameters were more abnormal than simple pure tone hearing. This patient spontaneously complained that he could hear but not understand speech. It thus appears that pure word deafness with bilateral temporal lesions may reflect a disorder of primary auditory function rather than a true language disorder.

Geschwind (51) postulated that pure word deafness could also result from a unilateral left temporal lesion, strategically placed so as to cut off the input to Wernicke's area from both primary auditory cortices. Well-documented cases of pure word deafness from such unilateral lesions are few (52), but a number of cases of Wernicke's aphasia have been reported in which auditory comprehension is affected much more severely than reading comprehension (18,20,21). Only the paraphasic speech of such patients distinguishes Wernicke's aphasia from pure word deafness. In fact, paraphasic speech has been present in most reported cases of pure word deafness (46). This feature may imply that the left temporal lobe damage extends into the classical Wernicke's area in the left superior temporal gyrus. The syndrome of pure word deafness thus overlaps both with the primary auditory disorders of cortical deafness and auditory agnosia and with Wernicke's aphasia.

GLOBAL APHASIA

Global, or "total," aphasia is often thought of as a simple sum of Broca's and Wernicke's aphasias, in that it comprises deficits of both expression and comprehension. This view of global aphasia is an oversimplification, since some global aphasics have islands of preserved functioning that must be sought carefully to find a way to communicate with these patients. The six basic language functions are usually all severely impaired: speech is nonfluent or completely absent; naming, repetition, and auditory comprehension are severely disturbed; and the patient cannot read or write. Global aphasia is thus easy to recognize at the bedside. Less severe deficits that affect all six language functions are sometimes called "mixed" aphasias. Such partial deficits, however, are rarely equal across language functions, and care should be taken to describe the patient's precise pattern of language impairments. With recovery, deficits in one area may improve faster or more completely than others, and patients may progress from a global or "mixed" category into a Broca's aphasia profile or, conversely, into a Wernicke's or anomic aphasia pattern. Even among patients with severe enough deficits to remain global aphasics, differences in performance have been found in individual modalities. For example, some patients with global aphasia become superior in written as compared to oral naming (53).

The associated deficits of patients with global aphasia are usually severe, including a dense right hemiparesis, hemisensory loss, and right homonymous hemianopsia. Occasional patients have no hemiparesis, usually implying separate lesions of Broca's and Wernicke's areas (54). Global aphasia without hemiparesis has also been seen in patients with internal carotid artery occlusion and with brain tumors (55).

The lesions of global aphasia are usually large, involving much of the perisylvian language cortex of the left frontal, temporal, and parietal lobes. In patients with stroke, global aphasia often indicates infarction of most of the territory of the middle cerebral artery, either from an embolus to the middle cerebral artery or from occlusion of the internal carotid artery in the neck. Large hemorrhages in the left basal ganglia may also produce global aphasia (56), but the patient is usually obtunded for the first few days after onset.

Naeser and colleagues (57) have studied the recovery of auditory comprehension in global aphasics. The most significant variable, as in Wernicke's aphasia, is the degree of direct damage to Wernicke's area; patients who have subcortical lesions involving the temporal isthmus but sparing Wernicke's cortical area have better improvement in comprehension than those

Table 3 Global Aphasia

1. Spontaneous speech	Nonfluent, mute, agrammatic
2. Naming	Impaired
3. Comprehension	Impaired
4. Repetition	Impaired
5. Reading	Impaired
6. Writing	Impaired
7. Associated signs	Right hemiparesis, right hemisensory loss, right hemianopsia
8. Lesion location	Left frontotemporoparietal

with involvement of Wernicke's area, despite large frontoparietal cortical lesions (see Chapter 5). In both global and Wernicke's aphasia, the cortical Wernicke's area appears crucial for auditory comprehension.

One difference between global aphasia and other aphasias is the extremely slow pace of recovery. While recovery is generally considered to be maximal in the first few months after a stroke, Sarno and Levita (58) have shown that recovery in global aphasics may actually be greater in the second 6 months after a stroke than in the first 6 months. This slow course of recovery must be considered in designing rehabilitation programs for these patients.

CONDUCTION APHASIA

Conduction aphasia is a relatively uncommon but theoretically interesting aphasia in which repetition is impaired out of proportion to all other language deficits. This syndrome has been the cornerstone of the disconnection theory, advanced by Wernicke (17) and reiterated by Geschwind (59); i.e., the concept that a neurobehavioral syndrome can result not from damage to a cortical center, but rather from disconnection of two intact centers. Because of the importance of this theory to aphasia, Chapter 6 is devoted to conduction aphasia and the disconnection model of aphasia; only a brief review is presented here.

Patients with conduction aphasia usually have fluent speech, often containing frequent literal paraphasic errors. Some patients pause repeatedly for self-correction, producing a less fluent speech pattern than that in Wernicke's aphasia. Naming may be deficient, and these patients make more literal paraphasias, or phonemically related errors, in naming as compared to Broca's and Wernicke's aphasics (60). Auditory comprehension is normal. Repetition, by contrast, is severely impaired, sometimes to seemingly impossible degrees. For example, a patient who could not repeat the word "boy" said "I like girls better." The ability to repeat words is more affected than the ability to comprehend or decode the words, or to produce words in response to a question (61). The impairment of repetition is the hallmark of conduction aphasia. Reading and writing are somewhat variable; reading aloud and writing to dictation often share some of the same abnormality as repetition.

Associated deficits in conduction aphasia include variable right hemiparesis, right hemisensory loss, and right hemianopia. Some patients have a severe ideomotor apraxia (see Chapter 21).

The lesions of conduction aphasia generally involve the left temporal or inferior parietal regions, but sparing much of Wernicke's area. Wernicke originally postulated that conduction aphasia results from a lesion that does not damage either Broca's or Wernicke's areas, but disconnects the two.

Table 4 Conduction Aphasia

1. Spontaneous speech	Fluent, literal paraphasic errors
2. Naming	± Mildly impaired
3. Comprehension	Intact
4. Repetition	Severely impaired
5. Reading	± Inability to read aloud
6. Writing	Variable
7. Associated signs	± Apraxia of limbs
	± Right hemiparesis, sensory loss, hemianopsia
8. Lesion location	Left temporal, parietal

A phrase is heard, decoded into language, and understood as language, but the patient cannot activate the motor plans for the utterance, stored in Broca's area. Geschwind (59) pointed to the arcuate fasciculus as the critical white-matter bundle connecting Wernicke's and Broca's areas. This bundle arises in the temporal cortex, arches around the sylvian fissure, and then turns forward above the extreme capsule and insula, deep to the inferior parietal lobule, to terminate in the left inferior frontal lobe (62). Benson et al. (63) have proposed that ideomotor apraxia accompanies conduction aphasia when the lesion lies in the left parietal lobe, while apraxia is absent with temporal lobe lesions. The arcuate fasciculus was affected in all six of the cases of Damasio and Damasio (62), but some cases also had damage in the insula, the cortical Wernicke's area, and the inferior parietal lobule. Brown (64) argued that no cases of conduction aphasia have had lesions restricted to the arcuate fasciculus, and a few cases have been reported in which this fasciculus was spared. Levine and Calvanio (65) also questioned the role of cortical damage rather than a simple disconnection.

The disconnection theory of conduction aphasia has been debated not only on anatomical grounds, but on behavioral grounds as well. A number of investigators have advocated a deficit of auditory short-term memory as the basis of the poor repetition in conduction aphasia. Several investigators have documented deficient auditory verbal short-term memory in patients with conduction aphasia (66–69). In these studies, visual short-term memory, as in recitation of a string of printed words, was superior to auditory short-term memory. Tzortzis and Albert (70) found that memory for sequences was specifically disrupted in patients with conduction aphasia, a deficit present in both the auditory and visual modalities, with both verbal and nonverbal stimuli. A specific memory for sequences, rather than auditory-verbal short-term memory, would thus represent the defect in conduction aphasia.

Heilman and colleagues (71) found that both Broca's and conduction aphasics had decreased span for digits, whether presented orally or visually. This finding might explain the difficulty with repetition seen in both types of aphasia, but it suggests that the memory defect is not specific to conduction aphasia. Strub (72) pointed out that errors in repetition reflect linguistic factors as well as auditory short-term memory. For example, subjects did better if the words were spoken more slowly, or when the task could be done by matching rather than oral production of the words. The repetition errors made by their subject were paraphasic. Subjects repeated single nonsense words less well than familiar phrases. According to Strub (72), the defect in conduction aphasia involves the linguistic processing and sequencing of phonemes, rather than a simple memory deficit.

Another line of research in conduction aphasia has involved the use of delayed auditory feedback, in which the patient's own speech is played back after a delay. While this feedback interferes with the speech of normal subjects and most aphasics, it paradoxically improves the speech output of conduction aphasics (73,74). This abnormal result of delayed auditory feedback implies that feedback of auditory stimuli from the patient's own speech may be abnormal in conduction aphasia and may be a factor in the language disorder.

The final theory of conduction aphasia involves a disorder of "inner speech" representations, postulated by Goldstein to be involved in the interaction between nonverbal thought and speech expression (75). Feinberg and colleagues (76) tested the ability of conduction aphasics to perform analyses of words and phrases that they could not repeat, such as estimating word length and judging whether words rhymed or were homophones (words with the same sound but different spelling). Only one of five patients tested had difficulty with these "inner-speech" operations. Deficits of inner speech thus do not appear to account for the syndrome of conduction aphasia.

ANOMIC APHASIA

Anomic aphasia is a syndrome in which difficulty in naming is the principal deficit. Spontaneous speech is fluent but often marked by word-finding pauses and circumlocutions. Auditory comprehension, reptition, reading, and writing are largely intact, except for difficulty in eliciting proper names.

Associated deficits of anomic aphasia are variable. Some patients have no hemiparesis, hemisensory loss, or visual-field defect. The lesion localization of anomic aphasia is likewise variable. Geschwind (51) pointed to the angular gyrus as a common site of lesions underlying anomic aphasia, but patients with angular gyrus lesions often have associated alexia, agraphia, fluent aphasia, and sometimes acalculia, right-left confusion, and finger

Table 5 Anomic Aphasia

1. Spontaneous speech	Fluent, word-finding pauses, circumlocutions
2. Naming	Impaired
3. Comprehension	Intact
4. Repetition	Intact
5. Reading	Intact
6. Writing	Intact, except for anomia
7. Associated signs	Inconsistent
8. Lesion location	Left temporal, left angular gyrus, or diffuse

agnosia (see Chapter 21). Some patients with otherwise pure anomic aphasia have other signs of cognitive impairment suggestive of a dementia (see
Chapter 13). The neuropathology underlying anomic aphasia includes localized strokes in the left hemisphere, tumors of the deep temporal lobe white
matter, and dementing disorders such as Alzheimer's disease. Geschwind
(51) concluded that anomic aphasia is of less localizing value than the other
aphasia syndromes.

Since naming is at the heart of all language syndromes, Chapter 7 is devoted to a discussion of naming and its disorders.

TRANSCORTICAL APHASIAS

The term *transcortical aphasia* was coined by Lichtheim (77) to refer to aphasias resulting from lesions outside the primary, perisylvian language circuit
from Wernicke's area to Broca's area. Lichtheim's idea was that an "area of
concepts," separate from the language cortex, projects the content of language discourse into the language circuit. The hallmark of transcortical aphasias, by this anatomical explanation, is the preservation of repetition, which
requires only this circuit and no other input. While contemporary neuroanatomy no longer contains an anatomical "area of concepts," the idea of

Table 6 Transcortical Aphasias

Feature	TC motor	TC sensory	Isolation syndrome
Speech	Nonfluent	Fluent	Nonfluent, echolalic
Naming	Impaired	Impaired	Impaired
Comprehension	Intact	Impaired	Impaired
Repetition	Intact	Intact	Intact
Reading	± Spared	Impaired	Impaired
Writing	Impaired	Impaired	Impaired

transcortical aphasias as caused by lesions outside the primary language circuit, and therefore leaving repetition intact, has survived to the present time. There are three classical transcortical aphasia syndromes: transcortical motor (TCMA), transcortical sensory (TCSA), and mixed transcortical aphasia (MTCA), also called the syndrome of the isolation of the speech area.

Transcortical Motor Aphasia

Transcortical motor aphasia may be thought of as the transcortical analog of Broca's aphasia (78). The patient speaks little, responding to questions hesitantly and in brief, softly uttered or whispered phrases, often interrupted by long pauses. Once speech is produced, however, it is generally appropriate in content and syntax. In contrast to spontaneous speech, repetition is normal in speed and content, even for long sentences. Naming is usually preserved, although hesitant. Auditory comprehension, reading comprehension, and oral reading are performed well. Writing may share the same hesitancy of expression as speech. Some aphasiologists have questioned whether TCMA represents a true aphasia, since most of the deficit involves decreased initiation rather than an actual language disturbance.

Patients with TCMA often have right-sided weakness but usually no sensory loss or hemianopia. If there is a hemiparesis, the leg is often weaker than the arm, and the shoulder weaker than the hand, a pattern typical of infarctions in the territory of the anterior cerebral artery (79). This pattern of hemiparesis is the reverse of the usual middle cerebral artery territory pattern of arm greater than leg and hand greater than shoulder paralysis, seen in both Broca's and global aphasia. Some patients have other frontal lobe signs such as forced grasping of the right hand. Patients with bilateral frontal lobe lesions often show a profound decrease in initiation of all behaviors, not restricted to speech. In this context, *akinetic mutism* or *abulia* can be considered frontal syndromes with decreased behavior of all types, while TCMA is a lack of initiation of speech alone. Luria and Tsvetkova (80) called this syndrome *dynamic aphasia*, again indicating a defect in the motor initiation of speech.

The lesions of TCMA, as proposed by Lichtheim, lie outside the traditional perisylvian language circuit. Most involve the frontal lobe, superior or anterior to Broca's area. Freedman and colleagues (81) found that all seven of their cases with TCMA had lesions in the left frontal white matter, anterolateral to the left frontal horn, without major damage to Broca's area. Three cases also had involvement of the medial frontal region, particularly the supplementary motor cortex. If the lesion extended into the subcortical white matter deep to the precentral gyrus, in the face area of the motor homunculus, articulation was impaired in addition to the other features of TCMA. If the lesion involved the head of the caudate, anterior putamen and anterior portions of the external capsule, claustrum, extreme capsule, and insula, impaired comprehension was also present. Three patients had associated stuttering; their lesions involved either Broca's area or the lower third of the premotor area. The supplementary motor area thus appears to play a prominent role in the initiation of speech, and the white-matter lesions adjacent to the frontal horn may disconnect fibers from the supplementary motor area to the frontal premotor cortex. Masdeu, Schoene, and Funkenstein (82) also reported transient mutism followed by good recovery of language functions in a patient with infarction of the left supplementary motor area. Electrical stimulation of the supplementary motor cortex produces speech arrest, further supporting the role of this area in speech initiation (82).

The medial frontal lesions of TCMA are in the territory of the anterior cerebral artery, while the lesions of Broca's, Wernicke's, conduction, and global aphasia all lie within the middle cerebral artery territory. The separation of these vascular territories results in a relatively pure clinical syndrome of TCM aphasia, as compared to the other aphasic syndromes.

Recently, Albert et al. (83) have advocated the use of the drug bromocriptine to help with initiation of speech in TCMA. While the efficacy of this treatment remains to be proved, it represents the first use of a drug to aid recovery of aphasia.

Transcortical Sensory Aphasia

Just as TCMA is an analog of Broca's aphasia with preserved repetition, so TCSA is an analog of Wernicke's aphasia with preserved repetition. Naming is paraphasic, as in Wernicke's aphasia, and auditory comprehension is severely disturbed. Reading and writing are also impaired; only repetition is preserved. Kertesz and colleagues (84) noted that phonological and syntactic operations are to a large extent preserved, as seen in repetition, while semantic operations, as seen in comprehension and naming, are impaired. Heilman and colleagues (85) reported a single case of TCSA with intact naming; the implication was that the patient had an intact semantic system with access to speech encoding, but without access to phonemic decoding for comprehension.

Associated deficits of TCSA include right hemianopsia, contralateral sensory loss or tactile agnosia, and occasionally visual object agnosia (84). TCSA is a relatively uncommon stroke syndrome, occurring occasionally in patients with lesions in the region of the left temporo-occipital junction, sometimes overlapping into the adjacent parietal lobe. A few cases have lesions located more superiorly in the left hemisphere, at the junction of the parietal and occipital lobes (84). These localizations lie either within the territory of the posterior cerebral artery or in the "watershed" area between the middle and posterior cerebral artery territories. Kertesz and colleagues (84) suggested that the preserved phonological and syntactic functions are mediated by the intact left temporal lobe, while semantic functions are affected by the more posterior lesions. Syndromes closely resembling TCSA have also been described in patients with Alzheimer's disease of middle to late stages (86); see Chapter 13 for a more detailed discussion of language in dementia.

Mixed Transcortical Aphasia

Mixed transcortical aphasia, also called by Goldstein (87) the "syndrome of the isolation of the speech area," is the transcortical version of mixed or global aphasia. These patients cannot produce any meaningful speech utterances except for repetitions. Naming, auditory comprehension, reading, and writing are all severely impaired. Only repetition is preserved, and often this takes the form of echolalic repetition of anything the patient hears. Geschwind and coworkers (88) reported a patient who not only repeated phrases but would complete poems begun by the examiner, such as "Roses are red . . ." This patient could even learn new lyrics to songs published after she became aphasic. The lesion in this patient was a large watershed infarction of both cerebral hemispheres, damaging much of the frontal, parietal, and occipital lobes, but sparing the immediate perisylvian language cortex. The ability to memorize new song lyrics was interpreted to mean that the circuit from Wernicke's to Broca's area was not only preserved but also connected to the limbic system for memory storage, although much of the rest of the thinking brain was destroyed. Less severe versions of mixed transcortical aphasia involve partially impaired speech output and comprehension, with intact repetition. Ross (89), for example, reported a patient with a large infarction in the territory of the anterior cerebral artery, extending from the medial frontal region into the parietal lobe.

While the theory of a spared perisylvian language circuit for repetition, in the context of widespread left-hemisphere damage, has appeared to fit the phenomena of mixed transcortical aphasia, not all cases have had complete left perisylvian sparing. Brown (64) cited cases of partial destruction of the language area, and Grossi and colleagues (90) recently reported two cases with massive destruction of the left middle cerebral artery territory in the left frontal, temporal, and parietal lobes. These authors suspected that the right hemisphere might somehow mediate repetition and echolalia in these patients, a hypothesis that remains to be proved. A single case of MTCA has also been reported with a thalamic lesion (91). This syndrome has also been reported in late stages of dementing conditions such as Alzheimer's disease (86,92).

SUBCORTICAL APHASIAS

Until recent years, aphasia was thought to represent damage to the language cortex in the left hemisphere in virtually all cases. The recent documentation of aphasic deficits from subcortical lesions has necessitated a new category of subcortical aphasia. As stated earlier, subcortical aphasias are defined more by the anatomy of the brain lesion than by specific language characteristics, but several patterns of language disorder have been defined in patients with subcortical lesions.

Thalamic aphasia refers to aphasia syndromes secondary to lesions in the left thalamus. Numerous cases have been reported linking aphasia to thalamic hemorrhages (93–95). The aphasia pattern usually associated with thalamic damage is fluent, often with paraphasic errors, but with better comprehension and repetition than Wernicke's aphasia. As with most subcortical aphasias, the syndrome does not match any of the classical cortical aphasia syndromes. Mohr and colleagues (94) have described a "dichotomous" state in which patients speak coherently while alert, then degenerate into an unintelligible, paraphasic mumble when sleepy. Luria (96) emphasized the role of the thalamus in alerting the cortex, calling thalamic aphasia a *quasiaphasic disturbance of vigilance*. Since language deficits are readily apparent, however, most would consider thalamic aphasia a true aphasia.

Cerebral hemorrhages are not the ideal source of cases for language analysis, in that they exert pressure on the overlying language cortex. More convincing evidence that the thalamus is important to language has come from cases of thalamic infarction. Bogousslavsky and colleagues (97) presented a detailed analysis of 40 cases of thalamic infarction, in four separate vascular territories. The closest association with aphasia was in the territory of the tuberothalamic artery, which supplies the anterior thalamus, including the ventral anterior and part of the ventral lateral nuclei. Left-sided lesions in this territory were associated with hypophonia, verbal paraphasias, impaired comprehension, and intact repetition. Similar aphasic deficits were seen in patients with paramedian thalamic infarcts, in the territory of the thalamoperforating artery, although most patients had an initially depressed level of consciousness. The other two thalamic syndromes—posterior choroidal artery infarcts with infarction of the lateral geniculate body, and ventroposterolateral infarcts in the territory of the inferolateral arteries—had hemianopia and hemisensory loss, respectively, without language disturbance. Graff-Radford and colleagues (98,99) reported studies of patients with thalamic infarcts, including descriptions of reduced spontaneous speech but a fluent pattern of expression, anomia, perseveration in spontaneous speech, reduced comprehension, preserved reading, and intact repetition. Other reported cases of paramedian thalamic infarction have had deficits in memory and attention, with fluent aphasia and perseveration (100,101).

Other reported causes of thalamic aphasia have included surgical thalamotomy (102,103), thalamic tumors (104), an arteriovenous malformation of the thalamus (96), a thalamic abscess (105), and electrical stimulation of the thalamus, which caused disruption of naming and memory (106,107). Crosson (108) reviewed the evidence regarding thalamic involvement in language, including the known projections of the thalamus to portions of the language cortex, as well as participation in memory storage and retrieval. A comprehensive model of the role of the thalamus in language function, however, remains to be achieved. Thalamic aphasia also has implications for cerebral dominance. A right thalamic hemorrhage can cause aphasia in a left-handed patient, indicating that language dominance extends to the subcortical level (109,110).

Lesions of other parts of the basal ganglia of the dominant hemisphere have also been reported to cause aphasia. As in thalamic aphasia, hemorrhages were the original cases described. Alexander and LoVerme (111) described 15 cases of aphasia related to hemorrhages of the deep basal ganglia, including nine thalamic and six putamenal hemorrhages. The patients with putamenal hemorrhage were often mute early in their recovery, but fluent, paraphasic speech usually emerged, with relatively preserved comprehension and repetition. The authors noted that aphasic deficits might have been related to pressure effects on the overlying cortex, to disconnections of the cortical centers, or to a direct role of the basal ganglia in language.

More recently, aphasia has been reported in ischemic strokes with localized damage to the basal ganglia. The most commonly reported lesion site is an infarction of the head of the caudate nucleus, anterior limb of internal capsule, and anterior putamen, in the territory of lenticulostriate branches of the middle cerebral artery. We shall refer to this syndrome as the *anterior subcortical aphasia syndrome* (see Fig. 1). Features of this syndrome include dysarthria and decreased fluency, but with longer phrase length than Broca's aphasia, and with associated paraphasias. Comprehension is usually only mildly affected, and repetition is spared (112,113). Many patients have an associated right hemiparesis and impaired attention and short-term memory. Recovery is typically quite good. The neuroanatomy of this syndrome likely involves disruption in the caudate nucleus or anterior limb of fibers projecting to the caudate from the auditory cortex, and from the caudate to the globus pallidus, ventrolateral thalamus, and premotor cortex. Damasio and colleagues (113) stated that lesions of the white matter anterior to the caudate and putamen produced a picture similar to that of TCMA, while lesions of the posterior caudate, posterior limb of internal capsule, and posterior putamen generally produced only dysarthria. Naeser and colleagues (112) delineated three syndromes: (1) the anterior syndrome described above, (2) a Wernicke-like syndrome with more posterior lesions (see below), and (3) a global aphasia syndrome with lesions involving both sites.

Alexander and colleagues (114) expanded this analysis with 19 new cases. Lesions restricted to the putamen or head of the caudate nucleus did not

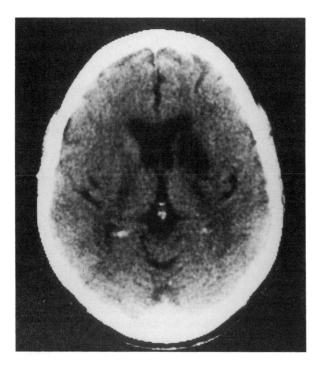

Figure 1 CT scan from a patient with the "anterior subcortical syndrome." The lesion is an infarction involving the left caudate head, anterior limb of internal capsule, and anterior putamen. The patient had dysarthria and nonfluent speech, with relatively preserved comprehension.

produce language disturbance, or at worst caused mild word-finding difficulty. Lesions involving the more posterior putamen were associated with hypophonia. There was still no language disturbance with involvement of the anterior limb of the internal capsule, except when this involved extensive injury to the caudate, putamen, and anterior limb of internal capsule, in which case the patients had the anterior subcortical aphasia syndrome described above. Dysarthria was also associated if the damage extended to the white matter of the periventricular region or the genu of the internal capsule. Lesions located more posteriorly, converging on the temporal isthmus, produced fluent aphasia, neologisms, and impaired comprehension. Lesions involving both areas, including the anterior caudate and putamen, internal capsule, periventricular white matter, and temporal isthmus, produced global aphasia. Finally, lesions more laterally placed, involving the insular cortex, extreme capsule, claustrum, and internal capsule, were associated with fluent aphasia, mild word-finding difficulty, and phonemic paraphasias that increased on repetition and reading aloud. This syndrome is identical to conduction aphasia.

The basis of subcortical aphasia likely involves connections between the basal ganglia and the cortex. The known feedback loop of cortex–striatum–globus pallidus–lateral thalamus–anterior limb of internal capsule–cortex has been implicated, with analogies to known relationships in movement disorders (114,115). These anatomical correlations apply to only small numbers of cases; other published cases of subcortical aphasia have suggested different anatomical relationships (116–120). Two reports have found disproportionate impairment of writing with subcortical lesions (119,120). Selective lesions of the caudate nucleus have also been reported (121); these produce "frontal lobe" syndromes involving poor attention and poor sequencing and planning. The study of subcortical lesions and their correlation with behavioral states is in an early phase, with considerable promise of new knowledge forthcoming.

APHASIA IN LEFT-HANDERS

The subject of hemispheric dominance for language is discussed in Chapter 1. Given the intense interest in language dominance, surprisingly few studies have investigated the specific language performance of left-handed patients with acquired aphasia. A few general statements can be made. More left-handers than right-handers develop aphasia after a stroke, regardless of the side of the stroke, suggesting that left-handed patients have some language representation in both cerebral hemispheres. Although aphasia is more common in left-handers, recovery may be better; hemisphere dominance may be less rigid, and either hemisphere can subserve recovery of language (122, 123). Naeser and Borod (124) reported a series of 31 left-handed aphasic patients, of whom 27 had left and four had right hemisphere lesions. The cerebral asymmetries measured on CT scan were not useful in predicting which hemisphere was responsible for aphasia. The majority of patients with aphasia and left-hemisphere lesions had aphasia syndromes similar to those of a matched group of right-handed aphasics with left-hemisphere lesions. Two patients, however, had destruction of the right frontal, temporal, and parietal cortices with nonfluent speech output but preserved comprehension, suggesting a left-hemisphere Wernicke's area but a right-hemisphere Broca's area. Most left-handers, like right-handers, have left-hemisphere dominance for speech and language, but some patients may have separate loci of dominance for handedness, motor speech, and auditory comprehension. A recent study by Basso and colleagues (125) found only slight differences between matched right-handed and non-right-handed patients with aphasia;

the one exception was a non-right-handed patient with conduction aphasia, whose matched right-handed patient with a similar lesion had global aphasia. In this study, recovery also differed little between non-right-handed and right-handed aphasic patients.

CROSSED APHASIA IN DEXTRALS

Another topic related to language dominance is the rare but well-documented occurrence of aphasia in right-handed patients with acquired right-hemisphere lesions. This pattern was first called *crossed aphasia* by Bramwell (126). Gloning and colleagues (127) estimated that 1% of right-handed patients with aphasia have right-hemisphere lesions, thereby implying that 1% of right-handed patients have language dominance in the right hemisphere. The reason for this "crossed" dominance is largely unknown.

Brown and Hecaen (123) reported that most right-handed patients with aphasia secondary to right-hemisphere lesions had nonfluent aphasia with agrammatism, regardless of the specific site of lesion within the right hemisphere. The authors likened this pattern to aphasia in children, who rarely have fluent aphasia, and postulated that the syndrome reflects a primitive or incomplete stage in the development of cerebral language dominance, in which language functions are more diffusely represented in the cortices of both hemispheres. Recent studies of crossed aphasia cases with detailed information on language functions and lesion localization, however, have not verified this pattern. Henderson (128) and Sweet et al. (129) reported cases of fluent aphasia secondary to lesions of the right-hemisphere analog of Wernicke's area. The intrahemispheric localization of language functions may thus be similar, regardless of which hemisphere is dominant for language. Basso and colleagues (130) reported seven crossed aphasics in whom the general pattern was comparable to expected aphasic deficits for analogous left-hemisphere lesions.

In a literature review of crossed aphasia, Alexander and colleagues (131) found that 22 of 34 cases with sufficient data had a "mirror-image" syndrome of aphasia, the syndrome expected with an analogous left-hemisphere lesion, while 12 cases had anomalous patterns of language impairment. A common "anomalous" aphasia syndrome was the preservation of fluent speech despite large suprasylvian, perirolandic lesions that would be expected to produce nonfluent aphasia if present in the left hemisphere. Interestingly, 11 of these 12 cases had greater impairment of written expression than of speech, a finding also present in four of seven of the cases of Basso and colleagues (130). In addition to these anomalies of language, nonlanguage functions are also atypical in these patients. For example, many lack the expected ideomotor apraxia seen so often in aphasic patients with left-hemisphere lesions, and many have neglect or visuospatial deficits, usually associated with right-hemisphere damage but not with aphasia (130,131). Alexander et al. (131) suggested that ideomotor apraxia may correlate with handedness more closely than with aphasia (see Chapter 21).

Overall, the "anomalous" cases suggest that dominance for different language functions may lie in separate hemispheres. For example, fluent speech production may be subserved by the left hemisphere, while language comprehension may be subserved by the right. Semantics and syntax may also be localized to different hemispheres in occasional patients (131). Further cases, with detailed lesion localization and language testing, will be needed to study these aspects of crossed aphasia.

New techniques such as Wada testing, SPECT, and PET functional brain imaging are beginning to be applied to crossed aphasia. Wada testing, in which sodium amytal is injected into the left carotid artery, has not worsened the language performance of right-handed "crossed aphasia" patients (132, 133), confirming the complete lateralization of language to the right hemisphere. Two studies of SPECT imaging have confirmed the atypical finding of reduced cerebral blood flow in the right hemisphere in association with a right-hemisphere lesion and aphasia (134,135). In one study (135), blood flow was also measured during activation tasks. Both frontal lobes showed activation during a test of phoneme detection, while only the right hemisphere showed activation during a mathematical task. Further research of this type should help to determine the atypical language dominance of patients with crossed aphasia.

APHASIA IN POLYGLOTS

The effects of acquired aphasia on different languages has been an area of interest to asphasiologists for generations. If a patient is fluent in more than one language, at least three questions can be raised with regard to the aphasia produced by an acquired left-hemisphere lesion: (1) will one language be less affected than another?, (2) will one recover faster or better than another?, and (3) will the aphasia type be the same in the different languages? Neurolinguists have also studied patterns of language breakdown in different languages to confirm theories of linguistic issues such as agrammatism (136). In the past, two principal theories predicted differential recovery of different languages. In 1895, Pitres (137) stated that the language the subject had used most before the onset of aphasia would be the first to recover. Eleven years later, Ribot (138) predicted that the native, or first-learned, language would be the most resistant to the effects of an acquired lesion. These two rules are now known as Pitres' and Ribot's laws. Minkowski (139) considered which language the subject has the most emotional investment in and the most motivation to recover. This will often be the language in which the patient speaks and works every day, usually the language also spoken by hospital personnel and speech pathologists. Lambert and Fillenbaum (140) examined bilingual Canadians and found another important variable to be the differential time of learning each language and the relative skill level. Canadians who learned French and English simultaneously in growing up (termed "compound bilinguals") had more similar patterns of language involvement than those who learned one language later than the other ("coordinate bilinguals").

Recent studies have not entirely resolved these issues regarding differential language involvement in aphasic polyglots. In one recent study (141), a patient who learned English, French, and Italian simultaneously in childhood showed a similar degree and pattern of aphasia in all three languages, while a second patient who grew up speaking Croatian but later learned Italian was more aphasic in Italian than in her native tongue. These authors postulated that compound bilinguals have similar representations for each language in neuroanatomical areas, while coordinate bilinguals might have different representations. Silverberg and Gordon (142) studied two Israeli aphasics who both learned Hebrew much later than a native language. The first had a moderately severe, nonfluent aphasia in Spanish and a milder, fluent aphasia in Hebrew. She recovered completely in Hebrew, incompletely in Spanish. The second patient, whose Hebrew was very limited, was globally aphasic in Hebrew, while he had only a mild anomia in Russian. These cases are interesting because they document that involvement of different languages in acquired aphasia can differ not only in degree, but also in aphasia type. These patients were both coordinate bilinguals, and in both the language that recovered better was the one used most by the patient at the time of the onset of aphasia.

Ojemann and Whitaker (143) studied disruption of naming by electrical stimulation in two bilingual patients. In both cases, naming in the more recently acquired language was disrupted by stimulation over a wider area than that in the native language, suggesting that the neuronal populations involved in elicitation of names differ depending on the specific language spoken. Different languages thus have different neuroanatomical underpinnings in the brains of bilingual patients. Obler and Albert (144) reviewed 106 cases from the literature and three of their own with polyglot aphasia. They found that Ribot's law applied no more than half of the time, while Pitres' rule appeared to apply more regularly in younger aphasic patients. No rule had consistent predictive value in the recovery of different languages.

REFERENCES

1. Broca P. Remarques sur le siège de la faculté du langage articulé, suivies d'une observation d'aphemie (perte de la parôle). Bull Soc Anat Paris 1861;6:330–357.

Reprinted in: Rottenberg DA, Hochberg FH, eds. Neurological classics in modern translation. New York: Hafner, 1977:136–149.

2. Benson DF, Geschwind N. The aphasias and related disturbances. In: Baker AB, Baker LH, eds. Clinical neurology. Ch 10. Philadelphia: JB Lippincott, 1989:1–34.

3. Alexander MP, Benson DF. The aphasias and related disturbances. In: Joynt RJ. Clinical neurology. Ch 10. Philadelphia: JB Lippincott, 1991:1–58.

4. Goodglass H, Kaplan E. Assessment of aphasia and related disorders. Philadelphia: Lea & Febiger, 1972.

5. Kertesz A. Western aphasia battery. New York: Grune & Stratton, 1982.

6. Goodglass H, Kaplan E, Weintraub S, Ackerman N. The "tip-of-the-tongue" phenomenon in aphasia. Cortex 1976;12:145–153.

7. Goodglass H, Blumstein SE, Gleason JB, Hyde MR, Green E, Statlender S. The effect of syntactic encoding on sentence comprehension in aphasia. Brain Lang 1979;7:201–209.

8. Heilman KM, Scholes RJ. The nature of comprehension errors in Broca's, conduction, and Wernicke's aphasics. Cortex 1976;12:258–265.

9. Benson DF. The third alexia. Arch Neurol 1977;34:327–331.

10. Robinson RG, Benson DF. Depression in aphasic patients: frequency, severity, and clinical-pathological correlations. Brain Lang 1981;14:282–291.

11. Mohr JP, Pessin MS, Finklestein S, Funkenstein HH, Duncan GW, Davis KR. Broca aphasia: pathologic and clinical. Neurology 1978;28:311–324.

12. Alexander MP, Naeser MA, Palumbo C. Broca's area aphasias: aphasia after lesions including the frontal operculum. Neurology 1990;40:353–362.

13. Alexander MP, Benson DF, Stuss DT. Frontal lobes and language. Brain Lang 1989;37:656–691.

14. Naeser MA, Palumbo CL, Helm-Estabrooks N, Stiassny-Eder D, Albert M. Severe nonfluency in aphasia. Role of the medial subcallosal fasciculus and other white matter pathways in recovery of spontaneous speech. Brain 1989;112:1–38.

15. Knopman DS, Selnes OA, Niccum N, Rubens AB, Yock D, Larson D. A longitudinal study of speech fluency in aphasia: CT correlates of recovery and persistent nonfluency. Neurology 1983;33:1170–1178.

16. Schiff HB, Alexander MR, Naeser MA, Galaburda AM. Aphemia: clinical-anatomic correlations. Arch Neurol 1983;40:720–727.

17. Wernicke C. Der Aphasische Symptomen Komplex. Breslau: Cohn & Weigert, 1874. Reprinted in: Eggert G, ed. Wernicke's works on aphasia. A source book and review. Vol 1. The Hague: Mouton, 1977:92–145.

18. Kirshner HS, Webb WG, Duncan GW. Word deafness in Wernicke's aphasia. J Neurol Neurosurg Psychiatry 1981;41:161–170.

19. Kirshner HS, Webb WG. Alexia and agraphia in Wernicke's aphasia. J Neurol Neurosurg Psychiatry 1982;45:719–724.

20. Kirshner HS, Casey PF, Henson J, Heinrich JJ. Behavioural features and lesion localization in Wernicke's aphasia. Aphasiology 1989;3:169–176.

21. Heilman KM, Rothi L, Campanella MS, Wolfson S. Wernicke's and global aphasia without alexia. Arch Neurol 1979;36:129–133.

22. Benson DF. Psychiatric aspects of aphasia. Br J Psychiatry 1973;123:555–566.

23. Bogen J, Bogen G. Wernicke's region – where is it? Ann NY Acad Sci 1976;280: 834–843.
24. Naeser MA, Helm-Estabrooks N, Haas G, Auerbach S, Srinivasan M. Relationship between lesion extent in "Wernicke's area" on CT scan and predicting recovery of comprehension in Wernicke's aphasia. Arch Neurol 1987;44:73–82.
25. Selnes OA, Niccum N, Knopman DS, Rubens AB. Recovery of single word comprehension: CT-scan correlates. Brain Lang 1984;21:72–84.
26. Kertesz A, Lau WK, Polk M. The structural determinants of recovery in Wernicke's aphasia. Brain Lang 1993;44:153–164.
27. Lesser RP, Luders H, Morris HH, Dinner DS, Klem G, Hahn J, Harrison M. Electrical stimulation of Wernicke's area interferes with comprehension. Neurology 1986;36:658–663.
28. Luria AR, Hutton A. A modern assessment of the basic forms of aphasia. Brain Lang 1977;4:129–151.
29. Blumstein SE, Baker E, Goodglass H. Phonological factors in auditory comprehension in aphasia. Neuropsychologia 1977;15:19–30.
30. Gainotti G, Caltagirone C, Ibba A. Semantic and phonemic aspects of auditory language comprehension in aphasia. Linguistics 1975;154(5):15–29.
31. Baker E, Blumstein SE, Goodglass H. Interaction between phonological and semantic factors in auditory comprehension. Neuropsychologia 1981;19:1–15.
32. Tallal P, Newcombe F. Impairment of auditory perception and language comprehension in dysphasia. Brain Lang 1978;5:13–24.
33. Blumstein SE. Phonological aspects of aphasia. In: Sarno MT, ed. Acquired aphasia. 2nd ed. San Diego: Academic Press, 1991:151–180.
34. Sherwin I, Efron R. Temporal ordering deficits following anterior temporal lobectomy. Brain Lang 1980;11:195–203.
35. Riedel K, Studdert-Kennedy M. Extending format transitions may not improve aphasics' perception of stop consonant place of articulation. Brain Lang 1985;24:196–207.
36. Albert M, Bear D. Time to understand. Brain 1974;97:373–384.
37. Weidner W, Lasky E. The interaction of rate and complexity of stimulus on the performance of adult aphasic subjects. Brain Lang 1976;3:34–40.
38. Blumstein SE, Katz B, Goodglass H, Shrier R, Dworetzky B. The effects of slowed speech on auditory comprehension in aphasia. Brain Lang 1985;24:246–265.
39. Boller F, Cole M, Vrtunski PB, Patterson M, Kim Y. Paralinguistic aspects of auditory comprehension in aphasia. Brain Lang 1979;7:164–174.
40. Ellis AW, Miller D, Sin G. Wernicke's aphasia and normal language processing: a case study in cognitive neuropsychology. Cognition 1983;15:111–144.
41. Caramazza A, Berndt RS, Basili AG. The selective impairment of phonological processing: a case study. Brain Lang 1977;18:128–174.
42. Lytton WW, Brust CM. Direct dyslexia: preserved oral reading of real words in Wernicke's aphasia. Brain 1989;112:583–594.
43. Sevush S, Roeltgen DP, Campanella DJ, Heilman KM. Preserved oral reading in Wernicke's aphasia. Neurology 1983;33:916–920.
44. Hier DB, Mohr JP. Incongruous oral and written naming. Brain Lang 1977;4:115–126.

45. Margolin DI. Cognitive neuropsychology. Resolving enigmas about Wernicke's aphasia and other higher cortical disorders. Arch Neurol 1991;48:751–765.
46. Goldstein MN. Auditory agnosia for speech ("pure word-deafness"). A historical review with current implications. Brain Lang 1974;1:195–204.
47. Coslett HB, Brashear HR, Heilman KM. Pure word deafness after bilateral primary auditory cortex infarcts. Neurology 1984;34:347–352.
48. Mendez M, Geehan GR. Cortical auditory disorder: Clinical and psychoacoustic features. J Neurol Neurosurg Psychiatry 1988;51:1–9.
49. Tanaka Y, Yamadori A, Mori E. Pure word deafness following bilateral lesions. A psychophysical analysis. Brain 1987;110:381–403.
50. Kanshepolsky J, Kelley JJ, Waggener JD. A cortical auditory disorder. Clinical, audiological and pathologic aspects. Neurology 1973;23:699–705.
51. Geschwind N. The organization of language and the brain. Science 1970;170:940–944.
52. Takahashi N, Kawamura M, Shinotou H, Kirayama K, Kaga K, Shindo M. Pure word deafness due to left hemisphere damage. Cortex 1992;28:295–303.
53. Mohr JP, Sidman M, Stoddard LT, Leicester J, Rosenberger PB. Evolution of the deficit in total aphasia. Neurology 1973;23:1302–1312.
54. Tranel D, Biller J, Damasio H, Adams HP, Cornell SH. Global aphasia without hemiparesis. Arch Neurol 1987;44:304–308.
55. Legatt AD, Rubin MJ, Kaplan LR, Healton EB, Brust JCM. Global aphasia without hemiparesis: Multiple etiologies. Neurology 1987;37:201–205.
56. Alexander MP, LoVerme S. Aphasia following left intracerebral hemorrhage. Neurology 1980;30:1192–1203.
57. Naeser MA, Gaddie A, Palumbo CL, Stiassny-Eder D. Late recovery of auditory comprehension in global aphasia. Improved recovery observed with subcortical temporal isthmus lesion vs Wernicke's cortical area lesion. Arch Neurol 1990;47:425–432.
58. Sarno MR, Levita E. Recovery in treated aphasia during the first year post-stroke. Stroke 1979;10:663–670.
59. Geschwind N. Disconnexion syndromes in animals and man. Brain 1965;88:237–294 and 585–644.
60. Kohn SE. The nature of the phonological disorder in conduction aphasia. Brain Lang 1984;23:97–115.
61. Kinsbourne M. Behavioral analysis of the repetition deficit in conduction aphasia. Neurology 1972;22:1126–1132.
62. Damasio H, Damasio AR. The anatomical basis of conduction aphasia. Brain 1980;103:337–350.
63. Benson DR, Sheremata WA, Bouchard R, Segarra JM, Price D, Geschwind N. Conduction aphasia: a clinicopathological study. Arch Neurol 1973;28:339–346.
64. Brown JW. The problem of repetition: a study of "conduction" aphasia and the "isolation" syndrome. Cortex 1975;11:37–52.
65. Levine DN, Calvanio R. Conduction aphasia. In: Kirshner HS, Freemon FR, eds. The neurology of aphasia. Amsterdam: Swets & Zeitlinger, 1982:79–112.
66. Warrington EK, Shallice T. The selective impairment of auditory short-term memory. Brain 1969;92:885–896.

67. Warrington EK, Logue V, Pratt RTC. The anatomical localisation of selective impairment of auditory verbal short-term memory. Neuropsychologia 1971;9: 377–387.
68. Shallice T, Warrington EK. Auditory-verbal short-term memory impairment and conduction aphasia. Brain Lang 1977;4:479–491.
69. Saffran EM, Marin OSM. Immediate memory for word lists and sentences in a patient with deficient auditory short-term memory. Brain Lang 1975;2:420–433.
70. Tzortzis C, Albert ML. Impairment of memory for sequences in conduction aphasia. Neuropsychologia 1974;12:355–366.
71. Heilman KM, Scholes R, Watson RT. Defects of immediate memory in Broca's and condution aphasia. Brain Lang 1976;3:201–208.
72. Strub RL. The repetition defect in conduction aphasia: mnestic or linguistic? Brain Lang 1974;1:241–255.
73. Boller F, Marcie P. Possible role of abnormal auditory feedback on conduction aphasia. Neuropsychologia 1978;16:521–524.
74. Chapin C, Blumstein SE, Meissner B, Boller F. Speech production mechanisms in aphasia: a delayed auditory feedback study. Brain Lang 1981;14:106–113.
75. Goldstein K. Language and language disturbances. New York: Grune & Stratton, 1948.
76. Feinberg TE, Gonzalez Rothi LJ, Heilman KM. 'Inner speech' in conduction aphasia. Arch Neurol 1986;43:591–593.
77. Lichtheim L. On aphasia. Brain 1885;7:433–484.
78. Rubens AB. Transcortical motor aphasia. Studies Neuroling 1976;1:293–306.
79. Alexander MP, Schmitt MA. The aphasia syndrome of stroke in the left anterior cerebral artery territory. Arch Neurol 1980;37:97–100.
80. Luria AR, Tsvetkova LS. The mechanism of 'dynamic aphasia.' Foundations Lang 1968;4:296–307.
81. Freedman M, Alexander MP, Naeser MA. Anatomic basis of transcortical motor aphasia. Neurology 1984;34:409–417.
82. Masdeu JC, Schoene WC, Funkenstein H. Aphasia following infarction of the left supplementary motor area. A clinicopathologic study. Neurology 1978;28: 1220–1223.
83. Albert ML, Bachman DL, Morgan A, Helm-Estabrooks N. Pharmacotherapy for aphasia. Neurology 1988;38:877–879.
84. Kertesz A, Sheppard A, MacKenzie R. Localization in transcortical sensory aphasia. Arch Neurol 1982;39:475–478.
85. Heilman KM, Rothi L, McFarling D, Rottmann AL. Transcortical sensory aphasia with relatively spared spontaneous speech and naming. Arch Neurol 1981; 38:236–239.
86. Appel J, Kertesz A, Fisman M. A study of language functioning in Alzheimer patients. Brain Lang 1982;17:73–91.
87. Goldstein K. Die transcorticalen Aphasien. Ergebn Neurol Psychiat 1917;2: 349–629.
88. Geschwind N, Quadfasel F, Segarra J. Isolation of the speech area. Neuropsychologia 1968;6:327–340.

89. Ross Ed. Left medial parietal lobe and receptive language functions: mixed transcortical aphasia after left anterior cerebral artery infarction. Neurology 1980;30:144–151.

90. Grossi D, Trojano L, Chiacchio L, Soricelli A, Mansi L, Postiglione A. Mixed transcortical aphasia: clinical features and neuroanatomical correlates. A possible role of the right hemisphere. Eur Neurol 1991;31:204–211.

91. McFarling O, Rothi LJ, Heilman KM. Transcortical aphasia from ischemic infarcts of the thalamus: a report of two cases. J Neurol Neurosurg Psychiatry 1982;45:107–112.

92. Whitaker H. A case of the isolation of the language function. In: Whitaker H, Whitaker HA, eds. Studies in neurolinguistics. Vol 2. New York: Academic Press, 1976:1–58.

93. Fisher CM. The pathological and clinical aspects of thalamic hemorrhage. Trans Am Neurol Assoc 1959;84:56–59.

94. Mohr JP, Watters WC, Duncan GW. Thalamic hemorrhage and aphasia. Brain Lang 1975;2:3–17.

95. Reynolds AF, Turner PT, Harris AB, Ojemann GA, Lavis LE. Left thalamic hemorrhage with dysphasia: a report of five cases. Brain Lang 1979;7:62–73.

96. Luria AR. On quasi-aphasic speech disturbances in lesions of the deep structures of the brain. Brain Lang 1977;4:432–459.

97. Bogousslavsky J, Regli F, Uske A. Thalamic infarcts: clinical syndromes, etiology, and prognosis. Neurology 1988;38:837–848.

98. Graff-Radford NR, Eslinger PJ, Damasio AR, Yamada T. Nonhemorrhagic infarction of the thalamus: behavioral, anatomic, and physiologic correlates. Neurology 1984;34:14–23.

99. Graff-Radford NR, Damasio H, Yamada T, Eslinger PJ, Damasio AR. Non-haemorrhagic thalamic infarction. Clinical, neuropsychological and electrophysiological findings in four anatomical groups defined by computered tomography. Brain 1985;108:485–516.

100. Stuss DT, Guberman A, Nelson R, Larochelle S. The neuropsychology of paramedian thalamic infarction. Brain Lang 1988;8:348–378.

101. Fensore C, Lazzarino LG, Nappo A, Nicolai A. Language and memory disturbances from mesencephalothalamic infarcts. A clinical and computed tomographic study. Eur Neurol 1988;28:51–56.

102. Bell DS. Speech functions of the thalamus inferred from the effects of thalamotomy. Brain 1968;91:619–1638.

103. Samra K, Riklan M, Levita E, Zimmerman J, Waltz J, Bermann L, Cooper I. Language and speech correlates of anatomically verified lesions in thalamic surgery for parkinsonism. J Speech Hear Res 1969;12:510–540.

104. Smythe GE, Stern K. Tumors of the thalamus: a clinico-pathological study. Brain 1938;61:339–360.

105. Megens J, van Loon J, Goffin J, Gybels J. Subcortical aphasia from a thalamic abscess. N Neurol Neurosurg Psychiatry 1992;55:319–321.

106. Ojemann G. Language and the thalamus: object naming and recall during and after thalamic stimulation. Brain Lang 1975;2:101–120.

107. Ojemann G, Fedio P, Van Buren J. Anomia from pulvinar and subcortical parietal stimulation. Brain 1968;91:99–116.

108. Crosson B. Role of the dominant thalamus in language: a review. Psychol Bull 1984;96:491–517.
109. Kirshner HS, Kistler KH. Aphasia after right thalamic hemorrhage. Arch Neurol 1982;39:667–669.
110. Chesson AL. Aphasia following a right thalamic hemorrhage. Brain Lang 1983;19:306–316.
111. Alexander MP, LoVerme SR. Aphasia after left hemispheric intracerebral hemorrhage. Neurology 1980;30:1193–1202.
112. Naeser MA, Alexander MP, Helm-Estabrooks N, Levine HL, Laughlin SA, Geschwind N. Aphasia with predominantly subcortical lesion sites. Arch Neurol 1982;39:2–14.
113. Damasio AR, Damasio H, Rizzo M, Varney N, Gersh F. Aphasia with nonhemorrhagic lesions in the basal ganglia and internal capsule. Arch Neurol 1982;39:15–20.
114. Alexander MP, Naeser MA, Palumbo CL. Correlations of subcortical CT lesion sites and aphasia profiles. Brain 1987;110:961–991.
115. Crosson B. Subcortical functions in language: a working model. Brain Lang 1985;25:257–292.
116. Cappa SF, Cavallotti G, Guidotti M, Papagno C, Vignolo LA. Subcortical aphasia: two clinical-CT scan correlation studies. Cortex 1983;19:227–241.
117. Aram DM, Rose DF, Rekate HL, Whitaker HA. Acquired capsular/striatal aphasia in childhood. Arch Neurol 1983;40:614–617.
118. Fromm D, Holland AL, Swindell CS, Reinmuth OM. Various consequences of subcortical stroke. Prospective study of 16 consecutive cases. Arch Neurol 1985;42:943–950.
119. Tanridag O, Kirshner HS. Aphasia and agraphia in lesions of the posterior internal capsule and putamen. Neurology 1985;35:1797–1801.
120. Basso A, Della Sala S, Farabola M. Aphasia arising from purely deep lesions. Cortex 1987;23:29–44.
121. Mendez MF, Adams NL, Lewandowski KS. Neurobehavioral changes associated with caudate lesions. Neurology 1989;39:349–354.
122. Goodglass H, Quadfasel F. Language laterality in left-handed aphasics. Brain 1954;77:521–548.
123. Brown JW, Hecaen H. Lateralization and language representation. Observations on aphasia in children, left-handers, and "anomalous" dextrals. Neurology 1976;26:183–189.
124. Naeser MA, Borod JC. Aphasia in left-handers: lesion site, lesion side, and hemispheric asymmetries on CT. Neurology 1986;36:471–488.
125. Basso A, Farabola M, Pia Grassi M, Laiacona M, Zanobio ME. Aphasia in left handers. Comparison of aphasia profiles and language recovery in non-right-handed and matched right-handed patients. Brain Lang 1990;38:233–252.
126. Bramwell B. On 'crossed' aphasia and the factors which go to determine whether the 'leading' or 'driving' speech-centres shall be located in the left or in the right hemisphere of the brain, with notes of a case of 'crossed' aphasia (aphasia with right-sided hemiplegia) in a left-handed man. Lancet 1899;i:1473–1479.

127. Gloning I, Gloning K, Haub G, Quatember R. Comparison of verbal behavior in right-handed and non right-handed patients with anatomically verified lesion of one hemisphere. Cortex 1969;5:43–52.
128. Henderson VW. Speech fluency in crossed aphasia. Brain 1983;106:837–857.
129. Sweet EWS, Panis W, Levine DN. Crossed Wernicke's aphasia. Neurology 1984;34:475–479.
130. Basso A, Capitani E, Laiacona M, Zanobio ME. Crossed aphasia: one or more syndromes? Cortex 1985;21:25–45.
131. Alexander MP, Fischette MR, Fischer RS. Crossed aphasias can be mirror image or anomalous. Brain 1989;112:953–973.
132. Zangwill OL. Two cases of crossed aphasia in dextrals. Neuropsychologia 1979;17:167–172.
133. Delreux V, de Partz MP, Kevers L, Callewaert A. Aphasie croisée chez un droitier. Rev Neurol (Paris) 1989;145:725–728.
134. Perani D, Papagno C, Cappa S, Gerundini P, Fazio F. Crossed aphasia: functional studies with single photon emission computerized tomography. Cortex 1988;24:171–178.
135. Walker-Batson D, Wendt JS, Devous M, Barton MM, Bonte FJ. A long-term follow-up case study of crossed aphasia assessed by single-photon emission tomography (SPECT), language, and neuropsychological testing. Brain Lang 1988;33:311–322.
136. Paradis M. Recent developments in the study of agrammatism: Their impact for the assessment of bilingual aphasia. J Neurolinguistics 1988;3:127–160.
137. Pitres A. Etude sur l'aphasie ches les polyglottes. Rev Med 1895;15:873–899.
138. Ribot T. Diseases of memory, an essay in the positive psychology. London: Kegan Paul, 1906:122.
139. Minkowski M. Klinischer beitrag zur aphasie bei polyglotten, speziell im hinblick aufs Schweizerdeutsche. Schweiz Arch Neurol Psychiatr 1927:21:43–72.
140. Lambert WE, Fillenbaum S. A pilot study of aphasia among bilinguals. Can J Psychol 1959;13:28–34.
141. Mastronardi L, Ferrante L, Celli P, Acqui M, Fortuna A. Aphasia in polyglots: report of two cases and analysis of the literature. Neurosurgery 1991; 29:621–623.
142. Silverberg R, Gordon HW. Differential aphasia in two bilingual individuals. Neurology 1979;29:51–55.
143. Ojemann GA, Whitaker HA. The bilingual brain. Arch Neurol 1978;35:409–412.
144. Obler LK, Albert ML. Influence of aging on recovery from aphasia in polyglots. Brain Lang 1977;4:460–463.

5

How to Analyze CT/MRI Scan Lesion Sites to Predict Potential for Long-Term Recovery in Aphasia

Margaret A. Naeser and Carole L. Palumbo

Boston University School of Medicine and Veterans Affairs Medical Center, Boston, Massachusetts

INTRODUCTION

This chapter presents a method of lesion site analysis that may be used to help understand a stroke patient's potential for language recovery in three areas of aphasia: (1) *recovery of auditory language comprehension* (after 6 months or 1 year post-onset), (2) *recovery of spontaneous speech* (i.e., which patients are likely to have nonfluent speech after 6 months or 1 year versus those likely to have no meaningful spontaneous speech—for as long as 9 years post-onset), and (3) potential for treatment with a *verbal treatment program* (melodic intonation therapy or some other verbal treatment program) versus potential for treatment with a *nonverbal treatment program* (computer-assisted visual communication [C-ViC] or some other nonverbal treatment program). The C-ViC treatment program trains nonverbal patients to use pictures and icons on a Macintosh computer screen to communicate their needs and ideas.

Most of our current information regarding lesion location and resulting language behavior was developed from CT scan studies published in the 1970s and '80s. These studies examined language behavior resulting from lesions in primarily cortical areas (1–15) and in primarily subcortical areas (16–22). These and additional studies have recently been reviewed by Alexander and Benson (23).

The CT scan studies have helped us learn about the location of neuro-anatomical structures and white-matter pathways, and their role in the production of aphasic language behavior when a lesion is present. This chapter focuses on the relationship between lesions in a few of these cortical areas and subcortical areas on CT scan, on recovery of comprehension and spontaneous speech, and on potential for treatment with verbal or nonverbal treatment programs, as mentioned above. The emphasis is not on aphasia *syndromes*, per se, but on recovery of specific aspects of language behavior. This chapter also explains how to examine a chronic CT scan of *any* aphasic stroke patient, to understand potential for recovery of specific aspects of language behavior in the chronic phase, post-stroke. The CT scans on which the predictions for recovery are based are performed at least 2 or 3 months post–stroke onset (MPO). The recovery of auditory comprehension or spontaneous speech is based on expected language behavior after at least 6 months or 1 year post-onset.

The method of lesion analysis presented in this chapter is, at this time, most easily applied to areas of infarction on chronic CT scans. There are special problems associated with lesion site analysis on MRI scans; these are addressed at the end of the chapter. Most material is based on our research at the CT/MRI Scan Aphasia Research Laboratory at the Boston University Aphasia Research Center, Boston Department of Veterans Affairs Medical Center.

The term *recovery* in this chapter usually refers to the actual late language scores, i.e., the language scores attained by a patient 6 MPO, or even 1–3 years post–stroke onset. The term does not usually refer to amount or rate of change from early, time 1 scores (1 or 2 MPO) to late, time 2 scores (6 MPO, or 1–3 years post-onset). These are different areas of investigation. The time 1 and time 2 scores – and therefore amount of change – are listed, however, in most of our published papers. All our CT scan recovery studies have been *retrospective*.

The latest post-onset language socres were always used for a patient – i.e., the longest post-onset scores, and thus the more stable, late scores. The early language scores at 1 or 2 MPO were also examined, but these individual scores were usually not useful for predictions of recovery in the chronic phase.

Lesion *size* analysis is discussed little in this chapter, because research from our laboratory and others has not found total lesion size to be helpful in making predictions for recovery, except in very large or very small lesions (4,8,12,13,24,25). For example, in our previous lesion size studies, the mean lesion size for transcortical motor aphasics was 5.7% left-hemisphere tissue damage (SD 3.3) and the mean lesion size for conduction aphasics was 3.6% (SD 2.4); there was no significant difference between these two aphasia types (26,27). The transcortical motor aphasics had primarily frontal lobe lesions, however, while the conduction aphasics had primary parietal lobe lesions. The two groups had very different language behavior characteristics, including excellent sentence repetition for the transcortical motor aphasics and poor sentence repetition for the conduction aphasics. In our experience, knowing only the percent lesion size, and not the exact lesion site, is not useful for predicting language recovery.

The mean lesion size for global aphasia patients with cortical and subcortical lesions is 28.1% left-hemisphere tissue damage (SD 11.2) (complete left middle cerebral artery territory ischemic infarction). The mean lesion size for global aphasia patients with primarily subcortical lesion is only 13.6% left-hemisphere tissue damage (SD 3.2) (28). The subcortical global aphasia patients have a total lesion size (13.6%) less than half of that observed in global aphasia patients with cortical and subcortical lesions (28.1%). The subcortical global aphasia patients have lesions primarily in the putamen and internal capsule area, with white-matter lesion extension in three directions: (1) *anterior* (across the anterior limb, internal capsule, and white matter near the frontal horn, deep to Broca's area), (2) *posterior* (across white matter in the temporal isthmus, deep to Wernicke's area), and (3) *superior*, into the white matter near the body of the lateral ventricle (18). These subcortical global aphasia patients have lesions that undercut the critical white-matter pathways for speech and comprehension. These small subcortical white-matter lesions may extend only a few millimeters in one direction and yet produce profound language deficits. Hence, over the last decade, our research has increasingly shifted away from overall lesion size analysis to precise CT scan lesion site analysis.

METHOD OF LESION SITE ANALYSIS

Most CT scans examined in our research are obtained at approximately 15–20° to the canthomeatal line, with 10 mm slice thickness and 3 mm slice overlap through the ventricles, beginning at the level of the suprasellar cistern. Our method of lesion site analysis includes examination of lesions in specific, separate cortical and subcortical language areas. These separate neuroanatomical areas are diagrammed on the CT scan slices shown in Figure 1b. Most of these neuroanatomical areas are listed in various CT scan atlases (29–31).

The extent of lesion (degree of infarction) within each neuroanatomical area in Figure 1b is visually assessed using a 0-to-5-point rating scale, where 0 = no lesion; 1 = equivocal lesion; 2 = small, patchy, or partial lesion; 2.5 = patchy—less than half of area has lesion; 3 = half of area has lesion; 3.5 = patchy—more than half of area has lesion; 4 = more than half of

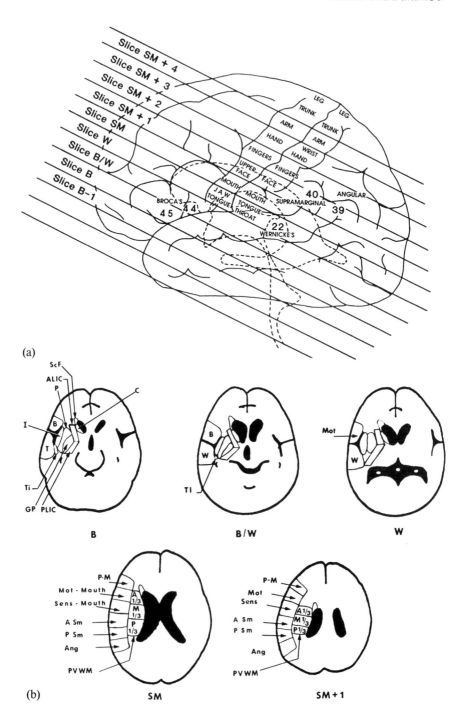

(a)

(b)

area has solid lesion; and 5 = total area has solid lesion. An extent-of-lesion rating is recorded for each cortical and subcortical area on the CT scan slices shown in Figure 1b.

An extent-of-lesion rating >3 for a specific neuroanatomical area is of special importance. Extent-of-lesion ratings >3 (indicating lesion in greater than half of a specific area) have been observed to correlate with increased severity of language deficit and reduced potential for recovery of auditory comprehension (13,32) and spontaneous speech (25). All scans were rated by at least two experienced raters, and conferenced data were used. In previous studies, we have observed an interrater reliability coefficient of 0.93 (33).

LESION SITE ANALYSIS AND RECOVERY OF AUDITORY LANGUAGE COMPREHENSION

Wernicke's Aphasia

This section explains how to analyze CT scan lesion sites to predict potential for long-term recovery of auditory comprehension in Wernicke's aphasia.

Ten male Wernicke's aphasia patients were studied who were classified after 6 MPO as mild, good-recovery cases (*n* = 5) or moderate-severe, poor-recovery cases (*n* = 5) (13). Each patient was right-handed and had suffered a single-episode left-hemisphere occlusive-vascular stroke between the ages of 47 and

---

Figure 1 (a) Lateral diagram of the location of cortical language areas in relationship to the ventricular system (dotted lines). The CT scan slices are marked at 20 degrees to the canthomeatal line, similar to the angle at which they are performed. Numbers refer to Brodmann's areas as follows: 44 and 45, Broca's area; 22, Wernicke's area; 40, supramarginal gyrus area; 39, angular gyrus area. The parts of the motor and sensory homunculi are labeled for each slice. Note that the motor/sensory cortex areas for the mouth are located on slice SM. (b) Location of specific neuroanatomical areas on CT scans that are visually assessed for extent-of-lesion ratings. The CT scan slices B, B/W, W, SM, and SM + 1 are labeled according to the system of Naeser and Hayward (2). Each neuroanatomical area is examined using 0–5-point scale (0 = no lesion; 3 = half of area has lesion; 5 = entire area has solid lesion; see text). B = Broca's area (45 on slice B, 44 on slice B/W): T = temporal lobe anterior-inferior to Wernicke's area on slice B; Ti = temporal isthmus; I = insular structures including insula, extreme capsule, claustrum, and external capsule; P = putamen; GP = globus pallidus; ALIC = anterior limb, internal capsule; PLIC = posterior limb, internal capsule; ScF = medial subcallosal fasciculus; C = caudate; W = Wernicke's area (22); Mot = motor cortex; P-M = premotor cortex; Sens = sensory cortex; A Sm = anterior supramarginal gyrus; P Sm = posterior supramarginal gyrus; Ang = angular gyrus; PVWM = periventricular white-matter area (A 1/3, anterior 1/3 PVWM; M 1/3, middle 1/3 PVWM; P 1/3, posterior 1/3 PVWM).

71 years ($x = 58.4$; SD 6.9), with no significant group differences. The CT scans used for lesion site analysis were performed between 3 and 36 MPO.

The auditory comprehension test scores from the Boston Diagnostic Aphasia Exam (BDAE) (34) were examined for two time periods. Time 1 (T1) scores were obtained 1 to 2 MPO; time 2 (T2) scores were obtained more than 6 MPO. The second test, to determine T2 scores, was administered 6 to 13 MPO for the mild group and 12 to 38 MPO for the moderate-severe group. The T2 scores for the moderate-severe group were taken as long after onset as possible, in order to extend the potential recovery period.

Patients were separated on the basis of T2 scores as follows (1) good-recovery cases scored above 0 (above the 50th percentile) on the BDAE Overall Auditory Comprehension z-score; (2) poor-recovery cases scored below 0 (below the 50th percentile) (see Fig. 2). The reader is referred to the original paper (13) for exact T1 and T2 test scores for all 10 Wernicke's aphasia patients.

The CT scans were analyzed with two methods: (1) lesion *site* analysis, as described above, in which the 0–5-point extent-of-lesion rating scale was used to visually rate the amount of infarction (degree of damage) within each

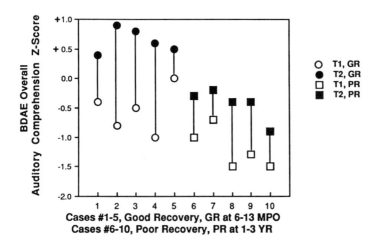

Figure 2 Times 1 (1–2 MPO) and 2 (6 MPO or 1–3 years). Overall Auditory Comprehension z-scores for 10 Wernicke's aphasia patients. The graph shows overlap in the T1 scores among some of the good-recovery (GR) and poor-recovery (PR) cases; thus, the T1 test scores could not be used on a case-by-case basis to predict GR or PR after 6 MPO. (From Ref. 91.)

specific cortical and subcortical area, and (2) total lesion *size* analysis, in which the total percent left-hemisphere temporoparietal lesion size was quantified using a computer-based technique (27,35).

Since the time of Wernicke, there have been multiple interpretations regarding the exact location and limits of Wernicke's area (36). For the purpose of this study, Wernicke's area was defined as the posterior two-thirds of the left superior temporal gyrus. On CT scans, the anterior half of Wernicke's area, i.e., the middle third of the superior temporal gyrus, was located lateral to the maximum width of the third ventricle on slice B/W (Fig. 1b). In addition, the posterior half of Wernicke's area, i.e., the posterior third of the superior temporal gyrus, was located lateral to the roof of the third ventricle on slice W (Fig. 1b). The supramarginal and angular gyrus areas in the parietal lobe were also analyzed on slices SM and SM + 1 (Fig. 1b).

All good-recovery Wernicke's patients with T2 Auditory Comprehension z-scores above 0 had lesions in only half, or less than half, of Wernicke's area. All poor-recovery Wernicke's patients with z-scores below 0 had lesions in more than half of Wernicke's area (see Fig. 3, top). The correlation between T2 BDAE Overall Auditory Comprehension z-scores and extent of lesion within Wernicke's area was -0.91 ($p < 0.001$).

The total percent left temporoparietal lesion size was not useful in distinguishing between good-recovery versus poor-recovery cases of auditory comprehension at T2 (Fig. 3, bottom). The correlation between the T2 Auditory Comprehension z-scores and total percent left temporoparietal lesion size was -0.56 (not significant). There was also no significant correlation between amount of change between T1 and T2 and extent-of-lesion rating within Wernicke's area ($r = -0.494$; n.s.). There was also no significant correlation between amount of change and total percent left-hemisphere temporoparietal lesion size ($r = -0.013$; n.s.).

There was a significant correlation, however, between total percent left temporoparietal lesion size and the T2 Visual Confrontation Naming scores from the BDAE (-0.88; $p < 0.001$). This latter finding (naming to pictures) is in general agreement with Kertesz (37), who found that the highest degree of correlation between total lesion size and severity of aphasia existed for anomic aphasia patients.

Case Examples

Figure 4 shows the CT scan of a Wernicke's aphasia patient with lesion in Wernicke's cortical area, only on slice W, and good recovery of auditory comprehension 7–10 MPO (lesion in about half of Wernicke's total area). Figure 5 shows the CT scan of a Wernicke's aphasia patient with complete lesion in Wernicke's cortical area on both slice B/W and slice W, and poor recovery of auditory comprehension 14 MPO (lesion in all of Wernicke's area).

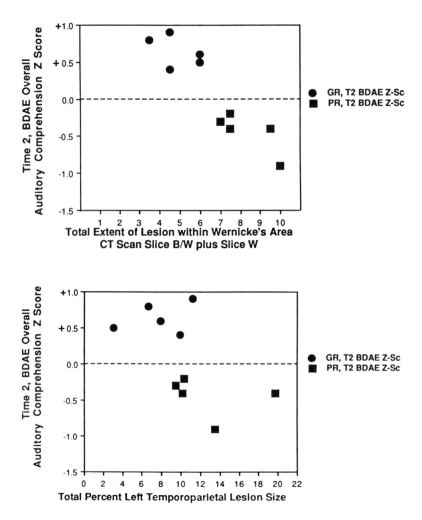

Figure 3 (Top) Graph showing a highly significant correlation ($r = -0.91$; $p < 0.001$) between the total extent-of-lesion ratings within Wernicke's area on CT scan slices B/W and W and T2 BDAE Overall Auditory comprehension z-scores for 10 Wernicke's aphasia patients. A total extent-of-lesion rating of 10 reflects a rating of 5 (complete solid lesion) in Wernicke's area on both slices B/W and W. Patients with total extent-of-lesion ratings ⩽6 have lesion in no more than half of Wernicke's area; these patients had good recovery after 6 MPO, and T2 BDAE z-scores above 0 or above the 50th percentile. Patients with total extent-of-lesion ratings >6 have lesion in more than half of Wernicke's area; these patients still had poor recovery more than 1–3 years post–stroke onset. (Bottom) Graph showing no significant correlation ($r = -0.56$, not significant) between total percent left temporoparietal lesion size on CT scan slices B, B/W, W, SM, and SM + 1 and T2 BDAE Overall Auditory Comprehension z-scores for 10 Wernicke's aphasia patients. There was overlap between the GR and PR cases around the 10% lesion size value. Total lesion size could not be used to separate all GR from PR cases at T2 testing. Only total extent-of-lesion ratings within Wernicke's area could be used to separate all GR from PR cases at T2 testing (see Figure 3, top).

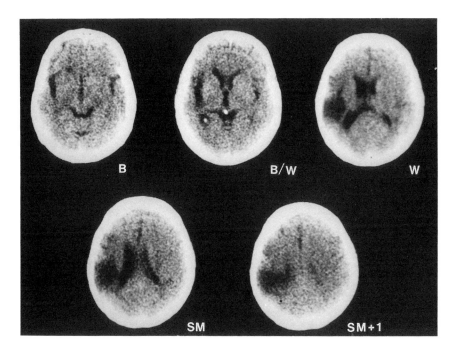

Figure 4 CT scan performed 24 MPO in a mild Wernicke's aphasia patient who had good recovery (+0.9 on BDAE Auditory Comprehension z-score) at T2 testing (7 MPO). Lesion was present only in the posterior half of Wernicke's area on slice W (extent-of-lesion rating 4.5). There was additional parietal lobe lesion in the anterior and posterior supramarginal gyrus areas, surface and deep. (From Ref. 13.)

Results from this study support the notion that extent-of-lesion ratings for Wernicke's area on a chronic CT scan (performed 2 or 3 MPO) may be useful in predicting long-term recovery of auditory comprehension in Wernicke's aphasia patients. Those patients with lesions in only half, or less, of Wernicke's area have a better prognosis for recovery of auditory comprehension within the first year post–stroke onset.

Global Aphasia

This section explains how to analyze CT scan lesion sites to predict potential for long-term recovery of auditory comprehension in global aphasia.

Fourteen right-handed stroke patients with global aphasia (12 men and two women, aged 50 to 66 years) who had unilateral left-hemisphere ischemic infarcts were studied (32). All patients had been tested at least twice with the BDAE (34). Time 1 testing ranged from 1 to 4 MPO. All patients had been classified as globally aphasic at T1 on the basis of the BDAE. All patients

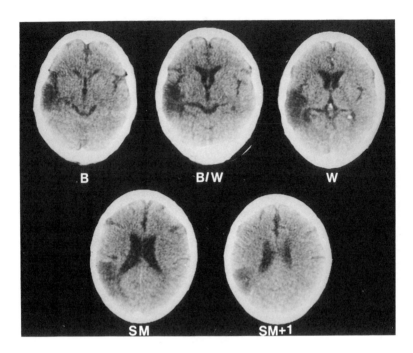

Figure 5 CT scan performed 7 MPO in a severe Wernicke's aphasia patient who had poor recovery (−0.9 on BDAE Auditory Comprehension z-score) at time 2 testing (14 MPO). Extensive lesion was present in Wernicke's area on both slices B/W and W (extent-of-lesion rating 5 on each slice = total extent-of-lesion rating of 10). Large temporal lobe lesion was also present on slice B (extent-of-lesion rating 4.5), anterior and inferior to Wernicke's area. There was additional parietal lobe lesion in anterior and posterior supramarginal gyrus areas, surface and deep. There was also some lesion in angular gyrus on slices SM and SM+1. (From Ref. 13.)

had BDAE Auditory Comprehension z-scores at T1 that were below −1.0, i.e., showing severe auditory comprehension deficits. Time 2 testing was approximately 1 to 2 years post–stroke onset.

All patients had CT scans obtained after 2 MPO (range 2 to 110 MPO). CT scan lesion site analysis was performed. Extent-of-lesion ratings were computed for the separate cortical and subcortical areas shown in Figure 1b. These included major frontal, parietal, and temporal lobe areas, as well as subcortical structures. Special emphasis was placed on analyzing the extent of lesion in Wernicke's cortical area (and immediate subjacent white matter) on CT scan slices B/W and W and the extent of lesion in the subcortical temporal lobe structure, the subcortical temporal isthmus area, on CT scan slices B and B/W (see Fig. 1b for location of these areas on CT scan slices B, B/W, and W). The subcortical temporal isthmus area contains auditory pathways from the medial geniculate nucleus of the thalamus to Heschl's gyrus. Lesion in the temporal isthmus area has been associated with auditory language comprehension deficits since the time of Nielsen (38). In the present study, its location was defined as the white matter inferior to the sylvian fissure/insular area and anterior to the temporal horn on CT scan slices B and B/W (18,38) (Fig. 6).

Nielsen (38) described the small subcortical temporal isthmus area: "It measures from 10 to 15 mm across and is in height nearly equal to that of the thalamus . . . The artery of supply of the isthmus is the anterior choroidal." In the present study, only the anterior half of the temporal isthmus was evaluated for extent of lesion in auditory pathways; the posterior half of the temporal isthmus contains visual pathways.

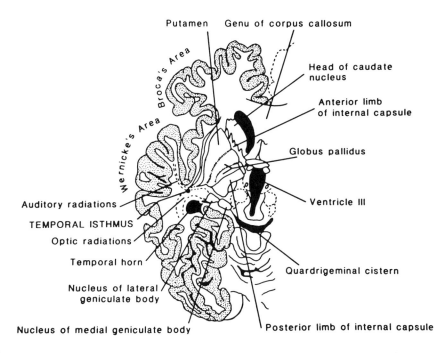

Figure 6 Schematic drawing of CT scan slice B/W (left hemisphere) showing location of the auditory radiations within the anterior half of the subcortical temporal isthmus area, which is located in the white matter inferior to the sylvian fissure and superior to the temporal horn. (From Ref. 32.)

On the basis of the lesion site analysis, the subjects were classified into two groups. Global aphasia cases in group 1 had cortical/subcortical lesions in the frontal, parietal, and temporal lobes, including Wernicke's cortical area. Each case in group 1 (n = 9) had lesion in at least half of Wernicke's cortical area. These are labeled FPT cases to reflect cortical/subcortical lesions in the frontal, parietal, and temporal lobes.

Group 2 global aphasia cases (n = 5) also had cortical/subcortical lesions in the frontal and parietal lobes, but only subcortical lesions in the temporal lobe, including the subcortical temporal isthmus area (Ti). These are labeled FPTi cases to reflect cortical/subcortical lesions in the frontal and parietal lobes, but only subcortical temporal lobe lesions, including the Ti. Both groups had similar mean extent-of-lesion ratings in frontal, parietal, and subcortical areas, including the subcortical Ti area. All cases in the FPT group had lesions in more than half of Wernicke's cortical area; none of the cases in the FPTi group had cortical lesions in Wernicke's area.

There was no significant difference in age at stroke onset between the two groups (FPT group: mean 58.2 years, SD 4.2; FPTi group: mean 57.8 years, SD 5.0). Each group had only one woman. There were no significant differences between the two groups in terms of MPO when T1 or T2 testing was performed.

In four of the five FPTi cases, the T2 Auditory Comprehension z-scores were above -0.5. In eight of the nine FPT cases, z-scores were below -0.5 (Fig. 7). There was a significantly greater increase ($p < 0.01$) in the amount of recovery that had taken place from T1 to T2 for the FPTi group versus the FPT group in the BDAE Overall Auditory Comprehension z-score. The mean change from T1 to T2 for the FPTi group was $+1.58$. The mean change from T1 to T2 for the FPT group was only $+0.65$.

The FPTi cases had a significantly greater ($p < 0.01$) amount of recovery from T1 to T2 at the single-word level of comprehension (Word Discrimination and Body-Part Identification subtests) versus the FPT cases. Patients in the FPTi group had significantly higher ($p < 0.01$) Body-Part Identification absolute scores at T2 than did patients in the FPT group (T2 FPTi mean 14.3; SD 3.6 vs. T2 FPT mean 5.7; SD 4.5).

Thus, most global aphasia cases with temporal lobe lesions that included at least half of Wernicke's cortical area had poor recovery of auditory comprehension 1 to 2 years post–stroke onset. Most global aphasia cases with only subcortical temporal lobe lesion, including the subcortical temporal isthmus area, had better recovery of auditory comprehension 1 or 2 years post–stroke onset.

There were no significant differences between the two groups in the amount of recovery that had taken place from T1 to T2 in the number of words per phrase length in spontaneous speech, single-word repetition, or naming.

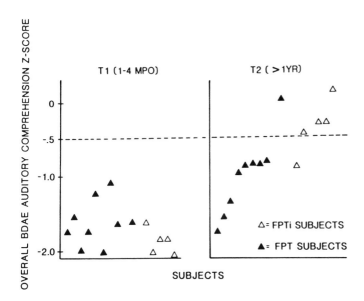

Figure 7 Graph of BDAE Overall Auditory Comprehension z-scores for all cases at time 1 (T1) and time 2 (T2) testing. Note that at T1 testing not one FPT case (cortical/subcortical lesion in the frontal, parietal, and temporal lobes, including Wernicke's cortical area) or FPTi case (cortical/subcortical lesion in the frontal and parietal lobes but only subcortical temporal lobe lesion including the temporal isthmus) achieved a z-score better than −0.1. At T2 testing, four of five FPTi cases achieved z-scores better than −0.5. At T2 testing, only one of nine FPT cases scored better than −0.5. (From Ref. 32.)

Most subjects in each group remained severely impaired in these three language functions at T2. See the original paper (32) for exact T1 and T2 scores.

Case Examples

Figure 8 shows the CT scan and BDAE Auditory Comprehension z-scores for an FPTi case with relatively good recovery of auditory comprehension more than 1 year after onset. Figure 9 shows the CT scan and BDAE Auditory Comprehension z-scores for an FPT case with poor recovery of auditory comprehension even 8 years post–stroke onset.

Results from this study suggest that CT scan lesion site analysis in global aphasia patients can be useful in predicting which subset of these severe patients has greater potential for recovery of some auditory language comprehension (especially single-word comprehension) 1 or 2 years post-onset. A majority of the patients (approximately 80%) with only subcortical temporal

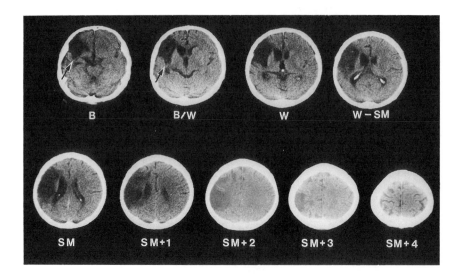

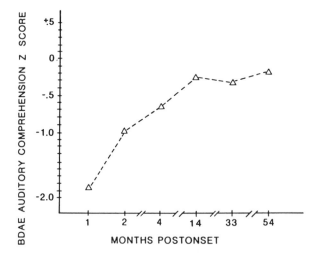

Figure 8 (Top) CT scan at 33 MPO of an FPTi case (age 61 years) showing exten-sive cortical/subcortical lesion in the frontal and parietal lobes but only subcortical temporal lobe lesion in the temporal isthmus area at slices B and B/W (arrows). Note complete sparing of Wernicke's cortical area on slices B/W and W. (Bottom) Graph showing this patient's BDAE Overall Auditory Comprehension z-scores over a period of several months post-onset. Note good recovery of auditory comprehension begin-ning 2 to 4 MPO. His BDAE Auditory Comprehension z-scores were −0.24, −0.33, and −0.18 at 14, 33, and 54 MPO, respectively. (From Ref. 32.)

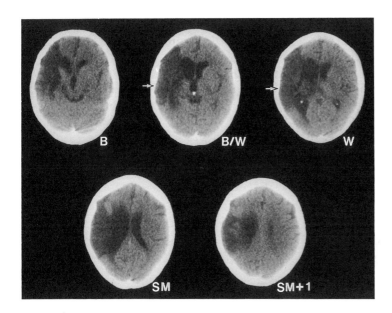

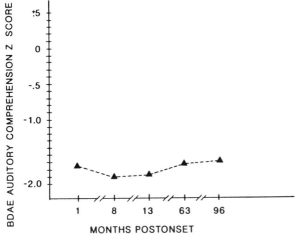

Figure 9 (Top) CT scan at 8 MPO of an FPT case (age 61 years) showing extensive cortical/subcortical lesion in the frontal, parietal, and temporal lobes, including Wernicke's cortical area, compatible with global aphasia. There was complete lesion in Wernicke's cortical area, including the immediately subjacent white matter on slices B/W and W (arrows). (Bottom) Graph showing this patient's BDAE Overall Auditory Comprehension z-scores over a period of several months post-onset. A severe auditory comprehension deficit was still present 8 years post-onset (z-score = −1.7). (From Ref. 32.)

isthmus lesions (versus cortical lesions in Wernicke's area in the temporal lobe) had good recovery of single-word comprehension more than 1 year post-onset.

The results from this study support the notion of Sarno and Levita (39, 40) that global aphasia patients are not a homogeneous group. Careful examination of the extent of cortical versus subcortical lesions in the temporal lobe thus may be useful in predicting a subset of global aphasia patients who have potential for greater recovery of auditory comprehension 1 or 2 years post–stroke onset. The extent-of-lesion ratings should be performed on CT scans obtained 2 or 3 MPO, because the exact borders of an infarct are not well visualized on CT scans performed earlier.

LESION SITE ANALYSIS AND RECOVERY OF SPONTANEOUS SPEECH

This section explains how to analyze CT scan lesion sites to predict potential for long-term recovery of spontaneous speech (i.e., which patients are likely to have nonfluent speech 6 months or 1 year post-onset versus those likely to have no meaningful spontaneous speech—even 9 years post–stroke onset).

Research in our laboratory and others (18,21,25,41) has demonstrated that the presence of lesions in subcortical white-matter areas can have a profound limiting effect on recovery of spontaneous speech. In our 1989 study, for example, we observed that recovery of spontaneous speech was related to extent of lesion in two deep, subcortical white-matter areas *combined*: (1) the medial subcallosal fasciculus area, which is located deep to Broca's area, *plus* (2) the middle one-third of the periventricular white-matter area, which is located deep to the motor/sensory cortex area for the mouth.

The medial subcallosal fasciculus (ScF) area, anterolateral to the frontal horn, contains, in part, projections from the supplementary motor area (SMA) and the cingulate gyrus, area 24, to the head of the caudate, and is believed to be involved, in part, with initiation of speech (see the area marked *ScF* on slices B and B/W in Fig. 1b). The middle one-third periventricular white-matter (PVWM) area, adjacent to the body of the lateral ventricle, contains, in part, motor/sensory projections for the mouth and is believed to be involved, in part, with motor/sensory aspects of speech production (see the area marked *M 1/3* on slice SM in Fig. 1b).

In our 1989 study, we observed that when extensive lesion was present in *both* of these two subcortical white-matter areas there was no recovery of nonfluent speech; the patient remained unable to produce any meaningful spontaneous speech, even as late as 9 years post–stroke onset. Additional neural connections contained within each of these two subcortical white-matter areas are described later in this section. The methodology and results from our 1989 study on recovery (or no recovery) of spontaneous speech are summarized below.

The CT scans and number of words per phrase length in spontaneous speech were examined for 27 right-handed aphasia patients (24 men and three women) with single-episode left-hemisphere occlusive-vascular strokes (thromboembolic infarcts) (25). The mean age at onset was 57.6 years (SD 7.6; range 35 to 69 years). Each patient had a CT scan performed 2 months to 9 years after stroke onset.

The number of words per phrase length for spontaneous speech was determined from the elicited spontaneous speech sample for description of the Cookie Theft Picture from the BDAE (34). These speech samples were obtained from the latest testing time available 6 months to 9 years after stroke onset. The speech samples were used to assign patients to one of four groups, based on severity of impairment of spontaneous speech. The classification of patients regarding deficit in speech-production ability was carried out independently from the CT scan lesion site analysis.

Group 1: No Speech or Only a Few Irrelevant Words

Group 1 consisted of seven patients (six men, one woman) who were able to produce either no speech, or only a few irrelevant words in describing the Cookie Theft Picture. The speech samples for these patients were obtained at a variety of times post-onset ranging from 9 months to 8 years. The BDAE Auditory Comprehension z-scores ranged from -1.60 to -0.11, the Word Repetition scores ranged from 0 to 8, and the Visual Confrontation Naming scores ranged from 0 to 19. Not all cases in this group were globally aphasic in all areas of language.

Group 2: Only Stereotypies

Group 2 consisted of 10 patients (all men) who were able to produce only stereotypies in describing the Cookie Theft Picture. Speech samples included phrases such as "Boom, boom," "morning, morning . . . boy, boy," or "1, 2, 3, 4, 5 . . . boom, boom." The samples for these patients were obtained at times ranging from 6 months to 9 years post-onset. The BDAE Auditory Comprehension z-scores ranged from -1.9 to $+0.09$, the Word Repetition scores ranged from 0 to 7, and the Visual Confrontation Naming scores ranged from 0 to 24. This group was similar to group 1 in that not all cases were globally aphasic in all areas of language.

Group 3: A Few Words and/or Some Overlearned Phrases

Group 3 consisted of five patients (four men and one woman) who were able to use a few words and/or some overlearned phrases in describing the Cookie

Theft Picture. One of these speech samples included such phrases as "there, too . . . there, too . . . um . . . I don't know . . . that's all I guess gee whiz. I don't know, that's all . . . well . . . that, too and there and there." Their spontaneous speech, which was more difficult to classify, was considered borderline between the most severe cases in groups 1 and 2 and the least severe cases in group 4. The speech samples for these patients were obtained from 7 months to 4.5 years post-onset. The BDAE Auditory Comprehension z-scores ranged from -2.1 to $+0.29$, the Word Repetition scores ranged from 0 to 9, and the Visual Confrontation Naming scores ranged from 0 to 42. This group was similar to groups 1 and 2 in that not all cases were globally aphasic in all areas of language.

Group 4: Nonfluent Broca's

Group 4 consisted of five patients (four men and one woman) who were able to provide verbal information relevant to the Cookie Theft Picture with reduced, hesitant, poorly articulated, agrammatical speech. One of these speech samples included such phrases as "The wady is doing her dishes. Sink undis over uh . . . The window is open and the w-won . . . a very funny day outside . . . ook children . . . a boy and a girl." The speech samples for these patients were obtained from 7 months to 6 years post-onset. The BDAE Auditory Comprehension z-scores ranged from $+0.38$ to $+0.93$, the Word Repetition scores ranged from 6 to 9, and the Visual Confrontation Naming scores ranged from 58 to 101. This group had milder deficits in all language modalities than the other three groups.

When t-tests were used to compare the two groups' BDAE scores, the patients in group 4 had significantly higher ($p < 0.005$) Auditory Comprehension z-scores and Visual Confrontation Naming scores than the patients in groups 1, 2, or 3. In addition, the patients in group 4 had significantly higher ($p < 0.005$) Word Repetition scores than the patients in group 2. There were no other significant differences in auditory comprehension, word repetition, or naming among the groups.

CT scan lesion site analysis was performed. An extent-of-lesion rating was recorded for each cortical and subcortical area on the CT scan slices shown in Figure 1b.

No significant differences (Mann-Whitney U-tests, $p < 0.01$ and beyond) were observed in the extent-of-lesion ratings for specific lesion site areas between the aphasia patients with no speech (group 1) and those with stereotypies (group 2). Therefore, the lesion site data from these two groups were combined, forming a no speech/stereotypies group ($n = 17$), for comparison with the nonfluent Broca's group ($n = 5$). (The lesion site data for patients who used only a few words and/or some overlearned phrases—group 3—are discussed later.)

When the extent-of-lesion ratings for each neuroanatomical area for all cases were examined, there was no single neuroanatomical area that alone could distinguish the 17 no speech/stereotypies cases from the five nonfluent Broca's cases. However, when the extent-of-lesion ratings were examined for two deep, subcortical white-matter areas, the *combined*, total extent-of-lesion ratings for these two areas showed no overlap between the no speech/stereotypies cases and the nonfluent Broca's cases. These two deep, subcortical areas were the medial ScF area (mean lesion extent across slices B and B/W) plus the middle one-third PVWM area on slice SM. The location of these two areas is marked in the shaded areas on CT scan slices, B, B/W, and SM, illustrated in Figure 10a.

The total extent-of-lesion ratings for these two deep, subcortical white-matter areas, combined, for each no speech/stereotypies case and each non-fluent Broca's case are shown in Figure 10b. Each no speech/stereotypies case had a total extent-of-lesion rating above 7, and each nonfluent Broca's case had a total extent-of-lesion rating below 6. No other lesion site combination could be used to divide these 22 cases into the two groups.

The mean extent-of-lesion ratings in the medial ScF area alone were not adequate to differentiate these two very different groups of patients. The extent-of-lesion ratings in the middle one-third PVWM alone were also not adequate to discriminate these two very different groups of patients. It was only when the extent-of-lesion ratings were *combined* for these two lesion site areas (mean extent-of-lesion rating for the medial ScF area across slices B and B/W plus the middle one-third PVWM area on slice SM) that the two groups were successfully discriminated on the basis of CT scan extent-of-lesion ratings. The neural connections contained within these two deep, subcortical white-matter pathway areas are discussed briefly below.

Medial Subcallosal Fasciculus Area

The medial ScF area is a narrow white-matter area surrounding the lateral angle of the frontal horn containing a pathway through which fibers pass from the supplementary motor area (SMA), and the cingulate gyrus area 24, to the caudate. The subcallosal fasciculus, which was first described by Muratoff (42) in the dog brain as the *Fasciculus subcallosus*, is located under the corpus callosum. Dejerine (43) has diagrammed it in the human brain and labeled the medial portion *substance grise sous-ependymaire* (Sge). The medial portion is very narrow; it is only one-tenth the distance from the lateral border of the frontal horn to the cortical mantle. (This represents only approximately a millimeter on a CT scan.) Yakovlev and Locke (44) have diagrammed these SMA and cingulate projections to the caudate in detail in the monkey brain. In their work the most medial portion of the subcallosal fasciculus is labeled the *stratum subcallosum* (see *St. Sbc.* in Figure 11).

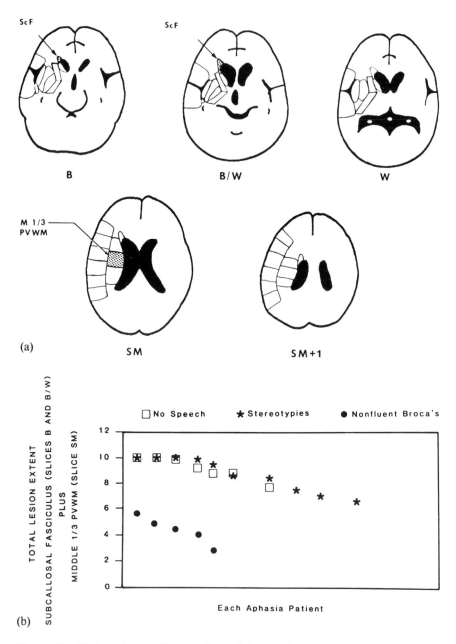

Figure 10 (a) Location on CT scan slices of the two deep, subcortical white-matter areas that, when examined for total extent of lesion *combined*, discriminated the cases with no speech or only stereotypies from those with nonfluent Broca's aphasia. These two deep, subcortical white-matter areas included (1) the medical subcallosal

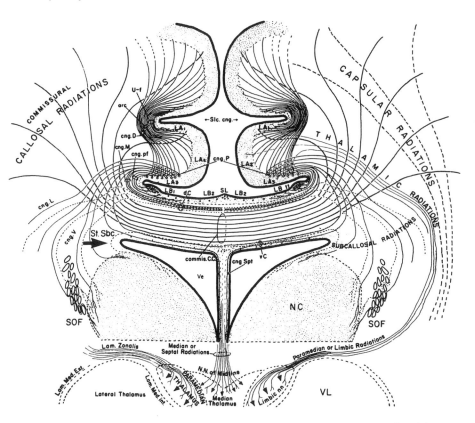

Figure 11 Drawing in coronal plane showing location of the medial subcallosal fasciculus (stratum subcallosum, St. Sbc) in the lateral angle of the frontal horn (arrow). Note that the connections from the cingulate gyrus and supplementary motor area to the head of the caudate are located within the St. Sbc area immediately lateral to the frontal horn. (From Ref. 44.)

---

fasciculus area, mean lesion extent at slices B and B/W, plus (2) the middle one-third PVWM at slice SM, the white matter deep to the lower motor/sensory cortex area for the mouth. (b) Total extent-of-lesion ratings on the CT scan in the two deep, subcortical white-matter areas *combined*: (1) the medial ScF area (mean extent-of-lesion rating across slices B and B/W) plus (2) the middle one-third PVWM area at slice SM, the white-matter area deep to the lower motor/sensory cortex area for the mouth, for individual cases in three groups. Note that all cases with the most severe limitation in speech (groups 1 and 2) had total extent-of-lesion ratings above 7; all cases with the least severe limitation in speech (group 4, Broca's aphasia) had total extent-of-lesion ratings below 6. The summed maximum extent-of-lesion rating on the graph represents maximum ratings of 5 (entire area has solid lesion) in each of the two deep subcortical white-matter areas combined. (From Ref. 25.)

Research by Benjamin and Van Hoesen (45) using horseradish peroxidase injections in monkey brains has shown strong reciprocal connections between cingulate gyrus area 24 and the SMA. The importance of the SMA in the "development of the intention-to-act" has been reviewed by Goldberg (46). Research by Barnes, Van Hoesen, and Yeterian (47) using the autoradiography technique in monkey brains has shown that a major entry point for direct projections from the cingulate gyrus to the caudate (and indirect projections from the SMA to the caudate due to strong cingulate-SMA reciprocal connections) is in the most medial white matter surrounding the lateral angle of the frontal horn in its most rostral portion. Jürgens (48) has observed direct connections from the SMA to the caudate. These mesial frontal cortex projections then spread to the ventral and lateral portion of the caudate and to the lateral portion of the putamen.

Thus, a lesion located in the most medial white matter surrounding the lateral angle of the most rostral portion of the frontal horn (medial ScF) would be interrupting pathways from the cingulate gyrus area 24 and SMA, leading into the caudate and putamen. This would have an effect on the initiation of and preparation for speech movements, and on the limbic aspects of spontaneous speech.

Middle One-Third Periventricular White-Matter Area

The middle one-third PVWM area adjacent to the body of the lateral ventricle on CT scan slice SM is believed to contain, in part, the subcortical white-matter fibers deep to the lower motor/sensory cortex area for mouth. These PVWM pathways are diagrammed coronally in Figure 12. The motor cortex projections for the mouth have recently been shown in an anterograde staining study with rhesus monkeys to project directly into the second quarter of the PVWM, adjacent to the body of the lateral ventricle (49). Thus, the middle one-third PVWM area probably contains the motor/sensory projections for the mouth, immediately superior to their descent into the genu of the internal capsule.

In addition to containing the motor/sensory projections for the mouth, the middle one-third PVWM area contains the body of the caudate nucleus, and numerous other intra- and interhemispheric pathways. These pathways include, in part: (1) the descending pyramidal tract pathways for the leg and arm (49,50), (2) the midcallosal pathways, (3) additional medial subcallosal fasciculus pathways with connections from the SMA and cingulate gyrus, to the body of the caudate (42–44), (4) the occipitofrontal fasciculus (43), and (5) the superior lateral thalamic peduncle, which includes projections from the dorsomedial nucleus and the anterior nucleus to the cingulate (51) and projections from the ventrolateral nucleus to the motor cortex.

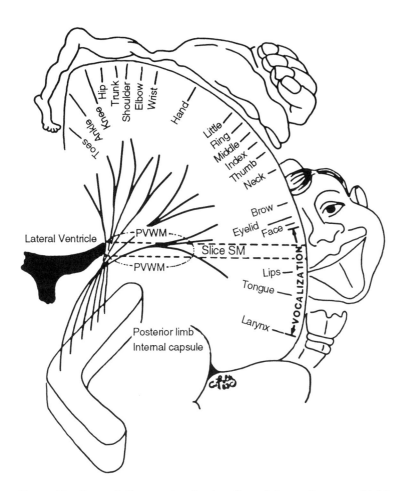

Figure 12 Coronal diagram showing location of descending pyramidal tract pathways in the deepest, subcortical periventricular white-matter (PVWM) area immediately adjacent to the body of the lateral ventricle (arrow). On CT scan these descending pyramidal tract pathways are located in the second and third quarters of the PVWM on slices SM and SM + 1. On the CT scan slices inferior to these, the pyramidal tract pathways are located in the posterior limb of the internal capsule (CT scan slices W, B/W, and B). (From Ref. 25.)

The lesion in the middle one-third PVWM area deep to the lower motor/sensory cortex area for mouth may have interrupted the pathways necessary for motor execution as well as, possibly, those pathways necessary for sensory feedback. Hence, we hypothesize that lesion in the *two* deep subcortical white-matter pathway areas—the medial ScF area and the middle one-third

PVWM area — *combined*, effectively prevents any relevant spontaneous speech because there are no available pathways for speech initiation, motor execution, or sensory feedback.

It is important to understand that the presence or absence of hemiplegia is not always a useful marker in predicting potential for long-term recovery of spontaneous speech (25, case 16). For example, the descending pyramidal tract pathways for the leg are most medial, within the second and third quarters of the PVWM area on CT scan, and immediately adjacent to the body of the lateral ventricle (slices SM and SM + 1) (49,52). The descending pyramidal tract pathways for the arm are slightly more anterior and lateral within the PVWM. Thus, if the paralysis is due to lesion in the PVWM, it will be directly related to the depth of the PVWM lesion, adjacent to the body of the lateral ventricle, assuming absence of lesion in higher cortical motor pathways for the leg and arm and in lower, subcortical motor pathways for the leg and arm (internal capsule and brainstem) (52).

A patient with no spontaneous speech may have lesion in the medial ScF and in more than half of the middle one-third PVWM area, but sparing the deepest portion of the middle one-third PVWM area, immediately adjacent to the body of the lateral ventricle, and have no paralysis. The CT scan of a patient without paralysis but who also had no spontaneous speech is shown in Figure 8, top (25, case 16). Thus, the severity of paralysis can be shown to have specific, separate lesion sites, and the severity of spontaneous speech can also be shown to have specific, separate lesion sites. Therefore, recovery from paralysis is often an issue separate from recovery of spontaneous speech.

In summary, the cases with the least recovery of spontaneous speech, i.e., those with no speech or only stereotypies (groups 1 and 2), had total extent-of-lesion ratings above 7 for the medial ScF area plus the middle one-third PVWM area. Those cases with better recovery of spontaneous speech, i.e., those with nonfluent Broca's aphasia (group 4), had total extent-of-lesion ratings below 6 for the medial ScF area plus the middle one-third PVWM area. Those cases who fell between these two groups in terms of severity of impairment of spontaneous speech, i.e., those with a few words and/or some overlearned phrases, basically also fell between the two groups in terms of combined extent-of-lesion ratings (ratings around 6). There were exceptional cases at either extreme within group 3. A few case examples and CT scans are presented below.

Case Examples

Case Example for Group 1 (No Speech or Only a Few Irrelevant Words). Case 3, H.J., is a 35-year-old man who at 9 months following stroke onset still had no speech, although he could phonate and produce grunt-like sounds.

The CT scan in Figure 13 shows a primarily subcortical infarct that included extensive lesion in the medial ScF area at slices B and B/W and extensive lesion in the middle one-third PVWM area at slice SM. The total extent-of-lesion rating in these two areas combined was 9.95. (On later follow-up testing, this patient continued to have no meaningful spontaneous speech 5 years post-onset.) He had a dense right hemiplegia with poor recovery (the second- and third-quarter PVWM lesion was immediately adjacent to the body of the lateral ventricle at slice SM).

H.J. had a moderate comprehension deficit (− 0.21 on the BDAE Auditory Comprehension z-score at 7 MPO). This moderate comprehension deficit is compatible with lesion in the anterior subcortical temporal isthmus area on slice B/W (see "Global Aphasia" above).

Case Example for Group 4 (Nonfluent Broca's Aphasia). Case 23, W.A., is a 50-year-old man who at 7 months following stroke onset produced non-

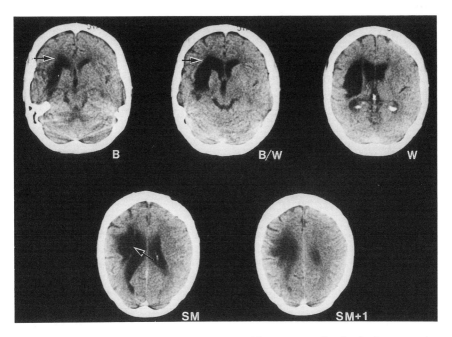

Figure 13 CT scan at 9 MPO for a 35-year-old man (case 3) who had no speech 7 MPO or even 2 years later (group 1). A dense right hemiplegia was present. The left-hemisphere lesion is on the left side of the CT scan. The extent-of-lesion rating for the medial ScF area at both slices B and B/W was 5 (see arrows), mean 5. The extent-of-lesion rating in the middle one-third PVWM area at slice SM was 4.95 (see arrows); total extent-of-lesion rating 9.95. Note that the entire lesion is primarily subcortical. (From Ref. 25.)

fluent, agrammatical speech that was compatible with Broca's aphasia. The CT scan in Figure 14 shows extensive lesion in the medial ScF area at slices B and B/W, but only minimal lesion in the middle one-third PVWM at slice SM (small, patchy lesion). The total extent-of-lesion rating in the two areas, combined, was 5.88. Mild hemiparesis was present initially, and there was good recovery (there was no lesion in the second and third quarter of the

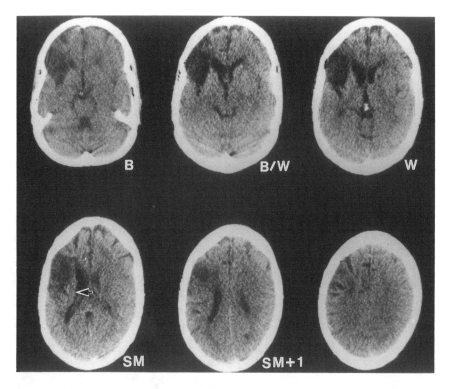

Figure 14 CT scan at 44 MPO for a 54-year-old man (case 23) who had nonfluent agrammatical speech and Broca's aphasia 7 MPO (group 4). A mild hemiparesis was present and there was good recovery. The extent-of-lesion rating in the medial ScF area at slice B was 4, slice B/W 3.75, mean 3.88. The extent-of-lesion rating in the middle one-third PVWM area at slice SM was only 2; the total extent-of-lesion rating was 5.88. The arrow at slice SM shows a minimal lesion in the middle one-third PVWM area that greatly reduced the combined total extent-of-lesion rating to below 6, a value compatible with his mild limitation in speech. The mild hemiparesis with good recovery in this case was compatible with sparing of the deepest PVWM area immediately adjacent to the body of the lateral ventricle at slices SM and SM + 1. This deepest PVWM area contains, in part, the descending pyramidal tract pathways. (From Ref. 25.)

PVWM area immediately adjacent to the body of the lateral ventricle at slices SM or SM + 1).

This case had a typical lesion distribution associated with longer-lasting Broca's aphasia that we have repeatedly observed in our laboratory. (The Broca's aphasics who were included in this study were still nonfluent and agrammatical at 7 months to 6 years following stroke onset.) This lesion distribution usually includes infarction in parts of Broca's area that extends across to the border of the frontal horn (including medial ScF area on slices B and/or B/W), plus superior lesion extension into the lower motor cortex area for the mouth (slices W and SM) that extends into the deep, anterior one-third PVWM area and sometimes part of the middle one-third PVWM area (slice SM). In some cases the lower motor cortex area lesion is absent (slices W and SM). The deep subcortical anterior one-third PVWM lesion, however, is usually always present. The cortical portions of this lesion are compatible with lesion sites in longer-lasting Broca's aphasia cases previously described by Mohr et al. (1).

Comparison of the CT scans for case 3 (Fig. 13), who had no speech 9 MPO, to case 23 (Fig. 14), who had functional nonfluent spontaneous speech 7 MPO, reveals that the latter — the less severe case — actually had more cortical damage (including damage in Broca's cortical area on slices B and B/W and the lower motor cortex area for the mouth on slice SM than did case 3, the more severe case, who had no cortical lesion in either Broca's cortical area or the lower motor cortex area for the mouth. Comparison of the CT scans for these two cases suggests that it is the extent of lesion (degree of infarction) within the two deep, subcortical white-matter areas (medial ScF area and middle one-third PVWM area) that is related to the severity of spontaneous speech output, not the extent of lesion within Broca's cortical area or the lower motor cortex area for the mouth. Case 3, with no spontaneous speech, had complete lesion in the medial ScF area at slices B and B/W and in the middle one-third PVWM area at slice SM. Case 23, with functional, nonfluent, spontaneous speech, had lesion in more than half of the medial ScF area at slices B and B/W but in only a small part (less than half) of the middle one-third PVWM area at slice SM.

Broca's Original Case, Leborgne. The results from the 27 cases examined in our 1989 study indicated that when extensive lesion was present in the medial ScF area and in the middle one-third PVWM area there was poor recovery of spontaneous speech with no meaningful speech produced even as long as 9 years post–stroke onset. These results are further supported by examination of the CT scan of Broca's original aphasia patient, LeBorgne.

Leborgne was 30 years old at the time of stroke onset, and he died 21 years later. His spontaneous speech was limited to the stereotypy "tan, tan." His auditory comprehension was reported to be good. He had a dense right hemiplegia. Broca attributed the poor speech to a lesion in the cortical region of the foot of the third left frontal convolution (53,54). Broca himself, however, never observed the depth of the lesion in Leborgne's brain because it was never cut, as was common practice at that time. Recently a CT scan was performed on the preserved brain 140 years post–stroke onset (55,56). Figure 15 shows slice B/W, W, SM, and SM + 1 of Leborgne's brain (no slice B was available). Examination of the deep subcortical white matter surrounding the lateral angle of the left frontal horn reveals extensive lesion in the medial ScF area at slice B/W. Because the lesion in the medial ScF area is so extensive at slice B/W, it is assumed there was a similarly extensive lesion in the medial ScF area at slice B. There is also extensive lesion in the middle one-third PVWM area at slice SM. The total extent-of-lesion rating for the two areas, combined, was estimated to be 9—a rating >7, hence compatible with no long-term recovery of spontaneous speech. As noted above, this patient was able to produce only the stereotypy "tan, tan" for 21 years following the stroke onset. The right hemiplegia may have been compatible with lesion in the deepest PVWM at slice SM + 1, or possibly some lesion in the posterior limb, internal capsule at slice W.

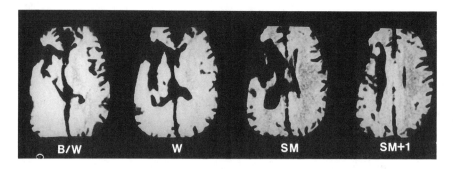

Figure 15 CT scan of Broca's original case, LeBorgne, who, at age 51 – 21 years after stroke onset – could produce only the stereotypy "tan, tan." This case was similar to the group 2 cases (only stereotypies) in the present study. A dense right hemiplegia was present. The extent-of-lesion rating in the medial ScF area at slice B/W was 5. Although slice B was not available, it was assumed that because the lesion was so extensive on slice B/W it was equally extensive on slice B (5); thus, the mean extent-of-lesion rating for the medial ScF area was 5. The extent-of-lesion rating for the middle one-third PVWM area at slice SM was 4, total extent-of-lesion rating 9. The total extent-of-lesion rating of 9 in these two deep subcortical white-matter lesion site areas was well within the range for cases with severe limitation in speech (total extent-of-lesion ratings greater than 7). (From Ref. 55.)

Our 1989 study focused on spontaneous speech; although all cases in groups 1 and 2 had severe limitation in spontaneous speech, not all these cases had complete cessation of speech. Ten of 17 cases in groups 1 and 2 could still repeat a few words, and four of 17 could correctly name some pictures upon visual confrontation. Research by Kirzinger and Jürgens (57) and others (58) has shown that lesion in the SMA has a direct effect on initiation of "spontaneous" motoric behavior patterns, which are triggered internally, and not on those triggered directly by external stimuli. Kirzinger and Jürgens (57) observed, for example, that after the SMA was ablated in squirrel monkeys and they were placed in isolation, the number of vocal "isolation calls" emitting from the monkeys was reduced, although the acoustic structure remained intact. Thus, the absence of internally generated (spontaneous) speech in the presence of some externally generated speech (word repetition and naming) may be compatible, in part, with lesions directly affecting projections from the SMA. Further, variation in word repetition and naming ability observed across those subjects who otherwise had no meaningful spontaneous speech may have been due, in part, to variation in the extent of lesion in the projections from the SMA, as well as other areas. This would require further study.

Results from this study suggest that careful examination of lesions in the medial ScF area and the middle one-third PVWM area is a starting point for assessing potential for long-term recovery of spontaneous speech in severely nonfluent stroke patients with infarction in the various branches of the left middle cerebral artery (LMCA). When working with patients who have lesions outside the distribution of the LMCA, especially in the left anterior cerebral artery (LACA), one must examine different structures. For example, in cases with LACA infarcts, it is possible that cortical lesions in the SMA and/or the cingulate gyrus area may combine with subcortical lesions in the middle one-third PVWM area to produce long-lasting impairment in speech, even if no lesion is present in the medial ScF area at slices B and B/W. Obviously, other cortical and/or subcortical lesion sites may also combine to produce severe limitation in spontaneous speech.

LESION SITE ANALYSIS AND TREATMENT IN APHASIA

We have recently completed two studies in which the method of CT scan lesion site analysis and results from the above-mentioned recovery studies were applied to treatment studies with aphasia patients who had limitation in spontaneous speech. The first study focused on lesion sites in patients with limited spontaneous speech who were treated with a verbal treatment program, Melodic Intonation Therapy (MIT) (59). The second study focused on lesion sites in patients with no spontaneous speech who were treated with a nonverbal treatment program, Computer-assisted Visual Communication (C-ViC) (60).

A Verbal Treatment Program: Melodic Intonation Therapy

Melodic Intonation Therapy (MIT) is a treatment program for aphasia patients with severely limited or nonfluent speech (61,62). In our study, CT scan lesion site analysis was used to examine the relationship between lesion sites and good versus poor response to MIT (59).

The MIT program uses phrases and sentences that are slowly intoned, with continuous voicing, using simple high-note, low-note patterns based on normal speech prosody (63). Two studies (64,65) have demonstrated that not all patients with limited verbal output respond positively to MIT. Positive response to MIT in these studies was defined as improvement in number of words per phrase as tested with the Cookie Theft Picture description from the Boston Diagnostic Aphasia Exam (BDAE) (66).

Language data were collected in a retrospective manner from files on patients treated with MIT in the Audiology and Speech Pathology Service, Boston D.V.A. Medical Center. Inclusion criteria for this study were the following: (1) patients enrolled in only one treatment program—the MIT treatment program—at a given time, (2) patients who had had only a single stroke, and (3) patients for whom a chronic CT scan was available for analysis, although no CT scan lesion site information was used at the time of treatment. All other patients were excluded from this study, especially those who were receiving more than the single treatment program. The decision to treat the patient with MIT was made by the speech–language pathologist treating the patient at that time.

A total of eight male stroke patients were included in the study. Each patient was right-handed and had suffered a single-episode left-hemisphere occlusive-vascular stroke between the ages of 24 to 65 years ($x = 49$; SD 14.2) (Tables 1 and 2). One patient (W.F.) had an additional small lesion in the right parietal lobe that was not extensive enough to be considered the primary cause of the aphasia. The scans used for CT scan lesion site analysis were performed between 3 to 36 MPO. All eight patients were treated with MIT during the chronic phase post-stroke, beginning 3–51 MPO.

All patients were separated into two groups: good response and poor response to MIT. Good response following a series of MIT treatments was defined as an increase of at least two words per phrase on the spontaneous speech characteristics rating scale as applied to the Cookie Theft Picture description. Poor response was defined as no increase in the number of words per phrase.

Four patients had good response with MIT; four patients had poor response (Tables 1 and 2). There were no significant differences between the

Table 1 Language Data for Patients with Good Response to Melodic Intonation Therapy

Case	Sex	Age at onset (yrs)	Tx. (MPO)	Dates in Tx.	No. Tx. sessions	Tx. level completed	Reason for discharge		BDAE No. wds./ phrase (7)	Artic. agility (7)	Gramm. form (7)	Aud. comp. z-score	Single wd. rep. (10)	No. of pre-MIT lang. behavior characteristics met (4)
M.E.	M	58	3	11/76–2/77	73	III	Completed	Pre-	1	3	1	+0.46	2	4/4
								Post-	3	2	1	+0.55	6	
W.A.	M	62	4	9/75–12/75	97	III	Completed	Pre-	5	1	6	+0.75	8	3/4
								Post-	7	3	7	+1.0	9	
T.H.[a]	M	41	10	3/73–9/73	81	III	Completed	Pre-	1	1	1	−0.46	0	4/4
								Post-	6	4	5	+0.45	7	
M.J.	M	37	18	9/75–12/75	51	III	Completed	Pre-	5	1	7	+1.0	10	3/4
								Post-	7	4	7	+1.0	10	
T.H.[a]	M	41	50	7/76–10/76	12	III	Completed	Pre-	2	2	2	+0.26	4	4/4
								Post-	4	5	5	+0.46	6	

[a]Patient received a second series of MIT treatments 4 years post-onset. The data from the second series are presented here for illustration only; they were not entered into any statistical analyses.

Table 2 Language Data for Patients with Poor Response to Melodic Intonation Therapy

Case	Sex	Age at onset (yrs)	Tx. (MPO)	Dates in Tx.	No. Tx. sessions	Tx. level completed	Reason for discharge		BDAE No. wds./ phrase (7)	Artic. agility (7)	Gramm. form (7)	Aud. comp. z-score	Single wd. rep. (10)	No. of pre-MIT lang. behavior characteristics met (4)
G.N.J.	M	49	4	1/88–2/88	9	I	Poor success	Pre-	0	0	0	−2.33	2	3/4
								Post-	0	0	0	NA	NA	
S.F.	M	65	5	10/88–12/88	6	I	Poor success	Pre-	0	0	0	NA	0	3/3[a]
								Post-	0	0	0	NA	0	
R.P.	M	57	5	1/89	7	Trial w/ level I, poor prog.	Poor success	Pre-	0	0	0	−1.48	4	3/4
								Post-	0	0	0	NA	NA	
W.F.	M	24	51	1/75–7/75	115	Level III, but no carryover	Completed	Pre-	1	2	1	−0.4	3	4/4
								Post-	1	3	1	−0.45	5	

[a]Data for fourth language behavior characteristic was not available.

good-response and the poor-response cases in age at onset or MPO when the MIT treatments were begun. The mean age at onset for the good-response cases was 49.5 years (SD 12.3), and they began MIT treatments at a mean of 8.75 MPO (SD 6.9). The mean age at onset for the poor-response cases was 48.75 (SD 17.75), and they began MIT treatments at a mean of 16.25 MPO (SD 23.17).

The language characteristics of aphasia patients who are good candidates for treatment with MIT have been under development since the first published papers (61,64). These pre-MIT language characteristics were recently summarized by Helm-Estabrooks and Albert (67) as follows:

1. Poorly articulated, nonfluent, or *severely restricted verbal output* that may be confined to a nonsense stereotypy (e.g., "bika bika")
2. At least *moderately preserved auditory comprehension*, exceeding the 45th percentile on the BDAE Rating Scale
3. *Poor repetition*, even for single words
4. Poorly articulated speech, earning a *rating of 3 or less for Articulatory Agility* on the BDAE Profile of Speech Characteristics

In this study, all patients treated with MIT had met at least three of four of these pre-MIT language characteristics (see Tables 1 and 2).

The MIT treatment program is hierarchically structured, and is divided into three levels. The decision to continue or terminate MIT treatment for a patient was made by the speech–language pathologist based on the patient's scores at each level of the program (63). A wide range for the total number of MIT treatments provided (6 to 115 treatments) was observed across the good-response and the poor-response cases (Tables 1 and 2). This wide range was due, in part, to the fact that if a patient could not complete level I, treatment was terminated.

Pre-MIT

Mann-Whitney U-tests were performed on the pre-MIT spontaneous speech data for the good-response versus the poor-response groups. The good-response group had significantly better pre-MIT spontaneous speech scores for number of words per phrase and grammatical form than the poor-response group (see Table 3, bottom). Although the good-response group had significantly better pre-MIT spontaneous speech scores, it should be remembered that each good-response case and poor-response case had met at least three of the four criteria for language characteristics associated with good candidacy for treatment with MIT (67).

Post-MIT

Mann-Whitney U-tests were also performed on the post-MIT spontaneous speech data for the two groups. As would be expected, the good-response

Table 3 Spontaneous Speech Statistics for Good- and Poor-Response Groups Treated with Melodic Intonation Therapy

	Pre-MIT		Post-MIT		Change	
	Mean	SD	Mean	SD	Mean	SD
Good response						
No. words/phrase	3.0	2.3	5.8	1.9	+2.8	1.5
Articulatory agility	1.5	1.0	3.3	1.0	+1.8	1.9
Grammatical form	3.8	3.2	5.0	2.8	+1.3	1.9
Poor response						
No. words/phrase	0.3	0.5	0.3	0.5	0	0
Articulatory agility	0.5	1.0	0.8	1.5	+0.3	0.5
Grammatical form	0.3	0.5	0.3	0.5	0	0

Mann-Whitney U-test comparisons for
the good-response versus the poor-response groups

	Pre-MIT		Post-MIT	
	z corrected for ties	*p*-level 1-tail	z corrected for ties	*p*-level 1-tail
No. words/phrase	2.14	0.016	2.38	0.008
Articulatory agility	1.52	0.064	1.95	0.025
Grammatical form	2.12	0.017	2.25	0.012

group had significantly better post-MIT spontaneous speech scores than the poor-response group (see Table 3, bottom).

Paired *t*-tests were performed on the spontaneous speech data at T1 versus T2 for the good-response cases. These patients showed significant improvement post-MIT in number of words per phrase ($p < 0.006$) and articulatory agility ($p < 0.03$). The poor-response group showed no significant improvement post-MIT on any of the spontaneous speech scores.

CT scan lesion site analysis was performed. The cortical and subcortical areas on CT scan examined for extent of lesion are shown in Figure 1b.

Relationship Between CT Scan Lesion Sites and Response to MIT

Each of the four good-response patients had a total extent-of-lesion rating of ≤7 (range 3.75 to 7) for the medial ScF area plus the middle one-third PVWM area (see Table 4, column headed "Total extent of lesion"). Each of the four poor-response patients had a total extent-of-lesion rating >7 (range 7.48 to 9.9). It is of interest to note that in this small study with eight patients, the good-response patients could be separated out from the poor-

Table 4 CT Scan Lesion Sites and Extent-of-Lesion Data for Patients with Good and Poor Responses to MIT

Case	CT scan (MPO)	Medial subcallosal fasciculus (mean B, B/W)	Mid. 1/3 PVWM (SM)	Total extent of lesion, med. ScF + mid. 1/3 PVWM[a]	Wernicke's area (mean B/W, W)	Temporal isthmus (mean B, B/W)[b]	Occipital length asymmetry
Good response							
M.E.	3.5	3	2	5	1	0.5	R
W.A.	44	3.25	2.5	5.75	0	0	L
T.H.	77	1.75	2	3.75	2	1.25	L
M.J.	72	5	2	7	0	0	=
Poor response							
G.N.J.	4	4	4.5	8.5	1.87	4.5	=
S.F.	3.5	5	4.9	9.9	2.87	4	L
R.P.	18	3.63	3.85	7.48	4.5	3.75	=
W.F.	100	4.9	4.8	9.7	5	5	R

[a] ≤7 = good response.
[b] <3 = good response.

response patients on the basis of the middle one-third PVWM area extent-of-lesion rating *alone*, in contrast to the lesion *combination* of medial ScF area plus the middle one-third PVWM area. All four good-response cases had middle one-third PVWM area extent-of-lesion ratings <3 (lesion in less than half of the middle one-third PVWM area). All four poor-response cases had middle one-third PVWM area extent-of-lesion ratings of >3 (lesion in more than half of the middle one-third PVWM area).

The extent-of-lesion ratings in Wernicke's area could not be used to separate the good-response from the poor-response cases, because although all four good-response cases had lesion in less than half of Wernicke's area, two of the four poor-response cases also had lesion in less than half of Wernicke's area (see Table 4, column headed "Wernicke's area").

All four good-response cases had extent-of-lesion ratings of <3 in the subcortical temporal isthmus area (lesion in less than half of this area). All four poor-response cases had extent-of-lesion ratings of >3 (lesion in more than half) in the subcortical temporal isthmus area.

There were no *cortical* language areas for which the extent-of-lesion ratings could be used to separate all the good-response cases from all the poor-response cases, including extent-of-lesion ratings in Broca's area, Wernicke's area, the supramarginal and angular gyrus areas, or the SMA.

In summary, chronic aphasia patients with good response to MIT had lower total extent-of-lesion ratings in the medial ScF area plus the middle one-third PVWM area than the chronic aphasia patients with poor response to MIT. Furthermore, there was no overlap between the two groups for total extent-of-lesion ratings in the two deep, subcortical white-matter areas. In addition, all patients with good response to MIT had lesion in less than half of Wernicke's area *and* the subcortical temporal isthmus area. All patients with poor response to MIT had lesion in more than half of the subcortical temporal isthmus area. In this small sample, the CT scan lesion site data could be used to separate all good-response from all poor-response cases.

Case Examples

The CT scan and extent-of-lesion ratings for one patient with good response to MIT are presented in Figure 16; those for one patient with poor response are presented in Figure 17.

The results from this study, using the method of CT scan lesion site analysis presented here, have expanded and revised the results from Naeser and Helm-Estabrooks' 1985 CT scan study with MIT (68). Results from the present study indicated that the total extent-of-lesion ratings in the medial ScF area *plus* the middle one-third PVWM area separated all good-response cases from all poor-response cases. The importance of these two deep, sub-

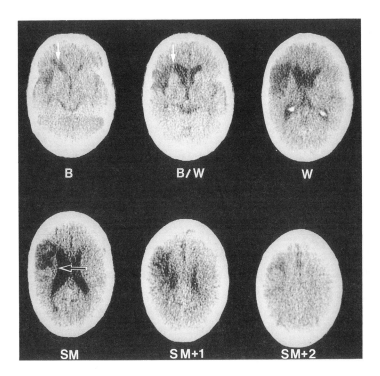

Figure 16 CT scan for a patient with good response to MIT, a 58-year-old man (M.E.). The total extent-of-lesion rating for the medial ScF area *plus* the middle one-third PVWM area was 5. This total extent-of-lesion rating was computed in the two deep, subcortical areas as follows: First area—medial ScF area at slice B = 2.5 (patchy lesion in less than half of the area, white arrow); medial ScF at slice B/W = 3.5 (patchy lesion in more than half of the area, white arrow); mean, medial ScF area at slices B and B/W = 3. Second area—middle one-third PVWM at slice SM = 2 (small, patchy, partial lesion, black and white arrow). Total extent-of-lesion rating for medial ScF area (3) + middle one-third PVWM area (2) = 5. Total extent-of-lesion rating <7 is compatible with good response to MIT. CT scan is 3.5 MPO. Note that this patient had almost no lesion in Wernicke's area on slices B/W and W (mean rating of 1) and almost no lesion in the subcortical temporal isthmus area on slices B and B/W (mean rating of 0.5). No lesion or only minimal lesion (<3) in Wernicke's area and the subcortical temporal isthmus area is compatible with good response to MIT. (See data for M.E. in Table 1.) (From Ref. 91.)

cortical white-matter areas to the production of nonfluent spontaneous speech (25) had not yet been recognized when our first CT scan study with MIT was published in 1985.

Results from the 1985 study had suggested that cases with bilateral lesions or extensive lesion including Wernicke's area or the subcortical temporal

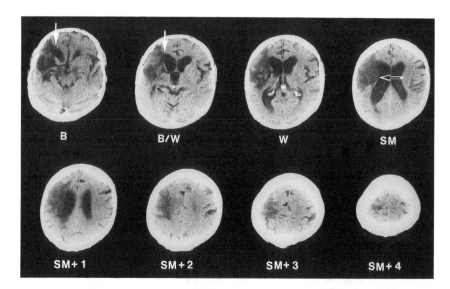

Figure 17 CT scan for a patient with poor response to MIT, a 65-year-old man (S.F.). The total extent-of-lesion rating for the medial ScF area *plus* the middle one-third PVWM area was 9.9. This total extent-of-lesion rating was computed in the two subcortical areas as follows: First area—medial ScF area at slice B = 5 (entire area has solid lesion, white arrow); medial ScF at slice B/W = 5 (entire area has solid lesion, white arrow); mean, medial ScF area at slices B and B/W = 5. Second area— middle one-third PVWM area at slice SM = 4.9 (almost the entire area has solid lesion, black and white arrow). Total extent-of-lesion rating for medial ScF area (5) + middle one-third PVWM area (4.9) = 9.9. CT scan is 3.5 MPO. Note that this patient had lesion in less than half of Wernicke's area. On slice B/W and W, there was only small, partial lesion in Wernicke's area (mean extent-of-lesion rating 2.87). Lesion was present in more than half of the subcortical temporal isthmus area, however, on slices B and B/W (mean 4). Lesion in more than half of the subcortical temporal isthmus area (>3) is compatible with poor response to MIT. (From Ref. 91.)

isthmus area would have poor response to MIT. In the present study, the only patient who had bilateral lesions had poor response to MIT. This patient, W.F., also had a total extent-of-lesion rating for the medial ScF area *plus* the middle one-third PVWM area that exceeded 7 (9.7). This rating fell within the total extent-of-lesion range for poor response to MIT, as well as no production of nonfluent spontaneous speech. Thus, from the results of the present study, it is not possible to comment on the relative importance of the right-hemisphere lesion contributing to poor response. It may be that a small right-hemisphere lesion has no negative effect in the MIT treatment process; we do not know. A discussion of the possible role of the right hemisphere in relation to good response to MIT was published in the 1985 study by Naeser and Helm-Estabrooks (68), and is not repeated here. The role of the right hemisphere in relation to recovery from aphasia in general, and in relation to recovery of spontaneous speech with MIT in particular, is an area that requires further research.

Other results from the 1985 study suggested that cases with extensive lesion in Wernicke's area or the subcortical temporal isthmus area would have poor response to MIT. The results from the present study tend to support that finding, because all good-response patients had lesion in less than half of Wernicke's area *and* the subcortical temporal isthmus area; however, two poor-response patients also had lesion in less than half of Wernicke's area. All poor-response cases in the present study, however, had lesion in more than half of the subcortical temporal isthmus area. Prior to MIT treatments, all four of the good-response cases had BDAE Auditory Comprehension z-scores better than -0.5; only one of the four poor-response cases scored better than -0.5. The relatively greater deficit in auditory comprehension for most of the poor-response cases was probably related to lesions in the subcortical temporal isthmus area in all of the four poor-response cases, and/or related to lesion in Wernicke's area in two of these cases (32).

The results from the present CT scan study support the 1989 study by Naeser et al. (25) regarding the role of the medial ScF area and the middle one-third PVWM area in relation to production of nonfluent spontaneous speech. Each of these two studies observed that most patients with total extent-of-lesion ratings >7 in the medial ScF area *plus* the middle one-third PVWM area did not recover spontaneous speech, even several years post-stroke onset. The poor-response patients in the present study without production of nonfluent spontaneous speech had a phrase length limited to zero words, or a one-word stereotypy. The severe limitation in spontaneous speech was present for all poor-response cases in the present study, both before and after the MIT treatments.

The mechanism underlying the effectiveness of MIT is unknown. The results from the present study suggest that the neural connections within the medial ScF area and the middle one-third PVWM area may be critical factors contributing, at least in part, to the production of spontaneous speech and to good response to MIT. The white-matter connections within the medial ScF area, located deep to Broca's cortical area, are believed to be important for the initiation of spontaneous speech. The white-matter connections within the middle one-third PVWM area, located deep to the motor/sensory cortex area for the mouth, are believed to be important for motor/sensory aspects of speech production.

The role of the temporal lobe structures in relation to good response to MIT is also unknown. The patients with good response to MIT had either no lesion or lesion in less than half of Wernicke's area *and* the subcortical temporal isthmus area. The lack of extensive damage to these temporal lobe structures is probably important for preserved ability to comprehend the verbal material presented for repetition and production during the MIT treatment process.

In summary, the aphasia patients with severely limited or nonfluent speech who appear to be the better candidates for treatment with MIT are those who meet at least three of four of the pre-MIT language characteristics listed above (67) and those patients who have total extent-of-lesion ratings of <7 for the medial ScF area *plus* the middle one-third PVWM area as well as lesion in less than half of Wernicke's area *and* the subcortical temporal isthmus area. The results from this study suggest that the method of CT scan lesion site analysis presented here may be an additional variable for speech–language pathologists to consider when conducting future research with other verbal treatment programs in aphasia.

A Nonverbal Treatment Program:
Computer-Assisted Visual Communication (C-ViC)

Almost 20 years ago, the first systematic attempts to utilize a substituted "language" based on representational and arbitrary icons were reported (69, 70). More recently, that iconic "language" has been further developed and adapted for use on a minicomputer (71–73). These investigators have demonstrated that severely aphasic patients can manipulate the computer "mouse" and button-click necessary for operation and can learn the rules of lexical organization. C-ViC enables patients with no spontaneous speech (or ability to read or to write) to use pictures and icons on a computer screen to communicate their needs and ideas (Fig. 18).

The patients learn to construct and comprehend complex sentences in the C-ViC pictorial "language." Not all severely aphasic patients, however, have been able to grasp the lexical and syntactic rules of the substituted language and use them to independently initiate communication.

The relationship between CT scan lesion sites and good response to C-ViC (ability to independently initiate communication) versus poor response to C-ViC (inability independently to initiate communication) was examined for seven severe aphasia patients with no ability to speak, read, or write (60). These patients were treated with C-ViC beginning in the chronic phase post-stroke. All seven patients had suffered a left-hemisphere cerebrovascular accident. The age at onset of stroke ranged from 43 to 65 years (mean 56; SD 7.5). One case was left-handed. All seven patients had severe right hemiplegia.

The Boston Assessment of Severe Aphasia (BASA) test (74) was performed immediately prior to C-ViC training and again at its termination. The BASA

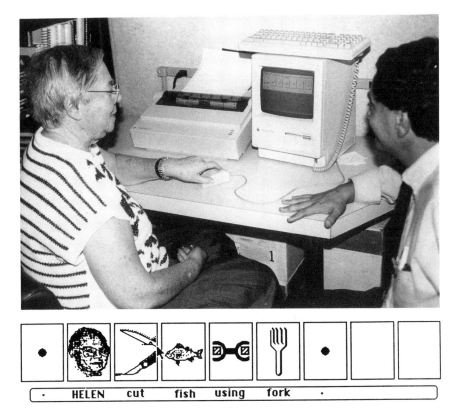

Figure 18 (Top) A severe nonverbal aphasia patient using the computer-assisted visual communication (C-ViC) program on the Macintosh computer. The patient has a right hemiplegia, and controls the mouse with the nonparalyzed left hand to select pictures and icons on the computer screen. (Bottom) Example of communication generated by a nonverbal aphasia patient in phase II of the C-ViC program. The patient's spouse has said that they ate at a fish restaurant over the weekend. When the clinician asked, "When you were at the restaurant, who cut your food for you?", the patient generated the above response. The C-ViC program is customized to individual patient needs, including photos of family members, hospital staff, etc. (The written labels, which are not usually provided because they tend to confuse the patient who cannot read or write, are provided here for purposes of illustration only.) (From Ref. 92.)

test, which was designed for severely aphasic patients, probes for even a very small improvement in auditory comprehension or language production. Most patients were also tested with parts of the Boston Diagnostic Aphasia Exam (BDAE) (66). Diagnosis prior to C-ViC treatment was severe aphasia with

Table 5 Patient Data and Language Test Scores for Patients Treated with the Computer-Assisted Visual Communication Treatment Program

						BDAE		BASA			C-ViC response
Case[a]	Sex	Age at onset (yrs)	MPO when C-ViC started	Months in Tx.		No. wds./ phrase (7)	Aud. comp. z-score	Auditory comp. raw score (16)	Total raw score (61)	Oral-gestural expression raw score (21)	phase II step 5 (PICA scale — 16)[b]
Good response											
B.J.[c]	M	43	7	3	Pre-	0	−0.8	13	49	14	
					Post-	1–2	+0.5	14	51	14	15.0
D.J.	M	54	6	6	Pre-	0	−1.75	8	36	9	
					Post-	0	NA[d]	7	39	14	14.5
S.H.	F	65	4	18	Pre-	0	NA[d]	7	26	3	
					Post-	0	NA[d]	10	37	5	14.0
C.A.	M	49	72	9	Pre-	0	−0.63	13	40	7	
					Post-	0	NA[d]	13	40	8	12.5
Poor response											
R.R.	M	59	21	28	Pre-	0	−0.61	6	25	3	
					Post-	0	NA[d]	6	38	13	9.0
F.W.	M	59	7	7	Pre-	0	−1.6	9	31	6	
					Post-	0	−0.33	13	41	7	8.5
S.M.	M	60	60	7	Pre-	0	−1.74	4	24	7	
					Post-	0	−1.61	8	29	7	8.0

[a]Patients are rank-ordered according to score in last column.
[b]The last step in phase II, step 5 of C-ViC requires the patient to independently initiate a question or command (score ⩾ 13).
[c]Left-handed but aphasic from left-hemisphere lesion.
[d]Not available.

no spontaneous output — spoken or written — in conversation or picture description. Auditory comprehension was also substantially impaired. Table 5 summarizes language capacity.

All seven cases had been previously treated with one or more traditional treatment programs without success. These included verbal treatment programs such as Melodic Intonation Therapy (61,62), and/or nonverbal treatment programs such as buccofacial visual action therapy, which trains patients with severe oral apraxia to produce representational gestures using the oral musculature (75) and/or limb–visual action therapy, which trains patients with severe aphasia and limb apraxia to produce representational, purposeful gestures with the hand and arm (76).

All patients were treated with C-ViC in the chronic phase >3 MPO, range 4 months to 6 years post-onset. The patients were seen as outpatients for half-hour treatment sessions, usually twice per week. All patients were able to match objects to pictured icons on a computer screen (and vice versa), and all were able to use the computer mouse easily with the nonparalyzed left hand.

The C-ViC training consists of two phases (77). In phase I, patients are trained to use the computer mouse to carry out commands presented in C-ViC (comprehension), to answer questions, and, finally, to compose descriptions of simple acts (production). Phase II focuses on real-life communicative acts, including expressing needs, making requests (giving commands), and asking questions (see Fig. 18). Variability in duration of C-ViC treatment in the present study reflected ongoing program development as well as patient availability. The C-ViC training now lasts approximately 9 months, including completion of phase II training.

The quality of the communications generated by patients using C-ViC in phases I and II were rated by the clinician, using the Porch Index of Communicative Ability (PICA) rating scale, which ranges from 1 to 16 (78). A PICA score of ≥ 13 represents independently initiated successful communication. Scores >13 were considered good C-ViC productions, scores <13 poor C-ViC productions.

To reach the criteria for continuation at the end of Phase I and to be considered a good-response case at the end of phase II, a patient's communications generated with C-ViC must reach scores of at least 13 on the PICA scale. A patient with a phase II C-ViC score of <13 was considered a poor-response case.

Three patients had good response, with phase II scores ranging from 14 to 15; one patient had borderline good response, with a score of 12.5; and three patients had poor response, with scores ranging from 8 to 9 (see Table 5, last column).

There was no significant correlation between the age at stroke onset and the phase II C-ViC score ($r = -0.482$), or between the MPO when entering the C-ViC program and the phase II C-ViC score ($r = -0.352$). There was also no significant correlation between the number of months for which a patient participated in the C-ViC program and the Phase II C-ViC score ($r = -0.275$).

S.H., one of the patients who had good response with C-ViC, was able to remain at home with her spouse instead of being transferred to a nursing home, as a result of the new communication ability provided through C-ViC. The necessity of a nursing home had been considered prior to C-ViC training because of severe difficulties in communication and management. As a result of this patient's success with the C-ViC program, a Macintosh computer was placed in the home, and she was able to use the system to communicate her needs to her husband, including when she felt there was a need for her prescriptions to be refilled.

Even patients with poor response to C-ViC by PICA scoring were able to use C-ViC for some interactions not possible with speech or writing. R.R. was considered to have poor response to C-ViC because he was not able to independently initiate communications with C-ViC following phase II training. He was, however, able to use C-ViC to answer specific questions posed by another person. For example, using the Macintosh computer in his home, R.R. can respond to his wife's spoken question, "What do you want for breakfast?"

The pre-C-ViC BASA scores had a general correspondence to good versus poor response with C-ViC. The four good-response cases had pre-C-ViC overall BASA scores of at least 26 correct items of the total 61 items; two of the three poor-response cases had scores of fewer than 26 correct items of the 61 (see Table 5). The four good-response cases had pre-C-ViC Auditory Comprehension BASA subtest scores of at least 7 correct items of the total 16 items; two of the three poor-response cases scored fewer than 7 of the total 16 items (Table 5). Thus, good response with C-ViC may be compatible with pre-C-ViC overall BASA scores of at least 26 and pre-C-ViC Auditory Comprehension BASA subtest scores of at least 7.

CT scan lesion site analysis was performed. The cortical and subcortical areas examined for extent-of-lesion ratings are shown in Figure 1b. The CT scans used for the lesion site analysis had been performed between 3 and 36 MPO.

Relationship Between CT Scan Lesion Sites and Response to C-ViC

There was no relationship between good response versus poor response to C-ViC and lesion extent in any single neuroanatomical area analyzed on CT scan. The 1989 study by Naeser et al. (25) had observed that extensive lesion in the medial ScF area plus the middle one-third PVWM area combined was compatible with no recovery of spontaneous speech. In fact, all seven cases in this C-ViC study had total extent-of-lesion ratings of >7 for the

Table 6 CT Scan Lesion Sites and Extent-of-Lesion Values for Patients Treated with the C-ViC Treatment Program

| | | | | | Extra areas | | | | | |
| | | | | | Extra area 1: supraventricular | | Extra area 2: temporal lobe | | | |
Case	CT scan (MPO)	Medial subcallosal fasc. (mean B, B/W)	Mid. 1/3 PVWM (SM)	Total extent of lesion, med. ScF + mid. 1/3 PVWM[a]	Supplem. motor area	Cingulate gyrus area 24	Wernicke's area (mean B/W, W)	Temporal isthmus (mean B, B/W)	Right-hemisphere lesion	Occipital length asymmetry
Good response										
B.J.[b]	12	5	4.9	9.9	0	0	0	0	No	=
D.J.	13	5	4.25	9.25	Deep	Deep	1	0	No[c]	=
S.H.	6	4.9	4.75	9.65	0	0	3.25	4.37	No	R
C.A.	72	3.5	5	8.5	0	0	4.55	4.5	No[d]	R
Poor response										
R.R.	49	4.75	4.9	9.65	Cortical and deep	Cortical and deep	2.5	4.5	No	L
F.W.	13	4.25	5	9.25	Cortical and deep	Cortical and deep	2.37	4.37	No	R
S.M.	60	2.37	4.75	7.12	Deep	Deep	4.9	5	No	L

[a] >7 = basic lesion, no recovery of spontaneous speech.
[b] Left-handed but aphasic from left-hemisphere lesion.
[c] Patchy low-density areas surrounding anterior and posterior borders of the body of the lateral ventricle present in right hemisphere.
[d] Shunt in right ventricle.

medial ScF area and the middle one-third PVWM area combined (see Table 6, column labeled "Total Extent of Lesion"). The good-response and poor-response cases had complete overlap of total extent-of-lesion ratings in these two white-matter areas.

Only one combination of additional lesion extension in two extra areas completely separated all good-response from all poor-response cases treated with C-ViC: extra area 1, the supraventricular area, including the SMA/ cingulate gyrus area 24 near the vertex, and extra area 2, the temporal lobe area, including Wernicke's area or the subcortical temporal isthmus area (deep to Wernicke's area). The poor-response patients had extensive lesion (extent-of-lesion ratings >3) in both of these two extra areas. The good-

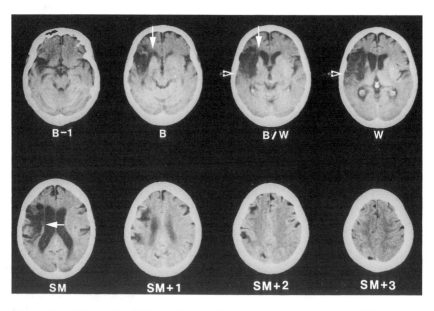

Figure 19   CT scan for S.H., a 65-year-old woman who entered the C-ViC program 4 MPO and had good response. The basic lesion site pattern associated with no recovery of spontaneous speech was present in the medial ScF area on slices B and B/W (white arrows), plus the middle one-third PVWM area on slice SM (white arrow). The total extent-of-lesion rating for the medial ScF area plus middle one-third PVWM area was 9.65. In addition, extensive lesion was present in only one of the two extra areas. Lesion was present in extra area 2, the temporal lobe area, including Wernicke's area on slices B/W and W (black and white arrows) and the subcortical temporal isthmus area on slices B-1 and B. No lesion was present in extra area 1, the supraventricular area including SMA/cingulate gyrus on slices SM + 2 or SM + 3. CT scan is 6 MPO. (From Ref. 92.)

response patients had extensive lesion (extent-of-lesion ratings >3) in none or only one of these two extra areas (Table 6).

Case Examples

The CT scan for one nonverbal patient who had good response to C-ViC training is shown in Figure 19; the scan for one nonverbal patient who had poor response is shown in Figure 20.

The results from this study suggest that CT scan lesion site analysis may be useful in identifying severe nonverbal aphasia patients who will probably not recover spontaneous speech but who can be trained to communicate

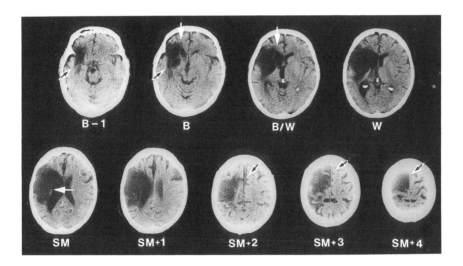

Figure 20 CT scan for R.R., a 60-year-old man, who entered the C-ViC program at 21 MPO and had poor response. The basic lesion site pattern associated with no recovery of spontaneous speech was present in the medial ScF area on slices B and B/W (white arrows), plus the middle one-third PVWM area on slice SM (white arrow). The total extent-of-lesion rating for the medial ScF area plus the middle one-third PVWM area was 9.65. In addition, extensive lesion was present in both of the two extra areas. Lesion was present in extra area 1, the supraventricular area, including SMA/cingulate gyrus near the vertex on slices SM + 2, SM + 3, and SM + 4 (black and white arrows); lesion was also present in extra area 2, the temporal lobe area, including the subcortical temporal isthmus area on slices B-1 and B (black and white arrows). CT scan is 4 years post-onset. (From Ref. 92.)

with the nonverbal C-ViC program. Patients with total extent-of-lesion ratings >7 for the medial ScF area plus the middle one-third PVWM area appear to be among the most appropriate patients for treatment with C-ViC. Furthermore, patients with extensive lesion in both of the two extra areas appear to be unable to independently initiate communication with C-ViC. They require assistance, such as repeated cues or repeated instructions.

The fact that some patients have poor response to C-ViC does not mean that they should not be trained to use C-ViC. *Poor response* refers to communications rated below 13 on the PICA scale and inability to independently initiate communications with C-ViC at the phase II level. The expectations of outcome with the C-ViC program may be lowered to accommodate patients who cannot independently initiate C-ViC messages but can use it with assistance to answer specific questions. Thus, practical use of C-ViC in the home, nursing home, or rehabilitation setting should be determined on an individual basis.

Sarno and Levita (40) have observed that the greatest recovery in severe aphasia patients occurs after 6–12 MPO. Therefore, it seems likely that with a severe, nonverbal aphasia patient, a chronic CT scan could be obtained after 3 MPO, and the results could be used to help with treatment decisions for the 6–12-MPO treatment period, and beyond. Of course, other treatment approaches should be used earlier, including helping the patient to use a basic communication board, drawing (79), or gesture (80–82).

Careful analysis of a chronic CT scan may help reduce the overall cost in long-term rehabilitation of severe, nonverbal aphasia patients by helping to identify potential for recovery (or nonrecovery) of spontaneous speech. Several factors should be considered, some of which are listed below:

1. The more complete borders of an infarct are best visualized on CT scans performed *after* 2 or 3 MPO. Acute CT scans performed earlier do not reveal the more complete borders of an infarct and are not useful in helping to make predictions for long-term recovery.
2. For the information in this chapter to be useful, the CT scan should be obtained at 20° to the canthomeatal line, without contrast, with 10 mm slice thickness and with 3 mm slice overlap, above the suprasellar cistern and through the ventricles. CT scans performed in this manner will conform to the CT scan slice images shown in Figure 1b, and the medial ScF area and the middle one-third PVWM area, as well as Wernicke's area and the temporal isthmus, can be easily located for detailed extent-of-lesion analysis.
3. If the total extent-of-lesion rating for the medial ScF area and the middle one-third PVWM area is <7, then it is likely the patient will recover some spontaneous speech. If the extent-of-lesion rating is also <3 for Wernicke's

area and the subcortical temporal isthmus area, then it is likely that the patient will have good response with a verbal treatment program such as MIT.

4. If the total extent-of-lesion rating for the medial ScF area and the middle one-third PVWM area is >7, then it is unlikely the patient will recover spontaneous speech. For these patients, a nonverbal treatment program might be considered such as C-ViC.

If the extent-of-lesion rating is also >3 for none or only one of the two extra areas observed in the C-ViC study, then it is likely the nonverbal patient will have good response with C-ViC and be able to independently initiate communication with C-ViC. The two extra areas on CT scan that must be examined regarding potential for good response with C-ViC are: extra area 1, the supraventricular area, including the SMA/cingulate gyrus area 24 near the vertex, and extra area 2, the temporal lobe area, including Wernicke's area or the subcortical temporal isthmus. If the extent of lesion is >3 for *each* of these two extra areas, then it is likely the nonverbal patient will have poor response with C-ViC and, although unable to independently initiate communication with C-ViC, will probably be able to answer simple questions with C-ViC.

LESION SITE ANALYSIS ON MRI SCANS

MRI scans are excellent at showing the presence of an infarction within 48 hours of stroke onset (83–86). The infarction is better visualized on MRI scans performed more than 3 MPO than on MRI scans performed 1 MPO (87). Even if chronic MRI scans are performed more than 3 MPO, however, there are unique problems regarding application of the method of lesion site analysis presented above.

This chapter presents a method of lesion site analysis that includes examination of deep, subcortical white-matter areas including the medial ScF area near the frontal horn and the middle one-third PVWM area near the body of the lateral ventricle. We have observed discrepancies regarding the depth of lesion on MRI scans versus CT scans especially near ventricle, including near the frontal horn. We have also observed discrepancies regarding the depth of lesion near ventricle on T1- versus T2-weighted MRI images. A case example showing some of these discrepancies is presented in Figures 21 and 22.

The patient (S.J.) was a 51-year-old man who was examined 3 years post-surgery for an aneurysm. This patient produced no substantive words for the BDAE Cookie Theft Picture description; i.e., he had no meaningful spontaneous speech 3 years post-onset. Based on the CT scan material presented

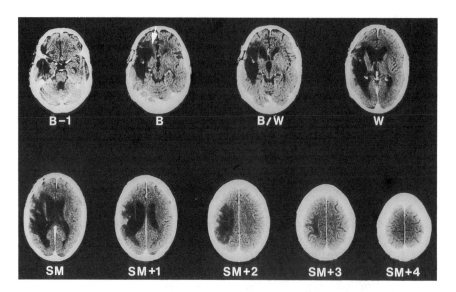

Figure 21 CT scan for S.J. performed 3 years postsurgery for an aneurysm. He had no spontaneous speech 3 years post-onset. This scan shows extensive lesion in the medial ScF area on slices B and B/W. In fact, the medial ScF lesion is so deep on slice B that it touches the frontal horn (white arrow). The extent-of-lesion rating for the medial ScF area on slice B was 4.9 (almost complete solid lesion), and the rating on slice B/W was 3.5 (patchy; more than half of the area has lesion). The mean extent-of-lesion rating for the medial ScF area across slices B and B/W was 4.2. The extent-of-lesion rating for the middle one-third PVWM area on slice SM was 3 (lesion in half of the area). The total extent-of-lesion rating for these two subcortical areas on CT scan was 7.2, a rating compatible with no recovery of meaningful spontaneous speech. (CT scan slice thickness was 10 mm, with a 3 mm overlap.) (From Ref. 93.)

earlier, the patient would be expected to have extensive lesion in the medial ScF area on slices B and B/W, plus extensive lesion in the middle one-third PVWM area on slice SM.

Figure 21, the CT scan for this patient performed 3 years post-onset, shows extensive lesion in the medial ScF area on slices B and B/W. In fact, the medial ScF lesion is so deep on slice B that it touches the frontal horn. The extent-of-lesion rating for the medial ScF area on slice B was 4.9 (almost complete, solid lesion); the rating on slice B/W was 3.5 (patchy; more than half of the area has lesion). The mean rating for the medial ScF area across slices B and B/W was 4.2. The extent-of-lesion rating for the middle one-third PVWM area on slice SM was 3 (lesion in half of the area). The total extent-of-lesion rating for these two subcortical areas on CT scan was 7.2, a rating compatible

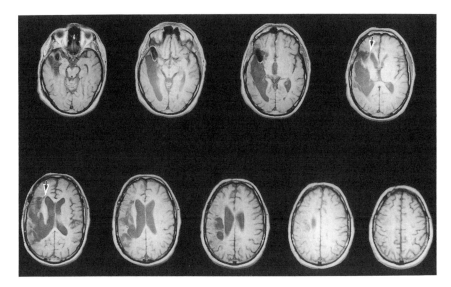

Figure 22a T1-weighted MRI images (TR 600, TE 200 ms) for S.J., also performed 3 years post-onset. These T1-weighted horizontal, axial images do *not* show the lesion in the medial ScF area to touch the frontal horn on either of the first two slices where frontal horns are present (black and white arrows). (MRI slice thickness was 5 mm, with a 2.5 mm gap.) The extent-of-lesion rating for the medial ScF area on the first two slices of these images would be only 0 or a 1. It has been our observation that the T1-weighted images underestimate the borders of the lesion, especially near the ventricle, as compared to a chronic CT scan performed at the same time post-onset. (From Ref. 93.)

with no recovery of meaningful spontaneous speech. (CT scan slice thickness is 10 mm, performed at 7 mm intervals.)

Figure 22a shows the T1-weighted MRI images (TR 600, TE 200 ms) for this same patient, also performed at 3 years post-onset. These T1-weighted horizontal, axial images do *not* show the lesion in the medial ScF area to touch the frontal horn on either of the first two MRI slices. (MRI slice thickness was 5 mm, with a 2.5 mm gap.) The extent-of-lesion ratings for the medial ScF area on the first two slices showing frontal horn on the T1-weighted MRI images would be only 0 or 1 (compared to extent-of-lesion ratings of 4.9 and 3.5, respectively, on the first two slices showing frontal horn on the CT scan images). It has been our observation that the T1-weighted images underestimate the borders of the lesion, especially near the ventricle, as compared to a chronic CT scan performed at the same time post-onset (88).

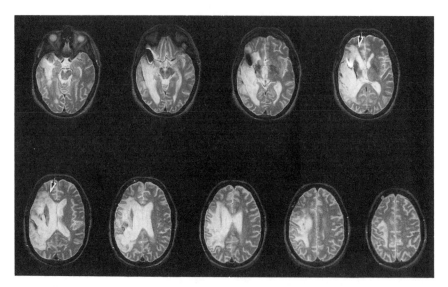

Figure 22b   T2-weighted images (TR 2000, TE 80 ms) for S.J. also performed 3 years post-onset. These T2-weighted horizontal, axial images show the lesion in the medial ScF area to touch the frontal horn on *both* of the first two slices where frontal horns are present (black and white arrows). The depth of the lesion in the medial ScF area on these images is not in agreement with that on the T1-weighted MRI images. If only the T1- and T2-weighted MRI images, and no CT scan images, were performed, we would not know which set of MRI images to use for the extent-of-lesion rating analysis. We have observed that the T2-weighted MRI images tend to exaggerate the borders of the lesion, especially near the ventricle. (From Ref. 93.)

Figure 22b shows the T2-weighted MRI images (TR 2000, TE 80 ms) for this same patient, also performed at 3 years post-onset. These T2-weighted horizontal, axial images *do* show the lesion in the medial ScF area to touch the frontal horn on *both* of the first two slices. The depth of lesion in the medial ScF area on these T2-weighted MRI images is not in agreement with that on the T1-weighted images. If only the T1- and T2-weighted MRI images, and no CT scan images, were performed, we would not know which set of MRI images to use for the extent-of-lesion rating analysis. We have observed that the T2-weighted MRI images tend to exaggerate the borders of the lesion, especially near the ventricle. The proton-density MRI images (TR 2000, TE 30 ms) also tend to exaggerate the borders of the lesion, especially near the ventricle (88).

Research from other laboratories (89) has shown that T2-weighted MRI images of chronic infarcts reveal borders that are larger than the corresponding areas of infarct that have been examined pathologically. Black et al. (90) have also observed larger areas of infarction on T2-weighted MRI images than on chronic CT scan.

In summary, the method of lesion site analysis presented in this chapter regarding potential for recovery in aphasia is best applied at this time only to CT scans that have been performed after 3 MPO, for the following reasons: (1) chronic T1-weighted MRI images tend to underestimate the borders of the lesion in relationship to the borders of the lesion on chronic CT scans (especially near ventricle) and (2) chronic T2-weighted MRI images tend to exaggerate the borders of the lesion in relationship to the borders of the lesion on chronic CT scans (especially near ventricle), and even in relationship to pathological findings.

ACKNOWLEDGMENTS

We would like to acknowledge the invaluable assistance of Malee Noelle Prete for assistance in CT scan analysis and data collection, and Claudia Cassano and Roger Ray for assistance with manuscript preparation. We also thank the Radiology Service of the Boston D.V.A. Medical Center, including Drs. A. Robbins and R. N. Samaraweera, and the Medical Media Service (John Dyke and Mary Burke), Boston D.V.A. Medical Center, for photography and illustrations.

This research was supported in part by the Medical Research Service of the Department of Veterans Affairs and by USPHS grant DC00081.

REFERENCES

1. Mohr JP, Pessin MS, Finkelstein S, Funkenstein HH, Duncan GW, Davis KR. Broca aphasia: Pathologic and clinical. Neurology 1978;28:311–324.
2. Naeser MA, Hayward RW. Lesion localization in aphasia with cranial computed tomography and the Boston Diagnostic Aphasia Exam. Neurology 1978;28:545–551.
3. Barat M, Constant PH, Mazaux JM, Caille JM, Arné L. Correlations anatomo-cliniques dans l'aphasie. Approt de la tomo densitometrie. Revue Neurologique 1978;134:611–617.
4. Kertesz A, Harlock W, Coates R. Computer tomographic localization, lesion size, and prognosis in aphasia and nonverbal impairment. Brain Lang 1979;8:34–50.
5. Damasio H, Damasio AR. The anatomical basis of conduction aphasia. Brain 1980;103:337–350.
6. Mazzocchi F, Vignolo LA. Localization of lesions in aphasia: Clinical CT scan correlation in stroke patients. Cortex 1980;15:627–654.
7. Damasio H. Cerebral localization of the aphasias. In: Sarno MT, ed. Acquired aphasia. New York: Academic Press, 1981:27–50.

8. Selnes OA, Knopman DS, Niccum N, Rubens AB, Larsen DL. Computed tomographic scan correlates of auditory comprehension deficits in aphasia: A prospective study. Ann Neurol 1983;13:558–566.

9. Knopman DS, Selnes OA, Niccum N, Rubens AB, Yock D, Larson D. A longitudinal study of speech fluency in aphasia: CT correlates of recovery and persistent nonfluency. Neurology (Cleveland) 1983;33:1170–1178.

10. Kertesz A. Localization of lesions in Wernicke's aphasia. In: Kertesz A, ed. Localization in neuropsychology. Orlando: Academic Press, 1983.

11. Freedman M, Alexander MP, Naeser MA. Anatomic basis of transcortical motor aphasia. Neurology 1984;34:409–417.

12. Selnes OA, Niccum N, Knopman DS, Rubens AB. Recovery of single word comprehension: CT scan correlates. Brain Lang 1984;21:72–74.

13. Naeser MA, Helm-Estabrooks N, Haas G, Auerbach S, Srinivasan M. Relationship between lesion extent in "Wernicke's Area" on CT scan and predicting recovery of comprehension in Wernicke's Aphasia. Arch Neurol 1987;44:73–82.

14. Alexander MP, Naeser MA, Palumbo CL. Broca's area aphasias: Aphasia after lesions including the frontal operculum. Neurology 1990;40:353–362.

15. Palumbo CL, Alexander MP, Naeser MA. CT scan lesion sites associated with conduction aphasia. In: Kohn SE, ed. Conduction aphasia. Hillsdale: Lawrence Erlbaum Associates, 1992.

16. Mazzocchi F, Vignolo AL. Localization of lesions in aphasia: Clinical CT scan correlations in stroke patients. Cortex 1979;15:627–654.

17. Alexander MP, LoVerme SR. Aphasia following left hemispheric intracerebral hemorrhage. Neurology 1980;30:1193–1202.

18. Naeser MA, Alexander MP, Helm-Estabrooks N, Levine HL, Laughlin SA, Geschwind N. Aphasia with predominantly subcortical lesion sites—description of three capsular/putaminal aphasia syndromes. Arch Neurol 1982;39:2–14.

19. Damasio AR, Damasio H, Rizzo M, Varney N, Gersh F. Aphasia with nonhemorrhagic lesions in the basal ganglia and internal capsule. Arch Neurol 1982; 39:15–20.

20. Cappa SF, Cavalloti G, Guidotti M, Papagno C, Vignolo LA. Subcortical aphasia: Two clinical-CT scan correlation studies. Cortex 1983;19:227–241.

21. Alexander MP, Naeser MA, Palumbo CL. Correlations of subcortical CT lesion sites and aphasia profiles. Brain 1987;110:961–991.

22. Alexander MP, Naeser MA. Cortical-subcortical differences in aphasia. In: Plum F, ed. Language, communication and the brain. New York: Raven Press, 1988:215–228.

23. Alexander MP, Benson DF. The aphasias and related disturbances. In: Joynt RJ, ed. Clinical neurology. Vol 1. Rev. ed. Philadelphia: JB Lippincott, 1991.

24. Vignolo LA. Lesions underlying defective performances on the Token Test: A CT scan study. In: Boller F, ed. Auditory comprehension: Clinical and experimental studies with the Token Test. Orlando: Academic Press, 1979:161–167.

25. Naeser MA, Palumbo CL, Helm-Estabrooks N, Stiassny-Eder D, Albert ML. Severe non-fluency in aphasia: Role of the medial subcallosal fasciculus plus other white matter pathways in recovery of spontaneous speech. Brain 1989; 112:1–38.

26. Naeser MA, Hayward RW, Laughlin SA, Zatz LM. Quantitative CT scan studies in aphasia. I: Infarct size and CT numbers. Brain Lang 1981;12:140–164.
27. Naeser MA, Hayward RW, Laughlin SA, Becker JMT, Jernigan TL, Zatz LM. Quantitative CT scan studies in aphasia. II: Comparison of the right and left hemispheres. Brain Lang 1981;12:165–189.
28. Naeser MA. CT scan lesion size and lesion locus in cortical and subcortical aphasia. In: Kertesz A, ed. Localization in neuropsychology. New York: Academic Press, 1983:63–119.
29. Hanaway J, Scott WR, Strother CM. Atlas of the human brain and the orbit for computed tomography. St Louis: WH Green, 1977.
30. DeArmond SJ, Fusco MM, Dewey MM. Structure of the human brain: A photographic atlas. 2nd ed. New York: Oxford University Press, 1976.
31. Matsui T, Hirano A. An atlas of the human brain for computerized tomography. Tokyo: Igaku-Shoim, 1978.
32. Naeser MA, Gaddie A, Palumbo CL, Stiassny-Eder D. Late recovery of auditory comprehension in global aphasia: Improved recovery observed with subcortical temporal isthmus lesion versus Wernicke's cortical area lesion. Arch Neurol 1990;47:425–432.
33. Borod JC, Carper M, Goodglass H, Naeser M. Aphasic performance on a battery of construction, visuo-spatial, and quantitative tasks: Factorial, structural, and CT scan localization. J Clin Neuropsychol 1985;6:189–204.
34. Goodglass H, Kaplan E. The assessment of aphasia and related disorders. Philadelphia: Lea & Febiger, 1972.
35. Jernigan TL, Zatz LM, Naeser MA. Semiautomated methods for quantitating CSF volume on cranial computed tomography. Radiology 1979;132:463–466.
36. Bogen JE, Bogen GM. Wernicke's region: Where is it? Ann NY Acad Sci 1976; 280:834–843.
37. Kertesz A. Aphasia and associated disorders: Taxonomy, localization and recovery. New York: Grune & Stratton, 1979.
38. Nielsen JM. Agnosia, apraxia, aphasia: Their value in cerebral localization. 2nd ed. New York: Hoeber, 1946:119–120.
39. Sarno MT, Levita E. Recovery in aphasia during the first year post stroke. Stroke 1979;10:663–670.
40. Sarno MT, Levita E. Some observations on the nature of recovery in global aphasia after stroke. Brain Lang 1981;31:1–12.
41. Hier DB, Davis KR, Richardson EP, Mohr JP. Hypertensive putaminal hemorrhage. Ann Neurol 1977;11:152–159.
42. Muratoff W. Secundäre Degeneration nach Durchschneidung des Balkens. Neurologisches Centralblatt 1893;12:714–729.
43. Dejerine J. Anatomie des Centres Nerveux. Vol 1. Paris: Rueff, 1895.
44. Yakovlev PI, Locke S. Limbic nuclei of thalamus and connections of limbic cortex. III. Corticocortical connections of the anterior cingulate gyrus, the cingulum, and the subcallosal bundle in monkey. Arch Neurol 1961;5:364–400.
45. Benjamin D, Van Hoesen GW. Some afferents of the supplementary motor area (SMA) in the monkey. Anatom Rec 1982;202:15A.
46. Goldberg G. Supplementary Motor Area structure and function. Review and hypothesis. Behav Brain Sci 1985;567–615.

47. Barnes CL, Van Hoesen GW, Yeterian EH. Widespread projections to the striatum from the limbic mesocortices in the monkey. Soc Neurosci Abstr 1980; 6:271.

48. Jürgens U. The efferent and afferent connections of the supplementary motor area. Brain Res (Amsterdam) 1984;300:63–81.

49. Schulz ML, Pandya D, Rosene D. The somatotopic arrangement of motor fibers in the periventricular white matter and internal capsule in the rhesus monkey. Ph.D. dissertation, Department of Behavioral Neuroscience, Boston University School of Medicine and Graduate School, 1993.

50. Ross ED. Localization of the pyramidal tract in the internal capsule by whole brain dissection. Neurology 1980;30:59–64.

51. Mufson EJ, Pandya DN. Some observations on the course and composition of the cingulum bundle in the rhesus monkey. J Comprehen Neurol 1984;225: 31–43.

52. Naeser MA, Alexander MP, Stiassny-Eder D, Galler V, Hobbs J, Bachman D. Real versus sham acupuncture in the treatment of paralysis in acute stroke patients – A CT scan lesion site study. J Neurolog Rehab 1992;6:163–173.

53. Broca P. Perte de la parole; ramollissement chronique et destruction partielle du lobe antérieur gauche du Cerveau. Bulletin de la Société d'Anthropologie de Paris 1861;2:235–238.

54. Broca P. Remarques sur le siège de la faculté du langage articulé, suivies d'une observation d'aphémie (Perte de la parole). Bulletin de la Société Anatomique de Paris 1861;36:330–357.

55. Castaigne P, Lhermitte F, Signoret JL, Abelanet R. Description et étude scannographique du cerveau de Leborgne: la découverte de Broca. Revue Neurologique 1980;136:563–583.

56. Signoret J-L, Castaigne P, Lhermitte F, Abelanet R, Lavoral P. Rediscovery of Leborgne's brain: Anatomical description with CT scan. Brain Lang 1984;22: 303–319.

57. Kirzinger A, Jürgens U. Cortical lesion effects and vocalization in the squirrel monkey. Brain Res (Amsterdam) 1982;233:299–315.

58. Smith AM, Bourbonnais D, Blanchette G. Interaction between forced grasping and a learned precision grip after ablation of the supplementary motor area. Brain Res 1981;222:395–400.

59. Naeser MA, Frumkin NL, Fitzpatrick P, Palumbo CL. Melodic intonation therapy with nonfluent aphasia patients as a new method of CT scan lesion site analysis. Submitted.

60. Naeser MA, Frumkin NL, Baker EH, Nicholas M, Palumbo CL, Alexander MP. CT scan lesion sites in severe nonverbal aphasia patients appropriate for treatment with a Computer-Assisted Visual Communication Program (C-ViC). Submitted.

61. Albert ML, Sparks R, Helm N. Melodic intonation therapy for aphasia. Arch Neurol 1973;29:130–131.

62. Sparks R, Holland AL. Method: Melodic intonation therapy for aphasia. J Speech Hear Disord 1976;41:287–297.

63. Helm-Estabrooks N, Nicholas M, Morgan A. Melodic intonation therapy program. San Antonio: Special Press, 1989.

64. Sparks R, Helm N, Albert M. Aphasia rehabilitation resulting from melodic intonation therapy. Cortex 1974;10:303–316.
65. Helm NA. Criteria for selecting aphasia patients for melodic intonation therapy. Paper presented at Language Rehabilitation in Aphasia, annual meeting of the American Association for the Advancement of Science, Washington, DC, 1978.
66. Goodglass H, Kaplan E. Assessment of aphasia and related disorders. 2nd ed. Philadelphia: Lea & Febiger, 1983.
67. Helm-Estabrooks NA, Albert ML. A manual of aphasia therapy. Austin, TX: Pro-Ed, 1991.
68. Naeser MA, Helm-Estabrooks N. CT scan lesion localization and response to Melodic Intonation Therapy with nonfluent aphasia cases. Cortex 1985;21: 203–223.
69. Baker E, Berry T, Gardner H, Zurif E, Davis L, Veroff A. Can linguistic competence be dissociated from natural language functions? Nature 1975;254:609–619.
70. Gardner H, Zurif E, Berry T, Baker E. Visual communication in aphasia. Neuropsychologia 1976;14:275–292.
71. Weinrich M, Steele R, Kleczewska M, Carlson GS, Baker EH, Wertz RT. Representation of "verb" in a computerized visual communication system. Aphasiology 1989;3:501–512.
72. Weinrich M, Steele R, Carlson GS, Kleczewska M, Wertz RT, Baker EH. Processing of visual syntax in a globally aphasic patient. Brain Lang 1989;36:391–405.
73. Steele RD, Weinrich M, Wertz RT, Kleczewska MK, Carlson GS. Computer-based visual communication in aphasia. Neuropsychologia 1989;27:409–426.
74. Helm-Estabrooks N, Ramsberger G, Morgan A, Nicholas M. Boston assessment of severe aphasia. San Antonio: Special Press, 1989.
75. Ramsberger G, Helm-Estabrooks N. Visual action therapy for bucco-facial apraxia. Clinical Aphasiology Conference proceedings. San Diego: College Hill Press, 1988.
76. Helm-Estabrooks N, Fitzpatrick P, Barresi B. Visual action therapy for global aphasia. J Speech Hear Disord 1982;47:385–389.
77. Baker EH, Nicholas M. Computer-assisted visual communication (C-ViC): An alternative communication system for severe aphasia. Am J Speech-Language Pathol J Clin Pract. In press.
78. Proch BE. Porch Index of communicative ability. Palo Alto: Consulting Psychologists Press, 1967.
79. Morgan A, Helm-Estabrooks N. Back to the drawing board: A treatment program for nonverbal aphasic patients. In: Brookshire RH, ed. Clinical Aphasiology Conference proceedings. Minneapolis: BRK Publishers, 1987:64–72.
80. Skelly M, Schinsky L, Smith R, Donaldson R, Griffin J. American Indian Sign (Amerind) as a facilitator of verbalization for the oral-verbal apraxic. J Speech Hear Disord 1974;39:445–456.
81. Skelly M, Schinsky L, Smith R, Donaldson R, Griffin J. American Indian Sign: Gestural communication for the speechless. Arch Phys Med Rehab 1975;56: 156–160.

82. Rao PR. The use of Amer-Ind Code with aphasic adults. In: Chapey R, ed. Language intervention strategies in adult aphasia. Baltimore: Williams & Wilkins, 1986:360–367.
83. Bydder GM, Steiner RE, Young IR, Hall AS, Thomas DJ, Marshall J, Pallis CA, Legg NJ. Clinical NMR imaging of the brain: 140 cases. Am J Radiol 1982; 139:215–236.
84. Buonnano FS, Kistler JP, DeWitt LD, Pykett IL, Brady TJ. Proton ('H) nuclear magnetic resonance (NMR) imaging in stroke syndromes. Neurolog Clin 1983;11:243–262.
85. Sipponen J. Visualization of brain infarction with nuclear magnetic resonance imaging. Neuroradiology 1984;26:387–391.
86. DeWitt LD, Buonanno FS, Kistler JP, Brady TJ, Pykett IL, Goldman MR, Davis KR. Nuclear magnetic resonance imaging in evaluation of clinical stroke syndromes. Ann Neurol 1984;16:535–545.
87. Alexander MP, Naeser M, Sweriduk S. Comparison of lesion profiles with CT and early and late MRI: Implications for aphasia research. Presented at the 29th annual meeting of the Academy of Aphasia, Rome, Italy, Oct 1991.
88. Naeser MA, Alexander MP, Palumbo CL, Samaraweera RN, Sweriduk S. Comparison of white matter infarcts on chronic CT scans versus chronic MRI scans: Why chronic CT scans correlate better with recovery of speech in aphasia. In preparation.
89. DeWitt LD, Kistler JP, Miller DC, Richardson EP, Buonanno FS. NMR-neuropathologic correlation in stroke. Stroke 1985;16:151.
90. Black S, Kertesz A, Nicholson L. Increased signal intensity in the border zone of chronic infarcts detected by T2-weighted NMR imaging. Neurology 1984; 34:116.
91. Frumkin NL, Palumbo CL, Naeser MA. Brain imaging and its application to aphasia rehabilitation: CT and MRI. In: Chapey R, ed. Language intervention strategies in adult aphasia, 3rd ed. Baltimore: Williams & Wilkins, 1994:47–79.
92. Naeser MA, Palumbo CL, Baker E, Nicholas M. CT scan lesion site analysis in severe aphasia—Relationship to no recovery of speech and treatment with the nonverbal Computer-assisted Visual Communication program (C-ViC). In: Helm-Estabrooks N, ed. Seminars in speech and language, New York: Thieme Medical Publishers, Vol 15(1), Feb. 1994.
93. Naeser MA, Palumbo CL. Neuroimaging and language recovery in stroke. J Clin Neurophysiol 1994;11(2):150–174.

6

Conduction Aphasia:
A Syndrome of Language Network Disruption

D. Frank Benson

UCLA School of Medicine, Los Angeles, California

Alfredo Ardila

Colombian Institute of Neuropsychology, Bogotá, Colombia

INTRODUCTION

Current attempts to comprehend the role of the brain in higher mental functions stress the interactions of multiple loci and connections, a network theory. Studies of language have long provided excellent arenas for network theories, dating to the original concepts of language formulation by Wernicke in 1874 (1). Basic to the network approach are two established concepts: the mosaic localizationist approach that stems from the hypothetical brain maps of Gall and the more recently established disconnection theories (2,3). Although described for over a century, disconnection has become widely recognized only in the past three decades (4). One venerable example of the disconnection process is conduction aphasia; this chapter approaches the underlying processes of the network theory through description of conduction aphasia.

Although initially described by Wernicke in 1874, conduction aphasia was long questioned and still remains among the more controversial of aphasic syndromes. Traditionally, three basic characteristics of conduction aphasia have been demarcated (5–11): (1) fluent, paraphasic (usually literal) conversational speech, (2) near-normal comprehension, and (3) repetition disturbances of a significant degree. In addition, the conduction aphasia syndrome often includes: (1) naming disturbances ranging from literal paraphasic contamination to total inability to produce the appropriate word, (2) a reading disturbance in which comprehension of written language is much better than reading aloud, (3) writing disturbances ranging from mild spelling difficulties to profound agraphia, (4) ideomotor apraxia of buccofacial and limb movements, and (5) minimal elementary neurological abnormalities (e.g., hemiparesis and cortical sensory loss).

The language disorder has been called afferent or kinesthesic motor aphasia (12,13), central aphasia (14), efferent conduction aphasia (11), reproduction conduction aphasia (15), repetition aphasia (*Nachsprache Aphasie*) (16), and conduction aphasia (1,5–7,17–20).

The most striking feature of the syndrome is the repetition disorder, a defect that has been explained in different ways. Wernicke's original postulation was in terms of disconnection (1) but many subsequent authors have interpreted the problem as an apraxic deficit (12,21–25). These interpretations consider conduction aphasia to be a verbal apraxia, an ideomotor apraxia of speech (23), or a kinesthesic apraxia of speech (24).

CLINICAL CHARACTERISTICS OF CONDUCTION APHASIA

Table 1 summarizes the main characteristics of conduction aphasia. Compared with other variations of aphasia, conduction aphasia patients display a particularly high number of literal paraphasias, highlighted by language repetition and naming tasks. Spontaneous language can fluctuate in the sense

Table 1   Characteristics of Conduction Aphasia

Basic language characteristics	
Conversational speech	Fluent, paraphasic
Comprehension of spoken language	Good to normal
Repetition of spoken language	Abnormal
Pointing	Good to normal
Naming	Abnormal
Reading	
Aloud	Abnormal
Comprehension	Good to normal
Writing	Abnormal
Associated neurological signs	
Motor system	Mild hemiparesis
Dysarthria	Absent
Cortical sensory loss	Present
Apraxia	Buccofacial and limb
Visual fields	Normal
Visual agnosia	Absent

that at times output is fluent and easily produced but at other times it is non-fluent, effortful, and paraphasic. Often the patient produces several words or even several sentences with ease but arrives at a particular word and becomes totally unable to continue. Self-corrections and successive phonological approximations to the target word (*conduit de approche*) are commonly observed (26). A few patients attempt to spell the word aloud when faced with word-production difficulties (27). Strictly speaking, the verbal output has characteristics of both fluent and nonfluent output but is traditionally classed as a fluent aphasia.

Although conduction aphasia patients occasionally present phonetic deviations and verbal paraphasias, the vast majority of alterations in their oral language correspond to the disturbance called literal paraphasia (substitution of an individual phoneme) or neologistic paraphasia (the substitution of multiple phonemes in a single word). Literal paraphasias are most frequently observed during repetition of low-frequency, phonologically complex words or non-words (logotomes). Automatic language is far better preserved, often totally free of paraphasia.

Some important language characteristics deserve emphasis. Conduction aphasia patients present approximations of the target word and self-corrections, suggesting that the acoustic image of the word is preserved. Furthermore, they easily differentiate correctly—from incorrectly—produced words. Although at times they are apparently unable to produce a word (in spontaneous or repetitive language), a moment later the word is produced without apparent effort.

The quantity of verbal output in conversation is notably smaller in conduction aphasia than in Wernicke's aphasia. There are many more pauses, usually hesitations for word-finding or difficulty in producing words so that the output has a broken, dysprosodic quality. Conduction aphasia is often interpreted as an "expressive aphasia" because of this disordered output. A number of features, however, differentiate conduction aphasia speech from the output of patients with Broca's aphasia. One or many different phrases are easily and correctly produced. These may be cliches (e.g., "I don't know if I can" or "What did you say?"), but the phrases are too numerous and variable to be classed as stereotypy. Broca's aphasia often contains output features best classed as phonetic deviations (dysarthria), a quality that does not characterize conduction aphasia, in which phoneme production is good, even to the level of adequate pronunciation of the wrong phoneme. The patient with conduction aphasia often performs adequately in series speech if given a start and will usually produce words better in singing than in conversational output.

Comprehension of spoken language is relatively, often strikingly, good in conduction aphasia. In some, comprehension appears virtually normal, and in others the difficulty appears limited to the understanding of complex grammatical structures or statements containing successions of key words or phrases. The comprehension of patients with conduction aphasia is fully adequate for normal conversation, and a significant degree of comprehension disturbance makes the diagnosis questionable.

In sharp contrast to the normal comprehension, patients with conduction aphasia have a serious problem repeating spoken language. This difference is an essential feature and is often considered the key finding. Characteristically the repetition disturbance features approximations contaminated with multiple literal paraphasias, but, if asked to repeat numbers or color names, the patient may produce a verbal paraphasic substitution (e.g., "the sky is blue" may be repeated as "the sky is green"). Repetition is usually more disturbed than conversational speech. When unable to correctly repeat a word or a phrase, the patient with conduction aphasia may produce an acceptable paraphrase (e.g., when asked to say the word "rifle," a soldier said "riffe, riddil, oh hell, I mean gun"). Similarly, even if unable to repeat a word or phrase, the patient may produce the same word or phrase with ease in a different conversational context.

Conduction aphasia patients present a distinctive dissociation between pointing and naming. Pointing ("show me . . .") is a very easy task for these patients, demonstrating good language comprehension. However, in naming, literal paraphasias tend to be abundant, about the same as in repetition. The name produced may have the correct number of syllables but will contain one or more literal paraphasias. An increased prevalence of phonologically oriented sequences (phonological resemblance to the target word) occurs sufficiently to have been proposed as a diagnostic criterion for conduction aphasia (28). Cues are of little help. Often, a patient states that a name is known but cannot be said correctly, a condition called "paraphasic anomia" (29). In addition, a true inability to find a word can occur in conduction aphasia, and in some cases anomia is a major feature.

Tests of reading can provide striking findings in many patients with conduction aphasia. Characteristically, reading out loud rapidly breaks down to a severely paraphasic output. Phoneme substitutions, omissions, additions, anticipations, and perseverations are observed. At times the patients will attempt to perform a literal (letter-by-letter) reading. Occasionally, neologisms (unrecognizable words) and verbal morphological paralexias are observed (30). In contrast, patients with conduction aphasia often comprehend written language with comparative ease. Some patients who are unable to read a three- or four-word newspaper headline aloud can read newspaper articles, novels, and even scientific textbooks with good comprehension.

The agraphia associated with conduction aphasia is complex and not well understood, but the ability to write is almost invariably disturbed to some degree. Spontaneous writing tends to be performed better than writing to dictation. Most patients produce well-formed letters, but the spelling is often incorrect, with additions, omissions, and substitution of letters (31). Words may be misplaced or omitted in a sentence. Because of right-hand sensory loss (32) or limb apraxia, letters may be poorly formed but recognizable. As a rule, letters are more accurately written to dictation than words that may be unrecognizable (neologisms) (30,33). The patient recognizes that the word is incorrectly written but cannot correct it; his attempts to correct often produce new mistakes. As a consequence, the written text tends to contain many corrections and crossed-out words. The patient often claims that he knows the right word (and even pronounces it) but cannot remember how it is written. Table 2 presents the relative frequency of different types of errors found in a sample of patients with conduction aphasia. Luria (12,13) termed this writing disorder "afferent motor agraphia," indicating a parallel in the errors in oral and written output and, therefore, a common underlying mechanism.

An additional complexity exists in the agraphia of conduction aphasia. Both an apraxia for writing (apraxic agraphia) and an agraphia correlated with the linguistic deficit (aphasic agraphia) may be evident. Apraxic agraphia has been defined as the inability to form normal graphemes, with inversions and distortions in their stead (19). In this situation, the patient fails to write letters, producing scribbles and nonletters. The agraphic deficit may be more severe than the aphasic deficit.

The basic neurological examination in cases of conduction aphasia varies considerably. In some, almost no neurological abnormality can be demonstrated; others will have considerable elementary neurological abnormality. Unilateral paresis may be totally absent, mildly present, or significant. When present, the weakness involves the face and arm to a greater degree than the

Table 2 Relative Frequency of Different Types of Writing Errors in Conduction Aphasia Patients

Error	Frequency (%)
Letter substitutions	25.0
Letter omissions	22.2
Neologisms (unrecognizible words)	20.8
Copying errors	13.9
Anticipations	6.9
Letter additions	5.6
Perseverations	5.6

Source: Ref. 30.

leg. Sensory findings are also variable, but some cortical sensory loss is often disclosed. During recovery from conduction aphasia a rather specific pain syndrome—called the "pseudothalamic pain syndrome" to suggest a resemblance to the classic thalamic pain syndrome—may develop (6,32,34). The pain is constant but less intense in degree and is not exacerbated by external stimuli. These patients have a cortical sensory loss and some decrease in pain realization and may have paresthesias and hyperalgesia. A few individuals with conduction aphasia show pain asymbolia (2,35), a disorder in which they respond considerably less to pain stimuli than would be anticipated. The pain asymbolia is bilateral, even though the pathology is limited to one (left) hemisphere. Pain asymbolia is not found in all conduction aphasia patients, but many tolerate more pain than other patients.

Variations occur in the examination of the visual system in conduction aphasia. Most often the extraocular movements and visual fields are normal, but some will have a visual field deficit, a quadrantanopsia or hemianopsia, probably reflecting involvement of fibers of the geniculocalcarine tract.

Ideomotor apraxia, another classic disconnection syndrome (2), is usually present in patients with conduction aphasia. When asked to perform buccofacial or limb movements on verbal command the patient may fail, even while protesting that he knows what he wants to do. The result is often an inappropriate movement that nevertheless demonstrates comprehension of the command. The incorrect movement on command (parapraxis) resembles the paraphasia that contaminates repetition. The association with buccofacial apraxia supports the postulation that conduction aphasia is a verbal apraxia, an apraxia involving the movements required for speaking (21,24), with errors in conduction aphasia verbalizations corresponding to apraxic movements. In this interpretation, conduction aphasia would represent a "segmentary ideomotor apraxia," an "ideomotor apraxia of speech" (23), or a "kinesthesic apraxia of speech" (24). Some authors emphasize the association of buccofacial apraxia and conduction aphasia (2,36), others the co-occurrence of literal paraphasias and buccofacial apraxia (37,38), and others the correlation between the conduction aphasia syndrome and ideomotor apraxia (8). Common underlying mechanisms are probable.

Finally, an association between conduction aphasia and acalculia deserves consideration. Patients with conduction aphasia often have a calculation deficit (39). They may fail mental mathematical operations and frequently make written errors. Serious impairment may be seen in the execution of serial operations and problem-solving tasks. Transcoding tasks, from verbal to numerical and numerical to verbal, are often failed. Many of these errors can be demonstrated to be based on verbal paraphasias, but they also fail in carrying and other tasks of the syntax of calculation and may even fail to recognize arithmetical signs (40). Structural damage underlying conduction aphasia may extend posteriorly to the anatomical area proposed for anarithmetia (41). Both syndromes (acalculia and conduction aphasia) can stem from closely associated left parietal areas (8) and are easily intermixed.

TOPOGRAPHY OF CONDUCTION APHASIA

The lesion in conduction aphasia tends to be limited in size, the smallest of the major varieties of aphasia. There is disagreement with regard to the location of the lesion, however. Wernicke (1) originally proposed that the crucial locus of damage in conduction aphasia was the insula, based on his belief that the pathways connecting posterior and anterior language areas coursed through the insula. Lichtheim's (3) case of conduction aphasia with postmortem data confirmed Wernicke's assumption, and additional cases suggested that when language repetition was disordered the insula was damaged (42). Dejerine (43,44), however, proposed that the arcuate fasciculus (a band of white matter originating in the posterior temporal lobe and coursing forward via the superior longitudinal fasciculus to the motor association cortex in the frontal lobe) was the main connecting pathway for the sensory and motor language areas. Supramarginal and/or parietal operculum damage involving the arcuate fasciculus was thus postulated as being crucial to the syndrome of conduction aphasia.

Dejerine's topography has come to be accepted (2,45,46), but Benson and colleagues (8,47) confirmed Kleist's (16) earlier demonstration that the clinical syndrome of conduction aphasia could result from damage in several different loci, including regions above, behind, or below the sylvian fissure (48). At least one case of transient conduction aphasia has been reported following putaminal hemorrhage (49), possibly resulting from mass effect of the hemorrhage on the surrounding brain structures. Conduction aphasia has been reported over a broad range of localized brain-damage sites (10, 11,47).

The classic (arcuate fasciculus) location was upheld by Damasio and Damasio (45,46), who reported CT studies of six cases, four of which had insula involvement. They proposed that the repetition disorder was based on disconnection of posterior sensory pathways from anterior motor areas, and further suggested that the repetition deficit followed damage in subinsular pathways. The cases reported by Murdoch et al. (50,51) also involved postrolandic structures, including subcortical structures under the middle portion of the insula. Ardila, Rosselli, and Pinzon (30) reported six cases of conduction aphasia with insula damage. Lesion extension to the underlying structures was variable, but in none was the cortex of the supramarginal gyrus, Broca's, or Wernicke's areas involved. Most reports in the literature suggest that brain damage in conduction aphasia follows pathology in the left parietal lobe (lower postcentral and supramarginal gyri) and/or the insula (5,7,8,10,11,30,32,45,46,52–54).

It has been recognized, however, that disturbed repetition of spoken language could follow damage to sites distant from the dominant insula/arcuate fasciculus. Based on cases of conduction aphasia following destruction of the dominant auditory association cortex, Kleist (16) conjectured that some individuals comprehended spoken language with the right temporal auditory cortex and produced language with the left motor speech area. The mechanism of damage in the left auditory association area producing a language disconnection was illustrated by Kleist (see Figure 1) and support for Kleist's demonstration came from Benson and colleagues' (8) case 3, a right-handed individual with conduction aphasia syndrome including good comprehension who, at postmortem, had total destruction of the left first temporal gyrus. Additional support was provided by Mendez and Benson (47), who reported three individuals with the conduction aphasia syndrome who had pathology outside the traditional dominant insula/arcuate fasciculus locus. In each case, a separation of the sites of auditory language comprehension and motor speech production could be postulated.

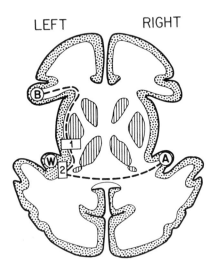

Figure 1 Kleist's diagrammatic explanation of conduction aphasia. A = right-hemisphere auditory association cortex; W = left-hemisphere auditory association cortex; B = left-hemisphere motor speech area; dashed lines indicate potential pathways connecting auditory association cortices with motor speech cortex; 1 = lesion in arcuate fasciculus producing repetition defect; 2 = lesion involving left auditory association cortex producing repetition defect. (From Ref. 6.)

MECHANISMS OF REPETITION ERRORS
IN CONDUCTION APHASIA

The ability to repeat accurately depends on a series of variables, including phonological composition, lexical status, length, syntactic form, predictability, and grammatical class (55–57). This holds true in normal people as well as aphasic individuals (58). While repetition defect is often considered the crucial clinical sign of conduction aphasia, it is also prominent in many other language disorders.

The possibility of several mechanisms, each capable of producing deficient repetition, has led to the postulation of different forms of conduction aphasia: efferent/afferent (10,11) or reproduction/repetition (15,59). The efferent-reproduction disturbance involves phonemic organization and the representation of words and follows parietal and/or insula damage; the afferent-repetition type involves short-term memory, affecting repetition of long passages of material, and is said to arise from temporal damage (60). Luria (24) held that conduction aphasia represented two different linguistic defects. His afferent motor aphasia resembled the efferent-reproduction, parietal type mentioned above. Luria considered this an inability to analyze, manipulate, or otherwise appreciate the featural composition of movements required to produce language sounds (*articulemes*), a kinesthesic apraxia of speech. The second type (afferent-repetition), which was considered a short-term verbal memory deficit, was included in Luria's acoustic-amnestic aphasia category. Benson et al. (8) distinguished two types, based entirely on anatomical locus of damage: suprasylvian (parietal) and subsylvian (temporal). Only the first was associated with ideomotor apraxia.

Despite the importance of repetition in aphasia, few studies have been devoted to analysis of repetition defects in aphasia (61,62). Goldstein (14) argued that repetition demands sensory perception, motor speech capacity, "inner speech," and understanding of the material to be repeated, and is also influenced by the attitude and educational level of the subject and the context in which the repetition occurs. Luria (12,24) noted that repetition required auditory (phonemic) analysis, control of speech articulation, and adequate audioverbal memory, and underlined that repetition of different types of materials required involvement of different neuroanatomical structures.

Gardner and Winner (61) analyzed repetition defects in 44 aphasic patients subdivided into eight groups (anomic, transcortical sensory, transcortical motor, isolation, Broca's, Wernicke's, conduction, and mixed anterior) using a test consisting of 11 items under two conditions (immediate and delayed repetition). Only short elements — from one to eight syllables — were included. In the immediate condition, the mixed anterior group produced the highest number of errors (almost 50%), followed by Broca's (35%), conduction (32%), Wernicke's (30%), transcortical motor (20%), transcortical sensory and isolation (10%), and anomic patients (3%). Performance was a product of the length and meaningfulness of the stimulus items; the delayed condition aided Broca's aphasics but impaired anomic aphasics.

Ardila and Rosselli (62) performed a similar analysis in 41 patients divided into seven groups (extrasylvian motor aphasia, Broca's aphasia, conduction aphasia, Wernicke's aphasia, anomic aphasia, alexia without agraphia, and global aphasia). Three repetition tests (words and high-probability and low-probability sentences) taken from the Boston Diagnostic Aphasia Examination (63) were presented. Errors were predominantly associated with perisylvian aphasias (Broca's, conduction, and Wernicke's), but in all aphasic groups some repetition errors were observed (Table 3). Errors were both quantitatively and qualitatively different between groups. In conduction aphasia, repetition errors were particularly evident in low-probability sentences; with meaningful words or sentences, performance was similar to that of Broca's and Wernicke's aphasia patients. Literal errors, self-corrections, and approximations to the target word were more common in conduction aphasia. There was a notable difference between high-probability and low-probability sentence-repetition scores. While scores in words and high-probability repetitions were better in conduction aphasia than in Broca's aphasia, the scores in the low-probability condition were only half the Broca's patients' scores.

Some general rules govern phonological switches in conduction aphasia (21,64). The first concerns *simplification*. Phonemes tend to be replaced by more easily produced language sounds. Jakobson's rule applies in that earlier-acquired phonemes (simpler from the articulatory point of view) tend to replace later-acquired phonemes (e.g., /r/ → /l/) (65). About 90% of the literal errors in conduction aphasia are due to *phoneme substitutions* and *phoneme deletions*. Second, *consonant changes* prevail (95% of the total number). In contrast, in other fluent aphasics (Wernicke's and extrasylvian), vowel changes are approximately six times more frequent than in conduction apha-

Table 3 Percentage Correct Repetition for Six Patient Groups in the Three Repetition Subtests of the Boston Diagnostic Aphasia Examination

	Anomic	Extrasylvian motor	Wernicke's	Conduction	Broca's	Global
Words	100.0	98.0	74.0	63.0	46.0	27.0
High-Probability sentences	71.2	95.0	45.0	53.7	50.0	0.0
Low-Probability sentences	52.5	67.5	22.5	21.2	45.0	0.0

Source: Ref. 62.

sia, and they are twice as frequent in Broca's aphasia. Phoneme substitutions represent about 70% of literal errors but phoneme deletions range up to 25%, suggesting attempts at articulatory simplification. Third, *phoneme additions* are minimal in conduction aphasia, and *phoneme exchanges* virtually non-existent (Table 4). The types of switches and the responsible mechanisms remain the same in spontaneous and repetitive language, but the frequency is higher in repetitive language. Kohn and Smith (66,67) suggested that conduction aphasia errors are disruptions at the stage of phonemic string construction; errors more often involve final consonants. In other types of aphasia, phonemic errors typically involve word-onsets. Odell et al. (68) emphasized that conduction aphasics display more substitutions than distortions, more errors in polysyllabic than monosyllabic words, and more errors in non-initial than initial syllabic positions in words. In contrast to Broca's aphasia, patients with conduction aphasia do not present syllabic stress errors or have difficulty initiating words.

It can be proposed that a variety of mechanisms underlie repetition deficits in the different types of aphasia: (1) limitations of the auditory-verbal short-term memory (prominent in anomic and Wernicke's aphasia), (2) difficulties in phonological production (Broca's and conduction aphasia), (3) defects in phoneme recognition (Wernicke's aphasia), (4) deficits in grammatical comprehension (Broca's aphasia), and (5) disturbed control of complex syntax (extrasylvian motor aphasia). Repetition is a multifaceted function; disordered repetition deserves careful analysis.

Table 4 Characteristics of Literal Paraphasias in Conduction Aphasia

	Percentage
Type of change	
Manner of articulation	56.9
Place of articulation	10.7
Manner and place of articulation	23.5
Voiced/voiceless (oral stops)	4.3
Vocalic	4.6
Mechanisms Utilized	
Substitution	52.6
Deletion	25.1
Reduplicative substitution	15.1
Addition	3.7
Reduplicative addition	2.7
Exchange	0.8

Source: Ref. 64.

SUMMARY

From the vantage points of history, clinical description, anatomy, linguistic breakdown, and cognitive network theories, conduction aphasia can be seen to represent a distinct disorder. The syndrome possesses unique properties and provides a valuable instrument for the investigation of brain/language relationship.

Clinically, conduction aphasia can be recognized by three prominent findings: fluent output, good comprehension, and poor repetition of spoken language. Both motor speech and repetition are contaminated by an excess of literal paraphasic substitutions. Anatomically, conduction aphasia most often occurs following damage in the anterior, inferior dominant parietal lobe (supramarginal gyrus), particularly when deep structures (insula, arcuate fasciculus) are involved. Important exceptions are recognized, however. These anatomically anomalous cases are almost always based on irregular loci for either motor speech or auditory language comprehension. The clinical syndrome is truly that predicted by Wernicke, a sensory/motor disconnection.

From a linguistic view, the syndrome is best characterized as a problem in phoneme sequencing, with a strong tendency to substitute simple for complex phonemes. Conduction aphasia differs from other aphasia syndromes in that, although the syndrome is clearly a language defect, both semantic and syntactic functions are relatively uninvolved (69).

Finally, as investigation of brain function enters a relatively new phase in which high-level cognitive acts including language are recognized as the products of complex blendings of individual brain functions, conduction aphasia stands as a relatively elementary, direct, and therefore valuable example. The cognitive function of language is disrupted, by damage not to a cortical area ("center") but to a connecting pathway, a disturbance within the neural network. Most aphasia syndromes contain both. Attempts to understand brain/language relationships demand unraveling of the neural networks active in a variety of language functions; conduction aphasia provides a prominent, readily defined embodiment of one dysfunction that involves cognitive circuitry.

Despite the fact that the theoretical interpretation and the exact site of pathology of conduction aphasia remains polemic, the syndrome of conduction aphasia is fully recognizable, occurs rather commonly, and offers excellent information for both clinicians and investigators of language.

REFERENCES

1. Wernicke C. Der Aphasische symptomenkomplex. Breslau: Cohn and Neigart, 1874.

2. Geschwind N. Disconnexion syndromes in animals and man. Brain 1965;88:237–294.
3. Lichtheim L. On aphasia. Brain 1885:7:433–484.
4. Absher JR, Benson DF. Disconnection syndromes: An overview of Geschwind's contributions. Neurology 1993;862–867.
5. Alexander MP, Benson DF. The aphasias and related disturbances. In: Joynt RJ, ed. Clinical neurology. Vol 1. Philadelphia: JB Lippincott, 1991.
6. Benson DF. Aphasia, alexia, and agraphia. New York: Churchill-Livingstone, 1979.
7. Benson DF. Classical syndromes of aphasia. In: Boller F, Grafman J, Rizzolatti G, Goodglass H, eds. Handbook of neuropsychology. Vol 1. Amsterdam: Elsevier, 1988:267–280.
8. Benson DF, Sheremata WA, Bouchard R, Segarra SM, Price D, Geschwind N. Conduction aphasia: A clinicopathological study. Arch Neurol 1973;28:339–346.
9. Damasio A. Aphasia. N Engl J Med 1992;326:531–539.
10. Kertesz A. Aphasia and associated disorders. New York: Grune & Stratton, 1979.
11. Kertesz A. Aphasia. In: Frederiks JAM, ed. Handbook of clinical neurology. Vol 45. Clinical neuropsychology. Amsterdam: Elsevier, 1985:287–331.
12. Luria AR. Higher cortical functions in man. New York: Basic Books, 1966.
13. Luria AR. Traumatic aphasia. The Hague: Mouton, 1970.
14. Goldstein K. Language and language disturbances. New York: Grune & Stratton, 1948.
15. Shallice T, Warrington EK. Auditory short-term memory impairment and conduction aphasia. Brain Lang 1977;4:479–491.
16. Kleist K. Gehirnpathologie. Leipzig: Barth, 1934.
17. Benson DF, Geschwind N. The aphasias and related disturbances. In: Baker AB, Baker LH, eds. Clinical neurology. Vol 1. Philadelphia: Harper and Row, 1976.
18. Benson DF, Geschwind N. The aphasias and related disturbances. In: Baker AB, Joynt RJ, eds. Clinical neurology. Vol 1. Philadelphia: Harper and Row, 1985.
19. Hecaen H, Albert M. Human neuropsychology. New York: Wiley, 1978.
20. Lecours AR, Trepagnier C, Naesser CJ, Lavelle-Huynh G. The interaction between linguistics and aphasiology. In: Lecours AR, Lhermitte F, Bryans B, eds. Aphasiology. London: Bailliere-Tindall, 1983:292–310.
21. Ardila A, Rosselli M. Conduction aphasia and verbal apraxia. J Neuroling 1990;5:1–14.
22. Brown JW. Aphasia, apraxia, and agnosia. Springfield, IL: Charles C Thomas, 1972.
23. Brown JW. The problem of repetition: A case study of conduction aphasia and the "isolation" syndrome. Cortex 1975;11:37–52.
24. Luria AR. Fundamentals of neurolinguistics. New York: Basic Books, 1976.
25. Vinarskaya EN. Clinical problems of aphasia. Moscow: Meditsina (in Russian), 1971.

26. Joanette Y, Keller E, Lecours AR. Sequences of phoneme approximations in aphasia. Brain Lang 1980;11:30–44.
27. Kohn SE. The nature of phonemic string deficit in conduction aphasia. Aphasiology 1989;3:209–239.
28. Kohn SE. The nature of phonological disorders in conduction aphasia. Brain Lang 1984;23:97–115.
29. Benson DF. Anomia in aphasia. Aphasiology 1988;2:229–236.
30. Ardila A, Rosselli M, Pinzon O. Alexia and agraphia in Spanish speakers: CAT correlations and inter-linguistic analysis. In: Ardila A, Ostrosky F, eds. Brain organization of language and cognitive processes. New York: Plenum, 1989; 147–175.
31. Benson DF, Cummings JL. Agraphia. In: Frederiks JAM, ed. Handbook of clinical neurology. Vol 45. Clinical neuropsychology. Amsterdam: Elsevier, 1985:457–472.
32. Hyman BT, Tranel D. Hemianesthesia and aphasia. An anatomical and behavioral study. Arch Neurol 1989;46:816–819.
33. Sgaramella TM, Ellis AW, Semenza C. Analysis of spontaneous writing errors of normal and aphasic writers. Cortex 1991;27:29–39.
34. Bogousslavsky J, Van Melle G, Regli F. Middle cerebral artery pial territory infarcts: A study of the Lausanne Stroke Registry. Ann Neurol 1989;25:555–560.
35. Biemond A. The conduction of pain above the level of the thalamus opticus. AMA Arch Neurol Psychiatry 1956;75:231–244.
36. De Renzi E, Pieczuro A, Vignolo LA. Oral apraxia and aphasia. Cortex 1966; 2:50–73.
37. Poeck K, Kerschensteiner M. Analysis of the sequential events in oral apraxia. In: Zulch KJ, Creutzfeldt O, Galbraith JC, eds. Cerebral localization. New York: Springer-Verlag, 1975:98–109.
38. Tognola G, Vignolo AL. Brain lesions associated with oral apraxia in stroke patients: A cliniconeuroradiological investigation with CT scan. Neuropsychologia 1980;18:257–272.
39. Ardila A, Rosselli M. Acalculias. Behav Neurol 1990;3:39–48.
40. Rosselli M, Ardila A. Calculation deficits in patients with right and left hemisphere damage. Neuropsychologia 1989;27:607–617.
41. Benson DF, Weir WS. Acalculia: Acquired anarithmetria. Cortex 1972;8:465–472.
42. Goldstein K. Uber die amnestische und centrale aphasia. Arch fuer Psychiatrie und Neurologie 1911;48:314–343.
43. Dejerine J. Anatomie des centres nerveux. Paris: Rueff, 1901.
44. Dejerine J. Semiologie des affections du système nerveux. Paris: Masson, 1914.
45. Damasio H, Damasio A. The anatomical basis of conduction aphasia. Brain 1980;103:337–350.
46. Damasio H, Damasio A. Localization of lesions in conduction aphasia. In: Kertesz A, ed. Localization in neuropsychology. New York: Academic Press, 1983:231–244.
47. Mendez MF, Benson DF. Atypical conduction aphasia: A disconnection syndrome. Arch Neurol 1985;42:886–891.

48. Hecaen H, Dell MB, Roger A. L'aphasie de conduction. L'Encephale 1955;2: 170–195.
49. Tuhrim S, Berndt RS, Joslyn JN. Transient conduction aphasia following putaminal hemorrhage. Cerebrovasc Dis 1991;1:113–116.
50. Murdoch BE. Computerized tomography scanning: Its contributions to the understanding of the neuroanatomical basis of aphasia. Aphasiology 1988;2: 437–462.
51. Murdoch BE, Thompson D, Fraser S, Harrison L. Aphasia following non hemorrhagic lesions in the left striato-capsular region. Austral J Hum Commun Disord 1986;14:5–21.
52. Damasio H. Cerebral localization in neuropsychology. In: Sarno MT, ed. Acquired aphasia. New York: Academic Press, 1981:27–50.
53. Demeurisse G, Capon A. Brain activation during a linguistic task in conduction aphasia. Cortex 1991;27:285–294.
54. Green D, Howes DH. The nature of conduction aphasia: A study of anatomical and clinical features and of underlying mechanisms. In: Whitaker H, Whitaker HA, eds. Studies in neurolinguistics. Vol 3. New York: Academic Press, 1977: 123–156.
55. Lecours AR, Lhermitte F, Bryans B. Aphasiology. London: Bailliere-Tindall, 1983.
56. Albert ML, Goodglass H, Rubens AB, Alexander MP. Clinical aspects of dysphasia. New York: Springer-Verlag, 1981.
57. Schuell H, Jenkins JJ, Jiminez-Pabon E. Aphasia in adults—diagnosis, prognosis and treatment. New York: Harper and Row (Hoeber Medical Division), 1964.
58. Berndt RS. Repetition in aphasia: Implications for models of language processing. In: Boller F, Grafman J, Rizzolatti G, Goodglass H, eds. Handbook of neuropsychology. Vol 1. Amsterdam: Elsevier, 1988:329–348.
59. Caplan DM, Vanier M, Baker C. A case study of reproduction conduction aphasia. I. Word production. Cog Neuropsychol 1986;3:99–128.
60. Caramazza A, Basili AG, Koller JJ, Berndt RS. An investigation of repetition and language processing in a case of conduction aphasia. Brain Lang 1981;14: 235–271.
61. Gardner H, Winner E. A study of repetition in aphasic patients. Brain Lang 1978;6:168–178.
62. Ardila A, Rosselli M. Repetition in aphasia. J Neuroling 1992;7:1–11.
63. Goodglass H, Kaplan E. The assessment of aphasia and related disorders. Philadelphia: Lea & Febiger, 1972.
64. Ardila A, Montanes P, Caro C, Delgado F, Buckingham HW. Phonological transformations in Spanish-speaking aphasics. J Psycholing Res 1989;18:163–180.
65. Jakobson R, Halle M. Two aspects of aphasia and two types of aphasic disturbances. In: Jakobson R, Halle M, eds. Fundamentals of language. The Hague: Mouton, 1956:55–82.
66. Kohn SE, Smith KL. Between-word speech errors in conduction aphasia. Cog Neuropsychol 1990;7:133–156.

67. Kohn SE, Smith KL. The relationship between oral spelling and phonological breakdown in a conduction aphasic. Cortex 1991;27:631–639.
68. Odell K, McNeil MR, Rosenbek JC, Hunter L. Perceptual characteristics of vowel and prosody production in apraxic, aphasic, and dysarthric speakers. J Speech Hear Res 1991;34:67–80.
69. Benson DF, Ardila A. Aphasia: A clinical perspective. New York: Oxford University Press. In preparation.

7

Naming and Naming Disorders

Victor W. Henderson

University of Southern California and the Los Angeles County/University of Southern California Medical Center, Los Angeles, California

Aphasia is usually defined as an acquired disorder of language. *Words* are the smallest independent units of language, and *naming* represents the assignment of a linguistic label to a word. "The naming of objects, their designation by words," according to Luria, "comprises one of the basic functions of language" (1, p. 397). For spoken language, this designation is phonological. If, rather than oral language, we consider written language or sign language, then naming would involve a graphemic label or a symbolic manual label. For oral language, it is clear that language difficulties affecting either the sounds of a language (phonology) or its meaning (semantics) will be manifest through a disturbance in naming. Naming disturbances are also referred to as *anomia* or *word-finding difficulty*. Of various performance measures, anomia correlates most highly with the severity of the communication impairment in aphasia (2). Indeed, naming deficits are so central to concepts of aphasia that most classification schemes depict anomia as the sine qua non of aphasia.

Naming disturbances are also identified with specific aphasic syndromes. In this sense, anomic aphasia is not synonymous with aphasic anomia. Moreover, anomia need not even be associated with aphasia. Nonlinguistic factors also influence the naming process, and murky boundaries between a language system and other cognitive domains are not always readily discerned.

HISTORICAL INTRODUCTION

Loss of Memory for Words

Anomia, especially word-finding difficulty affecting nouns and other substantive words, was well documented before epochal observations of Paul
Broca ushered in the modern era of aphasiology. A man who lost the "memory of all substantives" as well as the "power to name the substantives" was
reported in 1745 by Linnaeus (3), the Swedish botany taxonomist. In his 1812
Medical Inquiries and Observations upon the Diseases of the Mind, Benjamin
Rush, father of American psychiatry and a signer of the Declaration of In-
dependence, described a form of memory derangement that he characterized
as follows: "There is an oblivion of names and vocables, and a substitution
of a word no ways related to them. Thus I knew a gentleman, afflicted with
this disease, who, in calling for a knife, asked for a bushel of wheat" (4, p.
276). Chamberet (5) in 1818 reported the history of a 40-year-old artillery
officer who during the course of a febrile illness entirely lost the ability to
name persons or objects. Intelligence was not otherwise affected, but speech
was, by necessity, characterized by vague circumlocutions. Jean-Baptiste
Bouillaud, an important predecessor of Broca, noted in 1825 that the loss
of memory for words was one of the means by which speech could be impaired by cerebral lesions, and he cited an observation in which word loss
was confined largely to nouns (6). Larrey's case 3 years later was that of a
French soldier shot in the left frontal lobe who survived to resume his mili-
tary career but remained incapable of producing proper names or the names
of objects (7).

Word-finding difficulty was often conceptualized as being due to a circumscribed form of memory deficit. Based primarily on his own aphasic symptoms of 1825, Jacques Lordat (8,9) later distinguished *verbal amnesia* — which
indicated a loss of memory limited to word sounds and their oral usage —
from a more generalized loss of memory. Paraphasic errors were clearly described. In his initial reports beginning in 1861, Broca used the term *aphemia*
to describe the language disorder now known as Broca's aphasia (10–13)
but by 1867 (14,15) he had broadened his classification scheme to incorporate
Lordat's *verbal amnesia*. Broca's concept was similar to that of Lordat: verbal amnesia was the "loss of words as a result of the loss of the memory of
words" (15, p. 266). The same year, William Ogle extended their views in
describing *amnemonic aphasia* as an inability to "translate ideas into symbols. . . . In all cases . . . it appears to be a constant fact that grammatical
form is observed; only substantives are substituted for substantives, verbs
for verbs, numerals for numerals, proper names for proper names" (16, pp.
94,95). In his 1869 monograph *On Aphasia*, Bateman reported an instruc-
tive case and remarked that it was "singular that substantives and proper

names which are first acquired by memory in childhood should be sooner forgotten than verbs, adjectives, and other parts of speech which are of much later acquisition" (14, p. 69).

The term *paraphasia* was coined by Adolph Kussmaul in 1877 to indicate the "inability to properly connect word-images and the corresponding conceptions, so that, instead of the ones corresponding to the sense, misplaced or entirely incomprehensible word-images present themselves" (17, p. 749). He defined *amnesic aphasia* as "true aphasia" (p. 748) and as the "incapacity for the recollection of words as acoustic aggregates of sound" (p. 749). Elaborating, he stated, "the association between word and idea is interrupted" (p. 757). He noted that "[p]roper names and substantives in general are the words which are most frequently forgotten" (p. 758). This distinction between parts of speech was interpreted in terms of nouns being more concrete than other, more abstract, words: "We can conceive that the processes of excitation and the combinations in the cellular networks of the cerebral cortex must be much more numerous for the creation of an abstract than of a concrete conception, and the organic tracts which connect the former with its name must be correspondingly much more numerous than those of the concrete" (p. 759).

In considering patterns of anomic deficits under the rubric of *partial amnesia for signs*, Ribot in 1882 observed that the recollection of proper names is lost before that of substantives, and that the latter in turn precedes the loss of adjectives: "We see at first glance that the progress of amnesia is from the particular to the general. It first effaces proper names which are purely individual, then the names of concrete things, then substantives not formed from adjectives, and, finally, adjectives, and verbs which express qualities, states of being, and acts. Signs directly expressive of quality are the last to disappear" (18, p.166). He added, "other things being equal, a term has more chances of being repeated and fixed in the memory the greater the number of objects it represents, and the least chance of being repeated and fixed in the memory the smaller the number represented" (p. 167).

Varieties of Anomic Aphasia and Brain Localization

By the late nineteenth century, most writers on aphasia—e.g., Lichtheim (19), Wernicke (20), Bastian (21), and Freud (22)—had adopted the view that "concepts" were represented in a widespread manner within the cerebral cortex and did not assign a special role for naming to any discrete portion of the left cerebral hemisphere. Others, however, maintained that naming deficits could be especially prominent after circumscribed cortical damage. Two regions within the left cerebral hemisphere in particular came to be identified with anomic aphasia: the inferior temporal lobe and the inferior parietal lobule.

William Broadbent (23) in 1879 postulated the existence of a discrete "idea" or "naming" center, which he conjectured to be located on the posterior undersurface of the left temporal lobe. From clinical-anatomical observations in a woman with a temporal-lobe glioma, the Philadelphia neurologist Charles Mills (24) in 1895 also localized a naming center to the left inferior temporal gyrus. His patient was unable to name objects by sight or touch, although she promptly recognized the correct names when they were provided for her. Mills proposed that it was through actions of this center that "names are correlated with the concrete concepts of the objects named" (25, p. 375). In Sweden, Henschen's (26) exhaustive analyses led him to conclude that naming defects were especially associated with pathology in the left middle and inferior temporal gyri, a view adopted by Kinnier Wilson (27) in England and Johannes Nielsen (28) in Los Angeles. These authors also pointed out that anomia commonly arose from otic abscesses affecting this portion of the inferior temporal lobe. Of more recent note, selective anomia has been reported from electrical stimulation of the contiguous basal region of the left occipitotemporal gyrus (29).

One of those who distinguished among varieties of anomia was the preeminent English neurologist Henry Head, who described *nominal aphasia* as "essentially a loss of power to use names and want of comprehension of the nominal value or meaning of words and other symbols" (30, p. 414). Its "essential defect is inability to fit a name to an object or an object to a name" (p. 415). Based on a limited number of observations, Head believed that lesions of the left angular gyrus were particularly apt to cause nominal defects. He interpreted this localization in terms of the proximity of the angular gyrus to the visual cortex, with visual features being particularly important to word meaning. *Semantic aphasia*, characterized by a lack of recognition for the "ultimate significance and intention of words and phrases, apart from their direct meaning" (p. 416) was associated with lesions in the vicinity of the left supramarginal gyrus.

From their extensive analyses, Weisenburg and McBride identified *amnesic aphasia* as a clear-cut clinical syndrome consisting "essentially of a difficulty in evoking words as names for objects, conditions, or qualities" (31, p. 299). They found no precise localization of damage within the left hemisphere that was associated with amnesic aphasia. According to Kurt Goldstein, the principal symptom of amnesic aphasia was the "lack of nouns, adjectives, verbs and especially names for concrete objects in speech" (32, p. 246). These patients need not present any other disturbance in speech. Goldstein recognized that word-finding difficulty could be due to different causes, and he reserved the designation of amnesic aphasia for cases in which there were impairments in what he termed *abstract attitude*. The abstract attitude was required for more than a simple association between the sounds of a word and its object.

In Goldstein's view, the act of naming required that an object be experienced as representing a category. Goldstein believed that amnesic aphasia was uncommon and most often associated with tumors or abscesses in the left temporal-parietal region (32).

Luria (1) saw little localization value in anomia per se, but he also distinguished among several naming defects. Lesions of the left superior temporal lobe produced *acoustic aphasia*. Patients with this disorder lack a precise sound structure of words and produce frequent phonological paraphasias. Patients with *acoustic-mnestic* (amnestic or anomic) aphasia associated with lesions of the left middle temporal gyrus have word-finding difficulty characterized by circumlocutions and semantic paraphasias, but they do not evince phonological errors. Phonological cuing is of little benefit to these patients but can help amnestic aphasics whose lesion involves the left inferior parietal lobule. With lesions of the left frontal lobe, Luria (1) contended that patients could name concrete objects but had marked difficulties in recalling words during spontaneous speech, perhaps due to an executive dysfunction.

Geschwind (33) characterized patients with "classic" *anomic aphasia* as having difficulty in naming manifest by failure to produce a response, semantic and phonological paraphasias, or circumlocutory descriptions. This was viewed as a distinct syndrome. Understanding is spared, in that patients can usually choose the correct name if it is offered by the examiner and select a named object from a group of objects. In attributing anomic aphasia to lesions of the left angular gyrus, Geschwind (33,34) envisioned this region as a multimodal association area that contained "rules" for finding a specific word given its semantic attributes; here sensory information could be matched to the appropriate spoken word. Geschwind noted that lesions of both the left middle temporal gyrus and the left angular gyrus are associated with anomic aphasia. He argued that this dual localization is not necessarily conflicting; these two gyri are in fact anatomically continuous with each other, and they might serve similar functions (35).

Benson (36) distinguished three principle varieties of anomia. Articulatory difficulty or phonological paraphasias characterizes *word production anomia*, which accompanies Broca's aphasia or conduction aphasia. These patients benefit from phonological cues. Aphasics with *word selection anomia* can point to named objects that they are unable to name spontaneously, yet they do not benefit from phonological cues. Their lesion corresponds to the inferior temporal "naming center" described by previous writers. Individuals with *semantic anomia* also benefit poorly from prompts, but they are unable to select a correct item from an array when the name is offered. Benson suggested that the responsible lesion for his third variety lies in the left angular gyrus (36).

CLINICAL ASSESSMENT OF NAMING

The neurological basis of language can be inferred from analyses of patients with focal brain injury [e.g., gunshot wounds (37–40) or stroke (41,42)] or with more widely distributed alterations [e.g., Alzheimer's disease (43–47) or nonpenetrating traumatic brain injury (48–50)]. Recent techniques of direct cortical stimulation (51,52) and functional neuroimaging (53) have confirmed and expanded views of brain–behavior relationships derived from traditional methods. Naming impairments can affect any part of speech and different parts of speech can be differentially affected, but, as already indicated, most studies of naming have emphasized the production of nouns.

Naming abilities can be evaluated through an examination of a patient's speech or through more constrained naming tasks. Speech can be elicited conversationally or it can be assessed during structured discourse tasks. For example, a subject might be asked to produce a narrative account of what typically occurs at a birthday party, or to describe what is depicted in a drawing of a complex scene. More constrained naming tasks include categorical naming (e.g., "Tell me the names of tools that a carpenter might use") or naming to definition and responsive naming (e.g., "When I want to see my reflection, I look in the . . . ?). The most commonly employed naming task is confrontation naming, in which a patient is shown an object and asked to provide its name. According to Goodglass and Kaplan, "Naming to visual presentation is a universally used test for aphasia since virtually all aphasic patients have some loss of capacity to perform" (2, p. 40). Confrontation naming offers the virtue of offering a known target for naming without providing phonological cues as to the intended name. It can involve any sensory modality (auditory, gustatory, olfactory, tactile, or visual), but naming deficits in aphasia are usually independent of modality (54,55). Visual tasks are most often used in clinical and research settings. As explained by Head, "If I am asked to name an object placed before me, I recognize that it possesses certain characteristic qualities and attempt to find the verbal symbol which expresses them adequately. Now, in daily life the recognition of these qualities is mainly dependent on sight; detailed meaning . . . [is] largely based on visual impressions" (30, p. 502). Visual confrontation naming can involve real objects, photographs of real objects, or drawings of objects, but, for most aphasics, enhancing perceptual detail (e.g., photographs versus line drawings) does not augment naming performance (56–58). Consisting of 60 black-and-white line drawings that range in difficulty from bed to abacus, the Boston Naming Test (59) is one example of a visual confrontation naming task commonly used in clinical practice and research to assess naming performance.

Among aphasic patients, a *frequency effect* has been observed for naming errors. Word names less frequently encountered in a language, as estimated from standard word counts, are less likely to be produced correctly on visual confrontation naming tasks (60–62). Factors other than word frequency also influence naming. These include age at acquisition (63), grammatical class (64), imagibility, concreteness, and "operativity" (65). The last concept distinguishes discrete objects that can be manipulated or operated upon (e.g., vase or rock) from other objects that cannot (e.g., ceiling or cloud).

PROCESSES INVOLVED IN VISUAL CONFRONTATION NAMING

Although anomia is nearly ubiquitous among aphasics, it is important to emphasize that word-finding difficulty has both linguistic and nonlinguistic determinants. With regard to visual confrontation naming, several general stages can be heuristically identified [see discussions by Caramazza and Berndt (66), Goodglass (67), and Humphreys et al. (68)]. Such a categorization should not imply that a particular stage represents a discrete cognitive process identified with a circumscribed neurological substrate, that stages occur sequentially rather than in parallel, or that processing is unidirectional rather than bidirectional. Moreover, disturbances in other cognitive domains (e.g., attention) can impinge upon different aspects of the naming process.

An object to be named must first be perceived and perceptually analyzed. Perceptual parsing and object recognition is a complex process (69) that may benefit from feedback that occurs during lexical semantic processing (69, 70). Such perceptual features as color, shape, or motion may involve different neural substrates (71) and can be differentially affected by brain lesions. It remains controversial whether semantic memory is organized on the basis of verbal–nonverbal distinctions and according to different sensory modalities, or whether semantic representation is better conceptualized as a unified system (72–75).

Perceptual identification is followed by a search of semantic memory and lexical-semantic identification. Semantic memory may be accessed at different levels of semantic specification. For example, a picture of a robin, which is a typical exemplar from the superordinate category of birds, is likely to be named as *bird*, whereas an atypical exemplar such as ostrich is more likely to elicit *ostrich* as a response (76). Theoretically, phonology could follow semantic processing or be accessed directly after visual identification has occurred. It is likely, however, that phonological access normally occurs only after lexical semantic processing [but see cases of Schwartz et al. (77) and Silveri et al. (78)]. Finally, prior to overt speech production, a motor articulatory sequence must be activated, whose neural substrate includes premotor and motor cortices concerned with movements of the lips, tongue, palate, and respiration.

Incomplete semantic specification might occur because of an actual loss of lexical semantic information necessary to define a lexical item or word or because extant semantic information is not fully accessed, retrieved, and utilized. Defects in semantic processing could result in vague, circumlocutory responses or semantic paraphasic errors (e.g., "many-fingered fellow" or "sea urchin" for *octopus*). Phonological paraphasias (e.g., "occupus" for *octopus*) are attributed to deficits in phonological access or realization. This inference is supported by observations from aphasic patients with damage to the left cerebral hemisphere; those whose naming errors were predominantly phonological tended to perform well on semantic discrimination tasks (79). However, semantic errors might also occur when phonological specifications of the correct target word cannot be retrieved if those of a semantically related lexical item remain accessible (80). Indeed, semantic paraphasias are produced by most patients with aphasia due to damage of the left cerebral hemisphere, and this error type does not distinguish among diagnostic aphasic subgroups (81,82). Phonological paraphasias thus appear to represent defects in phonological access and processing, whereas semantic errors are associated with lexical deficits at either a semantic stage or (less commonly) at a phonological stage. As discussed below, perceptual misidentification can also lead to naming errors that sometimes share semantic (as well as perceptual) features with target items.

For some patients, naming deficits appear to be limited to discrete realms of semantic knowledge [e.g., errors might occur only for names of fruits and vegetables (83–87)]. The existence of category-specific anomia can be construed to indicate that semantic memory is represented or organized by categories, perhaps hierarchically within discrete neuroanatomical loci. However, other interpretations are plausible (88), and results from connectionist neural models of semantic representation argue that category-specific deficits require only that language processing involve information about functional, perceptual, and other attributes, and that these attributes be represented in a distributed fashion (89).

LEXICAL REPRESENTATION:
NEUROANATOMICAL CONSIDERATIONS

Naming depends on phonology, semantics, and nonlinguistic cognitive factors. Because of individual variability in the localization of language functions (51,90) and because processes involved in language tasks may involve widely distributed regions of the brain (53), it may not be possible to delineate rigid boundaries for brain regions responsible for specific aspects of naming. Naming errors are common after lesions that affect the left cerebral hemisphere (1,90–92) and most aphasiologists have long viewed regions of the left cerebral hemisphere abutting the Sylvian fissure as committed to language functions [e.g., Dejerine's concept of the *zone du langage* (93)]. Prior to Dejerine, Kussmaul (17), Lichtheim (19), and Wernicke (20) had already formulated the notion of so-called transcortical pathways—to use Wernicke's term (20)—which were deemed to be essential for concepts related to word meaning. The transcortical aphasias were considered to represent damage to these pathways or to association cortex from which they arose, and findings from patients with transcortical aphasia and other forms of aphasia help elucidate phonological and semantic processes involved in naming. Severe mixed transcortical aphasia (94-96) in the setting of border-zone ischemic injury that spares perisylvian cortical areas is postulated to reflect residual functions of a left-hemispheric perisylvian language zone bereft of input from encircling neocortical structures. In the face of profound impairments in propositional language, the striking preservation of oral repetition and serial speech implies that phonological knowledge is represented within residual perisylvian structures. One study of anomic patients with small lesions of the left hemisphere found phonological paraphasias to be particularly associated with lesions of the insula and subjacent putamen (90), and structures deep to the perisylvian cortex should also be considered in this anatomical formulation.

On the other hand, semantic knowledge is disrupted or lost in transcortical aphasia despite preservation of the perisylvian core, suggesting that lexical semantic representations involve brain regions other than the perisylvian cortex. Focal perisylvian damage might affect word-finding by disrupting phonological representations or by impeding retrieval of semantic information, but lexical semantic representation appears relatively spared when injury does not extend beyond the perisylvian core (97). Depending on the extent and location of injury, however, damage to cortex and transcortical pathways extrinsic to perisylvian regions could lead to an actual loss of semantic information, to an access or retrieval disturbance, or to both (96). Semantic knowledge is relatively preserved in transcortical motor aphasia (98) after damage to anterior regions of the left cerebral hemisphere, but it is disrupted in transcortical sensory aphasia (98-100) after more posterior damage. Other studies of aphasic patients support the view that semantic disturbances are more prominent after lesions of posterior rather than anterior regions of the left hemisphere (90-92,101,102). The general formulation that emerges is that phonological processing necessary for oral naming is a function of left-hemisphere perisylvian language areas, but that lexical semantic processing during a naming task depends on more posterior cortical association regions extrinsic to a central language core. For most adult right-handers, contributions of the right cerebral hemisphere to lexical semantic representation remain controversial.

LEXICAL SEMANTIC DISTURBANCES AND ANOMIA

Lexical semantic disturbances might entail impaired access to (or arousal within, or retrieval from) an intact semantic lexicon. Alternatively, disturbances might be due to an actual loss of semantic information that defines individual lexical items or words (103). Most theories of access dysfunction imply variable word-finding difficulty for individual words (103) (assuming that lexical access is not item-specific). An item misnamed on one occasion might be correctly named on another occasion or in a different context. For example, shown a wristwatch, a patient with an access disturbance might reply, "Oh, I have one at home," but be unable to provide the correct name. However, the same patient may later be able to name a watch. Alternatively, the examiner may have been able to elicit the correct response through responsive naming or by giving the initial sound of the intended target ("When I want to know what time it is, I look at my . . . ," or "The name sounds like *wa . . .*"). Here, the (arguable) assumption is that if the patient can arrive at the correct response, then the problem was one of lexical access rather than lexical loss (103,104).

Naming errors that consistently involve the same target items do not, in and of themselves, prove a loss of lexical information. Perceptual misidentification, for example, might also result in consistent errors (105). However, a profound loss of semantic information implies that a word not named on one occasion cannot be named on other occasions or in different contexts.

In aphasic patients with focal damage to the left cerebral hemisphere, anomia might be associated with a phonological or semantic disturbance, and these factors might differ among different patients. The ease with which cuing facilitates naming performance in aphasia (106) and the fact that many patients evince a "tip-of-the-tongue" phenomenon (107) support the view that lexical semantic organization is not disrupted in these patients. Some aphasics who produce semantic paraphasias also produce informative circumlocutions, and they can identify superordinate or functional information about unnamed target words (82); these results also imply at least some preservation of the knowledge about a target word. Gainotti et al. (108) distinguished between aphasics with and without semantic comprehension disorders. Although the severity of the naming deficits was comparable in the two groups, subjects with poor comprehension retained less knowledge of the phonological structure of the intended target word and produced more semantic paraphasias. Results were interpreted as suggesting that word-finding difficulty could result from different mechanisms, with the poor-comprehension subgroup experiencing difficulties in the lexical semantic system itself (108). Butterworth et al. (109) found a strong relationship between anomia and impairments in semantic comprehension. However, their aphasic subjects were as likely to name pictures that they had failed to identify as those with which they had made no errors, implying a variable inability to access or retrieve semantic knowledge. Their findings were partially supported by Huff et al. (110), who concluded that naming deficits in patients with left-hemisphere stroke implicated a lexical access disturbance as well as the loss of lexical semantic information.

Naming errors elicited on visual confrontation tasks are common in Alzheimer's disease (43–47,111–115). Most — but not all — errors appear to lie within a lexical semantic domain (43,45,111,113,116,117). Patients with Alzheimer's disease tend to make errors with the same items whose names are probed on different semantic tasks and to show a loss of knowledge about items they are unable to name (118,119), suggesting that the semantic impairment in this disorder, at least in part, involves a loss of information. In addition, naming errors in Alzheimer's disease tend to be consistent over time (110, 114,119), a finding that supports the semantic-loss hypothesis for Alzheimer's disease. When compared to aphasic stroke patients, patients with Alzheimer's disease were found by Margolin et al. (120) to be relatively less impaired on a lexical phonological task (controlled oral word association) than they were on a confrontation naming task, suggesting relatively greater semantic impairments in the demented group and phonological impairments for stroke patients.

Taken together, experimental findings imply that a loss of semantic information may play a larger role in the anomia of Alzheimer's disease than the word-finding difficulty that typically accompanies focal lesions of the left hemisphere. However, as with stroke patients, naming performance is enhanced when patients with Alzheimer's disease (44,47,104) are provided with phonological cues about target items. Because such prompts might aid in lexical retrieval, the improvement can be interpreted to indicate that a disturbance in lexical access or retrieval contributes to anomia. However, if lexical deterioration or lexical semantic loss represents a gradual erosion of knowledge about specific semantic attributes that define lexical items, then phonological cues might also improve performance by promoting the selection of a correct lexical item from among previously indistinguishable members of a semantic category (114,121). For example, residual semantic knowledge might permit a patient presented with a picture of a helicopter to identify it as "something that flies up above" but not to differentiate it from an airplane. The phonological cue *hel* could then facilitate retrieval of the correct phonological label from among semantically plausible targets. This scenario is compatible with a theory of lexical semantic loss in Alzheimer's disease in which cuing compensates for incomplete semantic specifications of some lexical items in addition to facilitating retrieval of residual lexical information (114).

NONLINGUISTIC DETERMINANTS OF ANOMIA

Both linguistic and nonlinguistic factors can affect influence naming. Two examples of nonlinguistic influences on visual confrontation naming are presented below, but these by no means exhaust the relevant possibilities.

Attention

The concept of attention encompasses both (1) general arousal, alertness, or vigilance and (2) selectivity, such that some stimuli (e.g., those in a certain spatial location or those having particular physical features) are processed more efficiently than others. The fact that inattention commonly affects naming was acknowledged a century ago by Freud, who remarked that "paraphasia observed in aphasic patients does not differ from the incorrect use and the distortion of words which the healthy person can observe in himself in states of fatigue or divided attention" (22, p. 13). An acute confusional state, or delirium, is characterized by primary deficits in the ability to maintain or shift attention and is often associated with systemic metabolic disturbances that diffusely affect the brainstem and the cerebral hemispheres. Confusion can also be prominent in patients with frank structural pathology (e.g., herpes encephalitis, infarction in the distribution of the right posterior cerebral artery, or traumatic brain injury). Word-finding difficulty is prominent in confusional states (122), but the underlying neural substrates for language need not be disrupted. As a consequence, inattentive or confused subjects remain linguistically competent, and an object misnamed on one occasion can be correctly named on another.

As argued above, a loss of lexical semantic information appears to disrupt naming performance in many patients with Alzheimer's disease. However, attentional deficits are common in this disorder and might also contribute to anomia. An attentional disturbance should imply lexical retrieval deficits and thus *inconsistency* in naming performance. Experimentally, this appears to be the case, as demented patients who are inconsistent in their naming performance have greater attentional deficits (123,124) and Alzheimer's disease patients who show behavioral evidence of poor attention benefit less well from semantic priming (125). Mildly impaired patients show greater naming consistency on naming tasks than do those who are moderately impaired (126). Findings suggest that the loss of lexical information may be an important determinant of anomia in Alzheimer's disease, but that superimposed attentional deficits, which presumably increase as a function of disease severity, may impair naming independently of informational loss (124).

Visual Perception

Defects at early, or "peripheral," stages of visual processing can, of course, impede visual confrontation naming. Thus, patients with senile macular degeneration or severe glaucoma might evince obvious naming difficulty confined to visually presented material. Confusion arises only when the examiner fails to consider ocular pathology in patients with acquired brain damage. The question of peripheral defects might also arise in patients with Alzheimer's disease, in which contributions of retinal ganglion degeneration (127) may be difficult to isolate from more central pathological alterations.

Impaired visual object recognition from cerebral lesions is referred to as visual *agnosia* (128). In the classical formulation of Lissauer (129), some patients with visual agnosia—those with so-called apperceptive agnosia—evince visual perceptual defects that impede object identification, for example, through a failure of shape discrimination (128) or through the failure to integrate information about shapes (130). Other patients, those with so-called associative visual agnosia (129), perceive normally (e.g., they can draw a picture of a presented object), yet they still cannot describe or mime its function and they cannot name it. Patients with visual agnosia will be unable to demonstrate knowledge about an object that they see but will be able to name the object perceived through another sensory modality.

The complex interplay between confrontation naming, perception, and attention is especially suggested by *simultanagnosia* (131–133) or impaired simultaneous perception. Patients with this disorder can identify individual parts of a complex visual array but cannot integrate isolated elements into a coherent whole. The patient of Thaiss and De Bleser (134), for example, was unable to name a line drawing of a refrigerator (drawn with its door open) but could name small items depicted on the refrigerator shelf. The primary defect may be a constriction of attention or an inability to shift attention from one visual feature to another.

Occasional patients with modality-specific naming impairments are of considerable theoretical interest. For example, patients with *optic aphasia* have naming deficits limited to visually presented objects; naming to touch or sound remains intact (135–139). The deficit differs from that of associative visual agnosia in that optic aphasics can sometimes show how to use objects that they are unable to name and thus show partial knowledge about the object, although some patients show features of both associative agnosia and optic aphasia (140). One interpretation of optic aphasia is that visual information does not permit access to other aspects of lexical semantic information (a visual–verbal disconnection) (136,137). Modality-specific misnaming has also been described for tactile (141,142) and auditory stimuli (143).

Perceptual misidentification may contribute to misnaming in Alzheimer's disease. For example, a patient may name a drawing of a pretzel as a *rope, chain, worm,* or *rattlesnake* (144). Errors that visually resemble target items are common in some studies (44,47,145–147), and naming is facilitated by allowing demented patients to handle as well as to see target objects (148).

Perceptually based naming errors are especially sensitive to visual degradation of the quality of the target (149). Error classification is at times problematic, and many errors share both visual and semantic features with the target item (e.g., a picture of a beaver variously misnamed as a *muskrat, platypus, mouse, rat, badger, squirrel, otter, groundhog, possum, chipmunk,* or *gopher*) (144). In patients with Alzheimer's disease, these so-called mixed errors are more strongly predicted by perceptually based errors than by semantically based errors with other naming items, implying a strong perceptual determinant for many mixed errors (147).

CONCLUDING NOTE

Because anomia occurs after impairments in different aspects of language, naming disorders are a sensitive indicator of aphasia, and naming performance should always be evaluated in the aphasic patient. However, the presence of anomia per se does elucidate underlying mechanisms for the aphasia. The foregoing discussion considers phonological and semantic contributions to naming errors, but aphasic deficits that affect word morphology or alter pragmatic aspects of communication might also be reflected in naming performance in certain tasks. Furthermore, other factors affect the naming process, some of which are considered above. Elucidation of how lingustic and nonlinguistic domains impact at the level of the single word can serve as a probe for normal cognitive functioning, and studies of naming will continue to be informative for the cognitive neuroscientist.

REFERENCES

1. Luria AR. Higher cortical functions in man. New York: Basic Books, 1966.
2. Goodglass H, Kaplan E. The assessment of aphasia and related disturbances. 2nd ed. Philadelphia: Lea & Febiger, 1983.
3. von Linné C. Glömska af alla Substantiva och i synnerhet namn. Kongl Swenska Wetenskaps Academiens Handlingar 1745;6:116–117. Cited in: Borenstein P. Forgetfulness of all substantives and especially names — Carl von Linné's description of case of aphasia from 1745. Presented at the 31st Annual Meeting of the Academy of Aphasia, Tucson, AZ, Oct 25, 1993.
4. Rush B. Medical inquiries and observations upon the diseases of the mind. Philadelphia: Kimber & Richardson, 1812:276–290. Fascimile reprint: New York: Hafner, 1962.
5. Chamberet, Perte de la mémoire des noms substantifs, survenu à la suite d'une fièvre intermittent. Journal Complémentaire du Dictionaire des Sciences Médicales 1818;2:364–367.
6. Bouillaud J. Traité clinique et physiologique de l'encéphalite, ou inflammation du cerveau. Paris: J-B Baillière, 1825:194–196,283–291.

7. Larrey. Wound of the brain, with loss of the memory of substantives. Journal de Physiologie de Magendie 1828;8. Cited in: Bateman F. On aphasia, or loss of speech, and the localisation of the faculty of articulate language. 2nd ed. London: J & A Churchill, 1890:186–187.

8. Lordat J. Analyse de la parole pour servir à la théorie de divers cas d'alalie et de paralalie (de mutisme et d'imperfection du parler) que les nosologistes ont mal connus. Journal de la Société de Médecine-Pratique de Montpellier 1843;7:333–353,417–433;8:1–17.

9. Henderson VW. Jacques Lordat's contributions to aphasiology. In: Rose FC, ed. Neuroscience across the centuries. London: Smith-Gordon, 1989:177–184.

10. Broca P. Remarques sur le siège de la faculté du langage articulé, suivies d'une observation d'aphémie (perte de la parole). Bull Soc Anat (Paris) 1861;6(2nd series):330–357.

11. Broca P. Sur le siège de la faculté du langage articulé. Bull Soc Anthrop (Paris) 1865;6:377–393.

12. Henderson VW. Alalia, aphemia, and aphasia. Arch Neurol 1990;47:85–88.

13. Henderson VW. Paul Broca's less heralded contributions to aphasia research. Historical perspective and contemporary relevance. Arch Neurol 1986;43:609–612.

14. Bateman F. On aphasia, or loss of speech in cerebral disease. London: JE Adlard, Bartholomew Close, 1868:63–78.

15. Broca P. Sur le siège de la faculté du langage articulé. Trib Med 1869;3:254–256,265–269.

16. Ogle W. Aphasia and agraphia. St George's Hospital Reports 1867;2:83–122.

17. Kussmaul A. Disturbances of speech. An attempt in the pathology of speech. In: von Ziemssen H, ed. Cyclopedaedia of the practice of medicine. Vol 14. New York: William Wood, 1877:581–875.

18. Ribot T. Diseases of Memory. An essay in the positive psychology. London: Kegan Paul, Trench, 1882:151–173.

19. Lichtheim L. On aphasia. Brain 1885;7:433–484.

20. Wernicke C. Einige neueren Arbeiten über Aphasie. Fortschritte der Medizin 1885;3:824 and 1886;4:371,463. In: Eggert EH, trans. Wernicke's works on aphasia. New York: Mouton, 1977:173–205.

21. Bastian HC. On different kinds of aphasia, with special reference to their classification and ultimate pathology. Brit Med J 1887;2:931–936,985–990.

22. Freud S. Zur Auffassung der Aphasien: Eine kritische Studie. Leipzig and Vienna: Franz Deuticke, 1891. In: Stengel E, trans. On aphasia: A critical study. New York: International Universities Press, 1953.

23. Broadbent WH. A case of peculiar affection of speech with commentary. Brain 1879;1:484–503.

24. Mills CK, McConnell JW. The naming centre, with the report of a case indicating its location in the temporal lobe. J Nerv Ment Dis 1895;22:1–7.

25. Mills CK. Aphasia and the cerebral zone of speech. Am J Med Sci 1904;43:375–393.

26. Henschen SE. Clinical and anatomical contributions on brain pathology. Arch Neurol Psychiatry 1925;13:226–249.

27. Wilson SAK. Aphasia. London: Kegan Paul, Trench, Trubner, 1926:70–79.
28. Nielsen JM. Agnosia, apraxia, aphasia. Their value in cerebral localization. Los Angeles: Los Angeles Neurological Society, 1936.
29. Lüders H, Lesser RP, Hahn J, et al. Basal temporal language area demonstrated by electrical stimulation. Neurology 1986;36:505–510.
30. Head H. Aphasia and kindred disorders of speech. Vol 1. Cambridge, England: Cambridge University Press, 1926:381–512.
31. Weisenburg T, McBride KE. Aphasia. A clinical and psychological study. New York: Commonwealth Fund, 1935:299–316.
32. Goldstein K. Language and language disturbances. New York: Grune & Stratton, 1948:246–291.
33. Geschwind N. The varieties of naming errors. Cortex 1967;3:97–112.
34. Geschwind N. Disconnexion syndromes in animals and man. Brain 1965;88:237–294,585–644.
35. Geschwind N. Problems in the anatomical understanding of the aphasias. In: Benton AL, ed. Contributions to clinical neuropsychology. Chicago: Aldine, 1969:107–128. Reprinted in: Geschwind N. Selected papers on language and the brain. Boston: D Reidel Publishing, 1974:431–451.
36. Benson DF. Neurologic correlates of anomia. In: Whitaker H, Whitaker HA, eds. Studies in neurolinguistics. Vol 4. New York: Academic Press, 1979:293–328.
37. Marie P, Foix C. Les aphasies de guerre. Rev Neurol (Paris) 1917;24:53–87.
38. Russell WR, Espir MLE. Traumatic aphasia. A study of aphasia in war wounds of the brain. London: Oxford University Press, 1961.
39. Newcombe F. Missile wounds of the brain. London: Oxford University Press, 1969.
40. Luria AR. Traumatic aphasia. Its syndromes, psychology and treatment. The Hague: Mouton, 1970.
41. Kertesz A. Aphasia and associated disorders. Taxonomy, localization, and recovery. New York: Grune & Stratton, 1979.
42. Tonkonogy JM. Vascular aphasia. Cambridge, MA: MIT Press, 1986.
43. Appell J, Kertesz A, Fisman M. A study of language functioning in Alzheimer patients. Brain Lang 1982;17:73–91.
44. Kirshner HS, Webb WG, Kelly MP. The naming disorder of dementia. Neuropsychologia 1984;22:23–30.
45. Bayles KA, Tomoeda CK. Confrontation naming impairment in dementia. Brain Lang 1983;19:98–114.
46. Cummings JL, Benson DF, Hill MA, Read S. Aphasia in dementia of the Alzheimer type. Neurology 1985;35:394–397.
47. Williams BW, Mack W, Henderson VW. Boston Naming Test in Alzheimer's disease. Neuropsychologia 1989;27:1073–1079.
48. Heilman KM, Safran A, Geschwind N. Closed head trauma and aphasia. J Neurol Neurosurg Psychiatry 1971;34:265–269.
49. Levin HS, Grossman RG, Kelly PJ. Aphasic disorder in patients with closed head injury. J Neurol Neurosurg Psychiatry 1976;39:1062–1070.
50. Levin HS, Grossman RG, Sarwar M, Meyers CA. Linguistic recovery after closed head injury. Brain Lang 1981;12:360–374.

51. Ojemann GA. Individual variability in cortical localization of language. J Neurosurg 1979;50:164–169.
52. Ojemann GA, Whitaker HA. Language localization and variability. Brain Lang 1978;6:239–260.
53. Posner MI, Petersen SE, Fox PT, Raichle ME. Localization of cognitive operations in the human brain. Science 1988;240:1627–1631.
54. Goodglass H, Barton MI, Kaplan EF. Sensory modality and object-naming in aphasia. J Speech Hear Res 1968;11:488–496.
55. Spreen O, Benton AL, Van Allen MW. Dissociation of visual and tactile naming in amnesic aphasia. Neurology 1966;16:807–814.
56. Corlew MM, Nation JE. Characteristics of visual stimuli and naming performance in aphasic adults. Cortex 1975;11:186–191.
57. Hatfield FM, Howard D, Barber J, Jones C, Morton J. Object naming in aphasics—the lack of effect of context or realism. Neuropsychologia 1977;15:717–727.
58. Seron X, Monsel J, Vanderlinden M, Vander-Kaa MA, Remitz A. Dénomination orale et aphasie: étude de trois contextes différents. Psychologica Belgica 1980;20:205–213.
59. Goodglass H, Kaplan E, Weintraub S. The Boston Naming Test. Philadelphia: Lea & Febiger, 1983.
60. Rochford G, Williams M. Studies in the development and breakdown of the use of names. Part IV. The effects of word frequency. J Neurol Neurosurg Psychiatry 1963;28:407–413.
61. Newcombe FB, Oldfield RC, Wingfield A. Object-naming in dysphasic patients. Nature 1965;207:1217–1218.
62. Kirshner HS, Casey PF, Kelly MP, Webb WG. Anomia in cerebral diseases. Neuropsychologia 1987;25:701–705.
63. Rochford G, Williams M. Studies in the development and breakdown of the use of names. The relationship between nominal dysphasia and the acquisition of vocabulary in childhood. J Neurol Neurosurg Psychiatry 1962;25:222–227.
64. Caramazza A, Hillis AE. Lexical organization of nouns and verbs in the brain. Nature 1991;349:788–790.
65. Gardner H. The contribution of operativity to naming capacity in aphasic patients. Neuropsychologia 1973;11:213–220.
66. Caramazza A, Berndt RS. Semantic and syntactic processes in aphasia: a review of the literature. Psychol Bull 1978;85:898–918.
67. Goodglass H. Disorders of naming following brain injury. Am Sci 1980;68:647–655.
68. Humphreys GW, Riddoch MJ, Quinlan PT. Cascade processes in picture identification. Cognit Neuropsychol 1988;5:67–103.
69. Biederman I. Recognition-by-components: a theory of human image understanding. Psychol Rev 1987;94:115–147.
70. Caramazza A, Berndt RS, Brownell HH. The semantic deficit hypothesis: perceptual parsing and object classification by aphasic patients. Brain Lang 1982;15:161–189.
71. Desimone R, Ungerleider LG. Neural mechanisms of visual processing in monkeys. In: Boller F, Grafman J, eds. Handbook of neuropsychology. Vol 2. New York: Elsevier, 1990:267–299.

72. Warrington EK. The selective impairment of semantic memory. Q J Exp Psychol 1975;27:635–657.
73. Shallice T. Specialisation within the cognitive system. Cognit Neuropsychol 1988;5:133–142.
74. Caramazza A, Hillis AE, Rapp BC, Romani C. The multiple semantics hypothesis: multiple confusions? Cognit Neuropsychol 1990;7:161–189.
75. Shallice T. Multiple semantics: whose confusions? Cognit Neuropsychol 1993; 10:251–261.
76. Jolicoeur P, Gluck MA, Kosslyn SM. Pictures and names: making the connection. Cognit Psychol 1984;16:243–275.
77. Schwartz MF, Marin OSM, Saffran EM. Dissociations of language function in dementia: a case study. Brain Lang 1979;7:277–306.
78. Silveri MC, Giustolisi L, Daniele A, Gainotti G. Can residual lexical knowledge concern word form rather than word meaning? Brain Lang 1992;43:597–612.
79. Gainotti G, Miceli G, Caltagirone C, Silveri MC, Masullo C. The relationship between type of naming error and semantic-lexical discrimination in aphasic patients. Cortex 1981;17:401–410.
80. Caramazza A, Hillis AE. Where do semantic errors come from? Cortex 1990; 26:95–122.
81. Kohn SE, Goodglass H. Picture-naming in aphasia. Brain Lang 1985;24:266–283.
82. Le Dorze G, Nespoulous J-L. Anomia in moderate aphasia: problems in accessing the lexical representation. Brain Lang 1989;37:381–400.
83. Yamadori A, Albert ML. Word category aphasia. Cortex 1973;9:112–125.
84. Warrington EK, Shallice T. Category specific semantic impairments. Brain 1984;107:829–854.
85. Hart J Jr, Berndt RS, Caramazza A. Category-specific naming deficit following cerebral infarction. Nature 1985;316:439–440.
86. Satori G, Job R. The oyster with four legs: a neuropsychological study on the interaction of visual and semantic information. Cognit Neuropsychol 1988;5: 105–132.
87. Sacchett C, Humphreys GW. Calling a squirrel a squirrel but a canoe a wigwam: a category-specific deficit for artefactual objects and body parts. Cognit Neuropsychol 1992;9:73–86.
88. Humphreys GW, Riddoch MJ. On telling your fruit from your vegetables: a consideration of category-specific deficits after brain damage. Trends Neurosci 1987;10:145–148.
89. Small SL, Hart J Jr, Nguyen T, Gordon B. Distributed representations of semantic knowledge in the brain. Soc Neurosci Abstr 1993;19:844.
90. Knopman DS, Selnes OA, Niccum N, Rubens AB. Recovery of naming in aphasia: relationship to fluency, comprehension and CT findings. Neurology 1984; 34:1461–1470.
91. Coughlan AK, Warrington EK. Word-comprehension and word-retrieval in patients with localized cerebral lesions. Brain 1978;101:163–185.
92. Newcombe F, Oldfield RC, Ratcliffe GG, Wingfield A. Recognition and naming of object-drawings by men with focal brain wounds. J Neurol Neurosurg Psychiatry 1971;34:329–340.

93. Dejerine J, Dejerine-Klumpke A. Anatomie des Centres Nerveux. Vol 2. Paris: J Rueff, 1901:247–252.
94. Geschwind N, Quadfasel FA, Segarra JM. Isolation of the speech area. Neuropsychologia 1968;6:327–340.
95. Assal G, Regli F, Thuillard F, Steck A, Deruaz J-P, Perentes E. Syndrome d'isolément de la zone du langage. Rev Neurol (Paris) 1983;139:417–424.
96. Henderson VW. Profound mixed transcortical aphasia: implications for language representation within the brain. Bull Clin Neurosci 1989;54:158–162.
97. Cappa S, Cavallotti G, Vignolo LA. Phonemic and lexical errors in fluent aphasia: correlation with lesion site. Neuropsychologia 1981;19:171–177.
98. Davis L, Foldi NS, Gardner H, Zurif EB. Repetition in the transcortical aphasias. Brain Lang 1978;5:226–238.
99. Brendt RS, Basili A, Caramazza A. Dissociation of functions in a case of transcortical sensory aphasia. Cognit Neuropsychol 1987;4:79–107.
100. Alexander MP, Hiltbrunner B, Fischer RS. Distributed anatomy of transcortical sensory aphasia. Arch Neurol 1989;46:885–892.
101. Lhermitte F, Derouesné J, Lecours AR. Contribution à l'étude des troubles sémantiques dans l'aphasie. Rev Neurol 1971;125:81–101.
102. Hart J Jr, Gordon B. Delineation of single-word semantic comprehension deficits in aphasia, with anatomical correlation. Ann Neurol 1990;27:226–231.
103. Gainotti G. The status of the semantic-lexical structures in anomia. Aphasiology 1987;1:449–461.
104. Neils J, Brennan MM, Cole M, Boller F, Gerdeman B. The use of phonemic cueing with Alzheimer's disease patients. Neuropsychologia 1988;26:351–354.
105. Shuttleworth EC, Huber SJ. A longitudinal study of the naming disorder of dementia of the Alzheimer type. Neuropsychiatry Neuropsychol Behav Neurol 1989;1:267–282.
106. Pease DM, Goodglass H. The effects of cuing on picture naming in aphasia. Cortex 1978;14:178–189.
107. Goodglass H, Kaplan E, Weintraub S, Ackerman N. The "tip-of-the-tongue" phenomenon in aphasia. Cortex 1976;12:145–153.
108. Gainotti G, Silveri MC, Villa G, Miceli G. Anomia with and without lexical comprehension disorders. Brain Lang 1986;29:18–33.
109. Butterworth B, Howard D, McLoughlin P. The semantic deficit in aphasia: the relationship between semantic errors in auditory comprehension and picture naming. Neuropsychologia 1984;22:409–426.
110. Huff FJ, Mack L. Mahlmann J, Greenberg S. A comparison of lexical-semantic impairments in left hemisphere stroke and Alzheimer's disease. Brain Lang 1988;34:262–278.
111. Martin A, Fedio P. Word production and comprehension in Alzheimer's disease: the breakdown of semantic knowledge. Brain Lang 1983;19:124–141.
112. Skelton-Robinson M, Jones S. Nominal dysphasia and the severity of senile dementia. Brit J Psychiatry 1984;145:168–171.
113. Flicker C, Ferris SH, Crook T, Bartus RT. Implications of memory and language dysfunction in the naming deficit of senile dementia. Brain Lang 1987; 31:187–200.

114. Henderson VW, Mack W, Freed DM, Kempler D, Andersen ES. Naming consistency in Alzheimer's disease. Brain Lang 1990;39:530-538.
115. Mack W, Williams BW, Freed DM, Henderson VW. Boston Naming Test: shortened version for use in Alzheimer's disease. J Gerontol 1992;47:P154-158.
116. Smith SR, Murdoch BE, Chenery HJ. Semantic abilities in dementia of the Alzheimer type. 1. Lexical semantics. Brain Lang 1989;36:314-324.
117. Hodges JR, Salmon DP, Butters N. The nature of the naming deficit in Alzheimer's and Huntington's disease. Brain 1991;114:1547-1558.
118. Huff FJ, Corkin S, Growdon JH. Semantic impairment and anomia in Alzheimer's disease. Brain Lang 1986;28:235-249.
119. Chertkow H, Bub D. Semantic memory loss in dementia of Alzhemer's type. What do various measures measure? Brain 1990;113:397-417.
120. Margolin DI, Pate DS, Friedrich FJ, Elia E. Dysnomia in dementia and in stroke patients: different underlying cognitive deficits. J Clin Exp Neuropsychol 1990;12:597-612.
121. Wingfield A, Goodglass H, Smith KL. Effects of word-onset cuing on picture naming in aphasia: a reconsideration. Brain Lang 1990;39:373-390.
122. Chédru F, Geschwind N. Disorders of higher cortical functions in acute confusional states. Cortex 1972;8:395-411.
123. Kempler D, Andersen E, Hunt M, Henderson VW. Linguistic and attentional contributions to anomia in Alzheimer's disease. J Clin Exp Neuropsychol 1990;12:398.
124. Henderson VW, Mack W, Kempler D, Andersen ES, Petrucco CM. Lexical loss and retrieval deficits in the anomia of Alzheimer's disease. Ann Neurol 1990;30:239.
125. Hartman M. The use of semantic knowledge in Alzheimer's disease: evidence for impairments of attention. Neuropsychologia 1991;29:213-228.
126. Knotek PC, Bayles KA, Kaszniak AW. Response consistency on a semantic memory task in persons with dementia of the Alzheimer type. Brain Lang 1990;38:465-475.
127. Hinton DR, Sadun AA, Blanks JC, Miller CA. Optic-nerve degeneration in Alzheimer's disease. N Engl J Med 1986;315:485-487.
128. Warrington EK. Agnosia: the impairment of object recognition. In: Vinken PJ, Bruyn GW, Klawans HL, Frederiks JAM ed. Handbook of clinical neurology. Vol 45. Clinical neuropsychology. Amsterdam: Elsevier, 1985:333-349.
129. Lissauer H. Ein Fall von Seelenblindheit nebst einem Beitrag zur Theorie derselben. Archiv für Psychiatrie und Nervenkrankenheit 1890;21:222-270. In: Jackson M, trans. A case of visual agnosia with a contribution to theory. Cognit Neuropsychol 1988;5:157-192.
130. Riddoch MJ, Humphreys GW. A case of integrative visual agnosia. Brain 1987;110:1431-1462.
131. Wolpert I. Die Simultanagnosie—Störung der Gesamtauffasung. Zeitschrift für die gesamte Neurologie und Psychiatrie 1924;93:397-415.
132. Kinsbourne M, Warrington E. Disorder of simultaneous form perception. Brain 1962;85:461-486.
133. Levine DN. Calvanio R. A study of the visual defect in verbal alexia—simultanagnosia. Brain 1978;101:65-81.

134. Thaiss L, De Bleser R. Visual agnosia: a case of reduced attentional "spotlight"? Cortex 1992;28:601–621.
135. Freund CS. Über optische Aphasie und Seelenblindheit. Archiv für Psychiatrie und Nervenkrankheiten 1889;20:276–297;371–416. In: Beaton A, Davidoff J, Erstfeld U, trans. On optic aphasia and visual agnosia. Cognit Neuropsychol 1991;8:21–38.
136. Poeck K. Neuropsychological demonstration of splenial interhemispheric disconnection in a case of "optic anomia." Neuropsychologia 1984;22:707–713.
137. Lhermitte F, Beauvois MF. A visual-speech disconnexion syndrome. Report of a case with optic aphasia, agnosic alexia and colour agnosia. Brain 1973; 96:695–714.
138. Gil R, Pluchon C, Toullat G, Micheneau D, Rogez R, Lefevre JP. Disconnexion visuo-verbale (aphasie optique) pour les objects, les images, les couleurs et les visages avec alexie "abstractive." Neuropsychologia 1985;23:333–349.
139. Riddoch MJ, Humphreys GW. Visual object processing in optic aphasia: a case of semantic access agnosia. Cognit Neuropsychol 1987;4:131–185.
140. Iorio L, Falanga A, Fragassi NA, Grossi D. Visual associative agnosia and optic aphasia. A single case study and a review of the syndromes. Cortex 1992; 28:23–37.
141. Beauvois MF, Saillant B, Meininger V, Lhermitte F. Bilateral tactile aphasia: a tacto-verbal dysfunction. Brain 1978;101:381–401.
142. Endo K, Miyasaka M, Makishita H, Yanagisawa N, Sugishita M. Tactile agnosia and tactile aphasia: symptomatological and anatomical differences. Cortex 1992;28:445–469.
143. Denes G, Semenza C. Auditory modality-specific anomia: evidence from a case of pure word deafness. Cortex 1975;11:401–411.
144. Logan C, Buckwalter JG, Henderson VW. Boston Naming Test error analysis in Alzheimer's disease (abstr). Soc Neurosci Abstr 1992;18:736.
145. Rochford G. A study of naming errors in dysphasic and in demented patients. Neuropsychologia 1971;9:437–443.
146. Cormier P, Margison JA, Fisk JD. Contribution of perceptual and lexical-semantic errors to the naming impairments in Alzheimer's disease. Perceptual Motor Skills 1991;73:175–183.
147. Henderson VW, Logan CL, Buckwalter JG. Semantic and perceptual predictors of "ambiguous" confrontation errors in Alzheimer's disease. Presented at the 31st Annual Meeting of the Academy of Aphasia, Tucson, AZ, Oct 26, 1993.
148. Barker MG, Lawson JS. Nominal aphasia in dementia. Brit J Psychiatry 1968; 114:1351–1356.
149. Tweedy JR, Schulman PD. Toward a functional classification of naming impairment. Brain Lang 1982;15:193–206.

8

PET in Aphasia and Language

E. Jeffrey Metter

Gerontology Research Center, National Institute on Aging,
National Institutes of Health, Baltimore, Maryland

INTRODUCTION

A major interest in behavioral neurology is to understand the organization of language in the brain. Two approaches are used in such studies: to study language function in normal individuals and to study changes that occur in language performance in the presence of brain damage. Although the two approaches focus on very different kinds of processes, the resulting conclusions about language organization and the role of the brain are quite similar. To carry out such studies, methods are needed to understand the anatomy and physiology of the brain under normal and abnormal conditions.

Current approaches to studying brain–behavior relationships are dependent on modern tomographic imaging techniques including x-ray computed tomography (CT), magnetic resonance imaging (MRI), positron emission tomography (PET), and single-photon emission tomography (SPECT). The first two techniques are used to study structural anatomy, while the latter two focus on physiological measures. The structural anatomy is particularly valuable in studying brain–behavior relationships through experiments of nature: subjects who develop focal or diffuse brain damage. Anatomical techniques are less useful for studying language in normal subjects. The structural damage in patients is assumed to cause the behavioral problems, although lesions may also have functional effects on other, nondamaged brain regions.

PET and SPECT make it possible to explore the consequences of structural damage on other regions by measuring the physiology of nondamaged parts of the brain. The physiology of the damaged brain under resting conditions is compared to that of normal controls. A second approach is to use PET and SPECT to examine physiological changes during the activation of the brain with specific controlled tasks. Such activation studies compare the subject in at least two states controlled by the experimenter.

This chapter examines the current understanding of brain physiology in relation to language as derived from PET and SPECT. The focus is on studies that have been done in aphasia, but a discussion of activation studies in normals is also included.

BRAIN IMAGING: GENERAL CONSIDERATIONS

PET and SPECT are emission tomographic methods based on the detection of gamma-ray emissions from intravenously injected radioisotopes. They are able to measure physiological parameters such as regional cerebral blood flow (rCBF), oxygen and glucose metabolism, and other biochemical processes. The two methods are distinguished by the type of radiopharmaceuticals and equipment employed.

PET uses positron-emitting isotopes, which have very short half-lives, necessitating the availability of a cyclotron. When emitted positrons collide with electrons, both are annihilated, creating two photons that travel 180° in opposite directions. By locating both photons using a pair of detectors, a line of origin can be established for the annihilation. By detecting a large number of such annilations, a computer can establish a map of the concentration of the radionuclide, much as is done for x-ray transmission using CT. Current PET equipment has a spatial resolution on the order of 3 to 4 mm, which does not approach that of CT or MRI. In the future, the resolution should improve to approximately 1 to 2 mm. The disadvantage of lower resolution is that most deep structures are not well resolved because of their smaller size, variable shapes, and nearness to other structures (1,2). The limitations are not so great as to negate the usefulness of the approach, but they must be considered in any interpretation.

A number of radionuclides are available that can be used to create isotopes that model physiological and biochemical processes, including (18F)-fluorodeoxyglucose (FDG) for glucose metabolism, (15O)-oxygen to measure oxygen metabolism, (15O)-water to measure cerebral blood flow, (18F)-DOPA for L-DOPA uptake, and (18F)-N-methylspiperone or 11C-raclopride for dopamine receptors. Techniques are being developed to study a number of brain receptors and other processes.

SPECT also employs isotopes injected intravenously. It differs from PET in that the radionuclides emit one gamma photon, which is located by using a collimator that acts as a filter, allowing only those photons within a specific path to be detected. Spatial resolution depends on the number of gamma counts and the diameter and length of the holes in the collimator. A resolution of 7 to 9 mm has been obtained with newer rotating three-headed gamma cameras. At present two radioisotopes are available to measure cerebral blood flow: N-isopropyl-p-iodoamphetamine (IMP) and 99mTc hexamethylpropylene amine oxide (HMPAO). These radiotracers have longer half-lives than positron emitters and do not require an on-site cyclotron.

What is measured by PET and SPECT is dependent on underlying physiological models. Two models are primarily used with PET: FDG to study glucose metabolism and oxygen-15 to study blood flow. FDG is a competitive inhibitor of glucose in mammalian cells. It is transported into the cell and phosphorylated in the same manner as glucose, but it cannot be processed further. Thus, the uptake of FDG parallels the cell's utilization of glucose, making FDG a marker of glucose uptake and metabolism. When used clinically, FDG is injected intravenously into the subject, who lies quietly for a period of about 40 minutes while the FDG is taken up by cells and equilibrium is reached. During this time, repeated arterialized venous blood samples are taken to describe the blood curve for the isotope. After 40 minutes, the brain is scanned to measure the distribution of 18F. Models have been developed that allow for the calculation of glucose metabolism based on the blood curve and the distribution of 18F uptake (3).

The accuracy of the FDG method is dependent on the number of photons detected, the stability of the model under pathological conditions, and the kinetic and lump constants used in the calculations. The major advantage of FDG over other PET methods currently used to examine blood flow and metabolism is that multiple high-resolution images can be obtained with 18F because of its approximate 2-hour half-life (as compared to the short, several-minute half-life of oxygen-15). The long half-life, however, makes FDG less than ideal for studying the activation of the brain during mental activities. Activation studies have been done with FDG, but interpretation can be difficult because of the 40-minute uptake period, and only one scan a day can be done. Activation studies are more appropriate with cerebral blood flow studies, in which the scan is completed in less than 10 minutes. This is part of the quandary in PET studies. The ideal isotopes for most studies use radionuclides with short half-lives, but to optimize the resolution of the resulting tomographs, a large number of counts is required, necessitating longer scanning times, a longer isotope half-life, or larger doses.

Oxygen-15 has a short half-life that allows for scanning over minutes. The shorter scanning time comes at the price of fewer radioactive counts, limiting resolution. A variety of models have been developed to measure cerebral blood flow using oxygen-15 (4–6). Models vary in how the oxygen is delivered, i.e., injected or inhaled. To obtain accurate measures of blood flow, an arterial line is necessary to determine a blood curve. Frequently, such arterial samples are not collected, and regional counts of oxygen-15 are obtained and expressed in relationship to some standard measure. The latter approach gives a relative index of regional cerebral blood flow. In normal subjects, changes in cerebral blood flow are closely associated with changes in cerebral metabolic rates and with neuronal activity (7–9).

MEANS OF STUDYING BRAIN-BEHAVIOR RELATIONSHIPS

Glucose metabolism and cerebral blood flow are highly state-dependent. An active brain utilizes more energy and requires greater blood flow than a resting brain. Two general approaches have been used to study the brain. One is to examine subjects in a resting state, with no attempt to regulate brain function. What the subject thinks about is uncontrolled and may affect the images. This approach has been used most commonly to study specific brain diseases. Resting studies are frequently done with room lights dimmed and with minimization of noise. In addition, some labs attempt sensory deprivation by plugging the ears and/or covering the eyes. These changes alter the pattern of glucose metabolism. Without such sensory deprivation, cerebral glucose metabolism is symmetrical in the left and right hemispheres (10–12).

The second approach is to use specific activations to control the thinking processes or to inject drugs to alter brain function. The subject is asked to complete specific tasks during the procedure. Duara et al. (13) believe that using a controlled task reduces the intersubject variability, making for more valid analyses, although Cameron et al. disagree (14). The activation approach is typically used to compare the effects of a task on a baseline state. Most functional activation studies use cerebral blood flow rather than metabolism. The advantage is that the scans take only a few minutes to complete, but at a sacrifice of spatial resolution. Techniques to subtract one set of images from a second set allow for the direct comparison of two brain states, such as the difference in brain function in seeing a word and naming a word. At present, it is not unusual to have three or four stepped tasks, with each succeeding task showing increasing complexity. The analysis consists of subtracting each scan from the one preceding it in the sequence. The resulting image represents regions specifically activated in response to the differences in the two tasks.

Such comparisons assume that energy utilization increases in a linear fashion as the involvement of a region in a task increases. If a brain region is important for a specific behavioral task, then that region should show greater energy utilization while the subject is doing the task than while he is not. The difference between the region activated by the task and the region at baseline can be analyzed by parametric statistics. This assumption is critical to the activation models, based on how the data are handled statistically. The assumption does not allow a region to participate in a task at the same energy utilization level as in the comparison state, nor does it specify how small a difference in energy utilization is critical for a specific region. It is possible that a 1–2% change might be critical for one region, while another region may require a 20% increase or decrease to be judged critical.

Few studies have examined this critical assumption in the human brain, and there has been no systematic effort to demonstrate that it is true in all brain regions or under all reported conditions. Fox and Raichle (15) examined the change in cerebral blood flow in visual cortex during varying rates of photic stimulation. They found a linear increase in rCBF in visual cortex from 0 to 7 kHz, but at rates above 15 kHz there was a gradual decline in level of activation. Linear activation occurred only over a limited range of stimuli. Furthermore, they were unable to demonstrate a significant increase in rCBF at 1 kHz as compared to 0 Hz. The warning from the study by Fox and Raichle is that true activation, if small, may be missed, and that, over some ranges of increasing stimulation, increases in rCBF may not occur, even if the region is actively involved in the processing. I am unaware of similar studies involving other brain regions. Some regions, such as visual, primary auditory, and sensory cortices, may be expected to show linear activation, but this may not be the case in more complex association areas where multiple tasks may be performed at the same level of metabolic activity.

Other factors may also be important for differential activation during task performance. Gur et al. (16) used easy and hard verbal analogy problems to explore the effects of anxiety state on global cerebral blood flow. Both easy and hard tasks showed approximately 20% increases in global blood flow as compared to the resting states, while the two tasks differed by only 5 to 10%. Most strikingly, the effect of anxiety was greater than the activation by the analogy problem.

Activation Studies: Normal Subjects

Activation studies seem to demonstrate several patterns of brain activation. The first is a relatively general increase in blood flow and metabolism that appears to be associated with the difficulty of the task and the degree of attention required. It is not unusual to find an increase in global blood flow and/or metabolism in response to a task associated with increase in many brain regions. The presence of such generalized activation makes it difficult to compare some pathological conditions with normal responses. For example, an anomic aphasic patient who is given a naming task may well activate many brain regions not activated by a normal subject, based purely on the increased difficulty of the task because of the anomia. A normal subject given a more demanding (but as difficult for the subject as the standard naming task is for the anomic patient) naming task might show the same activation pattern as the anomic patient. Similarly, using multiple detectors and xenon injection to measure surface cerebral blood flow, Ryding et al. (17) demonstrated a generalized increase in blood flow over much of the cerebral cortex with automatic speech and humming.

The second type of activation patterns are areas that tend to show little activation, even to tasks traditionally associated with the area. For example, it appears to be difficult to activate the supramarginal and angular gyri with many language-related tasks (Table 1, IPL column). This could represent a lack of a role for the regions, the limitations of the activation assumption, or difficulty with regional definition because of the convolutional nature of the gyri in these regions.

The third type of activation pattern involves focal areas of increased or decreased activity that appear to be task-dependent. The activation of visual cortex to visual tasks is an example of such changes.

Table 1 summarizes reported activation studies involving speech, language, and related tasks. The table is not meant to be comprehensive. The references include those in which a large number of specific regions were reported in a form convertible to the table. The key point is that a number of different strategies have been used in these studies. In some, the goal is to determine overall levels of brain activation between two behavioral states. In others, the goal is to find differential regional brain activation between two states. As mentioned earlier, the inferior parietal lobule, which includes the supramarginal and angular gyri, was seldom differentially activated in these paradigms. Additionally, the prefrontal regions and the supplementary motor area were frequently activated for a variety of activities associated with speech and language.

The earliest studies to examine rCBF in language used multiple detectors and xenon to examine cortical blood flow. The resulting maps were of low resolution and were not tomographic in nature. Different speech and language tasks, such as reading, word perception, and speaking, were found to activate different patterns of rCBF in both the left and right cerebral cortex (18). The presence of superior frontal and right-hemisphere activation, which could not be predicted from previous anatomical studies, indicated the potential value of the approach in broadening our understanding of brain-behavior relations. Auditory processing tasks in normal subjects produced significant increases over the left posterior sylvian region, with a trend for the verbal task to evoke a wider area of activation than the nonverbal task (19).

The same task handled by different mental strategies was found to result in different patterns of brain activation. Mazziotta et al. (20) found that, for tone sequences, individuals using highly analytical strategies showed greater left posterior temporal activations, while subjects using a nonanalytical strategy had right-sided activation. They also found that listening to a story produced generalized brain activation, with the greatest changes in the left hemisphere, whereas nonverbal stimuli with musical chords produced predominant right-hemisphere activation. Using SPECT, Goldenberg et al. (21) found that the pattern of rCBF activity in a word-memory task was dependent on the memory strategy. Subjects using a visual imagery strategy activated the left superior temporal regions and bilateral superior frontal regions, while a no-imagery strategy was associated with right-hemisphere activation. All word-memory tasks were associated with the activity of bilateral hippocampal and inferior temporal regions. Lang et al. (22), also with SPECT, found that an imagery task resulted in rCBF increase in both superior frontal lobe regions.

More recent studies have examined word naming using oxygen-15 water. These reports have shown that visual word recognition activates the left occipital lobe and left frontal region but does not specifically activate the parietal lobe, arguing against a role for the angular and supramarginal gyri in the processing of words (23,24). Such observations are at odds with aphasia research, in which focal parietal lesions are typically associated with deficits on such tasks. Steinmetz and Seitz (25) argue that the problem may be in averaging intersubject data rather than in focusing on intrasubject findings. I would suggest that the failure of activation of the left parietal lobe may result from the organization of the parietal association cortex, which behaves like the occipital lobe at 15 kHz of visual activation (15), i.e., where increased activity is associated with little activation.

Frith, Friston, Liddle, and Frackowiak (26) found that a word-fluency task (self-generation of lists) primarily activated prefrontal cortex. They attributed this to "intrinsic generation". The task also demonstrated a decline in activity in superior temporal cortex. An "extrinsic generation" task (deciding if a presented word is or is not a real word) activated the superior temporal gyrus but produced no change in prefrontal cortex. Many studies have indicated the clear importance of prefrontal regions in the generation of responses to word-related tasks. The specificity of the role is less clear.

Bartlett et al. (27) found no clear activation to a phoneme-discrimination task. Using a different conceptual approach, to examine the degree to which regional metabolism changes in relationship to other regions, they found an increase in the number of strong interregional correlations in the left hemisphere, and particularly Broca's region during the phoneme task.

Sergent, Zuck, Terriah, and MacDonald (28), in a sophisticated study of professional musicians, found a systematic increase in regional brain activity as the musical tasks became more complex. Sight-reading and playing on the

Table 1 Summary of Regional Brain Activation in a Selected Series of Reports

Ref.	Task	Baseline	MF	SFG	MFG	IFG	PrG	PoG	SPL	IPL	STG	MTG	ITG	LO	CO	Cin
Xenon inhalation studies: cerebral blood flow																
18	Automatic speech	Rest	−	+/+		+/	+/+	/+			+/+	+/+	/+			
76	Internal math	Rest	−	+/+	+/+	/+				+/+						
76	Internal jingle	Rest	−	+/+	+/+	+/+				+/			/+			
76	Interal route	Rest	−	+/+	+/+	+/+			+/+	+/+			+/+	+/+		
77	Visual symbols	Fixation	−	+/+		+/+			+/+	/+	+/+	/+	/+			
78	loudness	Rest	−								+/					
78	Word meaning	Rest	−								/+					
78	Word rhyme	Rest	−							/+	+/	+/+				
78	Word recognition	Rest									/+	/+				
FDG PET studies: glucose metabolism																
20	Listen story	Rest				+/					+/+	+/+				
20	Timbre	Rest		/+						/+	/+	/+				
79	Non-English words: L ear	Rest			+/+					/+	/+	+/+	/+			
79	Non-English words: R ear	Rest								/+	+/	/+				
Oxygen-15 PET: cerebral blood flow																
80	Visual symbols	Fixation												+/+		
80	Visual letter strings	Fixation	+/											+/+		

80	Visual non-words	Fixation													+/+	+/+
80	Visual words	Fixation	+/											+/+	+/+
23	Visual words	Fixation												+/+	+/+
23	Repeat words	Visual words	+/	+/	+/	+/+									+
23	Say uses words	Repeat	+/	+/											+
23	Auditory words	Fixation					+/+								
23	Repeat words	Auditory words	+/	+/	+/+										+
23	Say uses	Repeat words		+/											
81	Listen non-words	Finger move					+/+								
81	Noun-noun	Finger move					+/+								
81	Verb-noun	Finger move					+/+								
81	Verb list	Finger move	+/	+/			+/								
81	Word fluency	Other	+/				+/	+/							
26	Auditory word/non-word	Other					+/		+/						
24	Noise	Silence	+/+	+/	+/		+/+								+
24	Syllables	Noise		+/			+/	+/							
24	Phonetic	Syllable		+/	/+		+/		/+						/+
24	Pitch	Syllable	+/												+/+

Data presented as left-hemisphere region/right-hemisphere region. A blank means that no significant activation (or decline) was observed. + means a significant change was observed. − means that the region was not measured. MF = mesial frontal; SFG = superior frontal gyrus; MFG = middle frontal gyrus; IFG = inferior frontal gyrus; PRG = precentral gyrus; POG = postcentral gyrus; SPL = superior parietal gyrus; IPL = inferior parietal lobule; STG = superior temporal gyrus; MTG = middle temporal gyrus; LO = lateral occipital; CO = calcarine occipital.

keyboard activated cortical areas adjacent to but not the same as those activated by similar verbal tasks. Based on the activated regions, they argued that note recognition occurred through the spatial location of the notes. Interestingly, the supplementary motor and prefrontal cortex did not appear to be activated during the playing task, or during visual fixation (the baseline condition). The absence of supplementary motor activation during the motor part of the study raises the question as to its role in initiation of movements by professional musicians. The lack of prefrontal activation may reflect the lack of choice decision in the tested tasks. Subjects played what was written and did not improvise (i.e., make decisions on what they played).

Activation Studies: Aphasia

Soh et al. (29) examined rCBF using intracarotid xenon injections with multiple detectors during a speaking task in aphasic subjects. Variations in performance were found based on the nature of the aphasia and the location of flow abnormalities in the resting state. Normal subjects showed activation in the lower rolandic mouth area, the superior frontal region in the area of the supplementary motor cortex, and the posterior temporal area. With nonfluent aphasia, poor speech was associated with a lack of activation in the lower rolandic mouth area and the superior frontal gyrus, but activation did occur in the posterior temporal region. With fluent aphasia, no activation was seen in the posterior temporal region. In global aphasia, no activation was seen in the posterior temporal or rolandic regions, but increased flow was observed in the superior temporal gyrus.

Walker-Batson et al. (30,31), using SPECT, studied rCBF of normal and aphasic subjects during rest, a passive listening task (subjects listened to a series of consonant-vowel syllables), and a phoneme-detection task (subjects identified a particular phoneme when heard). Normal subjects demonstrated bilateral medial frontal activation to the phoneme detection task, while the aphasic patients showed no distinct cortical or subcortical activation, but ipsilateral or contralateral cerebellar activation during phonemic detection. These findings suggest that the frontal-motor system or the corticocerebellar loop was activated during the phoneme-detection task.

Summary

The future for understanding brain performance in specific language tasks is bright, owing to available imaging techniques and activation paradigms. The approach is clearly the wave of the future. Unfortunately, the zeal for the approach has led to the "wow" factor, with many mesmerized by the technology and what it can accomplish. To accomplish genuine advances, however, more effort has to be given to understanding the fundamental assumptions regarding what it means for blood flow or metabolism to increase in a brain region in response to a task, or for the response to be linear. Using subtraction techniques, researchers attempt to remove sequentially layers of brain activation to identify regions specific to a task. Using this approach they argue for distributed functional systems, but little has been done to integrate the resulting zones to confirm the distributed nature of the task in the brain.

RESTING BRAIN STUDIES IN APHASIA

Resting brain metabolism and flow studies have raised a number of new issues regarding the role of brain damage on the pathophysiological status of the brain. In the study of the effects of stroke on brain–behavior relationships (with the emphasis on aphasia), the following has been learned and is discussed in the sections below.

1. Focal brain lesions are associated with widespread, but in some instances predictable, changes in brain metabolism and presumably brain functioning.
2. Focal brain lesions that are clinically silent, defined through anatomical imaging, may lack distant metabolic effects.
3. In aphasia, metabolic changes occur in the temporoparietal regions in essentially all subjects, regardless of the location of the structural lesion.
4. Deep extension of the lesion into subcortical regions, or focal lesions in these areas, damage cortical-subcortical communication with disruption of cortical-basal ganglia-thalamic loops.
5. Correlations of behavioral performance are stronger to regional metabolism than to structural lesion location.
6. Associations exist between brain metabolism and functional recovery in aphasia.

Remote Brain Effects from Focal Brain Lesions in Stroke

Early PET studies in stroke confirmed the findings of remote brain metabolic and blood-flow changes that exceeded the size of the structural lesion, as first noted by xenon blood-flow studies (32). Cortical brain lesions were found to cause metabolic abnormalities in other brain regions, primarily in the ipsilateral hemisphere basal ganglia and thalamus, and in the contralateral cerebellum. Lacunar lesions in the subcortical areas were associated with predictable metabolic abnormalities in cortical regions. Figure 1 shows an example of the distant effects that may be seen with cerebral infarction (33). In this case, the CT and FDG PET studies were done 1 week before death. The CT showed several lacunar infarcts in the left and right internal

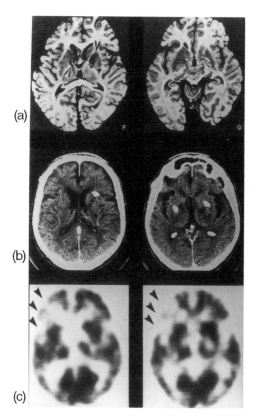

Figure 1 Comparison of (a) gross pathology, (b) CT, and (c) 18-FDG PET from a 69-year-old man with multiple cerebral infarctions who died 10 days after being studied. A metabolic abnormality was found in the left frontal region (left brain is on the left side of the figure) with no gross structural lesion in the area. A lacunar infarct was present in the genu of the left internal capsule with destruction of the anterior limb of the internal capsule. The left frontal hypometabolism appeared to result from the destruction of the anterior limb of the internal capsule. Lacunar infarcts were found in the right corpus striatum, which were not associated with any apparent remote metabolic abnormalities. Thus, slight differences in lesion location were associated with very different metabolic effects. (From Ref. 33.)

capsule/basal ganglia regions, and the same lesions can be seen on the gross section of the brain. The most striking structural lesion was degeneration of the anterior limb of the left internal capsule. The FDG scan shows similar changes in the regions of structural damage. In addition, there was prominent metabolic depression in the overlying left frontal region. No evidence of structural changes on CT, on the gross brain specimen, or on histological examination were found in this part of the frontal lobe. The case demonstrated the consequence to frontal lobe metabolism of a disconnection of the left frontal region from its input and output through the internal capsule. The infarcts in the right lenticular region did not damage the internal capsule and were not associated with remote metabolic effects.

Remote metabolic changes have been found in all symptomatic stroke cases we have studied. These have included decreased activity in the ipsilateral thalamus in both acute and chronic stages following stroke, ipsilateral cortex adjacent and at a distance from the lesion, cerebellar hemisphere contralateral to the cortical lesion, and the hemisphere contralateral to supratentorial infarctions (32,34–40). The presence of distant regions with hypometabolism suggests that function in undamaged tissue may be aberrant, possibly accounting for some aspects of the aphasic language disturbance. Furthermore, the presence of remote metabolic effects in all aphasic patients we have studied argues that remote metabolic changes may be required for persistence of chronic symptoms following a stroke.

In the chronic state, ipsilateral hemispheric hypometabolism is much greater than any change in the contralateral hemisphere. This is true even for lesions interrupting both intrahemispheric and transcallosal nerve fibers. The findings suggest that the impact of intrahemispheric neurons on ipsilateral regions is greater than the effect of transcallosal neurons on the contralateral hemisphere. Remote metabolic changes can clearly be transsynaptic, as is frequently seen when hemispheric lesions cause contralateral cerebellar hypometabolism. Such observations argue that different neuronal connections have distinct distant physiological and biochemical effects.

In acute infarction, areas of reduced rCBF appear earlier and usually larger than lesions seen on CT, and show more prominent contralateral changes than remain in chronic stages (41–44). As the infarct matures, two zones of abnormalities can be identified: a central zone with markedly reduced rCBF, which is the infarcted area seen on CT, and an area of hypoperfusion immediately surrounding the central zone called the *ischemic penumbra*. The ischemic penumbra is not seen on CT and is probably a result of deafferentation (45). Occasionally, an area of hyperemia (increased blood flow) is observed in an area surrounding the cerebral infarction (46).

Structural Brain Lesions with No Remote Metabolic Effects

In a number of subjects, small structural lesions were found by CT in the basal ganglia, internal capsule, and cerebral cortex that were not associated with known clinical findings (47,48). On FDG PET, no glucose metabolic abnormalities were found other than at the site of structural damage for these lesions. As an example, one right-handed woman who had volunteered as a normal control was found to have a lesion in the right hemisphere by CT, bordering on the right posterior putamen and posterior limb of the internal capsule (47). The FDG PET study was totally normal except for the area of the focal lesion. Detailed neuropsychological and memory evaluations in this woman were normal. The observation that asymptomatic focal structural lesions show no evidence of remote metabolic changes in the brain raises the hypothesis that, for a focal structural brain lesion to be symptomatic, it must have a functional effect on other brain areas outside the locus of structural damage. Such observations argue that lesion location and perhaps size may be critical.

Noncritical parts of the putamen may be damaged with little consequence. How lesions and remote metabolic effects in these asymptomatic subjects differ from symptomatic lesions is critical to the understanding of the remote metabolic abnormalities identified by PET.

Temporoparietal Metabolic Abnormalities in Aphasia

Models of the pathoanatomy of aphasia have been based on the correlation of the language disruption following a stroke with the areas of the brain damaged by infarction or hemorrhage. The observation that symptomatic focal brain lesions are associated with remote metabolic changes suggests that focal brain lesions have clear effects on other parts of the brain, and that such remote effects may play important roles in the resulting symptoms. Such observations appear to allow for unifying concepts regarding the development of aphasia following stroke, since not only can the lesion be studied, but also its consequences on other brain regions.

We examined the distribution of glucose metabolic abnormalities in 44 aphasic patients (49). In an initial analysis of 16 brain regions, 100% of subjects were found to have metabolic abnormalities in the temporoparietal region, regardless of the type of aphasia. This was associated with structural damage in the parietal lobe in 67%, Wernicke's area in 67%, and the posterior middle temporal region in 58%. Using a more detailed anatomical approach, 97% of subjects showed metabolic abnormalities in the angular gyrus, 89% in the supramarginal gyrus, and 87% in the lateral and transverse superior temporal gyrus (Table 2).

Table 2 Percentage of 44 Aphasic Patients[a] with Abnormal Metabolism for Each Reported Region

	Hemisphere	
	Left	Right
Precentral gyrus	78	6
Laterosuperior frontal gyrus	59	0
Middle frontal gyrus	59	0
Inferofrontal gyrus	54	0
Medial prefrontal gyrus	24	2
Superoparietal lobule	38	—
Supramarginal gyus	89	13
Angular gyrus	97	13
Posterocentral gyrus	63	4
Laterosuperior temporal gyrus	87	4
Transverse superior temporal gyrus	87	4
Middle temporal gyrus	2	2
Inferotemporal gyrus	70	70
Occipitotemporal gyrus	9	6
Laterosuperior occipital gyrus	70	10
Lateroinferior occipital gyrus	38	9
Caudate head	69	12
Caudate body	31	13
Putamen	71	0
Thalamus	85	9

[a]Distribution of aphasia type: 8 conduction aphasia, 19 anomic aphasia, 10 Broca's aphasia, 5 Wernicke's aphasia, 1 global aphasia, and 1 transcortical aphasia.
Source: Ref. 49.

The consistent finding of glucose hypometabolism in the left angular, supramarginal, and posterior superior temporal gyri suggests that these areas are essential (but not necessarily specific) for the development of aphasia and supports the concept of a unitary locus of functional abnormality in aphasia. The nature and extent of the aphasia, as argued later, appear to be dependent on a complex interplay between the structural damage and its effects on temporoparietal function and on the remainder of the brain. Although there may be a constant pathophysiology, the complex changes in the brain cause individual differences in the severity and characteristics of the aphasia.

Remote Effects of Subcortical Damage

Metabolic patterns associated with subcortical lesions have been reported by our group (34,50), summarized by Metter (51), and by Baron and his colleagues (52,53), who have more experience with thalamic lesions. We have observed five patterns associated with subcortical lesions. The first involves structural lesions in the basal ganglia and internal capsule that are asymptomatic, as described previously in this chapter (47,48). The other four patterns agree well with the "subcortical aphasia" syndromes discussed in Chapter 4. The second involves small lesions in the left posterior putamen, posterior part of the posterior limb of the internal capsule, or thalamus, resulting in glucose hypometabolism in the left temporoparietal cortex, sometimes associated with aphasia (34). The posterior putamenal lesions appear to disrupt thalamic innervation to the temporoparietal region. The aphasias in the few subjects we have seen with this pattern tend to be mild, with anomia. The third pattern involves anterior lesions in the putamen, internal capsule, and caudate nucleus associated with frontal lobe hypometabolism, including the prefrontal cortex (Figure 1) (33). The structural lesions appear to disrupt corticospinal and corticobulbar pathways, as well as frontal feedback loops that include frontal cortex, striatum, globus pallidus, and thalamus.

The fourth pattern comprises subcortical lesions associated with both frontal and temporoparietal hypometabolism. The lesions tend to be larger, involving both anterior and posterior aspects of the lenticular nuclei, as well as the internal capsule (50). The pattern represents the sum of patterns 2 and 3. The fifth pattern occurs in some patients with thalamic lesions, in whom the metabolic abnormality consists of a mild (5–15% decline) hypometabolism involving most of the hemisphere (50,51,54). We have not found this pattern in any aphasic patients. One hypothesis is that this diffuse hypometabolism results from damage to the nonspecific thalamic activating system (54). Other researchers (52,55,56) have made similar observations in a larger series of subjects with thalamic lesions. Others (57,56) have demonstrated that the cortical patterns are dependent on the damaged thalamic nuclei. The hypometabolism may be related to an abnormality in the maintenance of the overall cortical metabolic environment.

These five patterns are determined by the location of the lesion in the subcortical structures and are associated with cortical hypometabolism, arguing that the behavioral consequences of subcortical structural damage can be explained by the secondary effects of the lesion on cortex. The observations do not answer the question of whether subcortical structures have a direct role on the resulting behavior, independent of the indirect effects on the cortex. To address this question, we modeled the relationship of subcortical structural damage with cortical hypometabolism on behavior using path analysis (57). The models demonstrated that subcortical structural damage had a direct effect on fluency but not on comprehension. In addition, subcortical structures influenced the behavior indirectly through their actions on the frontal lobes. The internal capsule appears to be the most critical of the subcortical structures studied. Damage to the internal capsule may disrupt motor pathways, including the frontal-basal ganglia feedback loop involved with the control and management of speech production. Correlations between lesions of the head of the caudate and behavioral measures indicate that the caudate operates at a level related to recognition or motor planning of simple and overlearned material, including simple syntax, low levels of abstraction, and identification or sequencing of phonetic and semantic material (58).

Behavioral Correlations Are Stronger to Metabolism than to the Structural Lesion

Metabolic patterns were compared between Wernicke's, Broca's, and conduction aphasias (Fig. 2) (59). All three syndromes showed metabolic abnormalities in the temporoparietal region, although conduction aphasia was associated with less hypometabolism than the other two. The three syndromes differed in the extent of metabolic abnormalities in the prefrontal cortex, a part of the brain not felt to be directly involved in aphasia. Broca's aphasia was associated with marked hypometabolism throughout the left frontal lobe, including the prefrontal cortex. Wernicke's aphasia showed a more modest degree of frontal lobe hypometabolism, with prefrontal changes in about 50% of subjects. Conduction aphasic patients in general had little hypometabolism in the prefrontal regions, while about half had hypometabolism in Broca's area (60).

These striking differences in prefrontal hypometabolism raise questions as to the role of the prefrontal cortex in aphasic syndromes. The constancy of metabolic abnormalities in the left temporoparietal regions indicate a role in the production of aphasia.

If the level of metabolic abnormality reflects the degree of functional impairment for a region, then correlations with performance on aphasia tests should reflect on regional brain–behavior relationships. Pearson product moment correlations were determined between regional glucose metabolism and scores from the Western Aphasia Battery (WAB) (Table 3) (49). Significant correlations ($p < 0.01$; $r = 0.38$) were found with most left-hemisphere regional metabolic measures except for the parietal-precuneus. The only WAB measure that distinguished frontal from temporoparietal regions was the correlation of comprehension with temporoparietal metabolism.

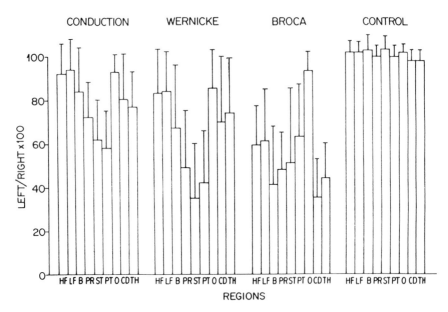

Figure 2 Comparison of regional left-hemisphere to right-hemisphere metabolic ratios for specific brain regions in seven Wernicke's, 11 Broca's, and 10 conduction aphasia patients. Regional abbreviations: HF = superofrontal (prefrontal); LF = inferofrontal (prefrontal); B = Broca's area; PR = inferior parietal lobule; ST = superior temporal (Wernicke's area); PT = posterotemporal; O = occipital; CD = head of caudate; TH = thalamus.

No significant correlations were found between the WAB scores and the right-hemispheric metabolic ratios, so these regions were not included in Table 3. In a previous study (61), we found that correlations of performance on the Boston Diagnostic Aphasia Battery were stronger to metabolic measures than to structural lesions. The major language-related subtests correlated with left temporoparietal metabolism. Likewise, Demonet et al. (55), using SPECT in 14 aphasic subjects, found that auditory comprehension correlated strongly with temporoparietal metabolism. Various regions showed correlations to the overall aphasia score.

Association of Brain Metabolism to Functional Recovery

The prognosis for aphasia recovery has shown a strong relationship to rCBF using xenon-inhalation measurements with multiple detectors during activation tests (62). Poor prognosis for recovery was associated with absence of

Table 3 Correlations Between Left-Hemisphere Regional Measures of Glucose and Scores on the Western Aphasia Battery

	AQ	Spont. speech	Comp.	Rep.	Naming	Read	Write
Lat. superior frontal g.	0.51[a]	0.65[a]	0.20	0.39[a]	0.45[a]	0.49[a]	0.52[a]
Medial superior frontal g.	0.31	0.38[a]	0.13	0.18	0.35	0.30	0.31
Middle frontal g.	0.53[a]	0.66[a]	0.18	0.41[a]	0.49[a]	0.48[a]	0.52[a]
Inf. frontal g.	0.57[a]	0.69[a]	0.25	0.48[a]	0.53[a]	0.51[a]	0.53[a]
Parietal-precuneus	0.22	0.26	0.18	0.14	0.20	0.19	0.30
Sup. parietal lobule	0.31	0.34	0.27	0.24	0.27	0.31	0.45[a]
Inf. parietal lobule	0.42[a]	0.47[a]	0.20	0.39[a]	0.38[a]	0.43[a]	0.52[a]
Supramarginal g.	0.42[a]	0.45[a]	0.29	0.41[a]	0.34	0.39[a]	0.41[a]
Angular g.	0.38[a]	0.31	0.46[a]	0.36	0.34	0.32	0.36
Lat. superior temporal g.	0.60[a]	0.59[a]	0.44[a]	0.58[a]	0.53[a]	0.50[a]	0.49[a]
Trans. superior temporal g.	0.47[a]	0.49[a]	0.30	0.46[a]	0.40[a]	0.36	0.31
Middle temporal g.	0.57[a]	0.47[a]	0.60[a]	0.53[a]	0.54[a]	0.53[a]	0.47[a]
Inf. temporal g.	0.46[a]	0.44[a]	0.45[a]	0.39[a]	0.41[a]	0.42[a]	0.38[a]

[a] $p < 0.01$ for $p = 0.01$ $r = 0.38$. The glucose measurements were regional to mean right-hemisphere glucose metabolism.

AQ = aphasia quotient; Spont. speech = spontaneous speech; Comp. = comprehension; Rep. = repetition.

The regional measures are the left-hemisphere region divided by the average right-hemisphere metabolic rate.

Source: Ref. 49.

increased flow in bilateral fronto-temporal regions during counting, conversation, and listening to music. Better aphasia recovery was associated with rCBF increases in the area homologous to Broca's area in the nondominant hemisphere. Knopman et al. (63,64), also using xenon inhalation with multiple detectors, found that aphasic patients with poor recovery developed increased activation of rCBF to a listening condition in the right inferior frontal region over a 3- to 9-month period that was not found in aphasic patients with good recovery. Walker-Batson et al. (65) studied a crossed-aphasic patient (i.e., aphasia in a right-hander resulting from a right-hemisphere lesion) who showed significant improvement over a 10-year period. rCBF was studied during a resting state, silently answering questions from the WAIS information subscale, and performing a mental arithmetic task and a phoneme-detection task. Cerebral activation occurred primarily in the right hemisphere, indicating that the patient was processing language information in this side of his brain. The findings from these studies argue that the nondominant frontal lobe becomes more active during activation procedures. The implications in recovery have been variable, but they may be important in predicting long-term prognosis.

SPECT has been used to predict recovery after cerebral infarction (66–72). The size of rCBF defect is inversely correlated with stroke recovery. Vallar et al. (40) studied the recovery of aphasia secondary to subcortical lesions with SPECT assessments within the first 33 days and at 3 months post-onset. All patients showed marked language improvement. Cortical hypoperfusion was seen for all patients in their initial study; 3-month scans showed significant increases of blood flow in cortical regions, indicating that recovery was likely due to improved cortical function. Bushnell et al. (68) studied 10 aphasic patients within 30 days and again at 3 months post-cerebral infarction. SPECT scans were obtained at the time of initial clinical testing to determine whether these images could predict aphasia recovery. Of all the parameters, only the volume of the defect was found to be predictive of recovery.

Tikofsky et al. (73) studied resting rCBF patterns using SPECT in five aphasic patients 1 year after stroke onset. Two patients with little change in their aphasia demonstrated large rCBF defects associated with infarcted tissue. The three remaining patients with improved aphasia showed reduced but not absent cerebral blood flow in the cortical language regions of the left hemisphere and slightly increased rCBF in regions of the right cerebral hemisphere. Tikofsky et al. (74), using the Boston Naming Test, found that improving aphasic patients showed greater rCBF activity in response to the naming task compared to normals, while the activity of the unimproved aphasic patients was lower than that of the normals.

We have studied eight aphasic patients at two points in time with FDG PET to determine if changes in comprehension were linked to improvement in temporoparietal regional glucose metabolism. Significant correlations were found between time-related changes of left and right temporoparietal regions and the change in the Western Aphasia Battery comprehension score (75).

CONCLUSIONS

The studies reviewed suggest that language requires the interaction of a number of highly integrated systems of the brain. This interaction involves both hemispheres as well as cortical and subcortical structures. Subcortical and prefrontal areas associated with various aspects of arousal, attention, and sequenced planning of response seem particularly important in language and speech. The contralateral cerebellum may also play an important but presumably indirect role. Future studies with SPECT, PET, and other imaging procedures should allow improved understanding of brain function in normal and diseased states.

The major direction of most studies is toward using activation procedures in both normal individuals and those with aphasia. The field is moving rapidly, and little concern is being given to the differences found between classical experiments of nature (studies of patients with focal brain lesions) and what is observed from activation procedures in normals. At some point, such differences will need to be understood, explored, and resolved.

The excitement from SPECT, PET, and xenon studies is the observation of the importance of brain regions other than the classical language cortex in normal language and aphasia. Studies are clearly showing the importance of frontal regions in normal and aphasic language. The role of the parietal lobe (angular and supramarginal gyri) is less clear at present. Aphasia studies argue for its importance, but this is not seen in activation studies (Table 1). Subcortical regions are also important in aphasia, but they are not as strokingly involved in normal activation studies. As such discrepancies are resolved, physiological brain imaging will clearly improve our understanding of normal and aberrant speech and language.

REFERENCES

1. Hoffman EJ, Huang SC, Phelps ME. Quantitation in positron emission tomography. 1. Effect of object size. J Comput Assist Tomogr 1979;3:299–308.
2. Mazziotta JC, Phelps ME, Plummer D, Kuhl DE. Quantitation in positron emission computed tomography. 5. Physical-anatomical effects. J Comput Assist Tomogr 1981;5:734–743.
3. Phelps ME, Huang SC, Hoffman EJ, Selin CS, Sokoloff L, Kuhl DE. Tomographic measurement of local cerebral metabolic rate in humans with F-18 2-fluoro-deoxyglucose: validation of method. Ann Neurol 1979;6:371–388.
4. Jones T, Chesler DA, Ter-Pogossian MM. The continuous inhalation of oxygen-15 for assessing regional oxygen extraction in the brain of man. Br J Radiol 1976; 49:339–343.
5. Frackowiak RSJ, Lenzi GL, Jones T, Heather JD. Quantitative measurement of regional cerebral blood flow and oxygen metabolism in man using ^{15}O and positron emission tomography: theory, procedure and normal values. J Comput Assist Tomogr 1980;4:727–736.
6. Huang SC, Carson RE, Phelps ME. Measurement of local blood flow and distribution volume with short-lived isotopes: a general input technique. J Cereb Blood Flow Metab 1982;2:99–108.
7. DesRosiers MH, Kennedy C, Potlak CS. Relationship between local cerebral blood flow and glucose utilization in the rat. Neurology (Minn) 1974;24:389.

8. Freygang WH, Sokoloff L. Quantitative measurement of regional circulation in the central nervous system by use of radioactive inert gas. Adv Biol Med Phys 1958;6:263-279.
9. Roy CS, Sherrington MB. On the regulation of the blood supply of the brain. J Physiol 1890;11:85-108.
10. Mazziotta JC, Phelps ME, Carson RE, Kuhl DE. Tomographic mapping of human cerebral metabolism: Sensory deprivation. Ann Neurol 1982;12:435-444.
11. Phelps ME, Kuhl DE, Mazziotta JC. Metabolic mapping of the brain's response to visual stimulation: Studies in humans. Science 1981;211:1445-1448.
12. Phelps ME, Mazziotta JC, Kuhl DE, Nuwer M, Packwood J, Metter J, Engel J. Tomographic mapping of human cerebral metabolism: Visual stimulation and deprivation. Neurology 1981;31:517-529.
13. Duara R, Gross-Glenn K, Barker WW, Chng JY, Apicella A, Loewenstein D, Boothe T. Behavioral activation and the variability of cerebral glucose metabolic measurements. J Cereb Blood Flow Metab 1987;7:266-271.
14. Cameron OG, Modell JG, Hichwa RD, Agranoff BW, Koeppe RA. Changes in sensory-cognitive input: effects on cerebral blood flow. J Cereb Blood Flow Metab 1990;10:38-42.
15. Fox PT, Raichle ME. Stimulus rate dependence of regional cerebral blood flow in human striate cortex, demonstrated by positron emission tomography. Neurophysiol 1984;51:1109-1120.
16. Gur RC, Gur RE, Skolnick BE, Resnick SM, Silver FL, Chawluk J, Muenz L, Obrist WD, Reivich M. Effects of task difficulty on regional cerebral blood flow: relationships with anxiety and performance. Psychophysiology 1988;25:392-399.
17. Ryding E, Bradvik B, Ingvar DH. Changes of regional cerebral blood flow measured simultaneously in the right and left hemisphere during automatic speech and humming. Brain 1987;110:1345-1358.
18. Larsen B, Skinhoj E, Lassen NA. Variations in regional cortical blood flow in the right and left hemispheres during automatic speech. Brain 1978;101:193-209.
19. Knopman DS, Rubens AB, Klassen AC, Meyer MW, Niccum N. Regional cerebral blood flow patterns during verbal and nonverbal auditory activation. Brain Lang 1980;9:93-112.
20. Mazziotta JC, Phelps ME, Carson RE, Kuhl DE. Tomographic mapping of human cerebral metabolism: auditory stimulation. Neurology 1982;32:921-937.
21. Goldenberg G, Podreka I, Steiner M, Willmes K. Patterns of regional cerebral blood flow related to memorizing of high and low imagery words—an emission computed tomography study. Neuropsychologia 1987;25:473-485.
22. Lang W, Lang M, Goldenberg G. EEG and rCBF evidence for left frontocortical activation when memorizing verbal material. In: Johnson R, Rohrbaugh JW, Parasuraman R, eds. Current trends in event related potential research. New York: Elsevier, 1987:328-334.
23. Peterson SE, Fox PT, Posner MI, Mintum M, Raichle ME. Positron emission tomographic studies of the cortical anatomy of single-word processing. Nature 1988;331:585-589.

24. Zatorre RJ, Evans AC, Meyer E, Gjedde A. Lateralization of phonetic and pitch discrimination in speech processing. Science 1992;256:846-849.

25. Steinmetz H, Seitz RJ. Functional anatomy of language processing: neuroimaging and the problem of individual variability. Neuropsychologia 1991;12:1149-1161.

26. Frith CD, Friston KJ, Liddle PF, Frackowiak RSJ. A PET study of word finding. Neuropsychologia 1991;29:1137-1148.

27. Bartlett EJ, Brown JW, Wolf AP, Brodie JD. Correlations between glucose metabolic rates in brain regions of healthy male adults at rest and during language stimulation. Brain Lang 1987;32:1-18.

28. Sergent J, Zuck E, Terriah S, MacDonald B. Distributed neural network underlying musical sight-reading and keyboard performance. Science 1992;257:106-109.

29. Soh K, Larsen B, Skinhoj E, Lassen NA. Regional cerebral blood flow in aphasia. Arch Neurol 1978;35:625-632.

30. Walker-Batson D, Devous MD, Bonte FJ, Oelschlaeger M. Single-photon emission tomography (SPECT) in the study of aphasia: A preliminary report. In: Brookshire RH, ed. Clinical aphasiology: conference proceedings. Minneapolis: BRK Publications, 1987:313-318.

31. Walker-Batson D, Devous MD, Millay KK, Reynolds S, Ajamani AJ, Grant DE, Bonte F. Tomographic regional cerebral blood flow activation during phoneme detection in normal and aphasic subjects. In: Prescott TE, ed. Clinical aphasiology. Vol 18. Boston: Little Brown, 1989:75-89.

32. Kuhl DE, Phelps ME, Kowell AP, Metter EJ, Selin C, Winter J. Effect of stroke on local cerebral metabolism and perfusion: Mapping by emission computed tomography of 18FDG and 13NH3. Ann Neurol 1980;8:47-60.

33. Metter EJ, Mazziotta JC, Itabashi HH, Mankovich NJ, Phelps ME, Kuhl DE. Comparison of x-ray CT, glucose metabolism and postmortem data in a patient with multiple infarctions. Neurology 1985;35:1695-1701.

34. Metter EJ, Wasterlain CG, Kuhl DE, Hanson WR, Phelps ME. 18FDG positron emission computed tomography in a study of aphasia. Ann Neurol 1981; 10:173-183.

35. Lenzi GL, Frackowiak RS, Jones T. Regional cerebral blood flow (rCBF), oxygen utilization (CMRO2) and oxygen extraction ratio (OER) in acute hemispheric stroke. J Cereb Blood Flow Metabol 1981;1(suppl 1):S504-S505.

36. Baron JC, Bousser MG, Comar D, Duquesnoy N, Sastre J, Castaigne P. Crossed cerebellar diaschisis: A remote functional depression secondary to supratentorial infarction in man. J Cereb Blood Flow Metabol 1981;1(suppl 1):S500-S501.

37. Martin WRW, Raichle ME. Cerebellar blood flow and metabolism in cerebral hemisphere infarction. Ann Neurol 1983;14:168-176.

38. Metter EJ, Kempler D, Jackson C, Hanson WR, Riege WH, Camras LR, Mazziotta JC, Phelps ME. Cerebellar glucose metabolism in chronic aphasia. Neurology 1987;37:1599-1606.

39. Bogousslavsky J, Miklossy J, Regli F. Subcortical neglect: Neuropsychological correlations with anterior choroidal artery territory infarction. Ann Neurol 1988;23:448-452.

40. Vallar G, Perani D, Cappa S, Messa C, Lenzi GL, Fazio F. Recovery from aphasia and neglect after subcortical stroke: neuropsychological and cerebral perfusion study. J Neurol Neurosurg Psychiatry 1988;51:1269-1276.

41. Ackerman RH, Correia JA, Alpert HM, Baron JC, Gouliamos A, Grotta JC, Brownell GL, Taveras JM. Positron imaging in ischemic stroke disease using compounds labelled with oxygen-15. Arch Neurol 1981;38:537-543.

42. Frackowiak RSJ, Wise RJS. Positron tomography in ischemic cerebrovascular disease. Neurol Clin 1983;1:183-201.

43. Hill TC, Magistretti PL, Holman BL, Lee RG, O'Leary DH, Uren RF. Assessment of regional cerebral blood flow (rCBF) in stroke using SPECT and N-isopropyl-1(I-123)-p-iodoamphetamine (IMP). Stroke 1984;15:40-45.

44. Hayman LA, Taber KH, Jhingran SG, Killian JM, Carroll RG. Cerebral infarction: Diagnosis and assessment of prognosis using 123 IMP-SPECT and CT. Amer J Nucl Res 1989;10:557-562.

45. Raynaud C, Rancurel G, Samson Y. Pathophysiologic study of chronic infarcts with I-123 isopropyl iodoamphetamine (IMP): The importance of peri infarct area. Stroke 1987;18:21-29.

46. Bushnell DL, Gupta S, Mlcoch AG, Romyn A, Barnes E, Kaplan E. Demonstration of focal hyperemia in acute cerebral infarction with iodine-123 iodoamphetamine. J Nucl Med 1987;28:1920-1923.

47. Metter EJ. Neuroanatomy and physiology of aphasia: evidence from positron emission tomography. Aphasiology 1987;1:3-33.

48. Metter EJ, Kempler D, Jackson CA, Riege WH, Hanson WR, Mazziotta JC, Phelps ME. Are remote glucose metabolic effects clinically important? J Cereb Blood Flow Metab 1987;7(suppl 1):S205.

49. Metter EJ, Hanson WR, Jackson CA, Kempler D, van Lancker D, Mazziotta JC, Phelps ME. Temporoparietal cortex in aphasia: evidence from positron emission tomography. Arch Neurol 1990;47:1235-1238.

50. Metter EJ, Jackson C, Kempler D, Riege WH, Hanson WR, Mazziotta JC, Phelps ME. Left hemisphere intracerebral hemorrhages studied by (F-18)-fluorodeoxyglucose PET. Neurology 1986;36:1155-1162.

51. Metter EJ. Role of subcortical structures in aphasia: Evidence from resting cerebral glucose metabolism. In: Vallar G, Cappa SF, Walesch CW, eds. Neuropsychological disorders associated with subcortical lesions. New York: Oxford University Press, 1992:478-500.

52. Baron JC, D'Antona R, Pantano P, Serdaru M, Samson Y, Bousser MG. Effects of thalamic stroke on energy metabolism of the cerebral cortex. Brain 1986;109:1243-1259.

53. Baron JC, Levasseur M, Mazoyer B, Legault-Demare F, Mauguiere F, Pappata S, Jedynak P, Derome P, Cambier J, Tran-Dinh S, Cambon H. Cortical hypometabolism and neuropsychological impairment in unilateral thalamic lesions. In: Vallar G, Cappa SF, Wallesch CW, eds. Neuropsychological disorders associated with subcortical lesions. New York: Oxford University Press, 1992:437-454.

54. Metter EJ, Riege WH, Hanson WR, Kuhl DE, Phelps ME, Squire LR, Wasterlain CG, Benson DF. Comparisons of metabolic rates, language and memory in subcortical aphasias. Brain Lang 1983;19:33-47.

55. Demonet JF, Celsis P, Puel D, Cardebat JP, Marc-Vergnes JP, Rascol A. Thalamic and non-thalamic subcortical aphasia: a neurolinguistic and SPECT approach. In: Vallar G, Cappa SA, Wallesch CW, eds. Neuropsychological disorders associated with subcortical lesions. New York: Oxford University Press, 1992:397–411.

56. Puel M, Demonet JF, Cardebat D, Berry I, Celsis P, Marc-Vergnes JP, Rascol A. Three topographical types of thalamic aphasia: a neurolinguistic, MRI and SPECT study. In: Vallar G, Cappa SF, Walesch CW, eds. Neuropsychological disorders associated with subcortical lesions. New York: Oxford University Press, 1992:412–426.

57. Metter EJ, Riege WH, Hanson WR, Jackson CA, Kempler D, van Lancker D. Subcortical structures in aphasias. An analysis based on (F-18)-fluorodeoxyglucose positron emission tomography, and computed tomography. Arch Neurol 1988;45:1229–1234.

58. Metter EJ, Riege WH, Hanson WR, Phelps ME, Kuhl DE. Evidence for a caudate role in aphasia from FDG positron computed tomography. Aphasiology 1988;2:33–43.

59. Metter EJ, Kempler D, Jackson C, Hanson WR, Mazziotta JC, Phelps ME. Cerebral glucose metabolism in Wernicke's, Broca's, and conduction aphasias. Arch Neurol 1989;46:27–34.

60. Kempler D, Metter EJ, Jackson CA, Hanson WR, Riege WH, Mazziotta JC, Phelps ME. Disconnection and cerebral metabolism: the case of conduction aphasia. Arch Neurol 1988;45:275–279.

61. Metter EJ, Riege WR, Hanson W, Camras L, Kuhl DE, Phelps ME. Correlations of cerebral glucose metabolism and structural damage to language function in aphasia. Brain Lang 1984;21:187–207.

62. Yamaguchi F, Meyer JS, Sakai F, Yamamoto M. Case reports of three dysphasic patients to illustrate r-CBF responses during behavioral activation. Brain Lang 1980;9:145–148.

63. Knopman DS, Rubens AB, Selnes O. Right hemisphere participation in recovery from aphasia: Evidence from xenon-133 inhalation rCBF studies. J Cereb Blood Flow Metab 1983;3(suppl 1):S250–S251.

64. Knopman D, Rubens A, Selnes O, Klassen AC, Meyer MW. Mechanisms of recovery from aphasia: Evidence from serial xenon 133 cerebral blood flow studies. Ann Neurol 1984;15:530–535.

65. Walker-Batson D, Wendt JS, Devous MD, Barton MM, Bonte FJ. A long-term follow-up case study of crossed aphasia assessed by single photon emission tomography (SPECT), language, and neuropsychological testing. Brain Lang 1988; 33:311–322.

66. Lee RG, Hill TC, Holman BL. Predictive value of perfusion defect size using N-isopropyl-(I-123)-p-iodoamphetamine emission tomography in acute stroke. J Neurosurg 1984;61:449–452.

67. Defer G, Moretti JL, Cesaro P. Early and delayed SPECT using N-isopropyl-p-iodoamphetamine iodine 123 in cerebral ischemia: A prognostic index for clinical recovery. Arch Neurol 1987;44:715–718.

68. Bushnell DL, Gupta S, Mlcoch AG, Barnes E. Prediction of language and neurologic recovery after cerebral infarction with SPECT imaging using N-isopropyl-p-(I123) iodoamphetamine. Arch Neurol 1989;46:665–669.

69. Giubilei F, Lenzi GL, Dipiero V. Predictive value of brain perfusion single photon emission computed tomography in acute ischemic stroke. Stroke 1990;21: 895–900.

70. Mountz JM, Modell JG, Foster NL, Dupree ES. Prognostication of recovery following stroke using comparison of CT and technetium-99m HMPAO SPECT. J Nucl Med 1990;31:61–66.

71. Limburg M, Royen EA, Hijdra A, Verbeeten B. rCBF-SPECT in brain infarction: When does it predict outcome? J Nucl Med 1991;32:382–387.

72. Gupta S, Bushnell D, Mlcoch AG, Eastman G, Barnes WE, Fisher SG. Utility of late N-isopropyl-p-(I 123)-iodoamphetamine brain distribution in the predictive recovery/outcome following cerebral infarction. Stroke 1991;22:1512–1518.

73. Tikofsky RS, Collier BD, Hellman RS, Sapena VK, Zielonka JS, Krohn L, Gresch A. Cerebral blood flow patterns determined by SPECT I-123 iodoamphetamine (IMP) imaging and WAB AQs in chronic aphasia: A preliminary report. Arch Neurol 1985;35:625–632.

74. Tikofsky RS. SPECT brain studies: Potential role of cognitive challenge in language and learning disorders. Adv Func Neuroimaging, Spring 1988:12–15.

75. Metter EJ, Jackson CA, Kempler D, Hanson WR. Temporoparietal cortex and the recovery of language comprehension in aphasia. Aphasiology 1992;6:349–358.

76. Roland PE. Cortical regulation of selective attention in man: a regional cerebral blood flow study. J Neurophysiol 1982;48:1059–1078.

77. Roland PE, Skinhoj E, Lassen NA. Focal activations of human cerebral cortex during auditory discrimination. J Neurophysiol 1981;45:1139–1151.

78. Knopman DS, Rubens AB, Klassen AC, Meyer M. Regional cerebral blood flow correlates of auditory processing. Arch Neurol 1982;39:487–493.

79. Kushner MJ, Schwartz R, Alavi A, Dann R, Rosen M, Silver F, Reivich M. Cerebral glucose consumption following verbal auditory stimulation. Brain Res 1987;409:79–87.

80. Petersen SE, Fox PT, Snyder AZ, Raichle ME. Activation of extrastriate and frontal cortical areas by visual words and word-like stumuli. Science 1990;249: 1041–1043.

81. Wise R, Chollet F, Hadar U, Friston K, Hoffner E, Frackowiak R. Distribution of cortical neural networks involved in word comprehension and word retrieval. Brain 1991;114:1803–1817.

9

Insights into Language Mechanisms Derived from the Evaluation of Epilepsy

Bassel Abou-Khalil

Vanderbilt University School of Medicine, Nashville, Tennessee

Our model of language organization in the brain was for a long time based solely on observation of "experiments" of nature. Patients with language deficits resulting from strokes, traumatic injury, or other insults had postmortem examination of the brain, and their language deficit was correlated with the location of the lesion (1,2). In 1870 Fritsch and Hitzig (3,4) established an important milestone when they used electrical current to stimulate the cerebral cortex of a dog and produced movements of the contralateral limbs. The findings were confirmed by Ferrier and others (5-8), leading to the eventual use of electrical stimulation in the human brain. Electrical stimulation of the human cortex was reported in the latter part of the nineteenth century, generally in subjects with epileptic seizures undergoing surgery (9-12). These reports concentrated on motor responses. Harvey Cushing (13) first demonstrated in 1909 that stimulation of the postcentral gyrus of conscious patients produced sensation in the opposite limbs, and Foerster (14) extended cortical stimulation beyond the sensorimotor cortex. Penfield and his associates (15-20) provided the most detailed reports of cortical stimulation, including stimulation of language cortex.

WILDER PENFIELD AND THE MAPPING
OF SPEECH CORTEX

Patients with refractory epilepsy requiring surgical treatment provided Penfield and his associates with a unique opportunity to study language and related cortical functions. Penfield and Roberts detailed their accumulated findings in their 1959 monograph *Speech and Brain Mechanisms* (20). The surgical treatment of epilepsy usually involves resection of the epileptogenic zone. Since this zone may include functional cortex, the elucidation of the cortical functions is necessary if they are to be preserved. Nevertheless, cortical functions including speech may be at least transiently disturbed if the resection approaches functional cortex. Roberts (20) listed the methods used to investigate speech mechanisms:

> Disturbances in speech with seizures, the results of electrical identification of cortical speech areas, the results of cortical excision with the evolution of transient aphasia during the postoperative period, similar studies when the nondominant hemisphere was involved, studies of handedness and of cerebral dominance (including the sodium Amytal aphasia test).

These remain the methods most often used in the evaluation of language functions in patients with epilepsy. The major contribution of Penfield and his associates (20) was a technique for electrical "interference" mapping of speech cortex.

Method of Cortical Stimulation

When planning electrical stimulation, Penfield carried out the initial craniotomies under local anesthesia. Prior to stimulation, electrocorticography was used to localize the epileptic abnormality, then the recording electrodes were left in place during the mapping. During the stimulation the surgeon and the patient could communicate verbally. The anesthetist usually served as an observer. The stimulation used bipolar or unipolar electrodes and started with determining the minimum voltage needed for a sensory response from the postcentral gyrus. This voltage was doubled for localizing speech areas. The language tests included confrontation naming, counting, and, less often, writing and reading aloud. Neither observer nor patient was aware of the time or location of stimulating electrode application. When a positive response was obtained, the area of cortex stimulated was labeled with a small ticket bearing a number. Stimulations associated with an epileptic afterdischarge were not included, because afterdischarges may produce interference in neighboring areas. Penfield (20) believed that negative results did not exclude an area from involvement in speech; he considered negative results more significant when they bordered an area where stimulation produced an aphasic arrest.

Results of Electrical Stimulation of Speech Cortex

Penfield observed that, whereas stimulation of some functional areas produced either activation or interference, interference was the only type of response with stimulation of language cortex. No intelligible words were produced by stimulation of the language cortex in a silent patient. Vocalization was produced in some regions, however, specifically the rolandic motor cortex and the supplementary motor cortex, in either the dominant or nondominant hemisphere. Roberts (20) pointed out that stimulation of the rolandic and supplementary motor areas might produce arrest through interference with motor control of speech organs. Speech arrest in these areas may occur with stimulation of either hemisphere and may be accompanied by movements of the face and tongue.

The regions producing interference with speech are shown in Figure 1A. The negative effects of stimulation were classified into the following categories: (1) total arrest of speech, (2) hesitation and slurring of speech, (3) distortion, (4) repetition of words and syllables, (5) confusion of numbers while counting, (6) inability to name with retained ability to speak, (7) misnaming with evidence of perseveration, (8) misnaming without perseveration. Although speech arrest could also result from motor interference with stimulation of either hemisphere, categories of interference 3–8 were seen almost exclusively with left-hemisphere stimulation and represented a specific interference with language (Figure 1B). In these language areas, electrical interference was effective only about 50% of the time. In addition, some patients never showed interference in speech, even though these patients later developed a postoperative transient aphasia. The language areas found were not necessarily homogeneous, and areas without interference sometimes separated contiguous points with interference (20). Three general language areas were identified in the dominant (usually left) hemisphere: inferior frontal (Broca's), posterior temporoparietal, and mesial frontal (supplementary motor). One striking and unexpected finding was the lack of any difference in the effect of electrical current on these three areas.

Aphasia Following Cortical Excision

The data derived from cortical stimulation were complemented by evaluation of language disturbances resulting from cortical excision, with analysis of the relationship of these disturbances to the location and size of resections (20). Postoperative aphasia occurred in 58% of left-hemisphere operations and 1% of right-hemisphere operations. The right-hemisphere patients

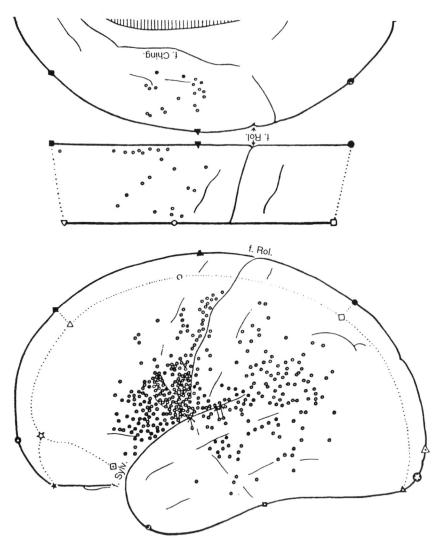

Figure 1A   Points in the left hemisphere where electrical stimulation interfered with speech. This includes interference with speech deemed secondary to interference with motor control of speech organs. (From Ref. 20.)

had less clear aphasia and were not well documented. This finding confirmed the dominance of the left hemisphere for language. Immediate postoperative aphasia occurred after 8% of left-hemisphere operations and did not occur after right operations. "Neighborhood" aphasia, defined as beginning one or more days after the operation, accounted for the vast majority of instances

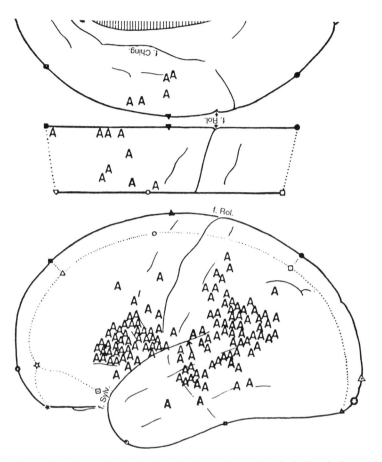

Figure 1B Points in the left hemisphere where electrical stimulation produced dysphasic or aphasic responses. (From Ref. 20.)

of postoperative aphasia. It frequently started 2–4 days after cortical resection, usually began to improve a week later, and subsided over several weeks. Despite its transient nature, it was sometimes profound. In the few exceptions when aphasia persisted, it seemed to be associated with persistent seizures. Aphasia was least frequent after removals in the anterior frontal region but followed resections in a wide variety of left-hemisphere locations. There was great variability between individuals; the same surgical lesion produced different language disturbances in different individuals. Nevertheless, Roberts and Penfield (20) suggested that the anterior 7 cm of the temporal lobe could be removed with only transient aphasia.

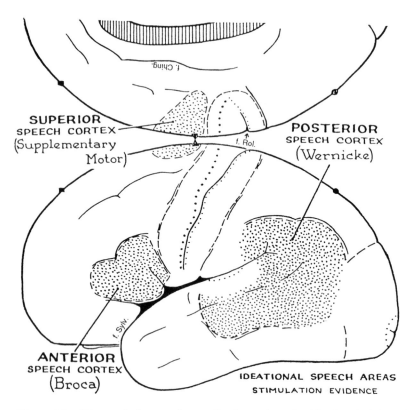

Figure 2A The cortical areas "normally devoted to the ideational elaboration of speech" as "derived exclusively from the evidence of electrical speech mapping." (From Ref. 20.)

Based on the combined evidence from electrical interference and surgical resection, Penfield and Roberts classified the language areas by importance: (1) the large posterior temporoparietal area, which Penfield felt was indispensable to normal speech, (2) Broca's area, which was considered second in importance, and (3) the supplementary speech area, located in the supplementary motor area, which was the most easily dispensable (Fig. 2). Penfield and Roberts quoted evidence of only transient aphasia after destruction of Broca's area; in one patient with an indolent tumor or hamartoma, complete removal of Broca's area did not produce aphasia. Aphasic disturbances resulting from ablations of the supplementary motor area disappeared within a few weeks.

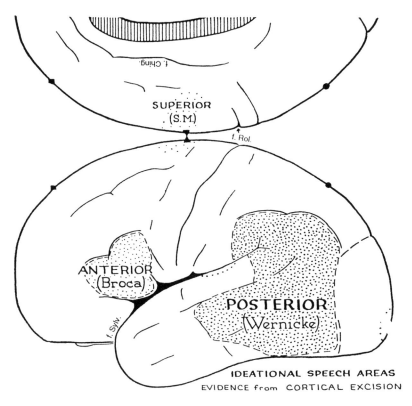

Figure 2B The cortical areas "devoted to the ideational elaboration of speech" as "derived exclusively from cortical excisions made around the speech areas." (From Ref. 20.)

CURRENT APPROACHES TO MAPPING OF LANGUAGE CORTEX

Intraoperative Mapping

Despite the pioneering work of Penfield and others (18,21,22), the surgical treatment of epilepsy remained confined for decades to a few academic medical centers in North America and Europe. In some centers, the mapping of language cortex prior to dominant temporal lobectomy was replaced by the use of other approaches to minimize the risk of aphasia. The most common approaches were to limit the temporal resection to the anterior 4–5 cm of the temporal lobe or to the cortex anterior to the vein of Labbé, and to spare the superior temporal gyrus (23–25). Because postoperative aphasia still occurred (26), some investigators continued to map language cortex prior to epilepsy surgery (27).

Ojemann and associates (28–32) have been the major proponents of intraoperative language mapping; through the use of this technique, they have made many contributions to the understanding of language functions. Ojemann modified the stimulation technique of Penfield. To have an alert and cooperative patient at the time of stimulation, Ojemann used local anesthesia and a very short-acting anesthetic, propofol, for the craniotomy. Prior to mapping language cortex, he determined the afterdischarge threshold for the area of interest and selected a subthreshold intensity. He then identified 10–20 sites for planned stimulation using numbered tickets. Language testing involved a naming task, in which the patient was asked to name pictures of common objects shown by a slide projector at a rate of one every 4 seconds. The electrical stimulus was a train of biphasic square-wave pulses, 1 ms in duration at a frequency of 60 Hz. The stimulus was applied with a pair of electrodes 5 mm apart, at the onset of an item presentation, and was held until the patient gave a correct response, or for a maximum of 4 seconds. All sites were stimulated at least three times. No site was stimulated twice in succession, and at least one slide without stimulation separated each stimulation. Only major errors or arrest of speech were considered; isolated hesitations were not. When a reading task was given, errors included slow effortful reading, or fluent reading with mistakes (27). Naming was chosen as the primary testing modality because naming deficits are present in virtually all aphasic syndromes (Chapter 4).

Ojemann and Dodrill (33) found that a left anterior temporal resection that came within 2 cm of a site with repeat naming errors on stimulation was associated with increased errors on a sensitive aphasia battery 1 month after the operation, whereas no changes occurred when the resection avoided naming sites by more than 2 cm. These findings validated the use of intraoperative electrical stimulation with a naming task to localize language areas in the lateral temporal cortex. Ojemann noted, however, that there was a high degree of functional specificity in the language cortex, with separation of functions. In a study of 55 subjects, both naming and reading were tested during cortical stimulation (32,34). There were 111 sites where stimulation disrupted either naming or reading; only one of the two functions was disrupted in 77% of these sites. In another study, separation of functions was also noted when naming, reading, short-term verbal memory, orofacial movement mimicry, and phoneme identification were tested during stimulation in 14 subjects. This separation of functions was true at frontal as well as temporal cortical sites. Language functions thus seemed to be compartmentalized into separate systems (32).

Ojemann made several additional important observations regarding the localization of language in the brain. In any one individual, sites with repeated evoked errors in one language measure are highly localized, but across the population of patients there is considerable variability in the location of these language sites (30,32,35). In a report of 117 patients, Ojemann et al. (30) found that most patients had essential language areas smaller than 2 cm². The margins of these areas were either sharp (surrounding cortex had no language function) or graded (stimulation of surrounding cortex produced single naming errors). The language areas were predominantly localized in the crown of gyri. In cases in which sulci or the sylvian fissure were explored, no independent language sites were found in the depth, but only continuation of language areas of gyri (30). Sixty-seven percent of patients had two or more distinct language areas in the perisylvian region, separated by "nonlanguage" cortex. In 24% of patients, three or more areas were identified. In patients with multiple areas, at least one language area was found in frontal cortex and another in temporoparietal cortex. Separate areas in the temporoparietal cortex were common, while in the frontal area they occurred less commonly (30,32).

The tremendous variability among individuals in the localization of language cortex is best illustrated by Figure 3. Any specific location in the temporal lobe showed language cortex in only a minority of patients. Although the percentages were higher in the frontal region, only one small area, immediately anterior to the motor cortex for the face, had language function in most individuals. In general, there was more variability in temporal lobe than frontal language cortex (30). Another important finding illustrated by Figure 3 is the presence of language cortex in parts of the temporal tip traditionally considered safe for surgical removal. This especially involved the superior temporal gyrus but was also found in the middle temporal gyrus. In the frontal region, naming areas were also noted well beyond the traditional boundaries of Broca's area, both anteriorly and superiorly (30). Some patients had no temporal language area. Naming sites were identified only in the frontal lobe in 17% and only in the temporoparietal region in 15% of the 90 patients with both frontal and temporoparietal mapping (30). The total combined area of language cortex was estimated to be 2.5 cm² or less in 50% of patients and 6 cm² or more in only 16% of patients.

Ojemann et al. found correlations between specific patterns of organization of naming sites and verbal IQ, or combined verbal IQ and gender categories. For example, those with larger language areas had a lower preoperative verbal IQ than those with small areas. In the subgroup of 55 patients in

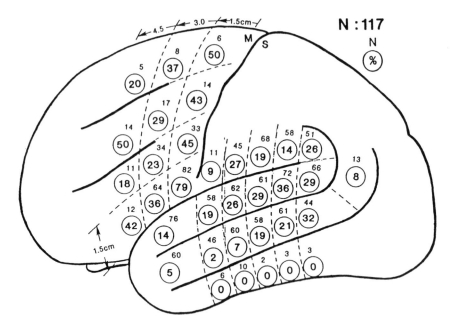

Figure 3 Variation in location of essential areas for language as assessed by electrical-stimulation mapping during object naming in 117 patients, all left-hemisphere-
dominant for language. Individual maps were aligned by the rolandic cortex and
the end of the sylvian fissure. The number above each circle is the number of patients with stimulation at that zone. The number inside the circle refers to the percentage of patients with an essential site for naming in that zone. (From Ref. 30.)

whom reading was also tested, a lower verbal IQ was associated with the
presence of sites in the superior temporal gyrus with only naming errors and
sites in the middle temporal gyrus with only reading errors. The reverse was
associated with a higher verbal IQ. Males with only temporoparietal and
no frontal naming sites tended to have a lower verbal IQ than males with
both frontal and temporoparietal sites. In addition, females may have been
overrepresented in the small subgroup of patients with only frontal naming
sites (30). Thus, there was a suggestion that the pattern of localization of
language is related to verbal abilities and gender. Ojemann did not find a
relationship between age and the localization of language areas. The distribution of language areas in a 4-year-old child was similar to that of patients
70 and 80 years old. There seemed to be no role for experience in the localization of language cortex (30).

Ojemann and colleagues also tested short-term verbal memory during lateral cortical stimulation. They demonstrated lateral temporal cortical regions essential for short-term verbal memory (36,37). Although supported by other investigators (38–40), this finding is in contradiction to the conventional view that memory functions reside in the hippocampus. Ojemann and colleagues noted that lateral temporal cortex was particularly related to the storage phase of recent verbal memory.

Ojemann et al. (41–45) used the opportunity of epilepsy surgery to study language processing with electrophysiological techniques, specifically electrocorticography and single-cell recordings. In one study, event-related potentials were recorded in six patients undergoing dominant hemisphere craniotomies. In response to silent naming, event-related potential changes were recorded simultaneously from premotor (slow potentials) and posterior temporoparietal (focal desynchronization) naming sites. This provided evidence of parallel processing of language in the brain (32).

Because of the invasive nature of microelectrode recordings, these recordings were obtained only from cortex included in the planned resection, not from essential cortex. The areas tested were preferentially at the resection margin, so as to study cortex relatively unaffected by the epileptic process. The recordings were obtained while the patients performed tasks related to naming, reading, recall, and a control task of visual perception. Many cells or cell populations located in temporal cortex not essential for language or verbal memory participated in language processes (41,44,45). The temporal cortex participating in language and memory thus appears to be substantially larger than that essential for those functions, as determined by electrical-stimulation mapping. In one study of 17 neuronal populations in the left temporal cortex of 13 patients, six cells or cell populations responded to short-term verbal memory only, one to reading only, and six to both (41). This finding provided further evidence for compartmentalization of language into separate systems. Changes related to language involved an increase in neuronal activity sustained throughout the task. Most cells that responded to memory typically showed increased activity during encoding and retrieval, but not during a distraction task. Some neuronal populations, however, showed relative inhibition of activity in relation to the memory task.

In another study, the activity of 41 neuronal populations in either left or right temporal cortex of 34 patients was monitored during presentation of words and sentences (44). No significant difference was seen between the left and the right temporal lobe. All neurons in the superior temporal gyrus responded to language but not to nonlinguistic sounds. Their responses seemed related to phonetic, not semantic aspects of language. Neurons in the middle and inferior temporal gyri were only slightly affected by listening to single words or sentences, but their responses disappeared during distorted or incomprehensible speech sounds. This suggested that these neurons may be involved in understanding language under certain conditions (44). The temporal cortex participating in language thus appears to be bilateral.

Ojemann's method of mapping language areas in the perisylvian cortex is convenient and provides substantial information about language, but it has limitations, as Ojemann himself admitted: the language areas based on intraoperative testing of naming in the primary language during perisylvian electrical stimulation do not define all cortex essential for language. This testing may miss cortical areas essential for reading, for verbal memory, and for naming in second languages. In addition, it does not evaluate the basal temporal cortex (30). There is recent evidence for the existence of a language area in this region of the cerebral cortex (46).

Extraoperative Mapping

Implanted intracranial electrode arrays were first utilized in the presurgical evaluation of epilepsy by Goldring (47,48), who advocated their use in children and those adults unable to tolerate local anesthesia for cortical mapping. Goldring used epidural electrodes to localize the sensorimotor cortex with somatosensory evoked potentials and cortical stimulation, as well as to record spontaneous seizures for better localization of the epileptic focus prior to surgical therapy. In patients with dominant hemisphere foci, Goldring (48) also used electrical stimulation of the grid to determine the "boundaries of the speech area."

The Cleveland Clinic epilepsy group made extensive use of subdural electrode arrays to record spontaneous seizures and evoked potentials, as well as to map cortical functions with electrical stimulation (49). A large variability was noted in the afterdischarge threshold of different electrodes, even ones only a centimeter apart, and in the same electrode on consecutive days (50). Based on this observation and the greater time available extraoperatively, the stimulation procedure was modified from that of intraoperative stimulations (49). The stimulus intensity was started at 1 mA and increased gradually until a definite response or interference was noted, an afterdischarge occurred, or the maximum of 15 mA was reached. The stimulation was generally performed in reference to an electrode overlying functionally silent cortex with a high afterdischarge threshold. The Cleveland Clinic group confirmed that positive effects usually occur with stimulation of primary motor and sensory cortex, whereas only negative effects usually occur with stimulation of association areas. At rest, neither patient nor observer will notice a negative effect. In fact, the patient may be unaware of the stimulation. However, if the patient performs a task that requires the stimulated cortex, the negative effect becomes obvious. To detect both positive and negative effects, reading was used as a screening test during stimulation of all electrodes. The observation was made that interference with reading may have more than one mechanism: it could be due to a positive motor effect when stimulating the primary motor cortex controlling speech-related muscles, a negative motor effect, an alteration of consciousness, or an interference with a language area.

The Cleveland Clinic group refined the identification of stimulation-defined language areas by the use of gradually increasing stimulus intensities, by testing for negative as well as positive motor effects, and by widening the language-testing repertoire. They identified the anterior and posterior language areas described by Penfield and collaborators and studied additional functions at these sites (51). They also described a new language area in the basal temporal region (50,52). They failed to confirm the presence of language function in the supplementary motor area (51). When speech arrest occurred with stimulation in that area, it was always associated with impairment of rapid tongue movements, suggesting that the supplementary motor area was not a true language area (Fig. 4).

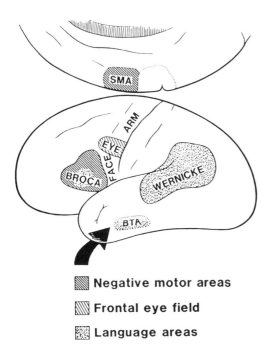

▨ Negative motor areas

▧ Frontal eye field

▨ Language areas

Figure 4 Language areas and negative motor response areas based on electrical-stimulation studies using implanted subdural electrodes. (From Ref. 51.)

Since the mapping technique used included a gradual increase in the current intensity, deficits could be graded according to intensity. The type of language deficit was found to be a function of stimulus intensity. At high stimulus intensities, a patient might have a global aphasia with speech arrest, but at lower intensities only very selective aspects of language processing were affected, with appearance of only anomia or only difficulty understanding complex oral commands (49).

These studies confirmed the marked variation across individuals in organization of language and other cortical functions (53). The Cleveland Clinic group did not reproduce the short-term verbal-memory deficits reported by Ojemann and colleagues with stimulation of the lateral temporal cortex, but the testing paradigms were different (54).

Lüders et al. (51) noted that stimulation of all language areas produces very similar findings, except that the anterior language area tends to be adjacent to sites with stimulation-evoked negative motor response. Negative motor responses were never evoked in the posterior language area or the basal temporal language area. The stimulation-defined language and negative motor areas are discussed in greater detail below.

Frontal Lobe Language Functions—Broca's Area

Lüders et al. (52) reported that language interference with stimulation of the prerolandic inferior frontal region corresponding approximately to Broca's area occurred in 15 of 22 patients (68%) with dominant hemisphere grids. Thus, most but not all patients had an inferior frontal language area demonstrated with electrical stimulation.

The frontal language area most often resided in the inferior frontal gyrus, but at times it extended to the middle frontal gyrus and even to the lower part of the superior frontal gyrus (54,55). In addition, not infrequently, language deficits similar to the ones elicited at the inferior frontal Broca's area were also elicited from the postrolandic suprasylvian region (49).

Lesser et al. (54) examined stimulation-induced alteration in motor output alone in three patients with subdural grid electrodes over the left frontal region. They considered an alteration in output to have occurred if the rate of speech or writing decreased by at least 50% as compared with baseline, but absolute arrest was usually found. The authors found areas of isolated stimulation-induced language disturbances in the posterior and inferior frontal lobe, but there were adjacent electrodes where speech arrest was associated with impaired rapid alternating movements of the tongue and/or fingers. Agraphia was also elicited from neighboring regions; it was always associated with impairment of other complex motor acts (54). Broca's area thus appears to include specific language cortex as well as a specialized negative motor response area probably responsible for the integration and planning of language-related motor function such as speech and writing (49). These results are consistent with previous observations that lesions in this area may produce oral apraxia and apraxia of writing (54).

Speech arrest was also produced with stimulation of the right inferior frontal region, but this was always associated with positive motor effect or impairment of rapid movements. Areas with interference with language alone were seen only on the left (51).

More recently, Schäffler et al. (55) reported three patients in whom stimulation of Broca's area produced language-comprehension deficits. These were most prominent in response to more complex auditory verbal instructions and visual semantic material. The processing of nonverbal material was not affected. This finding agrees with observations in Broca's aphasia indicating breakdown of auditory comprehension under stringent testing (56,57).

Negative Motor Area

A region of negative motor response was found surrounding Broca's area, as mentioned previously. A negative motor response was defined as an inability to perform a certain voluntary movement or to sustain a voluntary muscle contraction at a stimulation intensity that does not produce any symptoms or signs (51). Regions of negative motor response usually produce speech arrest with stimulation. Stimulation produces no symptoms or visible changes at rest, but results in an arrest of rapid tongue movements, which is the probable mechanism underlying speech arrest. These responses were usually seen immediately anterior to positive motor cortex, most often in the inferior frontal region anterior to motor face area, less often anterior to the frontal eye field or hand area, and frequently with stimulation of the supplementary motor area. Rarely they were noted with stimulation behind a sensory site. They were seen with the same incidence with stimulation of either hemisphere. The negative motor response affected mostly the tongue, followed by eyes and hands, then feet. In the extremities, distal movements were more affected than proximal ones. Not infrequently, several body parts were affected bilaterally simultaneously, but there was usually a contralateral predominance. In view of the selective involvement of areas essential for higher cortical functions, the authors speculated that the mechanism of negative motor response might involve interference with preparation of voluntary movements (51).

Posterior Language Area — Wernicke's Area

When stimulating the superior temporal gyrus behind the point where the rolandic and sylvian fissures meet (corresponding approximately to Wernicke's area), Lüders et al. (52) noted interference with language in only 14 of 22 patients (64%) with dominant hemisphere grids.

Lesser et al. (58) reported the results of electrical stimulation of Wernicke's area, located by finding reading arrest during stimulation over the superior temporal convolution. They demonstrated comprehension deficits with stimulation. At times comprehension was intact to simple tasks but impaired for more complex ones. Greater stimulus intensity also produced more pronounced and more consistent deficits. Lesser et al. (58) contrasted the stimulation-induced speech arrest with the fluent aphasia typically produced by structural lesions of Wernicke's area; they speculated that the acuteness of the interference may explain the difference. In one patient, longer duration of stimulation was associated with return of reading after initial muteness, suggesting that compensatory mechanisms may be engaged within seconds.

Basal Temporal Language Area

An unexpected observation derived from functional mapping with subdural grid electrodes was the finding of a basal temporal language area (BTLA) (46,49,51,52). The basal temporal cortex was not previously stimulated due to its inaccessibility. Lüders et al. (46) first reported a BTLA in a patient with subtemporal and lateral centrotemporoparietal convexity subdural electrode grids implanted as part of the presurgical evaluation of epilepsy. This patient underwent electrical stimulation of all grid electrodes while reading passages. Speech interference occurred with stimulation of an area in the lateral temporal cortex superiorly and posteriorly, corresponding to Wernicke's area. In addition, interference with speech occurred in a region of the basal temporal cortex, later found to be in the fusiform gyrus, 3.5 to 5.5 cm behind the temporal tip. Detailed testing of language function during electrical stimulation indicated that global aphasia occurred at high stimulus intensity and a relatively selective and severe dysnomia at lower intensity. The authors verified that there was no impairment of nonverbal skills and no negative motor effect (46). This cortical region was separated from Wernicke's area by at least 4 cm, and thus was clearly not an extension of that area.

In a later report (52), eight of 22 patients (36%) with dominant-hemisphere basal temporal grids demonstrated a basal temporal language area with electrical stimulation during a reading task. Interference with reading did not occur with nondominant basal temporal stimulation. Seven of the eight patients had a speech arrest during the reading task. Three patients had more detailed testing, indicating that confrontation naming was the most affected task, but repetition, writing, spelling, calculations, and verbal comprehension were also impaired. There was a clear dissociation between verbal and nonverbal tasks, which were completely preserved. The basal temporal language area was invariably located in the fusiform gyrus, starting 3-3.5 cm and ending 4-7 cm behind the temporal pole (52). The effects of stimulation were similar in the BTLA and Wernicke's area, suggesting a strong functional link between them. In addition, the preferential involvement of naming led Lüders et al. to speculate that the BTLA may be needed for access to verbal engrams, and may represent the *Wortschatz* ("word treasure," or vocabulary) area described by Wernicke.

The existence of a distinct BTLA defined by electrical stimulation was confirmed by other centers (59–63). Burnstine et al. (59) elicited language dysfunction in all of five consecutive patients studied with a large left basal temporal grid. They further characterized that area in its topography and functions. The rostrocaudal dimension of the BTLA was up to 63 mm. It started 11–35 mm and ended 39–74 mm behind the temporal tip. The BTLA included part of the fusiform gyrus in all patients, but, in addition, the parahippocampal gyrus was involved in three patients and the inferior temporal gyrus in one. The effects of stimulation were not identical for each patient, but the most consistently impaired tasks were spontaneous speech and passage reading. At the University of Michigan Medical Center, Kluin et al. (60,64) studied 10 patients with basal temporal strip electrodes implanted 4 cm behind the temporal tip. They elicited speech arrest in five patients and only slowing, hesitation, or paraphasias in two others when one or more basal temporal electrodes were stimulated during a passage-reading task. Among those with reading arrest, comprehension was impaired in three, intact in one, and not tested in one patient (60,64).

Abou-Khalil et al. (65) studied 16 patients with dominant basal temporal subdural electrodes implanted at Vanderbilt University Medical Center. Twelve patients had 16–20 electrode grids starting at 2.5 cm behind the temporal tip, and four had 4–5 electrode strips 4 cm behind the temporal tip. A BTLA was found in 11 of the 16 patients (69%). During passage reading there was a speech arrest in nine patients, slowing and paraphasias in two others. Auditory comprehension was impaired in seven, naming in nine (not tested in two). Writing was impaired in 50% and repetition in 8% of patients in whom they were tested (65). Spontaneous speech was not tested. There have also been two reports of patients with basal temporal lesions in the fusiform gyrus, a BTLA demonstrated by electrical stimulation, and simple partial seizures localized in the BTLA and characterized by global aphasia (61–63).

Whereas the demonstration of language functions in the basal temporal region by electrical stimulation is clear, the effects of ablation of the BTLA are not established. There is a discrepancy between the striking effects of stimulation and the much less impressive effects of ablation. In the first patient reported by Lüders et al. (46), the language area was not excised, but a Wernicke's aphasia was noted on the third postoperative day. This improved rapidly, but language function did not reach presurgical levels. Six months postoperatively he complained of difficulty remembering names and associating faces with names. Formal neuropsychological testing showed no change except for a 27-point decline in verbal memory. In their second report on the BTLA (52), Lüders et al. noted that five patients had the BTLA spared, two had it removed, and in one patient the BTLA was completely destroyed by a limited postsurgical infarct. This patient had a mild receptive aphasia in the immediate postoperative period, which disappeared completely 6 months later on formal testing. The language test battery obtained 6 months postoperatively showed no significant change in three patients, including two in whom the basal temporal language area was resected. Thus, there was no consistent difference in language outcome between those who had their BTLA resected and those who had it spared (52). In the series of Burnstine et al. (59), one patient had the BTLA removed and developed a postoperative dyslexia that lasted one year. The others, without BTLA resection, had no difficulties with language postoperatively.

Kluin et al. (60,64) tested language functions with the Boston Diagnostic Aphasia Exam before and after surgical therapy. All but one of their 10 patients had the basal temporal area removed. There was no increased language dysfunction postoperatively in the patient who had the area spared or in eight of the nine who had it removed. In our Vanderbilt series (65), we have also not seen a clear relationship between resection of the basal language area and decline in the verbal IQ or Boston Naming Test scores. The two patients with lesions of the fusiform gyrus reported by Abou-Khalil et al. and Suzuki et al. had removal of the BTLA. One developed difficulty with recalling and saying proper names that improved over several months. On a 4-month postoperative neuropsychological testing she had losses on verbal memory and Rey auditory learning (61,63). The other patient had mild naming difficulty immediately postoperatively but no decline in language functions tested 2 weeks postoperatively (62).

As one possible explanation for the discrepancy between stimulation and ablation effects, Lüders et al. (52) proposed that stimulation allows no time for compensation but ablative lesions are followed by recruitment of other areas to compensate for deficits. Burnstine et al. (59) suggested that the BTLA was not a primary language area but was connected to language areas by oligosynaptic chains, or that the BTLA was involved with memory retrieval necessary for language processing.

The BTLA is at least partly included in the typical anterior temporal resection for treatment of epilepsy. It is possible that BTLA ablation accounts for some of the language disturbances and decline in verbal memory often observed following dominant temporal lobectomy (26,66), but this needs to be clarified with a large study. Both immediate and long-term effects of BTLA ablation should be examined in patients with BTLA resection for treatment of epilepsy. Even when the BTLA is not restricted, the possibility that it has been undercut or disconnected should be considered.

Comparison of Intraoperative and Extraoperative Mapping Techniques

The relative advantages of extraoperative and intraoperative mapping have been discussed at length, without resolution regarding the preferred method (27,47,48,53,67). Goldring (47) argued that implanted electrode grids allow the recording of spontaneous seizures for better focus localization than is possible in the operating room and permit the mapping of functions in children and others who cannot cooperative for awake craniotomy. Extraoperative mapping obviates the need for patients to remain awake during craniotomies and provides greater time for testing, permitting delineation of the stimulation-induced impairment with greater precision. On the other hand, a separate operation is needed for implantation, and the electrode grids are associated with the risks of infection and mass effect.

Functional mapping with implanted electrode grids has some inherent limitations. The cortex is not directly visualized; therefore, the anatomical correlations are often indirect or have to be done when the electrodes are removed. The subdural plate may move, although suturing it to the dura reduces any movement. The electrodes are at fixed distances, and stimulation between them is not possible. The position and size of the electrodes limit the anatomical resolution. Finally, the afterdischarge thresholds may be more variable with epidural or subdural than with direct cortical stimulation, probably because of intervening membranes, cerebrospinal fluid, or vascular structures, or accumulation of blood. Thus, direct intraoperative stimulation may provide greater anatomical precision. Advocates of intraoperative stimulation also argue that it spares the patient an extra operation, the risk of infection, and great expense. However, it is associated with patient discomfort, and most children as well as some adults cannot tolerate an awake craniotomy. The limited time and limited testing repertoire in the operating room diminish the depth and precision of language evaluation, and some areas such as the basal temporal region are not readily accessible for direct intraoperative stimulation. Thus, the preferable method of functional mapping may depend on the need for intracranial recording of seizures in the presurgical evaluation, and on individual tolerance. The two techniques can be combined in selected cases (68,69).

Selected Aspects of Language Organization Addressed by Electrical Stimulation Mapping

Consistency and Stability of Stimulation-Defined Language Areas

Penfield and Roberts (20) noted that electrical stimulation of all speech areas causes disturbances 50% of the time. Ojemann and Whitaker (35) identified sites where naming errors occurred 100% of the time, and others where it occurred less consistently. However, Lesser et al. (54) reported that functional interference was consistent over repeated examinations using their stimulation technique. They suggested that one possible reason for inconsistency was the use of a fixed stimulus intensity for stimulation of all cortical sites. Studies with subdural electrodes indicated wide variability in the afterdischarge threshold even between adjacent electrodes, so that the optimal stimulus intensity (just below the afterdischarge threshold) had to be determined separately for each electrode. One should note, however, that Lesser et al. did not consider alterations significant if they were not consistent. Ojemann's findings may indicate a gradient between language cortex and cortex with no language function (32).

Regarding stability of language areas over time, Ojemann (27) noted that the location of essential language areas in adults did not change over time in the few cases in which remapping was undertaken without an intervening brain lesion.

Sensitivity and Specificity of Cortical Mapping in Localizing Language Areas

Penfield (20) noted that positive results are of real value in mapping language, but negative results do not exclude that the area stimulated is involved in speech. No interference in speech occurred in some patients, even though these patients later developed a postoperative transient aphasia. The later studies of Lesser et al. (50,54) suggested that failure to identify language cortex in some cases may be a result of the stimulation technique. The specificity of stimulation-induced language deficits may be highest when clear interference is noted in some areas, surrounded by functionally silent cortex (20,54). Ojemann (33) found that language deficits occurred if surgical resection approached within 2 cm of stimulation-defined naming sites, but not if a margin of 2 cm was maintained. This was a validation of both the sensitivity and the specificity of electrical stimulation in defining lateral temporal language areas. On the other hand, the presence of a basal temporal language area has not been shown to predict aphasia with ablation. The functional significance of a basal temporal language area is not yet clear (52).

Applicability of Findings to the General, Nonepileptic Population

Is the knowledge derived from language mapping with cortical stimulation in subjects with epilepsy applicable to those without epilepsy? This question cannot be answered definitively. However, there is evidence that language may be redistributed in the brains of people with epilepsy, but only under specific conditions.

Penfield and Roberts (20) suggested that lesions in infancy may produce displacement of the expected location of language areas. Large left-hemisphere lesions may displace language to the opposite hemisphere, whereas small lesions may displace language to a different area in the left hemisphere. Their conclusions were based predominantly on data from the intracarotid amobarbital test and from effects of surgical excision.

Others (70,71) have also suggested that migration of language may occur to the opposite hemisphere. The migration of language cortex in the same hemisphere is less well established. Ojemann (30) compared the patterns of language localization in 37 patients with lesions acquired in adulthood to those in 80 patients in whom the condition giving rise to epilepsy might have occurred perinatally. There were no statistically significant differences in the proportion of naming sites in the frontal, parietal, superior temporal, or middle temporal regions, even when the groups were matched by verbal IQ and gender. However, Ojemann did not report on the incidence of anterior temporal language areas in relation to age at onset of the condition/risk factor leading to epilepsy.

Devinsky and associates (72) studied 18 consecutive patients undergoing dominant temporal lobectomy and specifically evaluated the hypothesis that early age of seizure onset was associated with more anterior displacement of temporal language areas. They used language-testing paradigms adapted from Ojemann and Whitaker and tested confrontation naming, reading, and short-term verbal memory. They grouped responses occurring within 4.5 cm of the temporal pole as anterior and those at greater than 4.5 cm as posterior. They found that patients with naming deficits on stimulation of the anterior temporal lobe had an earlier mean onset of seizures (5.8 years) compared with those without naming deficits on stimulation of the anterior temporal lobe (12 years). This difference was most significant considering the superior temporal gyrus (3.2 years versus 13 years). There was a trend in the same direction when considering reading errors in the anterior temporal region. At surgery all the language areas were spared with at least a 1 cm margin. There were no significant differences in postoperative language functions between patients with and those without anterior temporal language. Devinsky et al. (72) postulated that seizure foci in the dominant temporal lobe during language development produced a more widespread or diverse pattern of language localization.

The question has also been raised that the BTLA might result from language redistribution due to the epileptic lesion. Burnstine et al. (59) argued that this is unlikely because the BTLA is often the seat of intense epileptiform activity, and language areas should migrate away from, not into, damaged cortex. The existence of the BTLA has not been demonstrated in normal people.

Thus, under certain circumstances, language redistribution may occur in patients with an epileptic lesion in the left hemisphere. However, additional evidence is required to determine whether redistribution occurs in individuals with epilepsy and no structural lesions, and in particular in individuals with

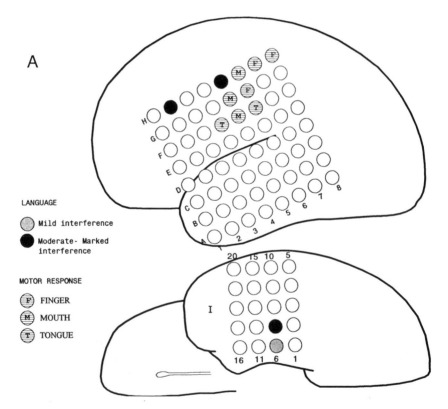

Figure 5 Four functional maps illustrating the variability in language localization in patients with epilepsy studied with implanted subdural grid electrodes. Patient C had a severe closed head injury with prolonged coma preceding his epilepsy. He "had to relearn to speak." His left frontal lobe has extensive areas of encephalomalacia.

amygdalohippocampal epilepsy, who constitute the majority of patients presenting for surgical treatment. To determine if language localization in normal controls differs from that of individuals with epilepsy, comparative studies are needed, using noninvasive testing such as positron emission tomography or functional magnetic resonance imaging (73–76).

Variability of Language Distribution

Most investigators involved in the presurgical evaluation of epilepsy have noted the marked variability in localization of language functions in the brain. The work of Ojemann and colleagues shows this variability best (Fig. 3). The maps of language areas drawn by Penfield and Roberts (Figs. 2A and B) represent combined data from a number of patients and thus do not express the variability. In this series, however, the posterior language area included parietal and middle temporal cortex. Figure 5 shows examples of variability in language distribution in four patients studied at Vanderbilt.

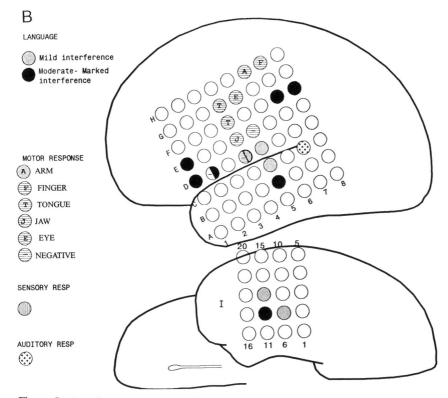

Figure 5 (continued)

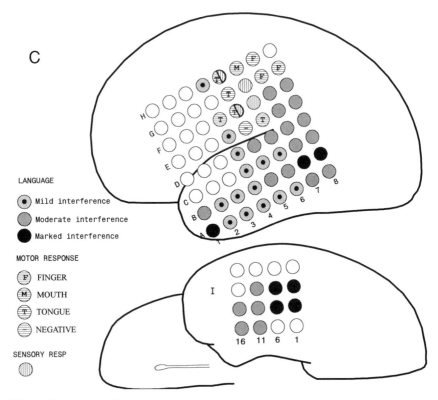

Figure 5   (continued)

It is possible that redistribution of language as a result of early onset of epilepsy contributes to this variability. However, there is evidence from lesion studies also indicating the presence of considerable variability in normal individuals; similar lesions can have vastly different consequences in different individuals (77,78). Despite this variability, the stimulation-defined language areas appear well defined in the individual patient.

Number of Language Areas

Penfield and Roberts concluded that there were three language areas (Figs. 2A and B): in rank of importance, the posterior (Wernicke's), the anterior (Broca's), and the superior (supplementary motor area) language areas. Ojemann showed that an individual patient may have more than one discrete temporoparietal or frontal language area, or one of them may be absent. Ojemann and his colleagues (79) supported Penfield and Roberts' view that

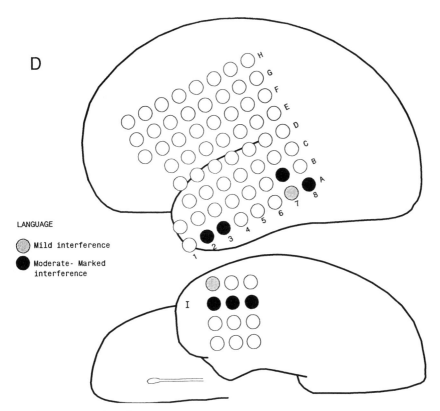

Figure 5   (continued)

the left supplementary motor area had language function, but language deficits with its resection were typically transient.

   Lüders and colleagues (46,49,51) consistently demonstrated a negative motor effect when stimulation of the dominant supplementary motor area produced a speech arrest. This suggested that apraxia was the basis for the speech disturbance. They concluded that the dominant supplementary motor area is not a primary language area. However, they described the basal temporal language area as a primary language area based on stimulation-induced deficits (46,52), but the effects of its ablation remain obscure. The data derived from stimulation of subdural grids concur with the findings by Ojemann et al. that any of the language areas may be absent in an individual patient (52). The exact proportion of individuals with specific language areas absent has varied among studies (30,32,52).

Specialization in the Language Areas

Penfield and Roberts (20) found no difference in the effect of electrical current on the three language areas they identified. In the concluding discussion, Penfield noted, "The aphasia of electrical interference does not seem to show such variety of pattern as that produced by brain lesions," although he admitted this may be an artifact of the testing administered.

Ojemann's work strongly suggested compartmentalization of language functions in separate systems. He found this to be most true of naming, reading, short-term verbal memory, and different languages (32). However, the two language functions traditionally separated in textbook diagrams — speech production and speech perception — did not show a clear separation. Electrical stimulation most frequently disrupted sequential orofacial movements used in speech production and the identification of speech sounds at the same sites, in both inferior frontal and temporoparietal regions (28,32). In addition, Ojemann et al. (30) found that attempts at localization of different types of naming errors were generally unproductive.

Lüders et al. (51,52) noted that stimulation of all language areas produces very similar findings. The frontal language cortex, however, was adjacent to or surrounded by areas producing a negative motor response with electrical stimulation. This suggested that the difference between Broca's and Wernicke's aphasias may be the involvement of "negative motor response" areas adjacent to the pure language cortex.

Thus, the evidence from electrical-stimulation mapping fails to distinguish different representations for "receptive" and "expressive" language. Other language functions may be compartmentalized based on Ojemann's work, but this specialization does not seem to follow anatomical guidelines.

Language Organization in Bilingual Individuals

The question most often asked in this regard is whether each language has a different representation in the brain of the bilingual individual, and whether there is greater participation of the right hemisphere.

Most lesion studies and series of Wada tests indicate that both languages are usually localized in the left hemisphere (80–82). After strokes and other lesions, however, there may be a differential involvement or differential recovery of languages (80).

Penfield disagreed with reports in the aphasia literature describing multilingual patients in whom aphasia following stroke affected one language and not another. He wrote (20):

After practicing for thirty years in the bilingual city of Montreal, I have examined many bilingual patients who were said in advance to be aphasic in only one language. In every case, careful testing showed defects in both languages . . . there is no basis for the supposition that one anatomical area of brain is used for one language and a separate area for another.

This assessment appeared to be based predominantly on observations of postoperative aphasia and was not accompanied by specific case presentations. Penfield and associates did not systematically test naming with different languages during cortical stimulation.

Ojemann and colleagues (32,83) gathered evidence during cortical mapping, as well as microelectrode recordings, suggesting anatomical separation of different languages into systems, just as was the case with naming, reading, and short-term verbal memory in one language. In a study of two bilingual patients (83), Ojemann and Whitaker found that the center of a language area was shared by the two languages, but that at many other surrounding sites naming with only one or the other language was affected. In addition, there seemed to be a wider cortical representation of the later acquired language in which the subjects were less competent. This suggested that the essential language areas might become smaller with increased facility with a language (83). These findings were confirmed with additional patients and alphabet-based languages, ideogram-based languages (such as Chinese), and manual communication systems (82,84). Somewhat specific for manual communication systems was the demonstration of a special role for the anterior temporal lobe (85,86). Microelectrode studies additionally showed that individual neurons responded to naming in one language but not the other (including sign language) (31,32,86). For further discussion of bilingual aphasia, see Chapter 4.

The Advantages Offered by Electrical Stimulation for Cortical Localization

Both intraoperative and extreoperative electrical stimulation have advantages over lesion studies (30,53). Lesions affect one area, whereas electrical stimulation can be applied anywhere in the surgical field, or where electrodes can reach. With electrical-stimulation mapping, alterations can be produced repeatedly to test the reliability of a particular finding, and patients serve as their own controls. Performance with the stimulus can therefore be compared to performance without the stimulus. The brief duration of electrical stimulation precludes functional reorganization or other compensatory mechanisms. Thus, electrical stimulation provides a window on the language function in its unaltered state, although epilepsy may have already altered it. With lesion studies it may be difficult to distinguish how much of the residual language function was initially spared by the lesion and how much was recovered as a result of functional reorganization. This last distinctive feature of stimulation studies may be an advantage when evaluating language mech-

anisms, but a disadvantage when predicting long-term outcome after ablation. Aphasia may be predicted should a certain area be resected, but its
expected pattern and extent of recovery cannot be foreseen.

THE INTRACAROTID AMOBARBITAL TEST

The intracarotid amobarbital (Wada) test is a method to inactivate tempor-
arily the regions of the brain supplied by the anterior and middle cerebral
arteries by injecting sodium amobarbital into the internal carotid artery. It
provides the opportunity to test the functions of the contralateral hemisphere
and other brain regions not inactivated by the amobarbital. The test was
originally intended to determine which hemisphere is dominant for language
prior to surgery (87). Milner et al. (88) modified the test to examine memory
and help predict the possibility of amnesia following hippocampal resection.
This discussion is limited to determining language dominance and functions
associated with it.

Intracarotid Amobarbital Test Procedure

Most epilepsy centers use the intracarotid amobarbital test as part of their
presurgical evaluation (89). The method of testing varies considerably (89–
93). We use a modification of the method used by the Montreal Neurological
Institute (94,95). The test is performed over 2 days, 1 day for each hemisphere,
to avoid residual amobarbital effects. Each session begins with an internal
carotid arteriogram with 3 cc of contrast injected at the same rate as amobarbital in order to visualize the cerebral vascular pattern and predict the
distribution of amobarbital. The contralateral anterior cerebral artery sometimes fills through the anterior communicating artery, and the ipsilateral
posterior cerebral artery sometimes fills through the posterior communicating artery. A persistent trigeminal artery precludes the test because the amobarbital would anesthetize the brainstem.

Baseline speech testing is done after the arteriogram to familiarize the
patient with the testing procedure and to serve as a control. Patients are
asked to name common objects, read single words aloud, count and recite
the days of the week forward and backward, spell single words, and follow
simple commands. They are also told a sentence to remember and shown two
line drawings to name and remember. Patients are asked to recall the items
after being distracted by reciting forward and backward and doing mental
arithmetic.

After this baseline assessment, the patients are asked to extend their arms
in the air and wiggle fingers and toes briskly while counting aloud. During
the counting, the examiner signals the radiologist to hand-inject 175 mg of

amobarbital diluted in 3 cc of saline over 2 to 3 seconds. Within a few seconds, the arm falls and the fingers and toes in the limbs contralateral to the side of injection stop wiggling. The patient stops counting if the hemisphere dominant for language is injected. Speech testing is repeated immediately after the injection while a second examiner tests tone and power in the contralateral hand and fingers. Muscle tone often persists in proximal but not distal muscles. When muscle tone reappears, the neuropsychologist presents new memory items before power returns to normal. Some centers begin memory testing when the patient is able to name objects (95), but this delays testing of the dominant hemisphere. After all neurological deficits have resolved, usually within 10 minutes, patients are asked to recall or recognize the memory items given under the effect of amobarbital.

Most centers first inject the side with the epileptic focus; some centers select the first side at random. Most test both hemispheres on the same day, 30–60 minutes apart, and use a smaller dose of amobarbital (75 to 125 mg) (71,96,97). The advantages of doing both sides on the same day are the need for only one femoral puncture and a reduced hospital stay. The disadvantage is that a residual amobarbital effect may bias the results. A few centers use sequential small injections (98,99). Some centers monitor the EEG during the procedure to detect seizures and encephalopathy and to determine the recovery of brain activity. The EEG may improve the understanding of unusual behavioral changes but is not necessary in most cases.

The clinical effects of intracarotid amobarbital include contralateral hemiplegia, hemianesthesia, homonymous hemianopia, and neglect. Aphasia occurs when the dominant hemisphere is injected. Patients are usually unaware of the deficits from amobarbital after they recover (100).

Determining cerebral dominance with the intracarotid amobarbital test is usually easy. The initial response to dominant-hemisphere injection is arrest of counting and global aphasia. It typically lasts 2 to 4 minutes but may last as long as 10. When the patient begins talking, an aphasic disturbance is evident, particularly in naming, with frequent paraphasic errors and perseverations. Language function and power usually return to baseline 7 to 10 minutes after injection. When the nondominant hemisphere is injected, the patient often continues counting, but dysarthria is common. Occasional patients are mute for 10 to 15 seconds, but when speech returns it is not aphasic. The response of patients with bilateral language representation is less dissimilar after left and right injections (101). The criteria for determining bilateral representation have not been established (89,93). Some centers require preservation of language functions after amobarbital is perfused in each hemisphere, others require language disturbances after both injections. Both may indicate bilateral language representation if technical failures and unusual amobarbital distributions can be excluded.

The selective intraarterial injection of amobarbital into the posterior cerebral artery (102) and the anterior selective Amytal procedure (103) are new techniques to evaluate memory functions more reliably in the mesial temporal structures. Since they do not involve language, they are not discussed here.

Findings on Language Organization from the Intracarotid Amobarbital Test

Several questions concerning language organization have been examined using the intracarotid amobarbital test. One of the earliest and most frequently addressed is the relationship of handedness to cerebral dominance for language. Other questions are the transfer of language dominance after cerebral injury, the patterns of language distribution in people with bilateral language representation, and the cerebral functions associated with language dominance.

Table 1A Cerebral Dominance for Language Determined by the Intracarotid Amobarbital Test in Right-Handed Patients

Author (ref.)	No. of patients	Hemisphere dominance (percentage)		
		Left	Right	Bilateral
Wada and Rasmussen (100)	6[a]	6 (100%)	0	0
Branch et al. (90)	48[a]	43 (90%)	5 (10%)	0
Rasmussen and Milner (70)	182[a]	168 (92%)	11 (6%)	3 (2%)
Mateer and Dodrill (101)	66	61 (92%)	1 (2%)	4 (6%)
Rausch et al. (71)	56	50 (89%)	4 (7%)	2 (4%)
Rey et al. (104)	29[a]	27 (93%)	0	2 (7%)
Silfvenius et al. (105)	50	47 (94%)	1 (2%)	2 (4%)
Woods et al. (96)	151[b]	137 (91%)	4 (3%)	10 (7%)
Zatorre (106)	38[a]	24 (63%)	2 (5%)	12 (32%)
Loring et al. (97)	91	73 (80%)	1 (1%)	17 (19%)
Wyllie et al. (107)	76	61 (80%)	5 (7%)	10 (13%)
Strauss et al. (108)	80[a]	61 (76%)	19 (24%)	
Charles et al. (109)	50	45 (90%)	1 (2%)	4 (8%)

[a]Selected for atypical features.
[b]Six patients with left hemiparesis not included.

Language Dominance in Right-Handed Individuals

All studies show that most right-handed people are left-hemisphere-dominant for language (Table 1). The percentage of right-handed people with right-hemisphere or bilateral language representation (atypical language representation) ranges from 0% to 37%. The two studies with the largest percentage of atypical language representation (24% and 37%) did not perform the intracarotid amobarbital test on all right-handed patients evaluated for surgical therapy, but rather selected those with hints of atypical language representation. Other series that studied unselected, consecutive patients showed 80–94% left-hemisphere language representation, 1–7% right-hemisphere dominance, and 4–19% bilateral language representation.

Table 1B Cerebral Dominance for Language Determined by the Intracarotid Amobarbital Test in Subgroups of Right-Handed Patients

| Author (ref.) | No. of patients | Hemisphere dominance (percentage) | | |
		Left	Right	Bilateral
No left-hemisphere insult preceding the age of 6 years				
Rasmussen and Milner (70)	140	134 (96%)	6 (4%)	0
With left-hemisphere insult preceding the age of 6 years				
Rasmussen and Milner (70)	42	34 (81%)	5 (12%)	3 (7%)
Left temporal lobe focus				
Rausch and Walsh (71)	26	20 (77%)	4 (15%)	2 (8%)
Right temporal lobe focus				
Rausch and Walsh (71)	30	30 (100%)	0	0
Without hemiparesis or extratemporal radiological abnormalities				
Woods et al. (96)	118	109 (92%)	4 (3%)	5 (4%)
Without hemiparesis, but with extratemporal radiological abnormalities				
Woods et al. (96)	33	28 (85%)	0	5 (15%)
Women				
Strauss et al. (108)	31	22 (71%)	9 (29%)	
Men				
Strauss et al. (108)	49	39 (80%)	10 (20%)	

Patients with epilepsy may not be typical of the general population with regard to language lateralization. The underlying cause of epilepsy and the presence of epileptiform activity may contribute to atypical language representation. To avoid this bias, several studies compared language representation in subgroups of patients (Table 1B). Rasmussen and Milner (70) studied 140 right-handed patients with no history or radiographic evidence of left-hemisphere injury before age 6 years. Ninety-six percent of right-handed patients were left-hemisphere-dominant for language, and the other 4% were right-hemisphere-dominant. Among 42 right-handed patients with evidence of injury to the left hemisphere before age 6, 81% were left-hemisphere-dominant for speech, 12% were right-hemisphere-dominant, and 7% had bilateral language representation. This study suggests that brain injury prior to age 6 years is a cause of atypical language representation. Woods et al. (96) showed that extratemporal radiographic abnormalities influence language dominance, but those restricted to the temporal lobe do not.

Rausch and Walsh (71) found that all right-handed patients with right temporal epileptogenic foci had left-hemisphere language dominance, but only 77% of those with left temporal foci had left-hemisphere language dominance. This finding extends the results of Rasmussen and Milner (70) to show that epileptic activity, in the absence of a definite cerebral injury, can also influence language lateralization.

Language Dominance in Left-Handed and Ambidextrous Individuals

The results of studies on language representation in left-handed patients have not been consistent (Table 2A). The probability of right-hemisphere dominance in non-right-handed people ranges from 8% to 50%, and right-hemisphere dominance or bilateral language (atypical language representation) from 36% to 86%. Most intracarotid amobarbital studies have only a small number of left-handed or ambidextrous subjects because they are less common than right-handed subjects. Studies from the Montreal Neurological Institute are an exception, because the intracarotid amobarbital test was used in all left-handed and ambidextrous patients, but only in selected right-handed patients. Overall, language representation is different in left-handed patients as compared to right-handed patients. Wada and Rasmussen (100) studied 12 left-handed individuals and found them equally divided between left- and right-hemisphere language dominance. Two additional patients with right infantile hemiplegia had right-hemisphere dominance. In contrast, all right-handed patients were left-hemisphere-dominant for language. The authors were probably not aware of the possibility of bilateral language representation. Subsequent studies from the Montreal Neurological Institute (70,90) found a similar incidence of left-hemisphere dominance among left-

Table 2A   Cerebral Dominance for Language Determined by the Intracarotid Amobarbital Test in Left-Handed or Ambidextrous Patients

Author (ref.)	No. of patients	Language dominance (percentage)		
		L hemisphere	R hemisphere	Bilateral
Wada and Rasmussen (100)	12	6 (50%)	6 (50%)	0
Branch et al. (90)				
Left-handed	51	22 (43%)	25 (49%)	4 (8%)
Ambidextrous	20	12 (60%)	2 (10%)	6 (30%)
Both	71	34 (48%)	27 (38%)	10 (14%)
Rasmussen and Milner (70)	214	112 (52%)	67 (31%)	35 (16%)
Mateer and Dodrill (101)	24	14 (58%)	8 (33%)	2 (8%)
Rey et al. (104)				
Left-handed	30	11 (37%)	15 (50%)	4 (8%)
Ambidextrous	14	7 (50%)	2 (14%)	5 (13%)
Silfvenius et al. (105)	11	7 (64%)	1 (9%)	3 (36%)
Woods et al. (96)	24	15 (62%)	5 (21%)	4 (17%)
Zatorre (106)	23	11 (48%)	2 (9%)	10 (43%)
Loring et al. (97)	12	6 (50%)	1 (8%)	5 (42%)
Strauss et al. (108)	14	2 (14%)	12 (86%)	

handed and ambidextrous patients (48–52%) but also noted a 14–16% incidence of bilateral language representation.

Two studies (90,104) had sufficiently large numbers of patients to determine handedness and language dominance separately in left-handed and ambidextrous subjects. Both studies showed that the percentage of patients with left-hemisphere dominance in the ambidextrous group was intermediate between the left-handed and right-handed groups. However, the proportion of bilateral language representation in ambidextrous individuals was higher than in right-handed or left-handed persons. The difference in bilateral language representation between left-handed and ambidextrous individuals was statistically significant by Fisher's exact test in the study by Branch et al. (90); association between mixed handedness and bilateral language representation was also seen in the smaller study by Rey et al. (104).

Left-handed and ambidextrous patients are a heterogeneous group, as demonstrated by examination of dominance in patient subgroups (Table 2B). Branch et al. (90) found that of left-handed or ambidextrous patients without injury to the left hemisphere before age 5, 64% had left-, 20% right-,

Table 2B Cerebral Dominance for Language Determined by the Intracarotid Amobarbital Test in Subgroups of Left-Handed or Ambidextrous Patients

Author (ref.)	No. of patients	Language dominance (percentage)		
		L hemisphere	R hemisphere	Bilateral
Patients without early injury to the left hemisphere				
Branch et al. (90)	44	28 (64%)	9 (20%)	7 (16%)
Rasmussen and Milner (70)	122	86 (70%)	18 (15%)	18 (15%)
Patients with early injury to the left hemisphere				
Branch et al. (90)	27	6 (22%)	18 (67%)	3 (11%)
Rasmussen and Milner (70)	92	26 (28%)	49 (53%)	17 (19%)
Patients with no extratemporal radiological abnormalities—no hemiparesis				
Woods et al. (96)	12	9 (75%)	1 (8%)	2 (17%)
Patients with abnormal extratemporal radiological studies—no hemiparesis				
Woods et al. (96)	12	6 (50%)	4 (33%)	2 (17%)
Patients with right hemiparesis				
Woods et al. (96)	10	1 (10%)	6 (60%)	3 (30%)

and 16% bilateral hemisphere dominance. These patients are similar to a normal left-handed or ambidextrous population; compared to right-handers, they are often atypical in their language representation. These findings were later confirmed by Rasmussen and Milner (70), who concluded that "the pattern of speech representation is less predictable in left-handed and ambidextrous subjects, and their speech functions are apt to be less strongly lateralized in the brain."

Woods et al. (96) were unable to show or exclude a relationship between handedness and language lateralization when patients with hemiparesis or radiographic evidence of brain injury outside the temporal lobes were excluded. The number of non-right-handed patients remaining after the above exclusion was insufficient to reach statistical significance.

Of left-handed or ambidextrous patients with history of early injury to the left hemisphere, 53–67% are right-hemisphere-language-dominant, and 11–19% have bilateral language representation (70,90). In the presence of right hemiparesis, atypical language representation is even more common (Table 2) (96).

Relation of Language Dominance to Other Lateralized Preferences

Handedness is the most commonly studied lateralized preference, but preferences also exist for one foot, eye, and ear. These preferences are often, but not always, the same side as for handedness. Many studies of language dominance either neglect foot, eye, and ear preference or factor them in the determination of handedness (90). Strauss and Wada (110) questioned patients separately about hand, foot, eye, and ear preference and correlated the findings with cerebral dominance. Among 73 individuals, 56% had congruent preference and 44% had a mixed pattern of preferences. Any right-sided preference was associated with left-hemisphere dominance in 94–95%. Right-hemisphere dominance was associated with left-handedness in 45%, left-footedness in 53%, left-eyedness in 68%, and left-earedness in 76%. Consistent left-sided preference for all four functions occurred in only 3% of patients with left-hemisphere language dominance but 50% of those with right-hemisphere dominance. Consistent right-sided preference for all four functions occurred in 53% of patients with left-sided language dominance, but only 10% of those with right-hemisphere dominance. Therefore, the assessment of all four indices together has a higher predictive value for cerebral language dominance than any index separately (110).

The Transfer of Language Functions Between Hemispheres

The findings of intracarotid amobarbital studies support the concept that language transfers to the right hemisphere after early left-hemisphere injury. Left-handed patients are more than three times as likely to be right-hemisphere-dominant for language if they had injuries to the left hemisphere in early childhood (70,90). Most left-handed patients with early left-hemisphere injury are right-hemisphere dominant for language (70,90). On the other hand, most right-handed patients with evidence of early injury to the left hemisphere are left-hemisphere-dominant for language (70). This suggests that early injuries that do not modify hand preference are unlikely to modify language representation. Nevertheless, right-handed patients with early left-hemisphere injury are three times as likely to have right-hemisphere language dominance, and almost five times as likely to have atypical language distribution, as compared to right-handed patients without a history of early left-hemisphere injury. Thus, language function may transfer even if hand preference does not. While hand preference (motor dominance) can shift independently of language dominance (104), they shift together in 68% of cases (111). A shift in language but not handedness is less common, and is more likely when brain injuries occur after infancy but before age 6 years (111).

   The probability that language will be transferred from the left to right hemisphere is influenced by the location of the injury. Rasmussen and Milner

(70) found that even large lesions that spared the primary speech zones (Broca's area and the temporoparietal language area) rarely affected subsequent lateralization of speech. Lesions of the frontal and parietal speech areas were more important than the posterior temporal language area. Among non-hemiparetic patients, abnormal extratemporal radiological findings are associated with a significant increase in left-handedness and in atypical speech representation (96). Almost one-third of patients with left-sided lesions have atypical speech representation, as compared to 5% with right-sided lesions. Abnormalities associated with atypical speech or left-handedness are more destructive or extensive than abnormalities associated with right-handedness and left-hemisphere speech representation. Both left-handedness and atypical language representation seemed to be markers for brain injury, and both together are a stronger marker than either alone. These findings suggest that left-handedness is associated with brain injuries that are likely to cause atypical speech representation. Woods et al. (96) found that radiological abnormalities restricted to the temporal lobe did not alter handedness or speech lateralization.

In contrast, Rausch and Walsh (71) studied 62 patients with temporal lobe epilepsy and found an unusually high incidence of right-hemisphere language dominance in right-handed patients with a left temporal lobe focus. They did not find right-hemisphere language dominance in right-handed patients with right temporal foci; they inferred that language dominance may transfer as a result of temporal lobe epileptiform activity alone, and without a transfer of handedness. It should be noted, however, that right-hemisphere dominance for language in right-handed individuals is not specific for people with epilepsy. Although rare, it occurs in nonepileptic people without history of early injury to the brain (112–114).

Most studies agree that the transfer of language to the right hemisphere is more likely if the left-hemisphere injury occurred before age 5 years, and that the probability of transfer increases with declining age below 5 (70,90, 110). The transfer of language dominance is most likely to occur when left-hemisphere injury or left seizure onset is in the first year (110). In a study of patients with left epileptogenic foci, the mean age at onset of neurological disorder in those with right-hemisphere dominance for language was 3.8 years, while the mean age at onset in a matched group with left-hemisphere dominance was 13 years (115).

Some language transfer may even occur in adults (116). Left intracarotid amobarbital injections did not affect residual language in three patients with severe, adult-onset aphasia that followed left-hemisphere injuries, but right-sided injections in two of the three resulted in complete speech arrest. However, this residual language was severely aphasic and not comparable to the normal or near-normal language function attained in patients with early left-hemisphere injuries.

There is evidence that gender may also influence transfer of language. Silfvenius et al. (105) suggested that women with left-hemisphere injuries are more likely than men to have bilateral or right-hemisphere language representation. This is consistent with the finding that the incidence of aphasia after left-hemisphere injury is lower in women than men (116). A small group of right-handed, left-hemisphere-dominant patients with epilepsy was studied by McGlone and Fox (117). They showed that the difference in oral fluency scores after left and right injections was smaller in women than in men. Strauss et al. (108) suggested that the window for transfer of language functions is narrow in women, with reorganization most likely during the first year, while in males the window may extend to adolescence. A shift in handedness was not affected by gender.

The transfer of some or all language functions to the right hemisphere may be associated with impairment on some language measures, especially naming and language comprehension, but many language functions do not suffer (118). Transfer of language functions, however, can occur at the cost of nonverbal functions (118,119). Patients who developed right-language dominance or bilateral language representation after early left-hemisphere injury had impaired performance on a variety of tests of nonverbal, visual-spatial ability, in comparison with those whose language functions remained in the left hemisphere (118).

Right-Hemisphere Language Dominance

Right-hemisphere language dominance is often not a simple reversal of the usual pattern. During the intracarotid amobarbital test, naming and reading errors are less strongly lateralized in patients with right-hemisphere language dominance (101). Both Branch et al. (90) and Wyllie et al. (107) reported patients in whom the intracarotid amobarbital test indicated pure right-language dominance but who were later found to have language function in the left hemisphere. Loring et al. (97) found that pure right language dominance was rare, and much less common than bilateral language representation. A limited repertoire of language testing may overlook bilateral hemispheric contributions to language.

Pattern of Bilateral Language Representation

Bilateral language representation is harder to show than complete unilateral language dominance. Variations in the technique of injecting amobarbital and the interpretation of responses may confound the results (89,93). The existence of bilateral language representation in some patients was pointed out by Branch et al. (90). They described a patient, studied early in their series, who had right-hemisphere dominance for language but proved to have some left language function when he developed an aphasia following resection of Broca's area on the left. This patient made them aware of the possibility of bilateral language representation. Serafetinides et al. (98) also noted evidence for bilateral language representation in some left-handed or ambidextrous patients. Aphasia usually developed after injection into either carotid, although the severity and duration of aphasia were often less on one side. In one patient, neither injection produced aphasia, yet transient aphasia followed a right temporal lobectomy (98).

An increased prevalence of mixed language dominance occurs in patients with early injuries of the left hemisphere who are left-handed or ambidextrous (70). In right-handed individuals, the incidence of bilateral dominance was 0% without early insult to the left hemisphere and 7% with such insult. In nonright-handed individuals the corresponding incidence was 15% and 19%. Rasmussen and Milner noted (70):

> In the 18 patients with evidence of bilateral speech representation the speech defects were mild, from both the left and right-sided injections, although the mean duration of contralateral hemiparesis was the same. In half of these patients speech was not arrested by either the right or left injection, but clear dysphasic responses were obtained with each.

The duration of speech arrest was significantly shorter in the other half. Nine patients showed a qualitative difference in the aphasia induced by right and left carotid injections. Injection of one side caused naming errors; injection of the other side (two-thirds right, one-third left) caused disturbances of serial repetition tasks, such as counting or reciting the days of the week. These findings were validated by cortical stimulation in some patients. Naming and serial tasks were dissociated in nine of 18 patients with no early left-hemisphere damage, and in eight of 20 with early left brain damage (70).

Mateer and Dodrill (101) compared patients with left, right, and bilateral language representation for neuropsychological functions and performance during the intracarotid amobarbital test. Patients with bilateral language representation had the greatest number of expressive errors on an aphasia screening test, suggesting that bilateral language presentation was disadvantageous for language functions (101). During the amobarbital test, naming errors tended to predominate when the right hemisphere was perfused and reading errors when the left hemisphere was perfused. Phonemic and grammatical errors were more frequent with left-sided injection.

Loring et al. (97) found that bilateral language representation was more common (21.4%) than exclusive right-sided language dominance, probably because several language functions were assessed during the test. Most patients with bilateral language had asymmetrical language representation (59% greater on the left, 18% greater on the right). No relative dominance was seen in 23%. In a survey of 55 epilepsy-surgery programs that perform Wada tests, the prevalence of mixed speech dominance varied from 0% to 20%, although one program reported 60% (36). Centers that reported a prevalence of 0–6% did not consider production of partial phonemes, serial rote speech (e.g., counting), or the expression of familiar words (e.g., a patient's own name) as indicative of speech control in the hemisphere contralateral to the injection. Other factors such as patient selection and the dose and manner of amobarbital administration also influenced the prevalence of speech dominance. Centers that tested all surgical candidates were likely to find a lower prevalence of bilateral language. The use of small doses of amytal may not completely suppress function in the injected dominant hemisphere, giving the impression that the contralateral hemisphere has language functions as well, and a large single dose of amobarbital or a series of injections may affect the contralateral hemisphere and suppress language on both sides.

Functions Associated with Cerebral Language Dominance

The intracarotid amobarbital test has been used to study several functions that are suspected to be lateralized in the human brain. We will discuss only memory, consciousness, and emotion.

The association of verbal memory and language in the same hemisphere has been reported by several investigators. Fedio and Weinberg (120) studied 12 patients during the intracortical amobarbital test with a continuous task that included naming objects, identifying and saying "and," then naming a new object and recalling the last response. The ability to say "and" was retained after the left injection and did not differ significantly between left and right injections. After the left injection, patients had a transient naming difficulty that persisted for 4 minutes after resumption of naming and a longer-lasting difficulty with verbal memory, which did not return to baseline after the end of the test. They concluded that amobarbital blocks consolidation and prevents entry of the memory trace into a short-term store.

Rausch et al. (121) found that recovery was slower for naming pictures of common objects; reading written words; matching to sample of pictures, written words, and, to a lesser extent, unfamiliar forms; and short-term recognition of pictures and written words after the left amobarbital injection. Performance was also decreased in a grand recognition test of written words and, to a lesser extent, pictures, but not unfamiliar forms. The effect was greater if the injection was contralateral to the epileptogenic focus.

An initial impaired arousal, unresponsiveness, or confusion has been reported after intracarotid amobarbital injections (98,100,122,123). Serafetinides et al. (98), using a gradual injection method in 15 patients with unilateral dominance, observed "loss of consciousness" after dominant-side injection in 87% of patients, after nondominant-side injection in 20%. The "loss of consciousness" typically lasted 30 to 150 seconds. Loss of consciousness after injection of the nondominant side was shorter in duration and never occurred only on the nondominant side. In three patients with bilateral language representation, consciousness was lost after left- and right-side injections but lasted longer after injection on the more dominant side. They concluded that the hemisphere dominant for language also has greater dominance for consciousness (98).

Other studies (120,124) have failed to reproduce these findings. Rosadini and Rossi used single injections of amobarbital and suspected impaired consciousness on clinical grounds in 22.5% of cases, but impaired consciousness was recorded in only 5.9% when a response-testing apparatus was used. There was no difference between left and right injections. Lesser et al. (125) also showed that the initial apparent "confusion" or inattentiveness following left-sided injection did not prohibit the formation of new memories, suggesting that consciousness was at least partially retained. Huh et al. (126) used a simple continuous performance task and demonstrated marked reduction in attention, more often with left injections. However, impairment of attention was associated with right-side injections in some and with left-side injections in others. The preponderance of evidence does not indicate that language dominance and consciousness are associated. A greater patient awareness of amobarbital-induced motor deficits has been noted following left, dominant-hemisphere injections (127,128).

Some studies report that euphoria is associated with nondominant-hemisphere injections and depression with dominant-hemisphere injections (123, 129,130). Rossi and Rosadini (130) reported emotional reactions in approximately 54% of tests. Dominant-hemisphere perfusions caused depression in 60% and euphoria in 40%; nondominant perfusions caused depression in 15%, euphoria in 76%, and components of both in 9%. Two patients with bilateral language representation developed euphoria after injections on both sides. These findings could not be reproduced by Milner and Branch (131), who found identical mood changes after left and right injections in 39% of 104 consecutive patients; 37% were more cheerful after left than right injection, and 24% more cheerful after right than left injection. Only five patients had depressive reactions; three after dominant- and two after nondominant-hemisphere perfusions. Fedio and Weinberg (120) also failed to associate hemisphere dominance and type of emotional reaction. More recently, however, Lee et al. (132,133) found evidence supporting specialized hemispheric roles in emotional processing. They examined emotional reactions after intracarotid amobarbital in 55 patients who had bilateral injections. Euphoric reactions occurred after left injection in five patients (9%) and after right injection in 15 patients (27%). Depression occurred in eight (15%) after left carotid injection and did not occur after right carotid injection.

Adequacy of the Intracarotid Amobarbital Test in Lateralizing Language

The intracarotid amobarbital test is the standard for lateralizing language functions (134,135), but its reliability depends on technical adequacy. Contralateral hemiplegia has been used to determine that amobarbital has reached its target. The thoroughness of the language testing may also affect the findings, especially when language functions are bilaterally represented.

The amobarbital test for language lateralization is based on three assumptions: (1) amobarbital in sufficient quantities will functionally deactivate the regions through which it flows, (2) the carotid injection reaches all brain areas of one hemisphere that are involved in language, and (3) there is no substitution for these language functions by ipsilateral or contralateral hemispheric regions during the test (136). These assumptions may not all be correct. Comprehension of word meaning, a task sensitive to dysfunction of the left posterior temporoparietal region, was intact in eight of 15 patients (53%) immediately after left intracarotid amobarbital injection. This is explicable by variable supply of the posterior temporoparietal region by the middle cerebral and the posterior cerebral arteries. These findings suggest that the intracarotid amobarbital test does not always specify the laterality of all language functions (136).

The intracarotid amobarbital test for language localization can be validated by electrical-stimulation mapping of the cortex, or by the presence or absence of aphasia following ablation. Branch et al. (90) reported misleading results in only one of 119 patients. This patient was thought to have speech representation in the right hemisphere alone, but excision of the left-hemisphere Broca's area caused a mild but definite aphasia. Wyllie et al. (107) analyzed 88 patients who had bilateral intracarotid amobarbital testing and unilateral extraoperative cortical stimulation using subdural electrode arrays. Among patients with intracarotid amobarbital evidence of left-hemisphere dominance, right-sided stimulation never showed language deficits and left stimulation caused language deficits in 96% of patients. However, a left-language area was found in 29% of patients who had right-hemisphere dominance by the intracarotid amobarbital test and then underwent cortical mapping on the left. Thus, errors of language lateralization with the Wada test are more likely when exclusive right cerebral dominance is indicated. Wyllie et al. (107) also found that patients with bilateral dominance on the Wada test had a language area detected more consistently with left stimulation (seven of seven) than right stimulation (two of seven). Despite these limitations, the intracarotid amobarbital test remains the procedure of choice for overall language lateralization.

Applicability of Findings to the Normal Population

Some findings from the intracarotid amobarbital test may not be applicable to the general population. Some studies have biased selection of right-handed individuals toward atypical language representation (70,90). The result of shift from early brain injury can affect language or handedness (70,71,104, 111,137,138). Left-handed patients may have transferred both motor and language dominance as a result of early injury to the left hemisphere. In patients with intractable epilepsy, both left-handedness and left-hemisphere or bilateral language distribution were found to be significant markers of extratemporal brain injury (96). Groups of consecutive left-handed or right-handed patients with no history of early brain injury and with late onset of epilepsy may be most representative of the normal population.

Correcting for the effects of transfer of function, the normal population is expected to have a lower incidence of right or bilateral language representation in people with left- or mixed-handedness, and possibly a lower incidence of atypical language representation in right-handed individuals.

FUTURE PROSPECTS FOR NONINVASIVE LOCALIZATION OF LANGUAGE IN SUBJECTS WITH EPILEPSY

Neuropsychological tests, such as divided visual tasks (e.g., divided visual field presentation of a verbal task) or dichotic listening paradigms (e.g., dichotic fused words), are not sufficiently reliable for language lateralization to replace the intracarotid amobarbital test (106,139,140).

Language localization will remain an important aspect of the presurgical evaluation of epilepsy. The intracarotid amobarbital test and electrical-stimulation mapping carry definite risks and cause patient discomfort. Efforts should continue to replace these tests with less invasive tests that provide equivalent data. Rapid-rate transcranial magnetic stimulation is a potential method for lateralizing language (141). An electric field is induced in the cortex, allowing electrical stimulation similar to that achieved with direct current. Ten-second, 8–25 Hz stimulus trains were applied to the frontal, central, temporal, and parietal regions on each side in six patients while they counted aloud. The intensity was increased if no speech arrest occurred. All six had a speech arrest with dominant left-hemisphere stimulation, but this was limited to a single stimulator position. The results of language lateralization were identical to those derived from the Wada test. This procedure seems promising but awaits validation in a larger group of patients, including some with atypical language representation. Rapid-rate transcranial magnetic stimulation is limited in that it cannot evaluate the distribution of memory functions.

Positron emission tomography (PET) and single photon emission computerized tomography (SPECT) have both been used for functional mapping (73–75,142–144). The images obtained with both techniques lack spatial resolution, but coregistration with magnetic resonance imaging (MRI) may improve their localizing power. Functional MRI may now be the most promising localizing imaging modality and is distinguished by its safety, potential to image repeatedly, and excellent spatial resolution (76). Functional MRI is currently limited to a single plane chosen in advance, but technical advances are likely to remove this obstacle.

Ojemann (32) noted that functional activation techniques generally demonstrate cortex that participates in the function tested, whereas interference testing demonstrates the cortex essential for that function. The areas participating in language functions extend beyond essential cortex. The purpose of language mapping prior to surgery is to identify essential cortex that should not be resected. Transient postictal aphasia remains common despite the identification of language cortex (20,145,146). This may be because of surgical manipulation and edema (20), or because the importance of some removed cortex was not identified by electrical stimulation. Some cortical areas may not be essential for language by themselves but become essential in combination with other parts. As much cortex participating in language functions should be spared as possible. Functional imaging with activation may provide the required data. Identification of the cortical areas essential for language is especially important when the epileptogenic zone encroaches on the language cortex; stimulation mapping may be the only choice in that situation.

APHASIA AND EPILEPSY

Ictal and Postictal Aphasia

Paroxysmal language disturbances have long been recognized in some patients with epilepsy (18,147–151). The patterns of these disturbances were carefully described in the French literature (150,152). Among patients with paroxysmal aphasic disturbances, a preponderance of left temporal epileptogenic foci was recognized. Hecaen and Piercy (148) noted, however, that left-handed patients had more frequent paroxysmal aphasia irrespective of the side of the focus. Alajouanine and Sabouraud (150) noted that patients often had aphasia at seizure onset, before loss of consciousness, and also postictally. Simple speech arrest was less predictive of the localization or lateralization of the epileptic focus, reflecting the possible motor nature of a speech arrest. Speech arrest occurred with left temporal as well as supplementary motor and bilateral rolandic foci, but it predominated with left-hemisphere foci (150,152). Paroxysmal verbal articulation deficits similarly occurred with foci in either hemisphere but predominated on the left.

Other paroxysmal speech disturbances described were auditory comprehension deficits, verbal amnesia, alexia, and agraphia, all predominating with left-hemisphere foci; "verbal automatisms," which occurred with either left or right temporal lobe foci (152); and palilalia and repetitive vocalizations, which occurred with left supplementary motor foci (152). Serafetinides and Falconer (151,153) also showed that in patients with temporal lobe epilepsy who were eventually helped by temporal lobectomy, ictal aphasia occurring during a period of awareness and later recalled by the patient was almost exclusively associated with left temporal foci. They carefully defined ictal speech automatisms as identifiable words or phrases that are linguistically correct, but for which the patient is subsequently amnestic. In a group of patients with temporal lobe epilepsy, speech automatisms occurred with either left or right foci, but slightly more often on the right (151,153). They divided these speech automatisms into "warning," "recurrent," "irrelevant," "emotional," and "perplexity" utterances. When warning and perplexity utterances (which may not be truly ictal) were excluded, the right-sided preponderance became more pronounced (151,153). King and Ajmone Marsan (154) did not find "verbal automatisms" to be related to the side of the focus, but postictal aphasia occurred in 65% of patients with a unilateral left temporal lobe focus, compared to 4% with a unilateral right temporal focus.

Earlier studies did not have the benefit of correlating the EEG with clinical observations of speech disturbances. Combined EEG and video monitoring permits reliable distinction of ictal and postictal manifestations, and provides repeated playback of seizures captured on video tape, for more accurate and reliable clinical observations. Advances in intracranial EEG recording techniques, in structural and functional imaging, and in the understanding of ictal semiology have also allowed improved localization of the epileptogenic focus. Recent studies have confirmed the correlation between postictal aphasia and a left temporal epileptogenic focus (155–158). In addition, Koerner and Laxer (156) did not find postictal aphasia in patients with extratemporal foci. Privitera et al. (157) used a simple test in which the time delay from the end of the seizure to correct reading of a test phrase was measured. The time delay was less than 54 seconds after right temporal lobe seizures and more than 68 seconds after left temporal lobe seizures. Devinsky et al. (159) found that only postictal global or nonfluent aphasia was specific for the left temporal lobe. Postictal paraphasic errors were also more common after left temporal seizures. Impaired comprehension with fluent but unintelligible speech, as well as anomia, occurred after seizures arising in either temporal lobe. These symptoms, however, may be hard to distinguish from confusion, impaired attention, or abulia. The postictal language disturbance in temporal lobe complex partial seizures seemed related to the hemisphere of seizure onset, not to the pattern of seizure spread to the contralateral hemisphere (157,159).

Ictal interpretable speech occurred almost exclusively in patients with right or nondominant temporal foci (155,156,158) and correlated very highly with intact postictal speech (156,158). Nonidentifiable speech occurred in both dominant and nondominant temporal lobe seizures (155). Bell et al. (160) described a patient with stereotypic ictal speech automatisms consisting of phonemic jargon and reiterative neologisms. Their patient had a temporoparietal vascular malformation in her dominant left hemisphere. We have also observed this phenomenon in a patient with a left temporal low-grade glioma (unpublished observation).

Aphasia is harder to study ictally than postictally because most seizures are brief and associated with altered awareness. Most reports of ictal aphasia are in people with episodes of simple partial status epilepticus (161–168) or very frequent, recurrent, simple partial seizures (169). Some cases have been tested in detail, with informative insights (167,169). For example, in the case described by Gilmore and Heilman (169), episodes of ictal speech arrest were associated with syntactic, but not lexical, comprehension errors, indicating an aphasic disturbance resembling Broca's aphasia. Others reported an ictal Wernicke's aphasia (163,166). Lecours and Joanette (167) demonstrated in their patient a variable aphasic profile during the course of single prolonged ictal aphasic episodes. Global aphasia evolved into Wernicke's aphasia, then conduction aphasia, then "amnesic aphasia." They perceived in this support for Pierre Marie's "oneness" doctrine of aphasia (170).

The anatomical basis of ictal and postictal aphasia is not known in most cases. Seizures that start with aphasic speech arrest, without altered consciousness or motor activity, are generally considered to originate in the dominant lateral-posterior temporal lobe (171–173). However, temporal lobe epilepsy is most often of amygdalohippocampal origin (172), and clinical or electrographic seizures limited to the amygdalohippocampal region are not usually associated with aphasia (157). There have been two reports of simple partial seizures with speech arrest and global aphasia, with an ictal discharge localized to the basal temporal area (61–63). In both cases, a basal temporal language area was demonstrated with electrical stimulation. Subdural electrode studies show that ictal activity originating in the hippocampus usually spreads to the basal temporal region before involving the lateral temporal electrodes (49). Therefore, it is quite likely that the basal temporal language area plays a role in ictal aphasia preceding loss of awareness. With spread of the seizure discharge to other temporal regions and to the frontal lobe, other language areas are likely to be involved. Postictal aphasia in most patients is probably caused by involvement of more than one language area (157).

The study of ictal and postictal aphasia has some of the advantages of electrical-stimulation mapping. The aphasia is very transient, and the patient can serve as an internal control. However, a major disadvantage is that the seizure spread may account for some seizure manifestations. The pattern of seizure spread may be variable and is not easily identified on scalp or even intracranial EEG.

Interictal Language Dysfunction In Epilepsy

Although clinical seizures are the most striking manifestation of epilepsy, there is evidence for functional cerebral disturbances interictally in most patients. The abnormal interictal EEG is one obvious example of this: patients with partial epilepsy may have focal epileptiform discharges (spikes or sharp waves), or less specific focal slow abnormalities. Functional imaging with PET or SPECT often reveals regional hypometabolism or hypoperfusion corresponding to the epileptogenic focus, another marker of interictal dysfunction (174–176). Neuropsychological and cognitive deficits have also been recognized in some patients with epilepsy (94,177). Some of these deficits have localizing or lateralizing significance, in particular if they are disproportionate to any global impairment. Specialized neuropsychological testing has become an important component of the presurgical evaluation of epilepsy. The reliability of neuropsychological tests in localizing epileptogenic foci has been challenged (178), but neuropsychological evaluation is useful in confirming or raising questions about localizations made with EEG and neuroimaging data. The usual approach is to sample cognitive abilities widely, then explore areas of selective impairment and contrast performance in different areas of cognition (179). Most commonly, skills involving language are compared to those involving visuospatial abilities. When the focus is suspected to be in the temporal lobe, as is most often the case, memory performance is closely inspected, especially the difference between verbal and visuospatial memory (179). In general, dominant-hemisphere epileptogenic foci are easier to identify with neuropsychological testing than nondominant foci (94).

Performance on the verbal portion of the Wechsler Adult Intelligence Scale has often been used as a measure of dominant hemisphere function in patients with epilepsy. Some studies have reported comparatively lower verbal IQ scores in patients with left temporal lobe epilepsy (180), but others found no group difference between those with left and right foci (181–182). Overall, a significantly reduced verbal as compared to performance IQ suggests a dominant-hemisphere focus (94).

The most studied language-related cognitive deficit in patients with epilepsy is verbal-memory loss. The incidence of verbal-memory impairment in epilepsy is not clear, as is true of other cognitive deficits, including language impairment. Most studies have compared groups without considering individual patient performance. The impairments are usually subtle (94,184), and some studies have even failed to document deficits (185,186). Nevertheless, there is a preponderance of evidence for the existence of verbal-memory deficit in patients with left dominant temporal lobe epilepsy and non-verbal-memory deficit with right temporal epilepsy (94,180,181,187–189). This impairment is seen in adults (94,190) and children (187). The verbal-memory deficit involves both encoding and delayed recall of verbal material (187, 190). Some studies found early recall of verbal material less differentially affected by left and right temporal foci (190,191). In one study (192), patients with left temporal lobe epilepsy performed more poorly on delayed than immediate recall and had a particularly poor performance on phonemic cued recall, while performance on semantic cued recall was relatively normal. Hermann et al. (188) found more impaired performance of left temporal lobe epilepsy patients on all measures of the California Verbal Learning Test, including immediate recall. Recall was strikingly impaired relative to recognition, suggesting specific difficulties with retrieval (188).

Less attention has generally been given to language disturbances in patients with epilepsy. Mayeux et al. (193) evaluated memory, verbal fluency, and naming in patients with generalized, right temporal, and left temporal epilepsy. The most discriminating measure was naming, which was significantly impaired in the left temporal lobe epilepsy group. Performance on several measures of verbal intelligence, learning, and memory were highly related with naming test performance (193). These results suggested that a naming deficit may play a role in poor performance on verbal-memory tasks. Hermann and Wyler (194) found that dominant temporal lobe epilepsy patients performed in a more impaired fashion than nondominant temporal lobe patients on six of the seven subtests of the Multilingual Aphasia Examination. This pattern was consistent and significant, yet none of the differences on the individual subtests reached statistical significance. Thus, there was evidence of mild generalized impairment of language function in dominant temporal lobe epilepsy patients (194). Reading may also be specifically affected in epilepsy. Children with epilepsy are more often delayed in reading than matched controls (195,196). A recent study (197) also found a history of dyslexia significantly more frequent in patients with epilepsy (9%) than in age-matched controls (2.3%). Stores and Hart (198) specifically demonstrated lower reading scores in children with left- as compared to right-hemisphere foci.

Neuropsychological deficits may be multifactorial in etiology. Structural lesions may be responsible for both the epilepsy and the neuropsychological disturbances. The seizure frequency may be so high that a postictal disturbance is often present in the interictal state. Antiepileptic drugs and other medications may affect cognitive functions adversely. The neuropsychological dysfunction may also be truly interictal and related to the epilepsy itself; interictal epileptiform discharges have been associated with a transitory cognitive impairment when sensitive testing is used (199–201). Aarts et al. (200) found left-sided discharges associated with transitory impairment on a verbal-memory task and right-sided discharges on a non-verbal-memory task. The impairment was noticeable when the discharge occurred during the stimulus presentation, but not if it occurred during the response. Shewmon and Erwin (201) demonstrated in two patients that transitory cerebral dysfunction was specifically related to the slow wave that follows a spike.

Landau-Kleffner Syndrome ("Acquired Aphasia with Convulsive Disorder")

Landau-Kleffner syndrome is characterized by the appearance of a language disorder usually between 3 and 7 years of age and an abnormal EEG with epileptiform discharges (202–206). Classically the disorder occurs in children with previously normal development (202). Less frequently, language development may be delayed before the onset of the aphasia (204,207). Epileptic seizures occur in only 70–80% of affected children and can be partial or generalized tonic-clonic, atypical absence, or myoclonic (203,205). Behavioral disturbances — most commonly, hyperactivity — have also been described (205,208).

The aphasic disturbance most often starts with an auditory verbal agnosia (204,209–211). Typically the parents suspect hearing loss, but the audiogram is normal (204). The disturbance progresses to a total loss of responsiveness to spoken language and to deterioration of verbal expression (203,206). Nonverbal skills are usually not affected, and children can be taught lip reading and writing (206). The course of the language disturbance is usually characterized by fluctuations, with eventual slow improvement (202,210,212,213).

The relationship of the language disorder to the EEG abnormalities and clinical seizures is not totally clear (205). It has been suggested that the EEG abnormality and the clinical seizures may be an epiphenomenon of underlying pathology in brain areas concerned with speech (214). However, most evidence favors that language dysfunction and its fluctuations are related to the "interictal" epileptiform EEG abnormality (202,205,215,216). A pattern of continuous spike waves has been reported during slow-wave sleep in patients with Landau-Kleffner syndrome (203,216), and improvement in language functions has been related to the disappearance of this pattern (205). The topography of the epileptiform discharges may also favor a relationship, since they usually predominate in the temporal or parietal regions

(215). In most cases, however, they are bilateral, or shift between the left and the right sides (203,206,215). The role of clinical seizures in the aphasic fluctuations is probably less important (202,217). The seizures are usually easily controlled, and sometimes nonexistent (203,217).

The etiology of this disorder is not known, and there is evidence of heterogeneity in its pathogenesis. A structural lesion has been reported only rarely (209,218). Vasculitis was suggested by arteriogram in one series of four patients (219). In one atypical case, a cortical biopsy suggested chronic encephalitis (220). However, only mild subpial gliosis was seen in two other patients who had a temporal lobectomy (215). An increased family history of seizures has suggested genetic factors in this condition. In addition, some EEG and clinical features of Landau-Kleffner syndrome are reminiscent of benign rolandic epilepsy, an epileptic syndrome with well-documented genetic predisposition (215,221).

The long-term outcome of Landau-Kleffner syndrome is variable. Most patients improve markedly but are left with moderate permanent deficits. Occasional patients show complete recovery or permanent, severe aphasia (204,205,212,213). The prognosis is worse when the condition starts at a very early age (221,222). A possible explanation is that the acquisition of some language and writing skills prior to onset makes re-education easier. An earlier onset may also indicate a more severe condition. Early recognition and institution of speech therapy may improve outcome. Treatment with antiepileptic drugs usually controls the seizures but does not clearly influence language function (206,223). Treatment with high-dose steroids may be effective (223). Surgical therapy with multiple subpial transections, a technique that disconnects horizontal cortical fibers while preserving functional vertical connections, also seems promising (224).

If the language disturbances in Landau-Kleffner syndrome are secondary to the epileptiform discharges, they may be an extreme, more durable form of the "transitory cognitive dysfunction" demonstrated in partial epilepsy (200). The bilaterality of the epileptiform abnormalities may explain the absence of compensatory mechanisms, and the worse prognosis with early onset. These, however, are speculations, and many questions about this condition remain unanswered.

Language and Verbal Memory Disturbances After Surgical Therapy of Epilepsy

Penfield and Roberts (20) observed language function closely after surgical resections for epilepsy. Their findings are summarized earlier in this chapter. Evidence from aphasia after resection helped them construct a map of language areas and assign a rank of importance to each area (Figure 2B).

Most studies since then have specifically assessed the neuropsychological effect of temporal resections, the most common epilepsy surgery, with a smaller number evaluating frontal resections. Left frontal resections were associated with impairment of word fluency (38,94). Temporal resections, on the other hand, specifically affected memory. Milner (94) pointed out that the postoperative deficits are usually an exaggeration of the mild deficits seen preoperatively, which are probably related to the epileptic process. She demonstrated that left dominant temporal resections impaired verbal memory whereas right temporal resections affected visuospatial memory (38,66,94). Milner indicated that the verbal-memory deficit was independent of aphasia, although if aphasia was present a verbal-memory disturbance could be part of it. Although it had been suggested that impairment was specific for auditory material (225), Milner showed it was the verbal nature of the material rather than the sensory channel that resulted in the difficulty (38,94). The extent of both hippocampal and lateral temporal resection influenced the severity of the verbal-memory deficit (38). Jones-Gotman (95) indicated that the extent of hippocampal resection affected performance on some verbal-memory tasks but not others. Thus, different aspects of verbal memory may be variably sensitive to left hippocampal injury. Saykin et al. (181) found that patients with onset of epilepsy prior to age 5 had less decline in verbal memory after left temporal lobectomy than those with later onset, suggesting redistribution of memory functions with an early insult. The decline in verbal memory was worse in patients who continued to have seizures. Interestingly, right temporal lobectomy was associated with improved verbal memory, suggesting that the epileptic activity on the right adversely affected left temporal function (180,226).

Less attention has been paid to the effect of temporal resections on language. Postoperative aphasia was common after dominant resections, according to Penfield and Roberts (20), but was almost always transient. Heilman et al. (26) reported four patients with anomic aphasia lasting longer than 6 months after left temporal lobectomy. Hermann and Wyler (227) also demonstrated a mild permanent postoperative anomia after dominant left temporal lobectomy, especially in patients who had not undergone preoperative mapping. They also reported a prospective controlled investigation of preoperative versus postoperative language function in patients who underwent anterior temporal lobectomy (194). In most patients, language was mapped intraoperatively. There was no significant loss in language ability 6 months postoperatively, and the group with dominant lobectomy actually showed significant improvement in receptive language comprehension and associative verbal fluency. This gain may be related to decreased interference from epileptic activity. Stafiniak et al. (145) examined naming before and 2–3 weeks after dominant temporal lobectomy. Patients with early risk factors (before age 5) for epilepsy did not show a decline in naming performance, whereas 60% of those without early risk factors demonstrated a significant decline. This difference was explained by an atypical representation of naming in patients with early risk.

In summary, verbal-memory disturbances are common after dominant temporal lobectomy and tend to persist, although they may improve with time. On the other hand, aphasia, and specifically anomia, is common in the acute postoperative period but usually disappears by 6 months after dominant temporal resection. Whether this aphasia is due to resection of the basal temporal language area, encroachment on lateral temporal naming sites, or another mechanism is not known (146).

CONCLUSIONS: EPILEPSY AND LANGUAGE

The observation, investigation, and treatment of epilepsy have contributed insights into the mechanisms of language functions. These insights have sometimes confirmed data from other sources, but often have also led to novel ideas. The textbook models of language function have been derived mostly from the study of lesions, particularly strokes. The input from epilepsy should be incorporated into these models. Further unique opportunities for language research lie in the evaluation of epilepsy. These opportunities are best capitalized on by collaboration of researchers in the fields of behavioral neurology and epileptology.

REFERENCES

1. Broca P. Remarques sur le siège de la faculté du langage articulé, suivies d'une observation d'aphémie (perte de la parole). Bull Soc Anat 1861;36:330–357.
2. Wernicke C. Der aphasische Symptomenkomplex. Breslau: Cohn & Weigert, 1874.
3. Fritsch G and Hitzig E. Über die elektrische Erregbarkeit des Grosshirns. Arch Anat Physiol Wiss Med 1870;37:300–332.
4. Hitzig E. Untersuchungen über das Gehirn. Berlin: A Hirschwald, 1874.
5. Ferrier D. Experimental researches in cerebral physiology and pathology. West Riding Lunatic Asylum Medical Reports 1873;3:30–96.
6. Ferrier D. The functions of the brain. 2nd ed. London: Smith, Elder, 1886.
7. Sherrington C. On the motor area of the cerebral cortex. In: Denny-Brown D, ed. Selected writings of Sir Charles Sherrington. London: Hamilton, 1939:397–439.
8. Franz SI. Variations in the distribution of the motor centers. Psychology Monographs 1915;19:80–162.
9. Devinsky O. Electrical and magnetic stimulation of the central nervous system: historical overview. In: Devinsky O, Berić A, Dogali M, eds. Electrical and mag-

netic stimulation of the brain and spinal cord. New York: Raven Press, 1993: 155-163.

10. Morgan JP. The first reported case of electrical stimulation of the human brain. J Hist Med Allied Sci 1982;37:51-64.

11. Horsley V. Remarks on ten consecutive cases of operation upon the brain and cranial cavity to illustrate the details and safety of the method employed. Brit Med J 1887;1:863-865.

12. Horsley V. The function of the so-called motor area of the brain. Brit Med J 1909;2:125-132.

13. Cushing H. A note upon the faradic stimulation of the postcentral gyrus in conscious patients. Brain 1909:32:44-53.

14. Foerster O. The motor cortex in man in the light of Hughlings Jackson's doctrines. Brain 1936;59:135-159.

15. Penfield W, Boldrey E. Somatic motor and sensory representation in the cerebral cortex of man as studied by electrical stimulation. Brain 1937;60:389-443.

16. Penfield W, Erickson T. Epilepsy and cerebral localization. Springfield, IL: Charles C Thomas, 1941.

17. Penfield W, Rasmussen T. The cerebral cortex of man. A clinical study of localization of function. New York: Macmillan, 1950.

18. Penfield W, Jasper H. Epilepsy and the functional anatomy of the human brain. Boston: Little, Brown, 1954.

19. Penfield W. Functional localization in temporal and deep sylvian areas. Res Publ Assoc Nerv Ment Dis 1956;36:210-226.

20. Penfield W, Roberts L. Speech and brain mechanisms. Princeton: Princeton University Press, 1959.

21. Penfield W. Epilepsy and surgical therapy. Arch Neurol Psychiatry 1936;36: 449-484.

22. Bailey P, Gibbs F. The surgical treatment of psychomotor epilepsy. JAMA 1951;145:365-370.

23. Falconer M. Anterior temporal lobectomy for epilepsy. In: Rob C, Smith R. Operative surgery. Vol. 14. London: Butterworths, 1968:142-149.

24. Jensen I. Temporal lobe surgery around the world. Acta Neurol Scand 1975;52: 354-373.

25. Crandall PH, Cahan LD, Sutherling W, Engel J Jr, Rausch R. Surgery for intractable complex partial epilepsy. In: Porter RJ, Morselli PL, eds. The epilepsies. London: Butterworths, 1985:307-321.

26. Heilman KM, Wilder BJ, Malzone WF. Anomic aphasia following anterior temporal lobectomy. Trans Am Neurol Assoc 1972;97:291-93.

27. Ojemann GA. Functional mapping of cortical language areas in adults: intraoperative approaches. In: Devinsky O, Berić A, Dogali M, eds. Electrical and magnetic stimulation of the brain and spinal cord. New York: Raven Press, 1993:155-163.

28. Ojemann GA, Mateer C. Human language cortex: localization of memory, syntax and sequential motor-phoneme identification systems. Science 1979;205: 1401-1403.

29. Ojemann GA. Brain organization for language from the perspective of electrical stimulation mapping. Behav Brain Res 1983;6:189-230.
30. Ojemann G, Ojemann J, Lettich E, Berger M. Cortical language localization in left-dominant hemisphere. J Neurosurg 1989;71:316-326.
31. Ojemann G. Organization of language cortex derived from investigations during neurosurgery. Semin Neurosci 1990;2:297-305.
32. Ojemann G. Cortical organization of language. J Neurosci 1991;11:2281-2287.
33. Ojemann GA. Electrical stimulation and the neurobiology of language. Behav Brain Sci 1983;6:221-230.
34. Ojemann GA. Some brain mechanisms for reading. In: Von Euler C, Lundberg I, Lennerstrand G, eds. Brain and reading. New York: Macmillan, 1989:47-59.
35. Ojemann G, Whitaker H. Language localization and variability. Brain Lang 1978;6:239-260.
36. Ojemann GA, Dodrill CB. Verbal memory deficits after left temporal lobectomy for epilepsy: mechanism and intraoperative prediction. J Neurosurg 1985;62:101-107.
37. Ojemann G, Dodrill CB. Intraoperative techniques for reducing language and memory deficits with left temporal lobectomy. In: Wolf P, Dam M, Janz D, Dreifuss F, eds. Advances in epileptology. Vol 16. New York: Raven Press, 1987:327-330.
38. Milner B. Brain mechanisms suggested by studies of temporal lobe. In: Darley FL, ed. Brain mechanisms underlying speech and language. New York: Grune & Stratton, 1967:122-145.
39. Fedio P, Van Buren JM. Memory deficits during electrical stimulation of speech cortex in conscious man. Brain Lang 1974;1:29-42.
40. Albert ML. Short-term memory and aphasia. Brain Lang 1979;7:145-163.
41. Ojemann GA, Creutzfeldt O, Lettich E, Haglund M. Neuronal activity in human lateral temporal cortex related to short-term verbal memory, naming and reading. Brain 1988;111:1383-1403.
42. Fried I, Ojemann GA, Fetz EE. Language related potentials specific to human language cortex. Science 1981;212:353-356.
43. Ojemann GA, Fried I, Lettich E. Electrocorticographic (ECoG) correlates of language. I. Desynchronization in temporal language cortex during object naming. Electroencephalogr Clin Neurophysiol 1989;73:453-463.
44. Creutzfeldt O, Ojemann G, Lettich E. Neuronal activity in human lateral temporal lobe. I. Responses to speech. Exp Brain Res 1989;77:451-475.
45. Creutzfeldt O, Ojemann G, Lettich E. Neuronal activity in human lateral temporal lobe. II. Responses to the subjects own voice. Exp Brain Res 1989;77:476-489.
46. Lüders H, Lesser RP, Hahn J, et al. Basal temporal language area demonstrated by electrical stimulation. Neurology 1986;36:505-510.
47. Goldring S. A method for surgical management of focal epilepsy, especially as it relates to children. J Neurosurg 1978;49:344-356.
48. Goldring S, Gregorie EM. Surgical management of epilepsy using epidural recordings to localize the seizure focus. Review of 100 cases. J Neurosurg 1984; 60:457-466.

49. Lüders H, Lesser R, Dinner D, et al. Commentary: Chronic intracranial recording and stimulation with subdural electrodes. In: Engel J, ed. Surgical treatment of the epilepsies. New York: Raven Press, 1987:297-321.

50. Lesser RP, Lüders H, Klem G, Dinner DS, Morris HH, Hahn J. Cortical afterdischarge and functional response thresholds: results of extraoperative testing. Epilepsia 1984;25:619-621.

51. Lüders H, Lesser RP, Dinner DS, Morris HH, Wyllie E, Godoy J. Localization of cortical function: new information from extraoperative monitoring of patients with epilepsy. Epilepsia 1988;29(suppl 2):S56-S65.

52. Lüders H, Lesser RP, Hahn J, et al. Basal temporal language area. Brain 1991; 743-754.

53. Lesser RP, Gordon B, Fisher R, Hart J, Uematsu S. Subdural grid electrodes in surgery for epilepsy. In: Lüders H, ed. Epilepsy surgery. New York: Raven Press, 1991:399-408.

54. Lesser RP, Lüders H, Dinner DS, Hahn J, Cohen L. The location of speech and writing functions in the frontal language area: results of extraoperative cortical stimulation. Brain 1984;107:275-291.

55. Schäffler L, Lüders HO, Dinner DS, Lesser RP, Chelune GJ. Comprehension deficits elicited by electrical stimulation of Broca's area. Brain 1993;116:695-715.

56. Adams RD, Victor M. Principles of neurology. New York: McGraw-Hill, 1989: 383.

57. Damasio AR. Aphasia. N Engl J Med 1992;326:531-539.

58. Lesser RP, Lüders H, Morris HH, et al. Electrical stimulation of Wernicke's area interferes with comprehension. Neurology 1986;36:658-663.

59. Burnstine TH, Lesser RP, Hart J, et al. Characterization of the basal temporal language area in patients with left temporal lobe epilepsy. Neurology 1990;40: 966-970.

60. Kluin K, Abou-Khalil B, Hood T. Inferior speech area in patients with temporal lobe epilepsy (abstr). Neurology 1988;38(suppl 1):277.

61. Abou-Khalil B, Welch L, Blumenkopf B, Newman K. Speech arrest with seizures starting in the inferior temporal region (abstr). Epilepsia 1991; 32(suppl 3):59.

62. Suzuki I, Shimizu H, Ishijima B, et al. Aphasic seizure caused by focal epilepsy in the left fusiform gyrus. Neurology 1992;42:2207-2210.

63. Abou-Khalil B, Welch L, Blumenkopf B, Newman K, Whetsell WO. Global aphasia speech arrest with seizure onset in the dominant basal temporal region. Epilepsia. In press.

64. Kluin K, Abou-Khalil B, Hood T. The basal temporal language area: changes in language functions after surgical ablation. In preparation.

65. Abou-Khalil R, Wertz RT, Abou-Khalil B, Welch L. Basal temporal language area: evidence from cortical stimulation and surgical ablation. In preparation.

66. Milner B. Psychological defects produced by temporal lobe excision. Res Publ Assoc Nerv Ment Dis 1958;36:244-257.

67. Ojemann GA, Sutherling WW, Lesser RP, Dinner DS, Jayakar P, Saint-Hilaire JM. Cortical stimulation. In: Engel J, ed. Surgical treatment of the epilepsies. New York: Raven Press, 1993:399-414.

68. Gordon B, Uematsu G, Lesser R, Schwerdt P, Fisher R, Vining EPG, Hart J. Utility of intraoperative neuropsychological testing with stepwise resection (abstr). Epilepsia 1991;32:87.

69. Sutherling WW, Lévesque MF. Comparison of chronic and acute cortical stimulations for localization and quantification of language cortex (abstr). Epilepsia 1991;32:25.

70. Rasmussen T, Milner B. The role of early left brain injury in determining the lateralization of cerebral speech functions. Ann NY Acad Sci 1977;299:355–369.

71. Rausch R, Walsh GO. Right-hemisphere language dominance in right-handed epileptic patients. Arch Neurol 1984;41:1077–1080.

72. Devinsky O, Perrine K, Llinas R, Luciano DJ, Dogali M. Anterior temporal language areas in patients with early onset of temporal lobe epilepsy. Ann Neurol 1993;34:727–732.

73. Ingvar D. Serial aspects of language and speech related to prefrontal cortical activity. A selective review. Hum Neurobiol 1983;2:177–189.

74. Petersen SE, Fox PT, Posner MI, Mintun M, Raichle ME. Positron emission tomographic studies of the cortical anatomy of single-word processing. Nature 1988;331:585–589.

75. Raichle M. Exploring the mind with dynamic imaging. Semin Neurosci 1990;2:307–315.

76. Belliveau JW, Kennedy DN, McKinstry RC, et al. Functional mapping of the human visual cortex by magnetic resonance imaging. Science 1991;254:716–719.

77. Basso A, Lecours AR, Moraschini S, Vanier M. Anatomoclinical correlation of the aphasias as defined through computerized tomography: exceptions. Brain Lang 1985;26:201–229.

78. Kirshner HS, Casey PF, Henson J, Heinrich JJ. Behavioral features and lesion localization in Wernicke's aphasia. Aphasiology 1989;3:169–176.

79. Rostomily RC, Berger MS, Ojemann GA, Lettich E. Postoperative deficits and functional recovery following removal of tumors involving the dominant hemisphere supplementary motor area. J Neurosurg 1991;75:62–68.

80. Paradis M. Bilingualism and aphasia. In: Whitaker H, Whitaker H, eds. Studies in neurolinguistics. New York: Academic Press, 1977;3:65–122.

81. Paradis M. Language lateralization in bilinguals: enough already! Brain Lang 1990;39:576–586.

82. Rapport RL, Tan CT, Whitaker HA. Language function and dysfunction among Chinese and English speaking polyglots: cortical stimulation, Wada testing and clinical studies. Brain Lang 1983;18:342–366.

83. Ojemann GA, Whitaker HA. The bilingual brain. Arch Neurol 1978;35:409–412.

84. Ojemann GA. Effect of cortical and subcortical stimulation on human language and verbal memory. In: Plum F, ed. Language, communication and the brain. New York: Raven Press, 1988:101–115.

85. Mateer CA, Polen SB, Ojemann GA, Wyler AR. Cortical localizaton of finger spelling and oral language: a case study. Brain Lang 1982;17:46–57.

86. Haglund MM, Ojemann GA, Lettich E, Bellugi U, Corina D. Dissociation of cortical and single unit activity in spoken and signed languages. Brain Lang 1993; 44:19–27.

87. Wada J. A new method for the determination of the side of cerebral speech dominance: a preliminary report on the intracarotid injection of sodium Amytal in man [in Japanese]. Med Biol 1949;14:221–222.

88. Milner B, Branch C, Rasmussen T. Study of short-term memory after intracarotid injection of sodium amytal. Trans Am Neurol Assoc 1962;87:224–226.

89. Rausch R, Silfvenius H, Wieser H-G, Dodrill CB, Meador KJ, Jones-Gotman M. Intraarterial amobarbital procedures. In: Engel J Jr, ed. Surgical treatment of the epilepsies. 2nd ed. New York: Raven Press, 1993:341–357.

90. Branch C, Milner B, Rasmussen T. Intracarotid sodium amytal for the lateralization of cerebral speech dominance: observations in 123 patients. J Neurosurg 1964;21:399–405.

91. Blume WT, Grabow JD, Darley FL, et al. Intracarotid amobarbital test of language and memory before temporal lobectomy for seizure control. Neurology 1973;23:812–819.

92. Raush R. Psychological evaluation. In: Engel J Jr, ed. Surgical treatment of the epilepsies. New York: Raven Press, 1987:181–195.

93. Snyder PJ, Novelly RA. Mixed speech dominance in the intracarotid sodium amytal procedure: validity and criteria issues. J Clin Exp Neuropsychol 1990; 12:629–643.

94. Milner B. Psychological aspects of focal epilepsy and its neurosurgical management. Adv Neurol 1975;8:299–321.

95. Jones-Gotman M. Commentary: psychological evaluation-testing hippocampal function. In: Engel J Jr, ed. Surgical treatment of the epilepsies. New York: Raven Press, 1987:203–211.

96. Woods R, Dodrill CB, Ojemann GA. Brain injury, handedness, and speech lateralization in a series of amobarbital studies. Ann Neurol 1988;23:510–518.

97. Loring DW, Meador KJ, Lee GP, Murro AM, et al. Cerebral language lateralization: evidence from intracarotid testing. Neuropsychologia 1990;28:831–838.

98. Serafetinides EA, Hoare RD, Driver MV. Intracarotid sodium amylobarbitone and cerebral dominance for speech and consciousness. Brain 1965;88:107–130.

99. Levin HS, Combs Cantrell DT, Soukup V, Crow W, Bartha MC. Preliminary results of an incremental intracarotid amobarbital procedure: evaluation of language and memory without sedation. J Epilepsy 1994;7:11–17.

100. Wada J, Rasmussen T. Intracarotid injections of sodium amytal for the lateralization of cerebral speech dominance. J Neurosurg 1960;17:266–282.

101. Mateer CA, Dodrill CB. Neuropsychological and linguistic correlates of atypical language lateralization: evidence from sodium Amytal studies. Hum Neurobiol 1983;2:135–142.

102. Jack CR Jr, Nichols DA, Sharbrough FW, Marsh WR, Peterson RC. Selective posterior cerebral artery Amytal test for evaluating memory function before surgery for temporal lobe seizures. Radiology 1988;169:787–793.

103. Wieser HG. Anterior cerebral artery amobarbital test. In: Lüders H, ed. Epilepsy surgery. New York: Raven Press, 1991:515–523.
104. Rey M, Dellatulas G, Bancaud J, et al. Hemispheric lateralization of motor and speech functions after early brain lesion: study of 73 epileptic patients with intracarotid Amytal test. Neuropsychologia 1988;26:167–172.
105. Silfvenius H, Christianson SA, Nilsson LG, Salsa J. Preoperative investigation of cerebral hemisphere speech and memory with the bilateral intracarotid amytal test. Acta Neurol Scand 1988;117:79–83.
106. Zatorre RJ. Perceptual asymmetry on the dichotic fused words test and cerebral speech lateralization determined by the carotid sodium amytal test. Neuropsychologia 1989;27:1207–1219.
107. Wyllie E, Lüders H, Murphy D, Morris H III, et al. Intracarotid amobarbital (Wada) test for language dominance: correlation with results of cortical stimulation. Epilepsia 1990;31:156–161.
108. Strauss E, Wada J, Goldwater B. Sex differences in interhemispheric reorganization of speech. Neuropsychologia 1992;30:353–359.
109. Charles D, Abou-Khalil R, Abou-Khalil B, et al. MRI asymmetries and language dominance. Neurology. In press.
110. Strauss E, Wada J. Lateral preferences and cerebral speech dominance. Cortex 1983;19:165–177.
111. Satz P, Strauss E, Wada J, Orsini DL. Some correlates of intra- and interhemispheric speech organization after left focal brain injury. Neuropsychologia 1988;26:345–350.
112. Habib M, Joanette V, Ali-Cherif A, Poncet M. Crossed aphasia in dextrals: a case report with special reference to site of lesion. Neuropsychologia 1983; 21:413–418.
113. Joanette V, Puel M, Nespoulous JL, Rascol A, Lecours AR. L'aphasie croisée du droitier. I. Revue de la littérature. Revue Neurol 1982;138:575–586.
114. Zangwill OL. Two cases of crossed aphasia in dextrals. Neuropsychologia 1979; 17:167–172.
115. Lansdell H. Laterality of verbal intelligence in the brain. Science 1962;135: 922–923.
116. Kinsbourne M. The minor cerebral hemisphere as a source of aphasic speech. Arch Neurol 1971;25:302–306.
117. McGlone J, Fox AJ. Evidence from sodium Amytal studies of greater asymmetry of verbal representation in men compared to women. In: Akimoto H, Kazamatsuri H, Seino M, Ward A, eds. Advances in epileptology: XIIIth Epilepsy International Symposium. New York: Raven Press, 1982:389–391.
118. Strauss E, Satz P, Wada J. An examination of the crowding hypothesis in epileptic patients who have undergone the carotid Amytal test. Neuropsychologia 1990;28:1221–1227.
119. Lansdell H. Verbal and nonverbal factors in right hemisphere speech: relation to early neurological history. J Comp Physiol Psychol 1969;69:734–738.
120. Fedio P, Weinberg LK. Dysnomia and impairment of verbal memory following intracarotid injection of sodium amytal. Brain Res 1971;31:159–168.

121. Rausch R, Fedio R, Ary CM, Engel J Jr, Crandall PH. Resumption of behavior following intracarotid sodium amobarbital injection. Ann Neurol 1984;15:31–35.
122. Gilman S, MacFadyen DJ, Denny-Brown D. Decerebrate phenomena after carotid amobarbital injection. Arch Neurol 1963;8:662–675.
123. Terzian H. Behavioural and EEG effects of intracarotid sodium amytal injections. Acta Neurochir 1964;12:230–239.
124. Rosadini G, Rossi GF. On the suggested cerebral dominance for consciousness. Brain 1967;90:101–112.
125. Lesser RP, Dinner DS, Lüders H, Morris HH. Memory for objects presented soon after intracarotid amobarbital sodium injections in patients with medically intractable complex partial seizures. Neurology 1986;36:895–899.
126. Huh K, Meador KJ, Loring DW, Lee GP, Brooks BS. Attentional mechanisms during the intracarotid amobarbital test. Neurology 1989;39:1183–1186.
127. Gilmore RL, Heilman KM, Schmidt RP, Fennel EM, Quisling R. Anosognosia during Wada testing. Neurology 1992;42:925–927.
128. Buchtel HA, Henry TR, Abou-Khalil BW. Memory for neurological deficits during the intracarotid amytal procedure: a hemispheric difference. Submitted for publication.
129. Perria L, Rosadini R, Rossi GF. Determination of side of cerebral dominance with amobarbital. Arch Neurol 1961;4:173–181.
130. Rossi FG, Rosadini G. Experimental analysis of cerebral dominance in man. In: Millikan CH, Darley FL, eds. Brain mechanisms underlying speech and language. New York: Grune & Stratton, 1967:167–184.
131. Milner B, Branch C. Reviewed in: Rossi FG, Rosadini G. Experimental analysis of cerebral dominance in man. In: Millikan CH, Darley FL, eds. Brain mechanisms underlying speech and language. New York: Grune & Stratton, 1967:177–184.
132. Lee GP, Loring DW, Meador KF, Brooks BS. Hemispheric specialization for emotional expression: a reexamination of results from intracarotid administration of sodium amobarbital. Brain Cogn 1990;12:267–280.
133. Loring DW, Meador KJ, Lee GP, Kin DW. Amobarbital effects and lateralized brain function: the Wada test. New York: Springer Verlag, 1992.
134. Dinner DS. Intracarotid amobarbital test to define language lateralization. In: Lüders HO. Epilepsy surgery. New York: Raven Press, 1991:503–506.
135. Petersen RC, Sharbrough FW, Jack CR. Intracarotid amobarbital testing. In: Wyllie E, ed. The treatment of epilepsy: principles and practice. Philadelphia: Lea & Febiger, 1993:1051–1061.
136. Hart J Jr, Lesser RP, Fisher RS, Schwerdt P, Bryan RN, Gordon B. Dominant-side intracarotid amobarbital spares comprehension of word meaning. Arch Neurol 1991;48:55–58.
137. Satz P, Orsini DL, Saslow E, Henry R. The pathological left-handedness syndrome. Brain Cogn 1985;4:27–46.
138. Satz P, Baymur L, Van Der Vlugt H. Pathological left-handedness: cross-cultural tests of a model. Neuropsychologia 1979;17:77–81.

139. Channon S, Schugens MM, Daum I, Polkey CE. Lateralisation of language functioning by the Wada procedure and divided visual field presentation of a verbal task. Cortex 1990;26:147-151.
140. Strauss E, Gaddes WH, Wada J. Performance on a free-recall verbal dichotic listening task and cerebral dominance determined by the carotid amytal test. Neuropsychologia 1987;25:747-753.
141. Pascual-Leone A, Gates JR, Dhuna A. Induction of speech arrest and counting errors with rapid-rate transcranial magnetic stimulation. Neurology 1991; 41:697-702.
142. Howard D, Patterson K, Wise R, Brown WD, Friston K, et al. The cortical localization of the lexicons. Brain 1992;115:1769-1782.
143. Leblanc R, Meyer E, Bub D, Zatorre RJ, Evans AC. Language localization with activation positron emission tomography scanning. Neurosurgery 1992; 31:369-373.
144. Damasio A, Bellugi U, Damasio H, Poizner H, Van Gilder J. Sign-language aphasia during left-hemisphere amytal injection. Nature 1986;322:363-365.
145. Stafiniak P, Saykin AJ, Sperling MR, et al. Acute naming deficits following dominant temporal lobectomy: prediction by age at 1st risk for seizures. Neurology 1990;40:1509-1512.
146. Pilcher WH, Roberts DW, Flanigin HF, et al. Complications of epilepsy surgery. In: Engel J Jr, ed. Surgical treatment of the epilepsies. 2nd ed. New York: Raven Press, 1993:565-581.
147. Jackson JH. On the scientific and empirical investigation of epilepsies. In: Taylor J, ed. Selected writings of John Hughlings Jackson. Vol 1. London: Hodder and Stoughton, 1931:163.
148. Hécaen H, Piercy M. Paroxysmal dysphasia and the problem of cerebral dominance. J Neurol Neurosurg Psychiatry 1956;19:194-201.
149. Ajmone-Marsan C, Ralston BL. The epileptic seizure. Springfield, IL: Charles C Thomas, 1957.
150. Alajouanine TH, Sabouraud O: Les perturbations paroxystiques du language dans l'épilepsie. Encéphale 1960;49:95-133.
151. Serafetinides EA, Falconer MA. Speech disturbance in temporal lobe seizures: A study in 100 epileptic patients submitted to anterior temporal lobectomy. Brain 1963;86:333-346.
152. Hécaen H, Angelergues R. Epilepsie et troubles du langage. Encéphale 1960; 49:138-169.
153. Falconer MA. Brain mechanisms suggested by neurophysiologic studies. In: Millikan CH, Darley FL, eds. Brain mechanisms underlying speech and language. New York: Grune & Stratton, 1967:185-203.
154. King DW, Ajmone-Marsan C. Clinical features and ictal patterns in epileptic patients with EEG temporal lobe foci. Ann Neurol 1977;2:138-147.
155. Gabr M, Lüders H, Dinner D, et al. Speech manifestations in lateralization of temporal lobe seizures. Ann Neurol 1989;25:82-87.
156. Koerner M, Laxer KD. Ictal speech, postictal language dysfunction, and seizure lateralization. Neurology 1988;38:634-636.

157. Privitera MD, Morris GL, Gilliam F. Postictal language assessment and lateralization of complex partial seizures. Ann Neurol 1991;30:391–396.
158. Fakhoury T, Abou-Khalil B, Peguero E. Differentiating clinical features of left and right temporal lobe seizures. Epilepsia. In press.
159. Devinsky O, Kelly K, Yacubian EMT, et al. Postictal behavior: a clinical and subdural electroencephalographic study. Arch Neurol 1994;51:254–259.
160. Bell WL, Horner J, Logue P, Radtke RA. Neologistic speech automatisms during complex partial seizures. Neurology 1990;40:49–52.
161. DePasquet EG, Gaudin ES, Bianchia A, DeMendilaharsu SA. Prolonged monosymptomatic dysphasic status epilepticus. Neurology (Minneapolis) 1976;26: 244–247.
162. Hamilton NG, Matthews T. Aphasia: the sole manifestation of focal status epilepticus. Neurology (NY) 1979;29:745–748.
163. Racy A, Osborn MA, Vern BA, Molinari GF. Epileptic aphasia: First onset of prolonged monosymptomatic status epilepticus in adults. Arch Neurol 1980; 37:419–422.
164. Dinner DS, Lüders H, Lederman R, Gretter TE. Aphasic status epilepticus: a case report. Neurology 1981;31:888–890.
165. Rosenbaum DH, Siegel M, Barr WB, Rowan AJ. Epileptic aphasia. Neurology 1986;36:822–825.
166. Knight RT, Cooper J. Status epilepticus manifesting as reversible Wernicke's aphasia. Epilepsia 1986;27:301–304.
167. Lecours AR, Joanette Y. Linguistic and other psychological aspects of paroxysmal aphasia. Brain Lang 1980;10:1–23.
168. Wells CR, Labar DR, Solomon GE. Aphasia as the sole manifestation of simple partial status epilepticus. Epilepsia 1992;33:84–87.
169. Gilmore RI, Heilman KM. Speech arrest in partial seizures: Evidence of an associated language disorder. Neurology 1981;31:1016–1019.
170. Marie P. Revision de la question de l'aphasie: la troisième circonvolution frontale gauche ne joue aucun rôle spécial dans la fonction du langage. Sem Médicale 1906;26:241–247.
171. Commission on Classification and Terminology of the International League Against Epilepsy. Proposal for classification of epilepsies and epileptic syndromes. Epilepsia 1985;26:268–278.
172. Commission on Classification and Terminology of the International League Against Epilepsy. Proposal for classification of epilepsies and epileptic syndromes. Epilepsia 1989;30:389–399.
173. Wieser HG, Müller RU. Neocortical temporal seizures. In: Wieser HG, Elger CE, eds. Presurgical evaluation of epileptics. Berlin Heidelberg: Springer-Verlag, 1987:252–266.
174. Engel JJr, Kuhl DE, Phelps ME, Mazziotta JC. Interictal cerebral glucose metabolism in partial epilepsy and its relation to EEG changes. Ann Neurol 1982;12:510–517.
175. Abou-Khalil BW, Siegel GJ, Sackellares JC, Gilman S, Hichwa R, Marshall R. Positron emission tomography studies of cerebral glucose metabolism in chronic partial epilepsy. Ann Neurol 1987;22:480–486.

176. Homan RW, Paulman RG, Devous MDSr, Walker P, Jennings LW, Bonte FJ. Cognitive function and regional cerebral blood flow in partial seizures. Arch Neurol 1989;46:964–970.

177. Deutsch CP. Differences among epileptics and between epileptics and non-epileptics in terms of some learning and memory variables. Arch Neurol Psychiat 1953;70:474–482.

178. Dodrill CB. Cognitive and psychosocial effects of epilepsy on adults. In: Wyllie E, ed. The treatment of epilepsy: principles and practice. Philadelphia: Lea & Febiger, 1993:1133–1140.

179. Jones-Gotman M, Smith ML, Zatorre RJ. Neuropsychological testing for localizing and lateralizing the epileptogenic region. In: Engel J Jr, ed. Surgical treatment of the epilepsies. 2nd ed. New York: Raven Press, 1993:245–261.

180. Ivnik RJ, Sharbrough FW, Laws ER Jr. Anterior temporal lobectomy for the control of partial complex seizures: information for counseling patients. Mayo Clin Proc 1988;63:783–793.

181. Saykin AJ, Gur RC, Sussman NM, O'Connor MJ, Gur RE. Memory deficits before and after temporal lobectomy: effect of laterality and age at onset. Brain Cogn 1989;9:191–200.

182. Schneider SK, Nowack WJ, Fitzgerald JA, Janati A. Souheaver GT. WAIS performance in epileptics with unilateral interictal EEG abnormalities. J Epilepsy 1993;6:10–14.

183. Camfield PR, Gates R, Ronen G, Camfield C, Ferguson A, McDonald W. Comparison of cognitive ability, personality profile, and school success in epileptic children with pure right versus left temporal lobe EEG foci. Ann Neurol 1984;15:122–126.

184. Reitan RM. Psychological testing of epileptic patients. In: Magnus O, Lorentz De Haas AM, eds. The epilepsies. In: Vinken PJ, Bruyn GW, eds. Handbook of clinical neurology. Vol 15. Amsterdam: North-Holland, 1974:559–575.

185. Small JG, Milstein V, Stevens JR. Are psychomotor epileptics different? Arch Neurol 1962;7:187–194.

186. Stevens JR, Milstein V, Goldstein S. Psychometric test performance in relation to psychopathology of epilepsy. Arch Gen Psychiatry 1972;26:532–538.

187. Fedio P, Mirsky AF. Selective intellectual deficits in children with temporal lobe or centrencephalic epilepsy. Neuropsychologia 1969;7:287–300.

188. Hermann BP, Wyler AR, Richey ET, Rea JM. Memory function and verbal learning ability in patients with complex partial seizures of temporal lobe origin. Epilepsia 1987;28:547–554.

189. Helmstaedter C, Durwen HF, Elger C. Verbal learning and memory test in 24 patients with complex partial seizures and right or left temporal focus. Epilepsia 1990;31:224.

190. Delaney RC, Rosen AJ, Mattson RH, Novelly RA. Memory function in focal epilepsy: a comparison of non-surgical unilateral temporal lobe and frontal lobe samples. Cortex 1980;16:103–117.

191. Delaney RC, Prevey ML, Mattson RH. Short-term retention with lateralized temporal epilepsy. Cortex 1982;22:591–600.

192. Mungas D, Ehlers C, Walton N, McCutchen CB. Verbal learning differences in epileptic patients with left and right temporal lobe foci. Epilepsia 1985;26: 340–345.

193. Mayeux R, Brandt J, Rosen J, Benson DF. Interictal memory and language impairment in temporal lobe epilepsy. Neurology 1980;30:120–125.

194. Hermann BP, Wyler AR. Effects of anterior temporal lobectomy on language function: a controlled study. Ann Neurol 1988;23:585–588.

195. Tizard J, Rutter M, Whitmore K. Education, health and behaviour. London: Longmans, 1969.

196. Rutter M, Graham P, Uyle W. A neuropsychological study in childhood. Clinics in developmental medicine 35/36. London: SIMP with Heineman, 1970.

197. Schachter SC, Galaburda AM, Ransil BJ. A history of dyslexia in patients with epilepsy. J Epilepsy 1993;6:267–271.

198. Stores G, Hart J. Reading skills of children with generalised or focal epilepsy attending ordinary school. Develop Med Child Neurol 1976;18:705–716.

199. Binnie CD, Marston D. Cognitive correlates of interictal discharges. Epilepsia 1992;33(suppl 6):S11–S17.

200. Aarts JHP, Binnie CD, Smit AM, Wilkins AJ. Selective cognitive impairment during focal and generalized epileptiform EEG activity. Brain 1984;107:293–308.

201. Shewmon DA, Erwin RJ. Focal spike-induced cerebral dysfunction is related to the after coming slow wave. Ann Neurol 1988;23:131–137.

202. Landau WM, Kleffner FR. Syndrome of acquired aphasia with convulsive disorder in children. Neurology. 1957;7:523–530.

203. Beaumanoir A. The Landau-Kleffner syndrome. In: Roger J, Dravet C, Bureau M, Dreifuss FE, Wolf P, eds. Epileptic Syndromes in infancy, childhood and adolescence. London: John Libbey Eurotext, 1985:181–191.

204. Deonna TW. Acquired epileptiform aphasia in children (Laundau-Kleffner syndrome). J Clin Neurophysiol 1991;7:288–298.

205. Paquier PF, Van Dongen HR, Loonen MCB. The Landau-Kleffner syndrome or "acquired aphasia with convulsive disorder": long-term follow-up of six children, and review of the recent literature. Arch Neurol 1992;49:354–359.

206. Aicardi J. Syndrome of acquired aphasia with seizure disorder (epileptic aphasia, Landau-Kleffner syndrome, verbal auditory agnosia with convulsive disorder), and continuous spike-wave during slow sleep ("electrical status epilepticus of slow sleep"). In: Aicardi J, ed. Epilepsy in children. 2nd ed. New York: Raven Press, 1994:207–216.

207. Echenne B, Cheminal R, Rivier F, Negre C, Touchon J, Billiard M. Epileptic electroencephalographic abnormalities and developmental dysphasias: a study of 32 patients. Brain Dev 1992;14:216–225.

208. Roulet E, Deonna T, Gaillard F, Peter-Favre C, Despland PA. Acquired aphasia, dementia, and behavior disorder with epilepsy and continuous spike and waves during sleep in a child. Epilepsia 1991;32:495–503.

209. Rapin I, Mattis S, Rowan AJ, Golden GG. Verbal auditory agnosia in children. Dev Med Child Neurol 1977;19:192–207.

210. Deonna T, Beaumanoir A, Gaillard F, Assal G. Acquired aphasia in childhood with seizure disorder: a heterogeneous syndrome. Neuropediatrics 1977;8:263–273.

211. Cooper JA, Jerry PC. Acquired auditory verbal agnosia and seizures in childhood. J Speech Hear Disord 1978;43:176–184.

212. Mantovani JR, Landau WM. Acquired aphasia with convulsive disorder: course and prognosis. Neurology. 1980;30:524–529.

213. Deonna T, Peter C, Ziegler AL. Adult follow-up of the acquired aphasia-epilepsy syndrome in childhood. Report of 7 cases. Neuropediatrics 1989;20: 132–138.

214. Holmes GL, McKeever M, Saunders Z. Epileptiform activity in aphasia of childhood: an epiphenomenon? Epilepsia 1981;22:631–639.

215. Cole AJ, Andermann F, Taylor L, et al. The Landau-Kleffner syndrome of acquired epileptic aphasia: unusual clinical outcome, surgical experience, and absence of encephalitis. Neurology 1988;38:31–38.

216. Hirsch E, Marescaux C, Maquet P, et al. Landau-Kleffner syndrome: a clinical and EEG study of five cases. Epilepsia 1990;31:756–767.

217. Gordon N. Acquired aphasia in childhood: the Landau-Kleffner syndrome. Dev Med Child Neurol 1990;32:270–274.

218. Otero E, Cordova S, Diaz F, Garcia-Teruel I, Del Brutto OH. Acquired epileptic aphasia (the Landau-Kleffner syndrome) due to neurocysticercosis. Epilepsia 1989;30:569–572.

219. Pascual-Castroviejo I, Martín VL, Bermejo AM, Higueras AP. Is cerebral arteritis the cause of the Landau-Kleffner syndrome? Four cases in childhood with angiographic study. Can J Neurol Sci 1992;19:46–52.

220. Lou HC, Brandt S, Bruhn P. Aphasia and epilepsy in childhood. Acta Neurol Scand 1977;56:46–54.

221. Dulac O, Billard C, Arthuis M. Aspects electro-cliniques et evolutifs de l'épilepsie dans le syndrome aphasia-epilepsie. Arch Fr Pediatr 1983;40:299–308.

222. Bishop DVM. Age of onset and outcome in "acquired aphasia with convulsive disorder" (Landau-Kleffner syndrome). Dev Med Child Neurol 1985;27: 705–712.

223. Marescaux C, Hirsch E, Finck S, et al. Landau-Kleffner syndrome: a pharmacologic study of five cases. Epilepsia 1990;31:768–777.

224. Andrews R, Morrell F, Whisler WW. Subpial cortical transection in Landau-Kleffner syndrome (abstr). Ann Neurol 1989;26:469.

225. Meyer V, Yates AJ. Intellectual changes following temporal lobectomy for psychomotor epilepsy; preliminary communication. J Neurol Neurosurg Psychiatry 1955;18:44–52.

226. Novelly RA, Augustine EA, Mattson RH, Glaser GH, et al. Selective memory improvement and impairment in temporal lobectomy for epilepsy. Ann Neurol 1984;15:64–67.

227. Hermann BP, Wyler AR. Comparative results of dominant temporal lobectomy under general or local anesthesia: language outcome. J Epilepsy 1988;1:127–134.

10

Alexias

Howard S. Kirshner

Vanderbilt University School of Medicine, Nashville, Tennessee

Alexias are acquired disorders of reading secondary to brain disease (1). As such, they are aphasias, in that reading is an aspect of language function. Alexias are distinguished from congenital disorders of reading, which are usually called *dyslexias*. In Europe and in the literature of cognitive neuropsychology and neurolinguistics, the two terms are often used synonymously.

Historically, alexias have been divided into three groups: (1) alexia with agraphia, (2) pure alexia without agraphia, and (3) aphasic alexia. The first two are classical syndromes described by the nineteenth century French physician Dejerine. New studies have contributed considerable insight into the neurolinguistic mechanisms of these disorders. Pure alexia without agraphia has remained a clear and distinguishable syndrome, little changed from Dejerine's original description, but the alexia with agraphia syndrome overlaps considerably with aphasic alexia, and both syndromes have undergone modification and reclassification in the light of new evidence of varying mechanisms of alexia. The new categories of alexia are discussed at the end of the chapter.

ALEXIA WITH AGRAPHIA

In 1891, Dejerine (2) described the syndrome of alexia with agraphia, in effect an acquired illiteracy. These patients have lost the ability to read and

277

write, without other language impairments. On a bedside examination, a patient with alexia with agraphia should have normal spontaneous speech, repetition, naming, and auditory comprehension. In fact, such pure cases of alexia with agraphia are rare; most patients have mild aphasic deficits, especially anomia and paraphasic errors in spontaneous speech (3). Some patients with alexia with agraphia may be considered to have a mild form of Wernicke's aphasia, with mildly paraphasic speech and lesser impairment of auditory comprehension than of reading comprehension. As discussed in Chapter 4, these Wernicke's aphasics may have localized lesions in the vicinity of the inferior parietal lobule, or supramarginal and angular gyri (4,5). Because alexia with agraphia is often mixed with aphasic deficits, Benson (3) has suggested the anatomical term *temporoparietal alexia* as the name for this syndrome.

The reading deficit of alexia with agraphia is variable, ranging from total inability to read—either aloud or for comprehension—to partial deficit patterns. Most patients cannot read single letters or words, but a few patients have been described who cannot read but can name letters, spell words aloud, and comprehend words dictated to them in spelled form (6–8). Other aspects of the reading deficit are discussed later in this chapter, in the context of the new neurolinguistic classifications of alexia. The writing disorder of alexia with agraphia varies from complete inability to write even single letters or words to partial ability to copy slavishly, without competence to write sentences either spontaneously or to dictation.

The neurological deficits most closely associated with alexia with agraphia are right visual field defects, such as right homonymous hemianopsia. Motor and sensory deficits on the contralateral side of the body are present in a minority. The other behavioral deficits of the Gerstmann syndrome or angular gyrus syndrome, discussed in Chapter 21, may also be associated with pure alexia with agraphia; these include calculation difficulty, right–left confusion, finger agnosia, and constructional impairment.

The anatomical area involved in alexia with agraphia is the inferior parietal lobule, comprising the supramarginal and angular gyri (2,3). Dejerine (2) conceived of the angular gyrus as a center for visual language, or "optical images of letters," much as Wernicke's area was the center for auditory word images. Since Dejerine considered these optical images of letters necessary for the initiation of writing, both reading and writing would be deficient after damage to the angular gyrus. Geschwind (9) rediscovered Dejerine's general explanations of the syndromes of alexia with and without agraphia, but in his model the angular gyrus was envisioned as a part of the association cortex responsible for transfer of information between sensory modalities such as vision and hearing. Since reading requires translation of visual into auditory language, the angular gyrus is essential to this function. Geschwind also pointed out that humans, as compared to experimental animals, are much more able to utilize information learned in one sensory modality to solve problems in another modality; the inferior parietal lobule is one of the cortical association areas that enlarged the most in the evolution from ape to man.

While some patients with alexia with agraphia have ischemic strokes in the territory of the posterior branches of the left middle cerebral artery, this syndrome also arises from mass lesions of the inferior parietal lobule, such as tumors, brain abscesses, and hemorrhages.

PURE ALEXIA WITHOUT AGRAPHIA

Dejerine (10) described the syndrome of pure alexia without agraphia, or "pure word blindness," in 1892. Although descriptions of acquired alexia had appeared earlier (11), Dejerine was the first to correlate alexia with focal damage to the left occipital lobe; his discussion of this syndrome, along with that of his 1891 case of alexia with agraphia, led to a model of the reading process that is still used today. Whereas pure alexia with agraphia is an acquired illiteracy, pure alexia without agraphia can be considered a "linguistic blindfolding," in which the patient can produce and understand spoken language and write normally but cannot read his own written productions. This inability to read one's own writing is the hallmark of the syndrome of pure alexia.

The syndrome of pure alexia without agraphia is much more frequently unassociated with other language deficits than is alexia with agraphia (hence the designation "pure"). Most patients have normal spontaneous speech, repetition, and auditory comprehension. Naming is usually adequate for objects, pictures, and body parts, but some patients have difficulty naming colors, an interesting phenomenon that we shall discuss later. Patients can write sentences spontaneously or to dictation, but they cannot read words or letters. Over time, recovery of letter naming is a frequent finding. The patient then becomes able to spell words aloud, letter by letter, and decipher the meaning. Eventually, the patient may be able to read silently, but very slowly; in these patients, unlike normal readers, the latency to read a word is dependent on the number of letters (12), suggesting that these patients have lost the ability to perceive a word as a whole, rather than through its component letters. While these patients may be able to read headlines and business items, they virtually never recover the ability to read for pleasure.

The associated deficits of pure alexia without agraphia are relatively consistent. Most patients have a right homonymous hemianopsia, or at least a loss of the right upper quadrant of both visual fields. Rare cases have been described with intact visual fields (13–16) or with loss of color vision only in the right field — "*hemiachromatopsia*" (10,17). Memory loss, especially for words, is quite frequent, and many older patients have a lasting loss of short-term memory. While unilateral lesions are thought to be unassociated with permanent memory loss, the patient of Mohr et al. (18) had persistent memory loss for 82 days until death, and autopsy confirmed normal right medial temporal structures. Memory loss has been well documented with this syndrome (19), often beginning as a confusional state (20) and then resolving into an isolated defect of short-term memory, with preserved immediate memory (digit span) and remote memory. Other cortical deficits are usually lacking. Calculations are normal. The disorder of reading does not involve spelling; patients can typically spell words properly in writing and in oral spelling, and they can understand words presented in dictated, spelled form. Other dysfunctions of the left parietal lobe, such as left–right confusion, finger agnosia, and constructional difficulty, are absent. Most patients also lack any primary motor deficit, although some have sensory loss on the right side of the body, and occasional patients have a right hemiparesis (21). The syndrome has been described with right occipital lesions in left-handed patients (22,23).

The difficulty in naming colors has been a controversial finding in pure alexia. Dejerine's original case had a right hemiachromatopsia, or loss of color perception in the right visual field, rather than a complete hemianopsia. Most patients, however, have intact perception of colors, as confirmed by performance on Ishihara color plates or in matching colored items (24). The color naming defect of pure alexia thus represents not a color blindness but an inability to match a perceived color with its name. While the term color anomia has been used for this phenomenon, patients can name the usual colors of objects or animals, indicating that there is no loss of the color names themselves. Color agnosia may be the best term for this disorder, since agnosias refer to perceptions that cannot be recognized or associated properly with meaning (see Chapter 21). Most patients with pure alexia without agraphia can name objects and pictures, although occasional cases have difficulty with naming of objects, or visual object agnosia (25). This difficulty may be more severe for two-dimensional drawings than for objects (26). As discussed in Chapter 21, visual object agnosia usually occurs in patients with bilateral occipital lobe lesions.

The localization of the syndrome of pure alexia without agraphia was delineated by Dejerine (10). The typical lesions involve damage to the left medial occipital lobe, affecting the right visual field, together with damage to the splenium of the corpus callosum. Both areas are supplied by the posterior cerebral artery, and most cases of pure alexia without agraphia result from strokes in this distribution. The patient has an intact right-hemisphere visual cortex and can see in the left visual field, but this visual information cannot be accessed by the left-hemisphere language centers for reading. Pure alexia without agraphia is thus an example of a disconnection syndrome

(9,10). The territory of the posterior cerebral artery includes branches to the midbrain; the thalamus; medial temporal structures, including the hippocampus; the splenium of the corpus callosum; and the occipital cortex. Those few cases with hemiparesis have involvement of the proximal branches to the midbrain (21), while thalamic involvement can account for right-sided sensory loss, memory loss, and even hemianopsia if the lateral geniculate body is affected (18). The medial temporal branches are the likely source of the verbal short-term memory deficits so common in this syndrome (19).

Damasio and Damasio (17) distinguished three subsyndromes of pure alexia. In type I, the entire medial temporal, splenial, and calcarine territory is affected, and deficits in memory, reading, and color naming are all present. In Type II, only the calcarine branches are involved, and the deficits involve right hemianopia and alexia but no memory or color naming difficulty. In Type III, the lesion involves the occipitotemporal white matter along the ventricle, including the optic radiations and visual association cortex, but sparing the splenium and calcarine cortex itself. These patients may have partial right visual field defects, especially right upper quadrantanopsia, or hemiachromatopsia, and some patients may even have normal visual fields and color vision. Color naming and memory deficits are absent in these patients.

Other lesions of the left occipital lobe have also been reported to cause pure alexia without agraphia. A patient with a left frontal tumor developed the syndrome, most likely from compression of the posterior cerebral artery secondary to transtentorial herniation (27). Cases of transitory or lasting alexia without agraphia have also been reported with a variety of other left occipital lesions, including tumors (13,28,29), intracerebral hemorrhages (16,30), surgical resections (31), and even head trauma (12,32,33).

Geschwind (9,24) explained the color agnosia along with the alexia by the disconnection mechanism. Colors are purely visual, while objects can elicit associations in other sensory modalities that might be accessible to the left-hemisphere language cortex via more anterior portions of the corpus callosum. Damasio and colleagues (26) found that the degree of difficulty in naming visual stimuli reflected the visual characteristics of the stimuli; drawings were not named as well as objects. With half of the normal visual field absent or deranged, and the remaining half unable to transmit its information properly to the left-hemisphere language centers, it is not surprising that some visual naming difficulties are found (26).

The disconnection theory of pure alexia is enticing in its simplicity, its ability to explain the major phenomena, and its service as an aid to remembering the syndrome. The disconnection theory, however, has a number of limitations in accounting for all the characteristics of pure alexia. First, not all cases of pure alexia have involvement of the splenium of the corpus callosum by CT or MRI scan. In fact, the syndrome has been reported as a transitory disturbance after left occipital lobectomy, in which no callosal lesion is present (31). Only two of Damasio's 16 cases of pure alexia had lesions involving the splenium (17). The argument can be made, however, that the white-matter tract coursing through the splenium is disconnected after its crossing, in the left occipital lobe or in the occipitotemporal connections to the angular gyrus, as in Damasio's type III cases (17) and those of Greenblatt (14) and Henderson (15).

In addition to the anatomical facts, some of the behavioral aspects of pure alexia are difficult to explain by a disconnection mechanism. For example, the ability of most subjects to read single letters but not words cannot be easily accounted for by a disconnection mechanism. Levine and Calvanio (30) showed that patients can identify only single letters flashed tachistoscopically into their left visual fields, while normal subjects can identify strings of at least three letters. This finding relates the alexia to other examples of *simultanagnosia*, or inability of patients with occipital lesions to identify more than one visual item at a time. Neuropsychologists have referred to pure alexia as "letter-by-letter reading," since the pattern of reading only single letters appears to be the central feature of the reading disorder (34).

A related concept is the inability of patients with pure alexia to read a word at a glance. Warrington and Rabin (35) have demonstrated that patients with left occipital lesions have a reduced "visual span of apprehension," or a reduced number of letters that can be perceived at a glance. This reduced visual span results in inability to recognize visual words without reading letter by letter; Warrington and Shallice (36) have referred to the pure alexia syndrome as "word-form dyslexia." In this context, it is interesting to note that the right hemisphere has ability to recognize words, as shown by experiments with patients with left hemispherectomy (37) or in patients who have undergone section of the corpus callosum (38), in whom words are flashed to the right hemisphere via the left visual field. Presumably, the right hemisphere is actively inhibited from participating in reading in patients with a left occipital lesion, but with an intact corpus callosum (at least the anterior portion). Warrington and Shallice (39) noted that a patient with pure alexia could categorize or partially comprehend words that he could not read aloud; they concluded that the basis of the alexia in their patient was a failure of access of this semantic information. Coslett and Saffran (40) reported similar semantic knowledge of printed words in four cases of pure alexia and suggested that the right hemisphere is able to perceive words and process their meaning, without the left hemisphere's having any conscious awareness of the words or ability to read them aloud. A last theory of the alexia of patients with left occipital lesions is the loss of visual verbal short-term memory, or a reduction in the span of letters that can be kept in active memory long enough to be processed for language comprehension (30). This explanation of pure alexia as a memory disorder is similar to the theory of conduction aphasia as a loss of auditory verbal short-term memory, discussed in Chapters 4 and 6.

APHASIC ALEXIA

As discussed in Chapter 4, most aphasic patients have some difficulty with reading; these patients can be classified as having *aphasic alexia*. Since the mechanisms of the reading disturbance in different aphasic syndromes are varied, the term aphasic alexia is no longer a very useful one. Modern neurolinguistic investigations of the reading process have led to more specific, mechanistic syndromes of alexia. Before discussing these syndromes, it is helpful to review the clinical features of the reading disturbance of Broca's and Wernicke's aphasia.

Alexia in Broca's Aphasia

Patients with Broca's aphasia, who comprehend spoken language relatively well, often have a surprising degree of difficulty with comprehension of written language. Benson (41) termed this syndrome the "third alexia," recognizing Dejerine's two, classical syndromes of alexia with and without agraphia. As pointed out by Henderson (42), Dejerine himself was aware of the presence of alexia in patients with Broca's aphasia and performed systematic investigations of reading in these patients. Of Benson's 61 Broca's aphasics, all but 10 had deficient reading, of varying severity. Patients with severe Broca's aphasia may have a nearly complete disruption of the grapheme-phoneme conversion necessary for reading. These patients have large lesions, involving not only Broca's area but major portions of the left frontal, parietal, and even temporal lobes; as discussed in Chapter 4, these patients may evolve over months from global to Broca's aphasia. Such patients cannot name single letters or read aloud nonsense syllables (43), and their reading is limited to recognition of familiar words.

The residual reading of severely aphasic patients is based on word recognition, precisely the function lost in the pure alexia with agraphia syndrome. The spared words are primarily nouns and verbs, usually short, picturable, and frequent in occurrence, as measured in random samples of the English language (43–48). They are recognized as complete letter strings; presumably, they can access semantics (meaning) without any intermediate translation into phonemes or auditory language. This residual reading may be mediated directly by the left occipital lobe or by the right hemisphere, while grapheme-to-phoneme conversion, the first-learned route to reading, is a function of the language cortex of the anterior left hemisphere. These different routes to reading are the basis of the neurolinguistic categories of alexia, discussed later.

Patients with Broca's aphasia and lesser degrees of alexia may have other mechanisms accounting for reading impairment. Benson (41) has pointed to disorders of saccadic eye movements from left to right, difficulty with the handling of sequential information, and a loss of the grammatical and syntactic function that is also evident in their speech production and comprehension of more complex auditory language.

Alexia in Wernicke's Aphasia

Patients with Wernicke's aphasia typically have severe impairments of both auditory and reading comprehension, in the setting of fluent, paraphasic speech output (see Chapter 4). Occasional patients with Wernicke's aphasia

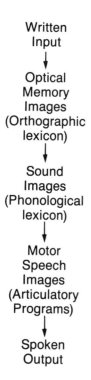

Written
Input

Optical
Memory
Images
(Orthographic
lexicon)

Sound
Images
(Phonological
lexicon)

Motor
Speech
Images
(Articulatory
Programs)

Spoken
Output

Figure 1   Diagram of the reading process, as envisioned by traditional interpretations of Wernicke's aphasia. The terms in parentheses are current, neurolinguistic versions of the original concepts.

recover auditory comprehension better than reading, such that their deficits evolve into the syndrome of alexia with agraphia (4,5). Benson has suggested the terms *central alexia* or *temporoparietal alexia* for these syndromes (3). According to Wernicke's original concept, the superior temporal area is a center for decoding spoken phonemes into words. Since reading was envisioned to take place via translation of printed words into auditory language, a lesion of Wernicke's area would be expected to disrupt reading in addition to auditory comprehension. A modern cognitive neuropsychologist might diagram the modules involved in reading, by Wernicke's system, as seen in Figure 1. Reading proceeds via a required series of stages from (1) the printed word input to (2) the lexicon of orthographic word images to (3) the sound images or "phonological lexicon" stored in Wernicke's area to (4) the "semantic store" of word meanings to (5) the Broca's area, where motor speech is encoded in a series of articulatory steps. The modern neuropsychologist, however, must also consider cases in which patients with Wernicke's aphasia

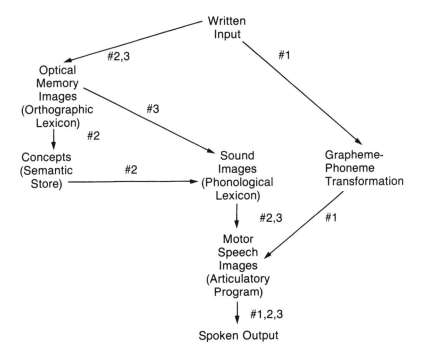

Figure 2 Modern version of the reading process. Note the existence of three separate routes to reading: #1 is the phonological (or grapheme-phoneme conversion) route, #2 the semantic (or lexical-semantic-phonological) route, and #3 the nonlexical phonological route. (Adapted from Ref. 56.)

have shown unusual preserved language skills, including: understanding of written language (5,49–51), reading aloud either without (52) or with comprehension (53,54), written naming and spelling (55), or auditory comprehension (4,5).

These variations in the deficit profile of Wernicke's aphasia require refinement of the model, as proposed by Margolin (56). This new model of the reading process, shown in Figure 2, is closely related to models developed from cognitive neuropsychological research on alexias, discussed below. A patient who can read aloud but not for meaning would have a lesion between the "optical memory images" and "concepts" boxes in the diagram, while the patient who can read for meaning but not aloud would have a lesion between the "concepts" or "semantic store" box and the "sound images" box. The model thus accounts for diverse clinical phenomena and explicates the cognitive processes involved in reading.

NEUROLINGUISTIC CATEGORIES OF ALEXIA

Working independently of the lesion-localization approach of clinical neurologists, cognitive neuropsychologists and linguists have described new categories of alexia (*dyslexia*), based on the stages of reading at which deficits arise. Of the classical syndromes discussed thus far, only pure alexia without agraphia has retained its status as a neuropsychological syndrome, under the designation *letter-by-letter dyslexia* (34). Other recently delineated reading syndromes include deep dyslexia, phonological dyslexia, and surface dyslexia.

Deep Dyslexia

Deep dyslexia, as defined by cognitive neuropsychology (55–59), conforms closely to the features described above under "Aphasic Alexia" of the type seen in patients with lasting, severe Broca's aphasia. The principal characteristics of deep dyslexia include: (1) intact reading of familiar words, (2) inability to read nonsense syllables or non-words, (3) semantic and visual errors in reading aloud, and (4) pronounced effects on reading ability based on word frequency, word imageability (picturability), and word class or part of speech. Imageable words are read more accurately than abstract words, while nouns and verbs are read more accurately than adjectives, adverbs, articles, and prepositions. Word reading, on the other hand, is not much affected by word length or by regularity of spelling (59). One such patient, cited by Patterson (59), could read "ambulance" but not "am". Semantic errors involve substitution of a word of related meaning to the intended word, often of no visual or phonemic resemblance to the intended word; examples given by Marshall and Newcombe (57) include "jail" for "prison" and "soccer" for "football". For Coltheart (58), semantic errors are the linchpin of deep dyslexia, since they imply that words are recognized with direct access to meaning rather than analyzed phonologically; deep dyslexia cannot be diagnosed without this central feature. Visual errors involve words that physically resemble the intended word, such as "perform" for "perfume" and "banish" for "blush". A third type of error occasionally seen in deep dyslexia is the "derivational error," such as "directions" for "directing".

Deep dyslexia involves the loss of reading by the "phonological" or grapheme-to-phoneme conversion route, with residual reading involving only recognition of familiar words (corresponding to reading route 2 in Figure 2). These patients are completely unable to sound out nonsense words, but they may recognize irregularly spelled words such as "yacht". Most cases have profound aphasia as well as reading deficit, and most have major damage to the left-hemisphere language centers (58). CT scan analyses of five patients with deep dyslexia revealed extensive left-hemisphere injury in all cases, including Broca's area and large areas of the left parietal lobe, as well as major damage to the frontal and parietal subcortical white matter. The left temporal lobe was damaged in only one case (60). Coltheart (61) has postulated that the residual reading of patients with deep dyslexia is accomplished by the right hemisphere. Indeed, a patient who underwent left hemispherectomy for intractable epilepsy had a deficit profile similar to that of deep dyslexia (62).

Phonological Dyslexia

Phonological dyslexia is similar to deep dyslexia, except that single-content words are read in a nearly normal fashion, and semantic errors are rare or absent (59,63,64). Table 1 summarizes the key differences among the four cognitive neuropsychological categories of alexia. As in deep dyslexia, there is poor reading of non-words. Both visual and derivational errors are seen, but somewhat less frequently than in deep dyslexia (59). Some patients with phonological dyslexia read individual words well, including both nouns and functor words, both imageable and nonimageable nouns, and both regularly and irregularly spelled words (63). Semantic judgments about the words, however, may be impaired; the patient can sometimes read words without access to meaning. The syndrome of phonological dyslexia, like deep dyslexia, involves the loss of the normal route of orthography (printed graphemes) to phonology (spoken phonemes), or grapheme-to-phoneme conversion. In deep dyslexia, only words whose meaning is recognized can be read aloud; only a semantics-to-phonology reading route can operate. In phonological dyslexia, another route is available to read words, independent of

Table 1 Features of Cognitive Neuropsychology Categories of Alexia

	Deep dyslexia	Phonological dyslexia	Letter-by-letter	Surface dyslexia
Word vs. non-word effect	+	+	−	−
Content vs. function word effect	+	+	−	−
Imageability/con-creteness	+	−	−	−
Word-length effect	−	−	+	+
Regularity of spelling	−	−	−	+

Source: Adapted from Ref. 59.

semantics; words are read via a lexical-phonological route (route 3 in Figure 2). Only the nonlexical-phonological route, by which non-words must be read, is inoperative.

Patients with phonological dyslexia vary as to the presence or severity of associated language disorders. Most have severe, nonfluent aphasia, although patients have been described with only partial aphasic syndromes such as anomic aphasia (65). A patient with Broca's aphasia and a category-specific auditory comprehension deficit for body parts, colors, numbers, and letters had otherwise typical phonological dyslexia (66). Lesions underlying phonological dyslexia may also be variable, in one case (64) involving only the left temporal lobe.

The importance of phonological dyslexia is that it reveals the presence of three separate pathways from printed letter strings to phonemes (orthography to phonology). These include the lexical-semantic-phonology, lexical-phonology, and nonlexical-phonology routes (see Figure 2). In deep dyslexia, the first two can operate, at least to some extent, and only the third route is impaired.

Surface Dyslexia

Surface dyslexia, a syndrome of disordered reading, is more or less the opposite of the deep dyslexia syndrome. In surface dyslexia, subjects can read laboriously by grapheme-phoneme conversion, but they cannot recognize words at a glance. They can read nonsense syllables but are completely unable to read words of irregular spelling, such as "yacht" or "colonel". They often pronounce words in a regularized fashion when reading aloud; in other words, their errors tend to be phonological rather than semantic or visual. An example would be to pronounce "pint" as if it rhymed with "lint".

These subjects often spell words in a phonological manner as well, such as "phurm" for "firm" (58). When a patient reads a word incorrectly, the meaning is then assumed to be that of the incorrect response; Marshall and Newcombe (57) cite the example of a subject who read the word "listen" as "Liston" and then interpreted it as: "that's the boxer." Reading in these patients is thus accomplished without any access to semantics until the word is pronounced. Individual graphemes are sounded out by the way they are most commonly pronounced in the language. This process inevitably leads to errors in reading aloud both irregularly spelled words and words that have regular spellings but atypical pronunciations; for example, the words "rough", "bough", "though", and "cough" have the same sequence of vowels but different pronunciations (59). A surface dyslexic reader might read all four words with the same pronunciation.

Detailed analyses of patients with surface dyslexia (67–69) have confirmed this pattern of reading, including the ability to read non-words as well as real words, the presence of mainly phonological errors, and the lack of semantic judgment until words are read aloud. These studies have also confirmed the existence of rules for the pronunciation of letter strings. These patients show a length dependency, reading shorter words more easily than longer ones (see Table 1). They may even read functors better than content words, the opposite pattern from deep dyslexia (68). Surface dyslexia thus represents a syndrome in which only one route of reading, the grapheme-phoneme route, is operative (route 1 in Figure 2), and patients cannot read words without pronouncing their component graphemes.

Recently, surface dyslexia has been reported in patients with progressive language deterioration secondary to neurodegenerative disease (see Chapter 14). These cases have included the primary progressive aphasia syndrome (70) and patients with *semantic dementia*, or progressive fluent aphasia with anomia and poor auditory comprehension and semantic memory (71).

CONCLUSION

The study of alexia has now progressed from classical descriptions of the three clinical syndromes of alexia with and without alexia and aphasic alexia toward a neurolinguistic classification of alexias based on precise mechanisms of reading function. In this format, only the alexia without agraphia syndrome has survived as a distinct entity, under the new name letter-by-letter alexia. The new syndromes of deep, phonological, and surface alexia will likely be further subdivided and correlated with more delimited lesion localizations. Implications also have been drawn from these syndromes, based on the separation of the three routes of reading discussed above, with regard to the development of reading in both normals and subjects with developmental dyslexia.

REFERENCES

1. Benson DF, Geschwind N. The aphasias and related disturbances. In: Baker AB, Baker LH, eds. Clinical neurology. Philadelphia: JB Lippincott, 1989:1-34.
2. Dejerine J. Sur un cas de cécité verbale avec agraphie, suivi d'autopsie. Mem Soc Biol 1891;3:197-201.
3. Benson DF. The alexias: a guide to the neurologic basis of reading. In: Kirshner HS, Freemon FR, eds. The neurology of aphasia. Amsterdam: Swets, 1982:139-161.
4. Kirshner HS, Webb WG. Alexia and agraphia in Wernicke's aphasia. J Neurol Neurosurg Psychiatry 1982;45:719-724.
5. Kirshner HS, Casey PF, Henson J, Heinrich JJ. Behavioural features and lesion localization in Wernicke's aphasia. Aphasiology 1989;3:169-176.
6. Albert ML, Yamadori A, Gardner H, Howes D. Comprehension in alexia. Brain 1973;96:317-328.
7. Mohr JP. An unusual case of dyslexia with dysgraphia. Brain Lang 1976;3:324-334.
8. Rothi LJ, Heilman KM. Alexia and agraphia with spared spelling and letter recognition abilities. Brain Lang 1981;12:1-13.
9. Geschwind N. Disconnexion syndromes in animals and man. Brain 1965;88:237-294, 585-644.
10. Dejerine J. Contribution à l'étude anatomo-pathologique et clinique des differentes varietés de cécité verbale. Mem Soc Biol 1892;4:61-90.
11. Broadbent WH. On the cerebral mechanisms of speech and thought. Medicochirugical Transactions 1872;55:145.
12. Staller J, Buchanan D, Singer M, Lappin J, Webb W. Alexia without agraphia: An experimental case study. Brain Lang 1978;5:378-387.
13. Greenblatt S. Alexia without agraphia or hemianopsia. Brain 1973;96:307-316.
14. Greenblatt S. Subangular alexia without agraphia or hemianopsia. Brain Lang 1977;3:229-245.
15. Henderson VW. Left hemisphere pathways in reading: inferences from pure alexia without hemianopia. Neurology 1985;35:962-968.
16. Caffarra P. Alexia without agraphia or hemianopia. Eur Neurol 1987;27:65-71.
17. Damasio AR, Damasio H. The anatomic basis of pure alexia. Neurology 1983;33:1573-1583.
18. Mohr JP, Leicester J, Stoddard LT, Sidman M. Right hemianopia with memory and color deficits in circumscribed left posterior cerebral artery territory infarction. Neurology 1971;21:1104-1113.
19. Benson DF, Marsden CD, Meadows JC. The amnestic syndrome of posterior cerebral artery occlusion. Acta Neurol Scand 1974;50:133-145.
20. Devinsky O, Bear D, Volpe BT. Confusional states following posterior cerebral artery infarction. Arch Neurol 1988;45:160-163.

21. Benson DF, Tomlinson E. Hemiplegic syndrome of the posterior cerebral artery. Stroke 1971;2:559–564.
22. Erkulvrawatr S. Alexia and left homonymous hemianopia in a non-right-hander. Ann Neurol 1978;3:549–552.
23. Pillon B, Bakchine S, Lhermitte F. Alexia without agraphia in a left-handed patient with a right occipital lesion. Arch Neurol 1987;44:1257–1262.
24. Geschwind N, Fusillo M. Color-naming defects in association with alexia. Arch Neurol 1966;15:137–146.
25. DeRenzi E, Zambolin A, Crisi G. The pattern of neuropsychological impairment associated with left posterior cerebral artery infarcts. Brain 1987;110:1099–1116.
26. Damasio AR, McKee J, Damasio H. Determinants of performance in color anomia. Brain Lang 1979;7:74–85.
27. Kirshner HS, Staller J, Webb W, Sachs P. Transtentorial herniation with posterior cerebral artery territory infarction. A new mechanism of the syndrome of alexia without agraphia. Stroke 1982;13:243–246.
28. Vincent FM, Sadowsky CH, Saunders RL, Reeves AG. Alexia without agraphia, hemianopsia, or color-naming defect: a disconnection syndrome. Neurology 1977;27:689–691.
29. Turgman J, Goldhammer Y, Graham J. Alexia without agraphia, due to brain tumor: a reversible syndrome. Ann Neurol 1979;6:265–268.
30. Levine DM, Calvanio R. A study of the visual defect in verbal alexia-simultanagnosia. Brain 1978;101:65–81.
31. Ajuriaguerra J, Hecaen H. La restauration functionelle après lobectomie occipitale. J Psychol (Paris) 1951;44:510–540.
32. Heilman KM, Saffran A. Geschwind N. Closed head trauma with aphasia. J Neurol Neurosurg Psychiatry 1971;34:265–269.
33. Lhermitte J, DeMassary J, Hugeuenin R. Syndrome occipital avec alexie pure d'origine traumatique. Rev Neurol (Paris) 1929;2:703–707.
34. Patterson K, Kay J. Letter-by-letter reading: Psychological descriptions of a neurological syndrome. Quart J Exp Psychol 1982;34A:411–441.
35. Warrington EK, Rabin P. Visual span of apprehension in patients with unilateral cerebral lesions. Quart J Exp Psychol 1971;23:423–431.
36. Warrington EK, Shallice T. Word-form dyslexia. Brain 1980;103:99–112.
37. Smith A. Speech and other functions after left (dominant) hemispherectomy. J Neurol Neurosurg Psychiatry 1966;29:467–471.
38. Gazzaniga MS, Sperry RW. Language after section of the cerebral commissures. Brain 1967;90:131–148.
39. Warrington EK, Shallice T. Semantic access dyslexia. Brain 1979;102:43–63.
40. Coslett HB, Saffran EM. Evidence for preserved reading in "pure alexia." Brain 1989;112:327–359.
41. Benson DF. The third alexia. Arch Neurol 1977;34:327–331.
42. Henderson VW. Jules Dejerine and the third alexia. Arch Neurol 1984;41:430–432.
43. Kirshner HS, Webb WG. Word and letter reading and the mechanism of the third alexia. Arch Neurol 1982;39:84–87.

44. Kapur N, Perl NT. Recognition reading in paralexia. Cortex 1978;14:439–443.
45. Saffran EM, Marin OSM. Reading without phonology: evidence from aphasia. Quart J Exp Psychol 1977;29:515–525.
46. Richardson JTE. The effect of word imageability in acquired dyslexia. Neuropsychologia 1975;13:281–288.
47. Goodglass H, Klein B, Carey P. Specific semantic word categories in aphasia. Cortex 1966;2:74–89.
48. Gardner H, Zurif E. Bee but not be: oral reading of single words in aphasia and alexia. Neuropsychologia 1980;18:219–223.
49. Kirshner HS, Webb WG, Duncan GW. Word deafness in Wernicke's aphasia. J Neurol Neurosurg Psychiatry 1981;41:161–170.
50. Caramazza A, Berndt RS, Basili AG. The selective impairment of phonological processing: a case study. Brain Lang 1977;18:128–174.
51. Ellis AW, Miller D, Sin G. Wernicke's aphasia and normal language processing; a case study in cognitive neuropsychology. Cognition 1983;15:111–144.
52. Lytton WW, Brust CM. Direct dyslexia: preserved oral reading of real words in Wernicke's aphasia. Brain 1989;112:583–594.
53. Sevush S, Roeltgen DP, Campanella DJ, Heilman KM. Preserved oral reading in Wernicke's aphasia. Neurology 1983;33:916–920.
54. Heilman KM, Rothi L, Campanella MS, Wolfson S. Wernicke's and global aphasia without alexia. Arch Neurol 1979;36:129–133.
55. Hier DB, Mohr JP. Incongruous oral and written naming. Brain Lang 1977; 4:115–126.
56. Margolin DI. Cognitive neuropsychology. Resolving enigmas about Wernicke's aphasia and other higher cortical disorders. Arch Neurol 1991;48:751–765.
57. Marshall JC, Newcombe F. Patterns of paralexia: a psycholinguistic approach. J Psycholing Res 1973;2:175–199.
58. Coltheart M. Deep dyslexia: a review of the syndrome. In: Coltheart M, Patterson K, Marshall JC, eds. Deep dyslexia. London: Routledge & Kegan Paul, 1980:22–47.
59. Patterson KE. Neuropsychological approaches to the study of reading. Br J Psychiatry 1981;72:151–174.
60. Marin OSM. CAT scans of five deep dyslexic patients. Appendix 1. In: Coltheart M, Patterson K, Marshall JC, eds. Deep dyslexia. London: Routledge & Kegan Paul, 1980:407–409.
61. Coltheart M. Deep dyslexia: a right hemisphere hypothesis. In: Coltheart M, Patterson K, Marshall JC, eds. Deep dyslexia. London: Routledge & Kegan Paul, 1980:326–380.
62. Patterson K, Vargha-Khadem F, Polkey CE. Reading with one hemisphere. Brain 1989;112:39–63.
63. Funnell E. Phonological processes in reading: new evidence from acquired dyslexia. Br J Psychol 1983;74:159–180.
64. Beauvois MF, Derouesne J. Phonological alexia: three dissociations. J Neurol Neurosurg Psychiatry 1979;42:1115–1124.
65. Rapcsak SZ, Gonzalez-Rothi LJ, Heilman KM. Phonological alexia with optic and tactile anomia: a neuropsychological and anatomical study. Brain Lang 1987;31:109–121.

66. Goodglass H, Budin C. Category and modality specific dissociations in word comprehension and concurrent phonological dyslexia. Neuropsychologia 1988; 26:67–78.

67. Shallice T, Warrington EK, McCarthy R. Reading without semantics. Quart J Exp Psychol 1983;35A:111–138.

68. Deloche G, Andreewsky E, Desi M. Surface dyslexia: a case report and some theoretical implications to reading models. Brain Lang 1982;15:12–31.

69. Bub D, Cancelliere A, Kertesz A. The orthographic reading route—evidence for algorithmic grapheme-phoneme conversion in a surface dyslexic. Presented at Academy of Aphasia, 1986.

70. Chiacchio L, Grossi D, Stanzione M, Trojano L. Slowly progressive aphasia associated with surface dyslexia. Cortex 1993;29:145–152.

71. Hodges JR, Patterson K, Oxbury S, Funnell E. Semantic dementia. Progressive fluent aphasia with temporal lobe atrophy. Brain 1992;115:1783–1806.

11

Disorders of Writing and Spelling

Marjorie Perlman Lorch

Birkbeck College, University of London and National Hospital for Neurology and Neurosurgery, London, England

OVERVIEW

Writing and spelling disorders are found in a variety of neurological conditions. The relatively limited use of writing in daily life and consequent lack of practice makes written language particularly susceptible to impairment (1). Significant brain damage, regardless of location, usually produces some degree of agraphia (2).

Typically, writing and spelling disorders occur in conjunction with reading disorders in the context of a central language disturbance of aphasia (3). Patients with right-hemisphere lesions may demonstrate disorganization of the visuospatial aspects of writing (4). Confused (5,6) and/or demented (7) patients with diffuse pathology often demonstrate selective difficulties in writing, reflecting a global cognitive impairment in organizing complex, integrative tasks. Many patients with motor disorders such as Parkinson's disease (8) lose the ability to produce legible writing. In addition, patients with temporal lobe epilepsy may demonstrate hypergraphic behavior, or excessive writing, between seizures (9).

This broad range of etiologies of writing difficulty derives from the multiplicity of processes that contribute to the successful execution of spelling and writing. Written language production involves both central and peripheral mechanisms, including: central language processes, additional functions dedicated to spelling, writing, and reading; mechanisms involved in visuospatial orientation; and motor planning and control of handwriting.

INTRODUCTION

This chapter reviews acquired disorders of writing and spelling that may occur concurrently with, or independently of, impairments in speech and reading. Consideration is given to clinicopathological correlations of the various symptoms and syndromes of agraphia. Assessment procedures are reviewed, along with some therapeutic techniques for specific deficits. Cognitive neuropsychological models of writing and spelling are outlined with specific reference to the quality and patterns of errors in specific syndromes of agraphia.

In this chapter, the terms *agraphia* and *dysgraphia* are used interchangeably to refer to acquired disorders of writing and spelling. The use of these terms does not imply any distinction in the degree of impairment or in the congenital or acquired nature of the disorder, as may be the case elsewhere. Rather, they reflect the North American (agraphia) versus European (dysgraphia) traditions in aphasiological terminology.

The production of writing involves four different levels of performance: the linguistic content, the spelling of individual words, the visuospatial organization of graphic symbols, and the motoric components of handwriting. These various components of the writing process are to some degree shared by other "higher" or complex cognitive behaviors. Agraphic disorders may thus be seen in conjunction with aphasia, alexia, agnosia, and apraxia, but agraphia can also occur in pure form; the neuropsychological status of agraphia is not entirely subordinate to other cognitive and linguistic skills.

DISSOCIATIONS IN SPEAKING, READING, WRITING, AND SPELLING

Dissociations between reading and writing can and do occur. The best known example is the syndrome of alexia without agraphia, discussed in Chapter 10. Conversely, agraphia can occur without an associated disturbance of reading, as in pure deep dysgraphia (10). Patients may also display nonparallel writing and reading disorders; examples include the combinations of phonological dyslexia and surface dysgraphia (11) and surface dysgraphia with letter-by-letter reading (12).

The ability to select and sequence letters to form words can also be demonstrated to dissociate according to modality of output; impairments of spelling can occur selectively in oral or written output. The use of anagram letters, Morse code, or other forms of letter production such as typewriters or word processors may be differentially affected. Kinsbourne and Warrington (13) first reported a case of preserved writing with impaired oral spelling. The patient had difficulty in both transforming heard words into spoken letter names (oral spelling) and transforming heard letter names into a spoken word. The ability to recognize orally spelled words has been shown to parallel visual reading rather than written spelling processes (14).

The converse of relatively preserved oral with impaired written spelling has also been described (15–20). In the case reported by Kinsbourne and Rosenfield (20), written spelling errors were independent of input modality and principally involved the intrusion of extraneous letters. The patient also had mild aphasia and the other symptoms of Gerstmann's syndrome (see Chapter 21). The lesion involved the left posterior parasagittal parietal lobe.

In contrast, Baxter and Warrington's patient (16) had no ability to write, while oral spelling showed a gradient of errors, greatest at the beginning of the word, improving toward the end of the word. This patient had a lesion in the right parietal lobe. The authors argued that the oral spelling problem reflected a disturbance of the patient's ability to image the word from which the letters could be "read," a rare symptom of left neglect referred to as *neglect dysgraphia* (21) (see below).

These cases exemplify the variation and range of symptoms and lesion localizations that can be evident in agraphia. To bring different aspects of spelling and writing impairments into focus, both clinical and cognitive classifications must be considered.

CLASSIFICATION

The classification of writing disorders has been subject to as many and varied distinctions and labels as the aphasias and alexias. The classification employed in this chapter was developed by Hécaen (22). It reflects the association of writing disturbances with major cognitive disorders: aphasic agraphia, apraxic agraphia, spatial agraphia. In addition, the designation of *pure agraphia* is used to indicate the absence of any other language, speech, or reading disorder arising from a focal lesion. *Isolated agraphia* is used to describe a severe writing disturbance arising from diffuse or multifocal pathology (5,6).

Another classification of the agraphias is that of Luria (23), who described sensory, afferent, sequential/motor, and visuospatial subtypes. I will heed Critchley's (24) caution that consideration of the numerous taxonomies that have been developed in the past for the agraphias is not warranted or rewarding.

In the following sections, the "central" and "peripheral" dysgraphic disorders are detailed. The distinction between central and peripheral in the context of the agraphias reflects cognitive metaphors rather than neuroanatomical facts; peripheral agraphias can arise from cortical lesions.

Central Agraphias

Central dysgraphias are disorders that affect lexical, semantic, and phonological processes up to and including the retrieval of the spellings of familiar words or the assembly of plausible spellings of unfamiliar words or nonwords. This is the point at which an abstract graphemic representation of the word is generated, according to cognitive models such as that of Ellis (25). Subsequent peripheral processes, including letter sequences of word forms, allographic selection, and motor output, are responsible for the production of orthography, whether in handwriting, oral spelling, typing, or letter arrangements. The impairment of this portion of the process is referred to as peripheral agraphia (25).

Aphasic Agraphia

J. Hughlings Jackson (26), and later Goodglass and Geschwind (27), believed that impairments of writing reflect the same linguistic deficiencies as those affecting speech and reading, and hence writing is always impaired to some extent in cases of aphasia. A recent historical review of agraphia has been presented by Leischner (28), and English translations of nineteenth-century German writings on agraphia have been published by De Bleser and Luzzatti (29).

For aphasic patients, writing is typically the most severely impaired modality when compared to verbal comprehension, verbal production, and reading (30,31). Writing tasks are in general more difficult for aphasics than either verbal or gestural tasks (32). Furthermore, performance on writing tasks is a poor predictor of overall language recovery (33). Writing is quite often the last skill to recover (30). A corollary of this fact is that writing performance is a highly sensitive measure of underlying, or partially recovered, aphasia in mildly impaired patients (34). A study of mildly impaired patients by Noll and Hoops (35) revealed an overall effect of spelling difficulty reflecting both central (grammatical word class) and peripheral factors (graphemic buffer effects), with "nonpropositional morphemes" (i.e., functors) being spelled more poorly relative to other parts of speech, and with greater spelling difficulty with long than with short words.

There are expected correlations between aphasic and agraphic disturbances. In nonfluent aphasias such as Broca's and transcortical motor aphasia, writing tends to resemble the features of expressive speech; written production is typically spare, effortful, clumsy in calligraphy, abbreviated, agrammatical, and poorly spelled (2). Agrammatism is often more pronounced in patients' written than spoken language. Broca's aphasics invariably have accompanying agraphia, but the association in transcortical motor aphasia is less consistent (2,36).

Detailed analysis of the spoken and written productions of Broca's and Wernicke's aphasics by Goodglass and Hunter (3) demonstrates significant parallels and contrasts. Both had longer grammatical runs in speech than in writing; however, the Wernicke's aphasic made more errors in speech than in writing, while the reverse was found for the Broca's aphasic [see also Frederici, Schoenle, and Goodglass (37)]. The pattern of lexical and syntactic errors typical of speech in these patients was also found in their writing, but in both aphasia types written productions contained more nouns than verbs and more specific than nonspecific lexical choices relative to their speech (3).

The relatively better-written-than-spoken production of language in conduction and Wernicke's aphasics has been amply documented (38–42). Dissociations between type of language impairment demonstrated in spoken-versus-written output have also been reported by Hier and Mohr (43) and by Patterson and Shewell (44). In both cases, speech was described as fluent but empty, yet written productions were agrammatical, consisting primarily of content words.

Aphemic patients are notable for their preserved ability to produce fluent written language in the face of almost no verbal output (see also Chapter 4). This sparing of written language production is taken as evidence for considering aphemia to be a motor-speech rather than true aphasic disturbance (22,45). However, writing and reading do show a range of dissociations with verbal language abilities, and lack of writing or reading impairment should not necessarily be taken as evidence against a central verbal language impairment. The larger lesions in cases of Broca's aphasia than in aphemia may be the source of the additional language and writing impairments (46).

Specific spelling-production impairments have been demonstrated to be associated with different types of aphasias. In a large group study of spelling disorders, Wapner and Gardner (47) asked aphasic patients to spell the names of objects in three conditions: oral, written, and using anagram letters. No differences were found in the overall number of words spelled correctly by the anterior versus posterior patients. Written spelling was found to be the easiest condition across all patient groups. Anterior aphasics had difficulty with oral spelling as expected, while the posterior aphasics performed consistently across the three different conditions. In analyzing the specific types of spelling that presented difficulties, it emerged that words with double consonants or silent letters were the source of more errors than other spellings. Letter substitutions were the most frequent type of spelling error, followed by omissions and additions. Wrong-word responses tended to begin with the same letter as the target, e.g., "knot" was written KNIFE, and KNOCK; "chalk" was written CHAIR and CALM. (In representing spelling performance the convention will be adopted that target words will be written with quotation marks and responses represented by uppercase letters.)

Wapner and Gardner (47) found that "mixed anterior" aphasics' spelling errors were characterized primarily by errors of omission. Anomic aphasics were most likely to add extraneous letters. Overall, anterior aphasics typically produced incomplete spellings (word fragments) or wrong words (semantic paragraphias). The posterior aphasics performed best at spelling regular words, and the majority of errors involved associated homonyms and omission of silent letters and the second letter of a vowel or consonant pair. Posterior aphasics were far more likely than anterior aphasics to produce letter strings that sounded like the target word. Examples of the different types of aphasic spelling errors: the target "doll" was spelled by posterior aphasics as DAWL or DOLLE, while anterior aphasics produced spellings of DOOL and DOG. Similarly, to the target "eraser" the posterior aphasics produced ERACER and ERASSOR, while the anterior aphasics produced ESAR, EAN, and ESARED (47).

Wapner and Gardner's finding for word regularity and phonologically plausible errors as features of spelling performance for posterior aphasics has been rediscovered in the more recent cognitive neuropsychology approach to writing and reading disorders. These features are currently considered a hallmark of the syndrome of lexical or surface agraphia.

Lexical (Surface, Orthographic) Agraphia

The initial description of lexical agraphia was the report of Beauvois and Derouesné (11) of a French patient with a left parieto-occipital angioma. The patient's ability to write a word correctly—whether spontaneously, in naming, or to dictation—was dependent on how frequent, how regular, and how unambiguous the sound-to-spelling (phoneme-to-grapheme) correspondence was. The patient substituted graphemes with identical phonological realizations, e.g., "Monsieur" → MESSIEU. Errors typically consisted of a phonologically plausible spelling. Novel words (non-words) were spelled successfully. This patient's reading did not mirror the writing deficit but rather reflected a phonological dyslexia (see Chapter 10). Two other cases of lexical agraphia with phonological dyslexia have been described (48).

English-speaking lexical or surface agraphic patients typically make errors in which words are misspelled but phonologically plausible: "spade" → SPAID and "flood" → FLUD (12). The term *surface dysgraphia* links it to the model of reading with its corresponding deep and surface dyslexic varieties developed by Marshall and Newcombe (49) (See Chapter 10).

Cases of lexical agraphia have figured in numerous clinical reports (12,50–54). All these cases of lexical agraphia are associated with temporo-parieto-occipital area lesions and posterior aphasia (i.e., Wernicke's, transcortical sensory, or anomic aphasia) (48). Roeltgen and Heilman (51) identified the junction of the posterior angular gyrus and the parietal-occipital lobe as the significant focus of pathology for lexical agraphia. Lexical agraphia has recently been reported in a patient with a left precentral gyrus lesion (55) and in a right-hander with a right posterior parieto-occipital lobe lesion (56).

The cognitive interpretation of this pattern of spelling is that an impairment in the ability to spell by access to word knowledge (i.e., the lexicon) results in spelling being carried out by a secondary skill based on knowledge of sound-to-spelling translation procedures.

Phonological Agraphia

In the second type of spelling impairment, phonological agraphia, defined by the cognitive description of the spelling process, irregular words or words with ambiguous spellings present no difficulty, but non-words cannot be spelled successfully. This failure to spell non-words (in contrast with the good performance of lexical agraphics with non-words) is the hallmark of phonological agraphia. In addition, patients cannot spell words that they do not comprehend or that they did not know premorbidly. The difficulty encountered in spelling non-words, new words, or non-comprehended words indicates a reliance on knowledge of the meaning of the word (semantic lexicon), with an inability to employ sound-to-spelling translations. Errors may have a high degree of visual resemblance to targets (48).

Numerous descriptions of cases of phonological agraphia have appeared in the last decade (40,51,57–61). Phonological agraphia is typically seen in patients with lesions that include the left supramarginal gyrus or underlying insula (58). A case of cross phonological agraphia has been presented in a left-handed patient with a lesion in the right supramarginal gyrus (62). The extent of the lesion varies greatly in cases of phonological agraphia, as does the type of co-occurring aphasic deficit (61). Phonological agraphia may be associated with Broca's, conduction, Wernicke's, or anomic aphasia (48).

The hallmark of phonological agraphia, difficulty in non-word spelling, may arise from three aspects of the process of assembled spelling: phonological segmentation, conversion of phonological segments to spelling patterns, and grapheme assembly (63). Consequently, various subtypes of phonological agraphia may exist.

The inability to spell non-words is important for information-processing models of normal reading but is not a significant clinical issue with regard to a patient's functional communication. However, the patient with phonological agraphia typically has some impaired ability to spell known words, in addition to the difficulties exhibited when tested with novel words. For example, the case reported by Bub and Kertesz (40) demonstrated 3% correct spelling of non-words and 79% correct spelling of words.

Deep Dysgraphia

The term *deep dysgraphia* is also linked to Marshall and Newcombe's (49, 64) model of dyslexia. Caplan (65) refers to this type of writing disturbance as a category-specific phonological agraphia, meaning that the writing impairment follows the pattern of phonological dysgraphia but affects specific word types. Both types of patients have difficulty spelling non-words, but deep dysgraphics also show deficits in spelling specific classes of words; in general, words with concrete meanings are spelled more successfully than those with abstract meanings, and words with syntactic functions such as prepositions and conjunctions present more difficulty than words with semantic functions such as nouns and adjectives. For example, a deep dysgraphic patient made the following errors in writing to dictation: "desk" → CHAIR; "yacht" → BOAT; "give" → TAKE (10). Words that cannot be spelled may be defined accurately, however, demonstrating that the meaning could be accessed but not the orthographic form (59). In the face of impaired phonological and semantic information, the visual form of the word representation may play a role in the spellings produced by deep dysgraphics. Patients may write individual letters of words in a noncanonical sequence (e.g., "dinner" → $D^6I^1N^2N^3E^4R^5$) or produce spellings with a similar overall word shape [e.g., "soul" written as SEAD (60)].

Numerous cases of deep dysgraphia have been described (10,39,44,58–60, 66). Extensive lesions are reported in the left posterior cortex, including the supramarginal gyrus or insula but sparing the angular gyrus (48). This anatomical feature has led Roeltgen to hypothesize that deep agraphia reflects residual writing abilities of the left hemisphere rather than the right hemisphere (4), as is argued for deep dyslexia (67).

Semantic Agraphia

Patients with semantic agraphia lose the ability to spell and write with meaning, although they can spell irregular words and non-words correctly. This semantic writing disturbance is seen in the context of general language comprehension difficulties associated with transcortical or subcortical lesion localizations (48).

Semantic agraphics confuse homophonic word spellings in writing to dictation despite disambiguating semantic contextualization (68). They are as likely to spell the correct word as its (often irregularly spelled) homophone, e.g., "not" as KNOT, "led" as LEAD, "doe" as DOUGH. The lexical phonological representation of homophones may directly address all its orthographic forms, e.g., "rein" → RAIN, REIN, REIGN. Such errors are also made by some surface dysgraphics (12), patients with dementia (17), and normal writers in slips of the pen (69).

Asemantic Writing

Patterson (70) described a patient who could not write spontaneously but could accurately produce writing to dictation, despite poor auditory comprehension and inability to spell nonwords. Writing to dictation was apparently being carried out through an auditory-graphemic whole-word correspondence, without recourse to meaning. This writing performance seems akin to the repetition ability in patients with isolation of the speech area.

Unilateral (Callosal, Disconnection, Hemiagraphia) Agraphia

In most cases of agraphia, the dominant and nondominant hand are equally affected, except in instances of hemiparesis or hemisensory disturbance (48). In instances of right hemiparesis due to left-hemisphere lesions, writing with the left hand is "automatic," and failure is thought to suggest interhemispheric (callosal) disconnection (2).

Typically, a right-handed patient suffering callosal disconnection due to surgical section or focal lesion will demonstrate unimpaired writing ability with the dominant hand but severe impairment with the nondominant (left) hand. Writing and spelling disorders may occur selectively in either the dominant or nondominant hand due to damage to the corpus callosum or associated pathways (71–73). The left hand's ability to write to dictation may be impaired yet produce better copies than the right (74).

The callosal fibers responsible for the integration of cognitive and linguistic tasks for motor production in the left and the right hand are distinct, although in close proximity. Various patterns of dissociation on performance of writing, drawing, tactile naming, and praxis have been described (75). In a case of demyelination of the corpus callosum due to Marchiafava-Bignami disease, a left-handed patient exhibited right unilateral apraxic agraphia and limb apraxia, left tactile anomia, and a drawing impairment with both hands (76).

Unilateral agraphia may be aphasic agraphia (74,77) or apraxic agraphia (78,79). Right-handers with left unilateral agraphia typically produce an illegible scrawl (72,79–81). In contrast, left-handed patients suffering from left unilateral agraphia may produce well-formed letter sequences (82–84).

The strong lateralization of written language in the left hemisphere for right-handers is underscored by the case studied by Burklund and Smith (85). They observed that writing was initially the most impaired of the language functions affected by left hemispherectomy for glioma, and that postoperatively it showed the least and slowest recovery. Hemispheric specialization for spelling and writing in left-handers is not consistent or predictable.

Lateralization of language, praxis, spelling, and writing may be selectively spared or impaired by left- or right-hemisphere lesions in non-right-handers, as in cases of crossed aphasia. Nonaphasic, peripheral agraphias occur in right-handers from nondominant-hemisphere lesions (4) (see "Spatial Agraphia" below).

The clinical manifestation of unilateral agraphia is assumed in aphasics with large left frontal lesions and right hemiparesis. In such patients, the written production mirrors the speech impairment (86). Due to the right hemiplegia, the agraphia is seen only with the left, nondominant, nonparalyzed hand, while the right hand is not examined for writing ability.

The quality of handwriting by the left and right hands of right-handed normal subjects has been studied (87,88). Mechanical details of penmanship differ widely from the dominant to nondominant hand. When testing the nondominant hand for agraphia, no assumptions can be made about its similarity to the mechanics of the dominant hand's productions premorbidly.

Over the past two decades, various writing prostheses have been developed to aid written productions with the right hemiplegic limb. Rehabilitation studies (89–94) reported that better written productions were achieved with the right hemiplegic limb plus prosthesis than with the left unimpaired and unaided limb in aphasic agraphic patients.

In a range of mild, moderate, and severe patients with various types of aphasia, the performance with the right (hemiplegic) hand was unexpectedly found to be superior in linguistic content rather than in allographic execution. This phenomenon of side differences in the writing of these aphasic patients therefore implicates "central" language processes rather than graphomotor programming. The agraphic writing in the motorically unimpaired left hand has been described by Leischner (92) as being due to a disconnection of the callosal pathways from the left to the right motor association area [c.f. Lebrun (95)].

The superior performance of the right limb in these studies is attributed to ability to control the writing prosthesis with the proximal muscles to produce handwriting. Brown and Chobor (90) argued that the ipsilateral innervation of the right nonpyramidal system might be responsible for the good performance of the right proximal arm, with poor performance of the left and right distal and left proximal muscles arising from the damaged left hemisphere.

Both Brown and his colleagues (89,90) and Leischner (92) suggested that nonpyramidal control of the proximal muscles employed in the use of the prosthesis was a source of compensation for the pyramidal impairment of the distal motor control normally required for writing. In a recent hemiplegic, agraphic patient with a subcortical lesion (93,94), however, treatment with a writing prosthesis succeeded in releasing the spasticity in the hemiplegic right limb, so that the patient could write with the unaided right hand. This patient used his distal musculature to produce linguistically superior writing with his right than with his left hand. Various theoretical explanations have been offered for this laterality effect in written production [for a critical review see Lorch (75)].

Peripheral Agraphias

Peripheral agraphias are distinct from the central agraphias detailed above. The processes affected in the peripheral agraphias occur subsequent to the successful retrieval of spelling and the creation of an abstract graphemic word representation. Deficits may reflect difficulty with the graphemic word representation held in a memory store (graphemic buffer) or subsequent stages of motor planning, programming, and output. The processes affected involve the externalization of a graphemic representation in handwriting, oral spelling, typing, or letter arranging (25,96).

One type of peripheral agraphia is related to disturbance in the operation of the graphemic buffer. Patients succeed or fail equally in writing words or non-words. Significantly, performance is the same in writing as in typing. Length is the variable most often affected in the spelling performance of peripheral agraphia, in both English (21) and Italian (97–99) patients. Errors may occur more frequently in the middle of the word than at the beginning or end, reflecting the nature of the memory store. Short words may be spelled correctly regardless of their regularity, abstractness, or frequency. The lesions typically involve the angular gyrus. Numerous descriptions of graphemic buffer impairments have recently appeared (21,52,66,98–101).

The graphemic buffer is thought to represent letter identities and letter positions in the sequence. Information for each of these two variables may be lost selectively. Kinsbourne and Warrington (102) documented a patient with loss of letter-position information. The spellings produced consisted of the correct letters in transposed order. Gersh and Damasio (73) reported a patient who could often indicate the correct number of letters in a word but not the individual letter identities.

There is evidence that the form of a word being produced has several levels of abstract representation, including graphemes, syllables, and morphemes (103). A patient described by Caramazza and colleagues (100) exhibited errors resulting from a faulty graphemic buffer that reflected morphological effects of word composition rather than single letters. This difficulty was evident in the middle portion of long words in both oral and written spelling. Letter-substitution errors in a peripheral agraphic patient with a graphemic buffer disturbance reported by Caramazza and Miceli (105) were composed almost entirely of consonants replacing consonants and vowels replacing vowels. Errors exclusively involving vowels with correct consonants have been documented in English (106) and Russian (107). [There is some evidence of the presence of phonological effects in the short-term buffer in a report of a Thai agraphic (108) and of lexical effects in the graphemic buffer (109).]

Katz (101) reported a patient who could write only the first two or three letters correctly regardless of the length of the target word; accuracy was closely related to the temporal order in which the letters were written. This pattern of performance suggests that information about letter identity rapidly faded from the graphemic memory store. The lesion was located in the left temporoparietal area involving the supramarginal gyrus, angular gyrus, and posterior limb of the internal capsule. The patient's speech was most typical of a conduction aphasia, and his reading showed phonological dyslexia. In addition, Katz's patient was unable to spell words aloud, indicating a deficit in letter naming. In his written productions, the patient often mixed upper- and lowercase letters within a word (see the following section for other letter-case difficulties).

Allographic (Ideational, Physical-Letter-Code) Agraphia

In cursive writing, word forms are composed of variable letter shapes whose individual forms are determined by the preceding and following letters, a phenomenon referred to as allographic variation. Patients have been documented to have difficulties at the allographic level, where letter shape is determined in the context of the whole word (20,110–113). These agraphic patients have intact oral spelling and can type or use block letters successfully. They may have difficulty remembering which letter shapes correspond to which letter identities, but when they do remember the writing of individual letters is fluent and well formed (25). The agraphia is thus not due to difficulty in producing graphomotor patterns. Well-formed writing is composed of words with letter omissions, substitutions, insertions, and reversals, indicating that the sequence of letter identities that comprises the word form is also affected (114). In some cases, the frequency of the letters in the language may also influence the type of error (105,113).

Patients may have both central and peripheral agraphic impairments. Goodman and Caramazza (52) described a patient with lexical agraphia affecting oral and written spelling and an allographic impairment in assigning visual shape to graphemes. High-frequency regular words and irregularly spelled words were unimpaired, but low-frequency irregular words were impaired. The errors were considered to occur after the graphic output form had already been retrieved and assembled, e.g., "pierce" → TIERCE (52). A left-handed patient has been described with central surface dysgraphia and unilateral left peripheral agraphia affecting the selection of allographs (83).

Kapur and Lawton (115) reported a left-handed woman with epilepsy secondary to a left occipital slow-growing glioma. The patient had no aphasia, alexia, or apraxia but showed difficulties in visuospatial constructional tasks. She could not write spontaneously or to dictation, producing incorrect but well-formed letters. Ability to spell orally and with plastic letter blocks was intact, as was copying. The patient could produce drawings of objects whose shape was analogous to a letter she was unable to produce, e.g., "rugby goals posts" but not H, 13 but not B. The successful performance in drawing these letter shapes to verbal cues suggests that she did not have a general impairment of visually guided motor behavior, but rather a specific deficit of the motoric codes for producing orthography.

Difficulties with selected letter cases have also been reported. These peripheral writing impairments are considered to reflect impairment of specific graphic images and/or motor patterns (38,115–119). Baxter and Warrington (116) reported a patient with a bilateral parieto-occipital tumor whose oral spelling ability was preserved, but writing of even individual letters was severely impaired. Lowercase letters were more impaired than uppercase in spontaneous written productions, but copying was accurate. There was no evidence of limb apraxia and good ability to produce drawings of objects from memory. Significantly, the patient could often describe the named letters while being unable to write them. This writing disturbance is called *ideational agraphia*, by analogy to ideational apraxia (116,120) (see Chapter 21).

Specific difficulty with letter formation affecting lowercase letters, with relative preservation of uppercase, has been described in the context of preserved spelling, independent of apraxia or visuoconstructional impairment (118,119,121). Allographic agraphia with spontaneous mixing of upper-and lowercase letters has also been reported (117). Critchley (24) noted that early reports of dysgraphia in German mention confusion of Gothic and Latin scripts.

In addition to letter identity and letter case, the allographic code also specifies the style of letter produced, such as cursive or printed script. Allographic agraphic patients may have selective impairments in each of these three aspects of the physical letter-code specification (109). A patient may mix upper- and lowercase letters and print and cursive writing within the same word (117).

Apraxic Agraphia

In patients with apraxic agraphia, writing to dictation or request is impaired, but copying and oral spelling are preserved, although sometimes without comprehension. Apraxic agraphia can be considered a peripheral agraphia, in which there is an impairment in the concrete realization of a sequence of letters as a series of pen strokes on the page (38). This type of written spelling disorder may also be described as a transitional agraphia, with reference to the transition from letter codes to graphomotor patterns (109,122). Letter-imagery deficits may also occur (19,123). Lesions typically include the left posterior parietal parasagittal region (112,124), but a recent case had surgical removal of a left-hemisphere tumor in Exner's area (posterior superior premotor cortex) (125). This patient also showed selective preservation of writing numbers.

In contrast to ideational agraphia, patients with apraxic agraphia may produce ill-formed individual letters, but the differences between cases and print and script are maintained (122). Individual letter strokes present difficulties (119); letters may be written on top of one another (125), and letter substitutions may be determined by physical similarity (e.g., *H* for K, *u* for y) (12,15,122).

Apraxic agraphia tends to occur in conjunction with unilateral limb apraxia. However, dissociations of apraxic agraphia from limb apraxia have been reported (22,116,122,125–127).

Spatial (Visuospatial, Afferent, Constructional) Agraphia

Spatial agraphia, arising from posterior right-hemisphere lesions in right-handers, is typically associated with spatial dyslexia and spatial dyscalculia. The difficulty is characterized by spatial disorganization of units of written language or calculation, without a disturbance in the coding or decoding of the units themselves (4). The production of a spatial array of letter or number sequences on a page is disturbed in spatial agraphia (128). Individual letters of words may be separated or malformed, with extra loops. Written lines may slant or undulate, or they may be crowded into the right side of the page (4). A "cascade phenomenon" may be demonstrated whereby an increasingly wide left-hand margin is used in successive lines (129).

Right parietal lobe deficits may produce a handwriting disturbance in which the motor programs for letters are not executed correctly; those letters involving recursive movement (e.g., *M, U, E*) cause particular problems. The strokes of the letters are often omitted or repeated (130). The frequency of omission or reduplication of letters and letter strokes are similar in writing to dictation and copying (131). This disturbance could be considered the agraphic form of constructional apraxia. These patients have difficulty not in oral spelling or sequencing letter forms, but rather in monitoring the production of the graphomotor program (65).

Lebrun (131) attributed the impairment to both visual and kinesthetic feedback, since the patients cannot identify letters with extra strokes, nor can they inhibit multiple perseverative loops. Writing may improve with eyes closed.

A specific form of spatial dysgraphia is seen in association with unilateral spatial agnosia (left neglect) and visual field defects arising from right posterior lesions (4,36). Writing is squeezed into the right side of the page, with a large left margin. Errors in writing the beginnings of words may occur. The patients seem to produce written spelling as if they were reading it off an "internal screen" (57). One such patient spelled with equally poor accuracy both forward and backward; the errors occurred at the beginning of words, regardless of the direction of the response (16). Right neglect agraphia has also been demonstrated to involve the right halves of words being produced in written, oral, and backward oral spelling (132). Spatial agraphia may appear in typing, where the left side of the keyboard is neglected (133).

Pure Agraphia

Agraphia usually co-occurs with aphasia, but pure agraphia is occasionally found. While some linguistic and cognitive processes are associated with functions not dedicated solely to writing and spelling, some components of written production are independent, dedicated processes. Impairment of these components produces different forms of pure agraphia. Many of the cases discussed above represent instances of pure agrapia [e.g., pure deep dysgraphia (10)]. *Pure agraphia* refers to writing disturbances arising from focal lesions, in contrast to the term *isolated agraphia*, which is reserved for writing disturbances arising from multifocal or diffuse disorders (see below).

Hécaen and Angelergues (cited in Ref. 38) reported a disproportionately large number of left-handers among patients with pure agraphia. These patients often demonstrated residual writing impairment after the resolution of a more general aphasia.

Pure agraphia is quite rare; indeed, some aphasiologists have doubted its existence (134). Vignolo (135) reported two cases of pure agraphia in a series of 90 right-handed patients with left-hemisphere strokes. The lesions involved the upper half of the "central region" in one case, and the upper part of the posterior inferior parietal lobule in the second. Basso, Taborelli, and Vignolo (86) analyzed 500 consecutive cases of left-hemisphere language disorders and found seven cases with predominant disturbances of writing. There were two cases of pure agraphia; both patients had surgery for parasagittal parietal lesions, involving a hematoma in one and a meningioma in the other. The authors suggested that this area is "crucial for the sensorimotor linguistic integration needed for writing" (p. 562). In addition, two cases had agraphia associated with mild alexia, and three cases had agraphia and mild nonfluent aphasia.

Shallice (38) suggested that selective writing impairments were rare in the series of Basso et al. (86) because the patients studied were Italian. The regularity of this language in its sound-to-spelling correspondences would make selective central writing deficits difficult to detect. Indeed, the copious reports of pure agraphia in Japanese include symptoms that specifically reflect the complexities of their heterogeneous writing system, e.g., pure agraphia for kanji (136) and pure agraphia for kana (137). Similarly, German agraphics have reportedly confused Latin and Gothic scripts (24). Although the basic cognitive processes involved in producing meaningful graphic language are considered universal, specific languages may show different patterns of agraphia.

Assal, Chapuis and Zander (138) reported a case of pure French agraphia with good oral spelling but poor copying, writing to dictation, and spelling by arranging alphabet blocks. Written words contained correct initial letters but increasing errors toward the end of the word, indicating difficulties in the graphemic buffer. Errors typically consisted of inversion and addition of incorrect letters. Calligraphic quality was not affected. This case might be considered to represent isolated rather than pure agraphia, since the writing impairment appeared against a background of mild, diffuse intellectual and memory impairments and calculation difficulty, but without evidence of aphasia, apraxia, alexia, or agnosia. The patient had stenosis of the left internal carotid artery, without description of the exact anatomical lesion, and little recovery was demonstrated after carotid endarterectomy or over 6 months.

Rosati and De Bastiani (110) reported a case of an Italian right-handed man, an ex-telegrapher who developed pure agraphia and could "read" but not transmit Morse code. The patient could copy but not transcode from upper- to lowercase (allographic dysgraphia). Writing to dictation or spontaneously consisted of words with omissions, additions, transposition, and perservation of letters. The letters themselves were well-formed but sometimes contained extra strokes, and the lines of script were arranged appropriately on the page. The patient reportedly had focal atrophy of the left temporal lobe due to a middle cerebral artery infarct.

Pure agraphia following superior parietal damage may be associated with a defect of visual guidance of hand movements. Auerbach and Alexander (139) reported a patient with impaired production of writing spontaneously, to dictation, and copying, with good oral spelling. Spelling errors involved omission, substitution, and repetition. Letters were poorly formed, with crossed lines and inappropriate loops. The lesion was in the left superior parietal lobe. This area is thought to be responsible for the integration of cross-modal sensory information and overlies white-matter pathways connecting visual association cortex (area 19) and motor association cortex (area 6) (139).

All the cases of pure agraphia described above involved posterior, temporoparietal lesions. Historically, the area associated with writing function was the so-called Exner's area, the second left frontal convolution (140,141). Hécaen and Consoli (46) analyzed 19 patients with lesions of the foot of the third frontal convolution (Broca's area), limited in extent by the rolandic gyri posteriorly and the sylvian fissure inferiorly. Of these, four patients had lesions that included the second frontal convolution (Exner's area) as well as Broca's area. Three of the four patients had no aphasia or agraphia. Five other subjects whose lesions were restricted to Broca's area showed mild agraphia with minimal dysprosody but no aphasia. Recent cases of pure agraphia (55) and alexia with agraphia (125) have been reported with lesions involving Exner's area (55). Other lesions associated with pure agraphia (142) have included a hematoma deep in the left centrum semiovale, sparing both parietal and frontal cortices, and a subcortical lesion of the left caudate and internal capsule (143). This wide range of lesion localizations that result in pure agraphias underscores the complexity of the processes involved in writing and spelling, independent of those involved in spoken language and reading.

Gerstmann's Syndrome

While agraphia can occur in association with various lesion localizations and neuropsychological impairments, agraphia as part of Gerstmann's syndrome (agraphia, dyscalculia, right–left confusion, and finger agnosia) is thought to have localizing value to the dominant inferior parietal region (144,145). Constructional apraxia, impaired memory, and alexia are frequently associated with Gerstmann's syndrome (see Chapter 21), and this larger constellation of symptoms reliably localizes to the area of the angular gyrus (146).

Agraphia in conjunction with autotopagnosia or impaired ability to point to body parts due to a left parietal glioma was thought to reflect a more severe disturbance of body scheme than specific finger agnosia and left–right confusion (147).

Isolated Agraphia

Isolated agraphia, in contrast to pure agraphia, refers to writing disturbances not caused by focal lesions. Varied etiologies can give rise to isolated agraphia, including confusional states associated with sodium amytal intoxication (5,6), migraine (24), and right middle cerebral artery infarctions (148). Impaired feedback due to the diffuse neurological impairment is considered the source of the agraphia.

Isolated agraphia in patients with confusional states has been investigated by Geschwind (5,6,149), who stated: "One of the most curious features of the confusional state is the dissolution of writing in even very mild cases . . . A patient with this very dramatic agraphia will typically have speech that is essentially normal . . . Indeed confusional states are probably the most common cause of pure agraphia" (p. 182). Chédru and Geschwind (6) studied acute confusional states induced experimentally with intravenous amytal. During the period of barbiturate intoxication, writing became spatially abnormal; it was scrawled in many directions on the page, and words had letters with perseverative loops, similar to those seen in afferent (constructional) agraphia secondary to right-hemisphere lesions. In other instances, incorrect words or misspellings were produced. In two cases of acute confusional states resulting from right middle cerebral artery infarctions, patients demonstrated agraphia without alexia, in conjunction with naming and calculation difficulties (148).

Dubois, Hécaen, and Marcie (150) studied six French patients with isolated, peripheral agraphia who were unimpaired in verbal and constructional ability but demonstrated co-occurring acalculia. Four of the six also showed general intellectual deterioration. Oral spelling and copying were unimpaired, but case-transcoding ability was affected. Spelling difficulties were manifested as combination and selection errors in the letters of written words. The majority of errors occurred in the middle rather than beginning or end of words, indicating some difficulty with the graphemic buffer.

Agraphia in Dementia

In dementia, as in confusional states, writing disturbances may affect linguistic and/or motoric aspects of spelling and writing. These disturbances are not homogeneous or distinctive. However, impairments in narrative writing have been found to correlate with severity of dementia, suggesting the utility of writing tasks for screening purposes (7). The writing and spelling disturbances in Alzheimer's dementia can be distinguished from those of posterior aphasic writing, but they show similarities to performance in very advanced, normal aging (151). Agraphia may often be found without parallel speech disturbance, as in the cases of isolated agraphia described above (5,6), containing both linguistic and extralinguistic features.

Agraphic features in Alzheimer's disease include shorter texts, letter and spelling errors, and selection of "content" words (i.e., nouns, verbs, adjectives) when compared to age-matched, normal controls (152). Specific impairment of lexical spelling and difficulty spelling irregular words with intact phonological spelling — i.e., lexical agraphia — has been demonstrated in patients with Alzheimer's disease (54,153,154). This pattern of spelling errors reflects localized pathology in the angular gyrus and adjacent parietal lobe, mimicking a focal syndrome.

Multi-infarct dementia may also give rise to isolated agraphia. A case described by Lesser (17) demonstrated spared but asemantic oral spelling with homophone confusions. Writing could proceed only after oral spelling of a word, otherwise consisting of a series of vertical strokes.

Afferent (constructional) dysgraphia may develop secondary to progressive posterior cortical dementia (155) or advanced subcortical dementia, as in progressive supranuclear palsy (156).

Other Graphic Disturbances

Motor disturbances including paresis, ataxia, dystonia, and disturbances of sensation and coordination of the upper limbs give rise to abnormalities of graphic production (nonaphasic agraphia). Peripheral nerve disturbances, in particular those involving the radial nerve, may disrupt the ability to write (2). A writing disturbance analogous to the dysarthria present in some nonfluent aphasics, due to deep subcortical damage, is manifest as a mechanical writing impairment secondary to a movement disorder.

Hypergraphia

Hypergraphia may be demonstrated as part of the interictal personality changes associated with temporal lobe epilepsy (157,158). This symptom was first described by Waxman and Geschwind (9), who reported seven cases of temporal lobe epilepsy with compulsive hypergraphic behavior. Patients wrote extensively and in a meticulous and highly ritualized manner, keeping circumstantial and pedantic notes of autobiographical information. Many patients were secretive about the contents of these writings. Words were defined and redefined with heavy use of parenthetical comments, underlining, uppercase lettering, and red ink for added emphasis. Many patients produced highly moral or religious writings. Schizophrenia may be associated with hypergraphia resembling that of temporal lobe epilepsy, including underlining and odd punctuation in addition to bizarre themes, idiosyncratic lexicon, and paragrammatic sentence constructions (2).

Evidence has been presented linking hypergraphia to right-hemisphere disorders. Hypergraphia may be more common in temporal lobe epileptics with right temporal foci (159). Yamadori (160,161) reported a distinctive type of "chaotic" hypergraphia due to right-hemisphere damage in the middle cerebral artery territory affecting the perisylvian cortex, subcortex involving the basal ganglia, or in the right thalamus. This symptom is typically manifest in the first month post onset of illness but may be lasting. This form of hypergraphic writing is also produced in copious amounts, but rather than being careful and precise as in cases of temporal lobe epilepsy, the writing is large, scrawling, chaotic, unconcerned, and sloppy. Calligraphy, lining, and spacing on the page are disorganized. Linguistic content is also somewhat metaphysical but semantically empty and lacking in text coherence. No spelling or grammatical errors are produced. This author has seen a case of "chaotic" hypergaphia due to a right temporal lobe tumor. The calligraphy was large and sprawling, the writing autobiographical, interwoven with mythic imagery. The text was incoherent and made use of idiosyncratic lexicon, showing similarities to schizophrenic writing (162).

Hypokinetic Agraphia, Micrographia

In contrast to the overly large scrawl produced by certain right-hemisphere-damaged patients, pathologically small writing is produced by patients suffering from extrapyramidal disturbances (2). Approximately one-third of patients suffering from Parkinson's disease exhibit micrographia. Handwriting disturbances may be the first sign of an extrapyramidal disorder and may antedate other symptoms by as much as 4 years (8). Patients are typically unable to increase writing size voluntarily. Writing diminishes in size as it proceeds along the line; writing that is uniformly small may be produced by corticospinal lesions (2). Automatic writing tasks such as the patient's signature, letters of the alphabet, or consecutive numbers will often reveal the progressive micrographia. Micrographia is not directly related to rigidity or tremor but is associated with increased movement time and subsequent difficulty in maintenance of force (163). The association with general bradykinesia is typical but inconsistent (8). It may be accompanied by progressive crowding or slant of letters, or a writing line that veers away from the horizontal.

While tremor associated with Parkinson's disease does not contribute to disturbances in handwriting, postural and cerebellar tremor gives rise to hyperkinetic agraphia. Chorea also produces graphic disturbances (2).

Mirror Writing

Writing may be produced from right to left with all the letters written backward. Mirror writing arises from diverse normal or pathological processes in adults and children as either an unconscious or deliberate performance. Some cases of natural facility to produce mirror writing are a result of left-handers' being forced to write with the right hand. Mirror writing may arise out of states with dissociations of consciousness or attention, such as concussion aftereffects, light anesthesia, intoxication, or hysteria (164).

The first modern report of pathological mirror writing is a case with associated jargonaphasia due to a left parietal tumor [Fox and Holmes, 1926, cited by Critchley (164)]. A second case with alexia and anarthria with left-hand mirror writing due to left sylvian artery occlusion was also reported at that time [Morlaas, cited by Critchley (164)]. Modern reports of acquired mirror writing from cortical lesions include those of patients with both left- and right-hand dominance (165). The underlying source of this deficit has been attributed to visuospatial disorientation (166) and graphomotor disturbances (167).

ASSESSMENT OF WRITING AND SPELLING

Testing written language function by asking for a patient's signature is a good initial test but is insufficient in itself and can be misleading (2). Quite often this automatic production can be performed in the absence of any other ability to produce propositional written language. Typical assessments of writing and spelling involve the following tasks: (1) signing one's name, (2) copying letters, numbers, words, and sentences, (3) transcoding scripts into print, cursive, uppercase and lowercase letters, and roman and arabic numerals, (4) writing to dictation of letters, numbers, words, and sentences, (5) writing the names of objects and demonstrated actions, and (6) spontaneous narrative writing of sequences and information.

Mechanical aspects of handwriting should be judged along with linguistic ones. Lined paper should not be used. Qualitative analysis of various characteristics of writing can be sensitive measures, including height and size of writing, placement on the page relative to the left and top margins, slope of lines, orientation, and spacing.

Premorbid level of attainment in writing skills and spelling must be ascertained and preferably verified by a family member. If possible, an earlier typical sample of the patient's writing should be obtained. Some individuals never master writing and do not use written skills in their daily adult lives (1). The specific language spoken by the patient is also important; in English the idiosyncratic nature of spelling rules and the nonphonetic orthography make the language more sensitive to agraphic disorders, as compared to a language such as Italian, in which spelling is regular and based directly on phonology, so that any word that is known should be spelled normally.

Linguistic analyses of the writing errors produced by different types of Italian and Spanish aphasics have recently been carried out (129,168). The study of patients who are speakers of such languages is useful in providing insight into graphemic production that is not confounded by the question of premorbid spelling knowledge due to the complete transparency and regularity of sound-to-spelling rules. Also illuminating, however, is the study of agraphia in languages with writing systems more complex than English, with inclusion of graphic codes for other levels of linguistic significance such as Japanese (169) and Thai (108).

REFERENCES

1. Parr S. Everyday reading and writing practices of normal adults: implications for aphasia assessment. Aphasiology 1992;6:273-283.
2. Benson DF, Cummings J. Agraphia. In: Frederiks J, ed. Handbook of clinical neurology. Vol 45. Clinical neuropsychology. New York: Elsevier, 1985.
3. Goodglass H, Hunter M. A linguistic comparison of speech and writing in two types of aphasia. J Commun Dis 1970;3:28-35.
4. Hécaen H, Marcie P. Disorders of written language following right hemisphere lesions: spatial dysgraphia. In: Dimond S, Beaumont J, eds. Hemispheric function in the human brain. London: Elek Science, 1974.
5. Chédru F, Geschwind N. Disorders of higher cortical functioning in acute confusional states. Cortex 1972;8:395-411.
6. Chédru F, Geschwind N. Writing disturbances in acute confusional states. Neuropsychologia 1972;10:343-353.
7. Horner J, Heyman A, Dawson D, Rogers H. The relationship of agraphia to the severity of dementia in Alzheimer's disease. Arch Neurol 1988;45:760-773.
8. McLennan JE, Nakano K, Tyler HR, Schwab RS. Micrographia in Parkinson's disease. J Neurol Sci 1972;15:141-152.
9. Waxman S, Geschwind N. Hypergraphia in temporal lobe epilepsy. Neurology 1974;24:629-936.
10. Bub D, Kertesz A. Deep agraphia. Brain Lang 1982;17:146-165.
11. Beauvois M-F, Derouesné J. Lexical or orthographic agraphia. Brain 1981;104:21-49.
12. Hatfield FM, Patterson K. Phonological spelling. Quart J Exp Psychol 1983;35:451-468.
13. Kinsbourne M, Warrington E. A case showing selectively impaired oral spelling. J Neurol Neurosurg Psychiatry 1965;28:563-566.
14. Katz RB. Recognizing orally spelled words: an analysis of procedures shared with reading and spelling. Brain Lang 1989;37:201-219.
15. Zangwill O. Agraphia due to a left parietal glioma in a left-handed man. Brain 1954;77:510-520.
16. Baxter D, Warrington E. Neglect dysgraphia. J Neurol Neurosurg Psychiatry 1983;46:1073-1078.
17. Lesser R. Selective preservation of oral spelling without semantics in a case of multi-infarct dementia. Cortex 1989;25:239-250.
18. Lesser R. Superior oral to written spelling: evidence for separate buffers? Cogn Neuropsychol 1990;7:347-366.
19. Friedman RB, Alexander MP. Written spelling agraphia. Brain Lang 1989;36:503-517.
20. Kinsbourne M, Rosenfield D. Agraphia selective for written spelling. Brain Lang 1974;1:215-225.
21. Hillis A, Caramazza A. The graphemic buffer and attentional mechanisms. Brain Lang 1989;36:208-235.
22. Hécaen H, Albert M. Human neuropsychology. New York: John Wiley, 1978.
23. Luria A. Traumatic aphasia. The Hague: Mouton, 1970.

24. Critchley M. Aphasiology and other aspects of language. London: Edward Arnold, 1970.
25. Ellis A. Normal writing processes and peripheral acquired dysgraphias. Lang Cogn Proc 1988;3:99–127.
26. Jackson J. On a case of loss of power of expression: inability to talk, to write and to read correction after convulsive attacks. Brit Med J 1866;192:326–330.
27. Goodglass H, Geschwind N. Language disorders (aphasia). In: Carterette EC, Friedman MP, eds. Handbook of perception. Vol VII. Language and speech. New York: Academic Press, 1976.
28. Leischner A. Agraphia. In: Vinken P, Bruyn G, eds. Handbook of clinical neurology. Vol 4. New York: John Wiley, 1969.
29. De Bleser R, Luzzatti C. Models of reading and writing and their disorders in classical German aphasiology. Cogn Neuropsychol 1989;6:501–585.
30. Smith A. Objective indices of severity of chronic aphasia in stroke patients. J Speech Hear Disord 1971;36:167–207.
31. Duffy R, Ulrich S. A comparison of impairments in verbal comprehension, speech reading and writing in adult aphasics. J Speech Hear Disord 1976;41: 110–119.
32. Porch D. The Porch index of communicative ability. Palo Alto: Consulting Psychologists Press, 1967.
33. Keenan T, Brassell E. A study of factors related to prognosis for individual aphasic patients. J Speech Hear Disord 1974;39:257–269.
34. Keenan T. The detection of minimal dysphasia. Arch Phys Med Rehab 1971; 52:227–232.
35. Noll J, Hoops H. Aphasic grammatical involvement as indicated by spelling ability. Cortex 1967;3:419–432.
36. Benson DF. Aphasia, alexia and agraphia. New York: Churchill-Livingstone, 1979.
37. Frederici AD, Schoenle PW, Goodglass H. Mechanisms underlying writing and speech in aphasia. Brain Lang 1981;13:212–222.
38. Shallice T. From neuropsychology to mental structure. New York: Cambridge University Press, 1988.
39. Assal G, Buttet J, Jolivet R. Dissociations in aphasia: a case report. Brain Lang 1981;13:223–240.
40. Bub D, Kertesz A. Evidence for lexicographic processing in a patient with preserved written over oral single word naming. Brain 1982;105:697–717.
41. Ellis A, Miller D, Sin G. Wernicke's aphasia and normal language processing: a case study in cognitive neuropsychology. Cognition 1983;15:111–144.
42. Levine DN, Calvanio R, Popovics A. Language in the absence of inner speech. Neuropsychologia 1982;20:391–409.
43. Hier D, Mohr J. Incongruous oral and written naming: evidence of a subdivision of the syndrome of Wernicke's aphasia. Brain Lang 1977;4:115–126.
44. Patterson KE, Shewell C. Speak and spell: dissociations and word-class effects. In: Coltheart M, Sartori G, Job R, eds. The cognitive neuropsychology of language. London: Erlbaum, 1987.

45. Benson DF, Geschwind N. Aphasia and related cortical disturbances. In: Baker AB, Baker LH, eds. Clinical neurology. New York: Harper & Row, 1971.
46. Hécaen H, Consoli S. Analyse des troubles du langage au cours des lesions de l'aire de Broca. Neuropsychologia 1973;11:377-388.
47. Wapner W, Gardner H. A study of spelling in aphasia. Brain Lang 1979;7:363-374.
48. Roeltgen DP. Agraphia. In: Heilman K, Valenstein E, eds. Clinical neuropsychology. 2nd ed. New York: Oxford University Press, 1985.
49. Marshall JC, Newcombe F. Patterns of paralexia—a psycholinguistic approach. J Psycholing Res 1973;2:175-199.
50. Coltheart M. The psycholinguistic analysis of acquired dyslexias. Philosophical Transactions of the Royal Society of London B 1982;298:151-163.
51. Roeltgen DP, Heilman KM. Lexical agraphia, further support for the two-strategy hypothesis of linguistic agraphia. Brain 1984;107:811-827.
52. Goodman R, Caramazza A. Dissociation of spelling errors in written and oral spelling: the role of allographic conversion in writing. Cogn Neuropsychol 1986; 3:179-206.
53. Newcombe F, Marshall JC. Reading and writing by letter sounds. In: Patterson KE, Marshall JC, Coltheart M, eds. Surface dyslexia: cognitive and neuropsychological studies of phonological reading. Hillsdale: Lawrence Erlbaum, 1985.
54. Baxter D, Warrington E. Transcoding sound to spelling: single or multiple sound unit correspondences. Cortex 1987;23:11-28.
55. Rapcsak SZ, Arthur SA, Rubens AB. Lexical agraphia from a focal lesion of the left precentral gyrus. Neurology 1988;38:119-123.
56. Gonzalez-Rothi L, Roeltgen R, Kooistra C. Isolated lexical agraphia in a right handed patient with a posterior lesion of the right cerebral hemisphere. Brain Lang 1987;30:181-190.
57. Shallice T. Phonological agraphia and the lexical route in writing. Brain 1981; 104:413-429.
58. Roeltgen D, Sevush S, Heilman K. Phonological agraphia: writing by the lexical-semantic route. Neurology 1983;33:755-765.
59. Baxter D, Warrington E. Category-specific phonological dysgraphia. Neuropsychologia 1985;23:653-666.
60. Hatfield F. Visual and phonological factors in acquired agraphia. Neuropsychologia 1985;23:13-29.
61. Alexander MP, Friedman RB, Loverso F, Fischer RS. Lesion localization of phonological agraphia. Brain Lang 1992;43:83-95.
62. Bolla-Wilson K. Speedie LJ, Robinson RG. Phonological agraphia in a left-handed patient after a right hemisphere lesion. Neurology 1985;35:1778-1781.
63. Barry C. Acquired disorders of reading and spelling: a cognitive neuropsychological perspective. In: Code C, ed. The characteristics of aphasia. New York: Taylor & Francis, 1989.
64. Newcombe F, Marshall JC. Transcoding and lexical stabilization in deep dyslexia. In: Coltheart M, Patterson KM, Marshall JC, ed. Deep dyslexia. London: Routledge and Kegan Paul, 1980.

65. Caplan D. Language: structure, processing and disorders. Cambridge, MA: MIT Press, 1992.
66. Nolan K, Caramazza A. An analysis of writing in a case of deep dyslexia. Brain Lang 1983;16:305–328.
67. Coltheart M. Deep dyslexia: a review of the syndrome. In: Coltheart M, Patterson K, Marshall JC, eds. Deep dyslexia. London: Routledge and Kegan Paul, 1980.
68. Roeltgen DP, Gonzalez-Rothi L, Heilman K. Linguistic semantic agraphia: a dissociation of the lexical spelling system from semantics. Brain Lang 1986;27:257–280.
69. Ellis A. Reading, writing and dyslexia. London: Erlbaum, 1984.
70. Patterson KE. Lexical but nonsemantic spelling? Cogn Neuropsychol 1986;3:341–367.
71. Sperry RW, Gazzaniga MS. Language following surgical disconnection of the hemispheres. In: Darley F, ed. Brain mechanisms underlying speech and language. New York: Grune & Stratton, 1967.
72. Geschwind N, Kaplan E. A human disconnection syndrome. Neurology 1962;12:675–685.
73. Gersh F, Damasio A. Praxis and writing of the left hand may be served by different callosal pathways. Arch Neurol 1981;38:634–636.
74. Bogen J. The other side of the brain: Dysgraphia and dyscopia following cerebral commisurotomy. Bull LA Neurol Soc 1969;34:191–220.
75. Lorch MP. Laterality of rehabilitation. Aphasiology. In press.
76. Rosa A, Demiati M, Carty L, Mizon JP. Marchiafava-Bignami disease, syndrome of interhemispheric disconnection and right-handed agraphia in a left hander. Arch Neurol 1991;48:986–988.
77. Botez MI, Crighel E. Partial disconnection syndrome in an ambidextrous patient. Brain 1971;94:487–494.
78. Heilman KM, Gonyea EF, Geschwind N. Apraxia and agraphia in a right hander. Cortex 1974;10:284–288.
79. Watson RT, Heilman KM. Callosal apraxia. Brain 1983;106:391–403.
80. Rubens AB, Geschwind N, Mahowald MW, Mastri A. Posttraumatic cerebral hemisphere disconnection syndrome. Arch Neurol 1977;34:750–755.
81. Yamadori A, Osumi Y, Ikeda H, Kanazawa Y. Left unilateral agraphia and tactile anomia. Arch Neurol 1980;37:88–91.
82. Gur RE, Gur RC, Sussman NM, O'Connor MJ, Vey MM. Hemispheric control of the writing hand: the effect of callosotomy in a left-hander. Neurology 1984;34:904–908.
83. Zesiger P, Mayer E. Left unilateral dysgraphia in a patient with an atypical pattern of handedness: a cognitive analysis. Aphasiology 1992;76:293–307.
84. Heilman KM, Coyle JM, Gonyea EF, Geschwind N. Apraxia and agraphia in the left hander. Brain 1973;96:21–28.
85. Burklund C, Smith A. Language and the cerebral hemispheres: observations of verbal and nonverbal responses during 18 months following left ("dominant") hemispherectomy. Neurology 1977;27:627–633.

86. Basso A, Taborelli A, Vignolo L. Dissociated disorders of speaking and writing in aphasia. J Neurol Neurosurg Psychiatry 1978;41:556-563.

87. Hansen AM, McNeil MR. Differences between writing with the dominant and nondominant hand by normal geriatric subjects on a spontaneous writing task: twenty perceptual and computerized measures. In: Brookshire R, ed. Clin Aphasiol 1986;16:116-122.

88. Hansen AM, McNeikl MR, Vetterm DK. More differences between writing with the dominant and nondominant hand by normal geriatric subjects: eight perceptual and eight computerized measures on a sentence dictation task. In: Brookshire R, ed. Clin Aphasiol 1987;17:152-158.

89. Brown J, Leader B, Blum S. Hemiplegic writing in severe aphasia. Brain Lang 1983;19:204-215.

90. Brown J, Chobor K. Therapy with a prosthesis for writing in aphasia. Aphasiology 1989;3:709-715.

91. Freidland J. Accessing language in agraphia: an examination of hemiplegic writing. Aphasiology 1990;4:241-257.

92. Leischner A. Side differences in writing to dictation of aphasics with agraphia: a graphic disconnection syndrome. Brain Lang 1983;18:1-19.

93. Lorch M, Whurr M. Hemiplegic writing with the use of a prosthesis in an aphasic agraphic patient. Grazer Linguistische Studien: Neuro- und Patholinguistik 1991;35:171-179.

94. Whurr M, Lorch M. The use of a prosthesis to facilitate writing in aphasia and right hemiplegia. Aphasiology 1991;5:411-418.

95. Lebrun Y. Unilateral agraphia. Aphasiology 1987;1:317-329.

96. Ellis A. Spelling and writing (and reading and speaking). In: Ellis A, ed. Normality and pathology in cognitive function. London: Academic Press, 1982.

97. Caramazza A, Miceli G, Villa G, Romani C. The role of the graphemic buffer in spelling: evidence from a case of acquired dysgraphia. Cognition 1987;26:59-85.

98. Miceli G, Silveri C, Caramazza A. Cognitive analysis of a case of pure dysgraphia. Brain Lang 1985;25:187-212.

99. Miceli G, Silveri C, Caramazza A. The role of the phoneme-grapheme conversion system and of the graphemic output buffer in writing. In: Coltheart M, Sartori G, Job R, eds. The cognitive neuropsychology of language. London: Erlbaum, 1987.

100. Caramazza A, Miceli G, Villa G. The role of the (output) phonological buffer in reading, writing, and repetition. Cogn Neuropsychol 1986;3:37-76.

101. Katz RB. Limited retention of information in the graphemic buffer. Cortex 1991;27:111-119.

102. Kinsbourne M, Warrington E. Disorders of spelling. J Neurol Neurosurg Psychiatry 1964;27:224-228.

103. Shallice T, Warrington E, McCarthy R. Reading without semantics. Quart J Exp Psychol 1983;35A:111-138.

104. Badecker W, Hillis A, Caramazza A. Lexical morphology and its role in the writing process: Evidence from a case of acquired dysgraphia. Cognition 1990;35:205-234.

105. Caramazza A, Miceli G. The structure of graphemic representations. Cognition 1990;37:243–297.
106. Cubelli R. A selective deficit for writing vowels in acquired dysgraphia. Nature 1991;353:258–260.
107. Simernitskaya EG. On two forms of writing defect following local brain lesions. In: Dimond SJ, Beaumont JG, eds. Hemisphere function in the human brain. London: Elek Science, 1974.
108. Gandour J, Darananda R, Holasuit S. Nature of spelling errors in a Thai conduction aphasic. Brain Lang 1989;41:96–119.
109. Margolin DI, Goodman-Schulman R. Oral and written spelling impairments. In: Margolin DI, ed. Cognitive neuropsychology in clinical practice. Oxford: Oxford University Press, 1992.
110. Rosati G, De Bastiani P. Pure agraphia: a discrete form of aphasia. J Neurol Neurosurg Psychiatry 1979;42:266–269.
111. Bub D, Black S, Howell J, Kertesz A. Damage to input and output buffers — What's a lexicality effect doing in a place like that? In: Keller E, Gopnick M, eds. Motor and sensory processes of language. Hillsdale: Lawrence Erlbaum, 1987.
112. Rothi L, Heilman K. Alexia and agraphia with spared spelling and letter recognition abilities. Brain Lang 1981;12:1–13.
113. Black S, Behrmann M, Bass K, Hacker P. Selective writing impairment: beyond the allographic code. Aphasiology 1989;3:265–277.
114. Papagno C. A case of peripheral dysgraphia. Cogn Neuropsychol 1992;9:259–270.
115. Kapur N, Lawton N. Dysgraphia for letters: a form of motor memory deficit? J Neurol Neurosurg Psychiatry 1983;46:573–575.
116. Baxter D, Warrington E. Ideational agraphia: a single case study. J Neurol Neurosurg Psychiatry 1986;49:369–374.
117. De Bastiani P, Barry C. A cognitive analysis of an acquired dysgraphic patient with an "allographic" writing disorder. Cogn Neuropsychol 1989;6:25–41.
118. Kartsounis L. Selective lower-case letter ideational dysgraphia. Cortex 1992;28:145–150.
119. Patterson KE, Wing A. Processes in handwriting: A case for case. Cogn Neuropsychol 1989;6:1–23.
120. Hermann K. Reading disability. Copenhagen: Munksgaard, 1959.
121. Kapur N, Gordon DS. Retraining of dysgraphia—a case study. J Neurol Neurosurg Psychiatry 1975;38:465–468.
122. Margolin DI. The neuropsychology of writing and spelling: semantic phonological, motor and perceptual processes. Quart J Exp Psychol 1984;34A:459–489.
123. Crary M, Heilman K. Letter imagery deficits in a case of pure apraxic agraphia. Brain Lang 1988;34:147–156.
124. Russell WR, Espir M. Traumatic Aphasia. Oxford: Oxford University Press, 1961.

125. Anderson SW, Damasio AR, Damasio H. Troubled letters but not numbers. Brain 1990;113:749–766.
126. Roeltgen DP, Heilman KM. Apractic agraphia in a patient with normal praxis. Brain Lang 1983;18:35–46.
127. Coslett HB, Rothi L, Valenstein E, Heilman K. Dissociations of writing and praxis: Two cases in point. Brain Lang 1986;28:357–369.
128. Critchley M. The Parietal Lobes. London: Edward Arnold, 1953.
129. Ardila A, Rosselli M, Pinzon O. Alexia and agraphia in Spanish speakers. In: Ardila A, Ostrosky-Solis F, eds. Brain organization of language and cognitive processes. New York: Plenum, 1989.
130. Ellis A, Young A, Flude B. "Afferant dysgraphia" in a patient and in a normal subject. Cogn Neuropsychol 1987;4:465–486.
131. Lebrun Y. Neurolinguistic models of language and speech. In: Whitaker H, Whitaker HA, eds. Studies in neurolinguistics. Vol 1. New York: Academic Press, 1976.
132. Caramazza A, Hillis A. Spatial representation of words in the brain implied by studies of a unilateral neglect patient. Nature 1990;346:267–269.
133. Valenstein E, Heilman KM. Apraxic agraphia with neglect-induced paragraphia. Arch Neurol 1979;36:506–508.
134. Kreindler A, Fradis A. Performances in aphasia. Paris: Gauthier-Villars, 1968.
135. Vignolo L. The anatomical and pathological basis of aphasia. In: Rose F, Whurr R, Wyke M, eds. Aphasia. London: Whurr Publ, 1988.
136. Soma Y, Sugishita M, Kitamura K, Maruyama S, Imanaga H. Lexical agraphia in the Japanese language. Brain 1989;112:1549–1561.
137. Tanaka Y, Yamadori A, Murata S. Selective kana agraphia. Cortex 1987;23: 679–684.
138. Assal G, Chapuis G, Zander E. Isolated writing disorders in a patient with stenosis of the left internal carotid artery. Cortex 1971;6:241–248.
139. Auerbach S, Alexander M. Pure agraphia and unilateral optic ataxia associated with a left superior parietal lobe lesion. J Neurol Neurosurg Psychiatry 1981;44:430–432.
140. Gordinier HC. Arguments in favour of the existence of a separate center for writing. Amer J Med Sci 1899;126:490.
141. Neilson JM. Agnosia, apraxia, aphasia. New York: Hoeber, 1946.
142. Croisile B, Laurent B, Michel D, Trillet M. Pure agraphia after deep left hemisphere haematome. J Neurol Neurosurg Psychiatry 1990;53:263–265.
143. Laine T, Martilla RJ. Pure agraphia: a case study. Neuropsychologia 1981; 19:311–316.
144. Levine DN, Mani RB, Calvanio R. Pure agraphia and Gerstmann's syndrome as a visuospatial-language dissociation: an experimental case study. Brain Lang 1988;35:172–196.
145. Mazzoni M, Pardossi L, Cantini R, Gioretti V, Arena R. Gerstmann syndrome: a case report. Cortex 1990;26:459–467.
146. Hier D, Gorelick P, Schindler A. Topics in behavioral neurology and neuropsychology. London: Butterworths, 1987.

147. DeRenzi E, Scotti G. Autotopagnosia: fiction or reality? Arch Neurol 1970; 23:221–227.
148. Mesulam M-M, Waxman S, Geschwind N, Sabin T. Acute confusional states with right middle cerebral artery infarctions. J Neurol Neurosurg Psychiatry 1976;39:84–89.
149. Geschwind N. Disorders of attention: a frontier of neuropsychology. Philosophical Transactions of the Royal Society London B 1982;298:173–185.
150. Dubois J, Hécaen H, Marcie P. L'agraphie "pure." Neuropsychologia 1969; 7:271–286.
151. Glosser G, Kaplan E. Linguistic and nonlinguistic impairments in writing: a comparison of patients with focal and multifocal CNS disorders. Brain Lang 1989;37:357–380.
152. Neils J, Boller F, Gerdeman B, Cole M. Descriptive writing abilities in Alzheimer's disease. J Clin Exp Neuropsychol 1989;11:692–698.
153. Rapcsak SZ, Arthur SA, Bliklen DA, Rubens AB. Lexical agraphia in Alzheimer's disease. Arch Neurol 1989;46:65–68.
154. Schwartz M, Marin O. Saffran E. Dissociation of language function in dementia: a case study. Brain Lang 1979;7:277–306.
155. Cipolotti L, Denes G. When a patient can write but not copy: a report of a single case. Cortex 1989;25:331–337.
156. Podoll K, Schwartz M, Noth J. Language functions in progressive supranuclear palsy. Brain 1991;114:1457–1472.
157. Bear DM, Fedio P. Quantitative analysis of interictal behavior in temporal lobe epilepsy. Arch Neurol 1977;34:454–467.
158. Sachdev HS, Waxman S. Frequency of hypergraphia in temporal lobe epilepsy. J Neurol Neurosurg Psychiatry 1981;44:358–360.
159. Roberts JKA, Robertson MM, Trimble M. The lateralizing significance of hypergraphia in temporal lobe epilepsy. J Neurol Neurosurg Psychiatry 1982; 45:131–138.
160. Yamadori A. Writing and hemispheric coordination. Aphasiology 1988;2: 427–432.
161. Yamadori A, Mori E, Tabuchi M, Kudo Y, Mitani Y. Hypergraphia: a right hemisphere syndrome. J Neurol Neurosurg Psychiatry 1986;49:1160–1164.
162. Perlman M. A case of autobiographical hypergraphia due to a right hemisphere tumor. Boston V.A. Aphasia Research Center. Unpublished manuscript, 1982.
163. Margolin DI, Wing AM. Agraphia and micrographia: Clinical manifestations of motor programming and performance disorders. Acta Psych 1983;54:263–283.
164. Critchley M. Mirror-writing. London: Kegan Paul, 1928.
165. Tankle RS, Heilman KM. Mirror writing in right-handers and left-handers. Brain Lang 1983;19:115–123.
166. Heilman KM, Howell G, Valenstein E, Rothi L. Mirror reading and writing in association with right-left spatial disorientation. J Neurol Neurosurg Psychiatry 1980;43:774–780.

167. Rodríguez R. Hand motor patterns after the correction of left-nondominant-hand mirror writing. Neuropsychologia 1991;29:1191–1203.
168. Sgaramella T, Ellis A, Semenza C. Analysis of the spontaneous writing errors of normal and aphasic writers. Cortex 1991;27:29–39.
169. Paradis M, Hagiwara H, Hildebrandt N. Neurolinguistic aspects of the Japanese writing system. New York: Academic Press, 1985.

12

Language, Communication, and the Right Hemisphere

Hiram Brownell,[1,2,3] **Howard Gardner,**[4] **Penny Prather,**[2,3,5] **and Gail Martino**[1]

[1]*Boston College, Chestnut Hill, Massachusetts*
[2]*Department of Veterans Affairs Medical Center, Boston, Massachusetts*
[3]*Boston University School of Medicine, Boston, Massachusetts*
[4]*Harvard Graduate School of Education, Cambridge, Massachusetts*
[5]*Brandeis University, Waltham, Massachusetts*

INTRODUCTION

This chapter seeks to correct an imbalance in the traditional view of language deficits associated with brain damage. Beginning with the seminal work of Paul Broca and Carl Wernicke in the nineteenth century, acquired language deficits resulting from brain injury have been associated with damage to the left cerebral hemisphere (1). During the following 130 years, the field of aphasiology has seen shifts of opinion regarding the precision with which linguistic function can be localized within the left hemisphere—e.g., ranging from Head (2) to Geschwind (3)—and concern with different levels of analysis from phonology and single-word meaning to sentences and connected text (4-7); however, one constant in the field has been the prevailing view that the left hemisphere mediates language in the vast majority of right-handed adults. This belief and the supporting literature on language deficits, which is reviewed in other chapters in this volume, represent critically important but incomplete information about the broader issue of communication, a topic that includes language and also paralinguistic and inferential components. The present chapter describes how communication ability requires the contribution of the right as well as left hemisphere and how right-sided injury limits patients' competence in this realm. This "right-hemisphere" research tradition, which has a shorter history dating back only a few decades (8-10), does not contradict earlier findings documenting the dominant role of the left hemisphere; rather, it complements those reports. The emerging consensus is that effective communication is the product of both hemispheres and can be impaired, in different ways, by injury to either hemisphere.

Patients with unilateral right-sided damage, even considerable damage, are typically not aphasic in the usual sense of the term. They retain a normal or nearly normal ability to form words that are phonologically correct, to name objects, and to unravel the syntax of complex sentences (e.g., "If the lion was killed by the tiger, which one was dead?"). At least at a superficial level, their linguistic performance seems unremarkable. Except in cases of gross attentional problems that impose a nonselective decrement on all performances, right-hemisphere-damaged (RHD) patients usually score well on tests of aphasia.

The absence of aphasia is not, by itself, a guarantor for successful communication. A moment's reflection shows that most communication requires much more than a sense of phonology, word definitions, or grammatical rules, as reflected in the following tasks required by a listener trying to understand what a speaker is saying. To understand completely and accurately a speaker's ironic comment, the point of a story, or the intended meaning of nonliteral language such as metaphor, the listener must go beyond exactly what is said. To apprehend a speaker's intended message, the listener must take note of the tone of voice and the context in which an utterance is produced; that is, the listener must evaluate what has transpired previously and determine how that has affected the mood of the speaker. In addition, he or she must apply the conventions governing polite conversation and the structure of narrative units such as stories and jokes. To extract the larger truth from one or several sentences, the listener must infer just how individual sentences fit together to form a larger whole. The point at which RHD patients have trouble is when communicating requires doing more than decoding the literal, denotative meaning of words and sentences and requires understanding the intended meaning of an utterance spoken in a certain way and in a specific social context. This extra level of understanding presents the most difficulty for these patients and imposes limits on a patient's effective interaction in natural settings.

This chapter starts with a composite description of patients who display what is sometimes referred to as the *right-hemisphere syndrome*. After a brief discussion of some methodological considerations relevant to studies of right-hemisphere dysfunction, the body of the review focuses on the effects of right-hemisphere brain injury on communication ability. The review outlines representative findings for those aspects of language (prosody, lexical semantics including metaphor and idioms, and narrative and conversational discourse) most often affected by right-sided injury: the goal is to illustrate the communication problems themselves and how they have been investigated and not to review exhaustively the literature on these aspects of language use, a task that has been undertaken by Joanette, Goulet, and Hannaquin (11) and others (12–15). The final section of the chapter considers general deficits that cut across cognitive domains (e.g., attention, integration ability) and that offer the promise of unifying accounts of many of the lexical and discourse deficits associated with RHD.

THE RIGHT-HEMISPHERE SYNDROME

Meeting a RHD patient during the acute stages of his or her illness, one often encounters an unkempt person who is likely to have poorly combed hair and to have dressed without much attention to detail. The patient will likely exhibit a combination of motoric, visuospatial, attentional, and affective problems. However, the expressed attitude toward these symptoms (and toward personal appearance) can seem apathetic, at times to the point of being anosognosic about even obvious physical symptoms such as hemiplegia, which might be explained as a limb being too tired to move or even belonging to someone other than the patient (16,17). Many of these symptoms are attenuated over time, rendering other deficits much more significant.

RHD patients' communication abnormalities persist in the chronic stages of their illness and recovery. Although not always immediately noticeable, these deficits become more apparent in extended conversation and when the scope of an "assessment" extends beyond the nuts and bolts of language and into the realm of natural communication. While talking to some RHD patients, one can detect a flat, robot-like voice quality due to a reduction in speech prosody. More often, one notices the patient's difficulty sticking to a topic; conversations change course abruptly and without warning; individual comments and activities often seem tangential to the topic at hand and at times frankly inappropriate.

Consider the following examples. A middle-aged male patient might interrupt formal testing to ask the female examiner about her romantic activities during the previous weekend. Or a patient might look up from a stimulus card (again during formal testing) to remark on something happening outside viewed through a window, or get up from the testing table to start making a snack. The same stimulus item might provide the basis for a rambling monolog based on some personal experience of the patient. A patient's sense of humor may also be changed in a variety of ways. After suffering RHD, patients may exhibit crudeness and simplicity in their attempts at humor. Comments that might be humorous in the context of a W. C. Fields film are produced at inappropriate times (e.g., referring to a spouse as "the old sow" in her presence).

RHD patients are often quite literal. In terms of comprehension, they can show superficially intact understanding of single sentences but still miss the thrust of an entire conversation. They often focus on a superficial, sometimes inappropriate level of interpretation for proverbs, idioms and metaphoric expressions, and many other types of sentences without full consideration of context that would support another interpretation. When asked by a physician during an exam, "How long have you been in here?," a patient might interpret the question as applying to the very immediate physical context and respond "about five minutes" rather than as referring to the intended more general frame of reference of how long the patient has been in the hospital. When presented with the sarcastic utterance "I am so glad that you have the television turned up so loud," a patient may miss the speaker's intended meaning and respond to the literal level of interpretation by saying "Good" rather than turn down the volume.

Left-hemisphere-damaged (LHD) aphasic patients offer a marked contrast. By definition, aphasic patients display obvious language problems with the mechanics of producing and understanding single words and sentences; however, they are very often very aware of their deficits and consciously try to compensate for them. (Exceptions can include severely impaired Wernicke's-type aphasic patients in the acute stage of their illness, who can appear oblivious to their deficits and almost euphoric.) As a rule, aphasic patients are far more likely than RHD patients to use context and other, nonlinguistic and paralinguistic channels (speech prosody, facial expression, prior context) to figure out at least the gist of what is being said. As a result, these patients may grasp an entire message without fully understanding any one sentence.

A major caveat that applies to the preceding syndrome description, and also to the results of the studies reviewed below, is that the characterizations apply to an abstract prototypical patient. A particular patient may not exhibit the full constellation of deficits and may even not exhibit any. Some patients will exhibit obvious impairments, while others show only subtle effects that require several carefully constructed stimulus items for detection. Some deficits are more appropriately viewed as abnormal tendencies: some RHD patients may retain the ability to process a certain kind of information but simply fail to do so as thoroughly as would most non-brain-damaged adults. The purpose of this review is not to list symptoms that will be present in all or even most patients with RHD; rather, the goal is to list the deficits that have been noted in significant numbers of RHD patients and that—singly or in combination—limit the prognoses of many patients.

METHODOLOGY

Some methodological characteristics of this literature should be noted. The first feature is the often imprecise description of lesion size and site. Most studies limit the subject populations to patients who have suffered unilateral damage due to stroke, and the model patient description specifies only unilateral damage in the distribution of the middle cerebral artery. Thus, relatively few patients used in studies have lesions restricted, for example, to the prefrontal lobes. Only occasionally are results reported separately for large groups of RHD patients subdivided into "frontal" (damage predominantly anterior to the Rolandic fissure) and "posterior" (damage predominantly temporal and/or parietal) categories. Less often described are the size and subcortical extent of damage.

One source for the lack of concern for localization within the right hemisphere is the generally held belief that the right hemisphere is less focally organized than the left (18). More precise lesion description would therefore contribute little. Intrahemisphere lesion localization may well be less critical for many of the cognitive and communicative functions discussed below. Some studies of communication ability have subdivided small samples of patients into anterior and posterior groups and have failed to note significant differences (19,20). However, until studies are designed specifically to assess the localization of the components of communication, it is premature to accept this null result of equipotentiality, especially since other functions such as prosody and attention to the left side of space have been consistently associated with specific regions (21,22).

A second consideration involves the demographic characteristics of subjects tested in typical studies and the nature of the research on communication. For historical reasons, a disproportionately large number of subjects in the studies have been male war veterans. Researchers and clinicians working with RHD patients should realize that the descriptions offered in past studies may need modification before being applied to specific subgroups or types of patients. For example, a tendency toward garrulously inappropriate comments may manifest differently in a female versus a male stroke patient. Understanding communication abnormalities involving the use of sarcasm or other conventions governing polite discourse will require consideration of educational and employment history as well as gender (23).

PROSODY

Shakespeare once wrote "I understand a fury in your words but not the words" (*Othello*, Act IV, Scene ii). This quote, as cited by Knapp and Hall (24), nicely captures the role of prosody in speech. By attending to an utterance's prosodic contour, which is characterized by variations in pitch (frequency), loudness (amplitude), time (duration), voice quality (timbre), and rhythm, a listener can extract considerable information about a speaker's communicative intention. Often, the "meaning" conveyed via prosody is affective in nature, indicating, for example, happiness, sadness, or anger. Used in this way, prosody is basic to communication and can often be understood by the listener even when speech itself is unintelligible or pronounced in a foreign language or in an unfamiliar cultural context (25,26).

In addition to affect, prosody is used to carry linguistic or pragmatic information that allows a listener to discriminate among questions, statements, and exclamations, or to perceive emphatic stress within sentences (e.g., to identify the most important new information in an utterance: "The BOY went to the store" versus "The boy went to the STORE"). Prosodic variation also carries lexical distinctions, e.g., "EN-trance" (an entry) versus "en-TRANCE" (to spellbind).

Monrad-Krohn (27) was among the first to characterize various types of prosodic disturbance. *Dysprosody* is a distortion of normal speech prosody, which can, for example, leave a patient speaking with what sounds like a foreign accent. In one such case, a Norwegian woman during World War II suffered left frontal damage, then developed what was perceived as a German accent and, as a result, was accused of being a Nazi (28). *Hyperprosody* is marked by an excessive or highly variable use of speech intonation.

More recent evidence suggests RHD can lead to either a decrease or an increase in intonational variation, the latter of which is called hypermelodicity or hyperprosody. This disorder is not readily apparent on listening to a patient but has been reliably documented using computer-based acoustic analysis (29,30). In a study by Colsher, Cooper, and Graff-Radford (29), patients with lesions affecting areas such as the Rolandic cortices, Brodmann's area 6, and the superior temporal gyrus in the right hemisphere were required to repeat semantically neutral sentences (e.g., "the bird flew away") with either a specific emotional (happy, sad, or angry) or linguistic (statement or question) prosody. Subjects' responses were recorded and subjected to acoustic analysis. The extremes in pitch (i.e., the peaks and valleys of fundamental voice frequency or F_0[31]) reflected an increased F_0 variability in RHD patients relative to controls.

The most common prosodic disturbance is termed *aprosody* or *aprosodia*, which is the absence of variation in tone or accent and is characterized by speech devoid of color, tone, or affect or the failure to make distinctions on this basis in comprehension. Although these impairments are often observed subsequent to right-hemisphere lesions due to stroke, production aprosodia is also a typical symptom of Parkinson's disease and schizophrenia (32). Following the practice in the neuropsychological literature, we will use the terms *affective* and *linguistic* prosody to reflect the kind of "meaning" conveyed, even though there are not clear acoustic differences between the two types.

Aprosodia for Affective Material

Patients suffering from affective aprosodia are unable to impart emotion to their speech, creating the impression that the patient suffers from a mood disorder. One contribution of research over the past decade has been to show that, despite outward appearances, affective aprosodia is separate from the mood disorders sometimes seen in RHD patients (33-36).

Affective aprosodia is a general label that includes different and separable components. Ross and Mesulam (35) have reported patients for whom prosodic production was impaired without obvious comprehension deficits. For example, following a lesion in the superficial right frontoparietal region (without significant subcortical extension), one patient, a schoolteacher, reported a marked inability to use variation in tone of voice to control the behavior of her students. Although she was unable to express emotion through speech prosody, this patient reported that she could still "feel" her emotions and that she was also able to perceive emotional prosody in others' speech. The production deficit extended beyond just language: she also reported feeling appropriately sad at her father's funeral, but at the same time she was unable to cry without effort. Eventually, this patient developed a compensatory strategy of adding explicitly worded mood indicators — "I am angry and mean it" (p. 144). Building on this and many other cases, Ross developed a taxonomy of affective aprosodias that could be demonstrated on bedside exam and that corresponded to classical teaching for aphasias associated with left-hemisphere lesions (34). Included in his set of eight types of aprosodias, Ross proposed a *motor aprosodia*, which was associated with right frontal damage and was analogous to motor or expressive aphasia associated with damage to Broca's area in the left hemisphere, and a *sensory aprosodia*, which was associated with right posterior damage and was analogous to sensory aphasia associated with damage to Wernicke's area in the left hemisphere.

Many other authors have confirmed the existence of prosodic abnormalities in both production and comprehension; however, the lesion localization for these and other symptoms defining Ross' taxonomy and the clear separation between production and comprehension deficits have not been treated consistently in the literature. In one recent study, for example, Cancelliere and Kertesz (21) tested prosodic expression, repetition, and identification (i.e., labeling stimuli as happy, sad, angry, or neutral), and also visual identification of emotional faces and emotional situations, in groups of LHD and RHD patients and control subjects. In general, aprosodias of different types were associated most often with lesions in the basal ganglia of either the left or right hemisphere and in the anterior temporal lobe and insula.

Impaired comprehension of emotional facial expressions and situations were also linked with destruction in the basal ganglia and the anterior temporal lobe. Finally, it is worth noting that the importance of the basal ganglia is consistent with evidence from patients with Parkinson's disease who exhibit aprosodia (37).

In many other studies of prosodic disturbances, mixed groups of RHD patients were tested such that both anterior and posterior lesions were represented. In one elegant study, Heilman, Bowers, Speedie, and Coslett (38) used filtered speech to separate prosodic from propositional dimensions of linguistic stimuli. For one condition, sentences produced by a male speaker to reflect happy, angry, or sad emotions were passed through acoustic filters that effectively made the words themselves unintelligible, thereby leaving only the prosodic contour as a cue. (In another condition testing comprehension of linguistic prosody, sentences were spoken as questions, statements, or exclamations and similarly filtered.) Subjects—including nonneurological controls and heterogeneous groups of RHD and LHD, aphasic patients—then listened to the intonation patterns and responded by picking the appropriate interpretation from an array. This task showed a clear comprehension deficit relative to the control subjects for the RHD group.

Aprosodia for Linguistic Material

Relatively fewer studies have assessed the right hemisphere's role in processing linguistic prosody. One of the first to do so was carried out by Weintraub, Mesulam, and Kramer (39), who used a variety of tasks including sentence–picture matching to assess discrimination of word stress. Subjects heard a stimulus such as "BLUEjay" and had to choose among pictures that included one of the familiar bird and another of the letter of the alphabet printed in blue ink. Also tested were same–different discrimination of emphatic stress ("STEVE drives the car" versus "Steve drives the CAR") and sentence contour (rising intonation indicating a question versus falling intonation indicating a statement), repetition of sentence prosody (question versus statement), and production. Relative to a non-brain-damaged control group, RHD patients showed significant impairments on all tasks. This general pattern of results has been replicated for Swedish-speaking stroke patients and Parkinson's patients (40,41), but there have also been some discrepancies in the assessment of production of linguistic prosody. Emmorey (42), for example, found significant disturbances in prosody production and comprehension for LHD, aphasic patients but not for RHD patients.

The variety of prosodic disturbances observed in RHD patients raises several questions about the underlying nature of the impairment(s). One issue is the link between these patients' affective abnormality and their prosodic disturbances. RHD patients often exhibit affective abnormalities (43); it is therefore tempting to attribute their prosodic disturbances—at least in part— to their affective disorder. If patients have trouble understanding or responding to emotions, then they will have trouble processing that content regardless of the mode of transmission (facial expression, speech prosody, or propositional speech). Affective deficit may increase or exacerbate RHD patients' prosodic disorders, but, as alluded to above, there is abundant evidence for a prosodic disorder that exists apart from the emotional realm. For example, the study by Heilman et al. (38) provided tests of both affective and linguistic prosody comprehension by groups of RHD and LHD patients. Relative to control subjects, RHD patients showed impaired comprehension of emotional prosody, while both RHD and LHD patients showed impaired comprehension of linguistic prosody. Thus, RHD patients' poor performance may be more notable with affective material due to the additional problem with affective content, but there still exists an impairment for linguistic material as well.

Similarly, not yet clear is the extent to which RHD patients' prosodic deficits can be accounted for at the level of acoustic sensation or perception rather than that of emotional or linguistic interpretation. An issue that applies mostly directly to the comprehension of both affective and linguistic prosody is the extent to which an underlying perceptual deficit precludes normal interpretation of prosodic contours. RHD patients' ability simply to discriminate emotional prosody is disturbed (44,45). Tucker, Watson, and Heilman (44), for example, have shown that when asked to judge whether two sentences were said with the same or different emotional tone, RHD patients showed significant impairment relative to an aphasic control group. If patients cannot even discriminate distinctions in perceptual tasks, the communicative function of that information will be lost.

LEXICAL IMPAIRMENTS INCLUDING METAPHOR AND IDIOMS

One compelling characteristic of RHD patients' language use is their tendency to be literal or concrete in the sense of being drawn to only one of two or more possible interpretations of a picture, word, phrase, proverb, or fable. This tendency, which has been documented repeatedly using a variety of stimulus types, highlights how a language-based abnormality can exist alongside the largely intact linguistic abilities of this patient population. One early demonstration of the limited range of possible interpretations was reported by Gardner and Denes (46). These authors asked subjects to match nonrepresentational line drawings (e.g., an *up* or a *down* arrow) with linguistic concepts such as "wealth" or "poverty" for which non-brain-damaged control subjects showed good agreement (at least 80%). As expected, LHD, aphasic patients performed worse on this task than control subjects. More interesting, though, was the reaction of the RHD patients tested: either they objected to the entire task as if they had not grasped the possibility of interpreting words in terms of other kinds of symbols or they performed roughly at the level of the LHD patients.

RHD patients' pervasive literalness similarly affects their interpretation of highly familiar idiomatic and metaphoric phrases with fixed meanings (e.g., "turning over a new leaf," "he has a heavy heart"). The rationale for treating highly familiar, conventionalized metaphoric phrases and idioms as lexical entities is that, for most speakers, such phrases are so overlearned that they are understood as unanalyzed wholes rather than as novel strings of words (47). The most common paradigm used to examine this form of non-literal language comprehension is sentence–picture matching in which subjects are asked to read or listen to a phrase, e.g., "he has a heavy heart," and to select an appropriate pictorial representation from a set of alternatives (48–50). In the study by Winner and Gardner (50), for example, the pictorial alternatives for the phrase "he has a heavy heart" included a correct metaphorical interpretation (a man crying), a literal, pragmatically odd interpretation (a man carrying an oversized heart), a depiction of the adjective used in the stimulus phrase (a barbell with lots of weight to represent "heavy"), and a depiction of the noun used in the stimulus phrase (a heart). As expected, a non-brain-damaged controls had no trouble choosing the correct metaphorical interpretation. The RHD patients, on the other hand, were often drawn to the literal interpretations (a man carrying an oversized heart); indeed, they chose the literal alternative almost as often as the correct, metaphorical alternative. What makes this result for the RHD patients particularly striking is that the effect of brain damage was to bias them *away* from the more common or familiar form of the phrase considered as a whole and toward a novel interpretation. Because of the relatively simple nature of the linguistic stimuli, LHD, aphasic patients were also tested and scored slightly better overall than the RHD patients, and were almost never drawn to the literal alternatives. Thus, despite their frank aphasia, the LHD patients performed more normally on this language-comprehension task in some respects than did the (nonaphasic) RHD patients.

Winner and Gardner (50) offered an additional observation about the RHD patients' performances. Although the RHD patients were, in a sense, captured by the literal alternatives in the picture-selection portion of the task, they responded better when asked to generate oral interpretations of metaphors in that, with some prodding, they were able to explain the metaphorical meaning. This comment suggests that with sufficient task structure provided by an examiner, RHD patients are capable of processing metaphorical meaning, although this level of meaning is not the level that occurs to them spontaneously.

Because RHD patients often have visuospatial problems and may have particular difficulty comparing linguistic and pictorial content, later studies of metaphor comprehension avoided pictorial stimuli and used exclusively lexical materials. Brownell, Potter, Michelow, and Gardner (51), for example, asked groups of RHD, LHD, and non-brain-damaged control subjects to judge relatedness among the following set of dimensional adjectives: "warm," "cold," "deep," "shallow," "loving," "hateful," "wise," and "foolish." In this task, a subject was given sets of three words (e.g., "warm"–"loving"–"cold") and asked to select the two that were most closely associated. The task forced subjects to choose among several alternative semantic dimensions as a basis for responding. Subjects might, for example, choose to group words on the basis of antonymic association (warm–cold), or they might group them preferentially on the basis of a metaphorical equivalence (e.g., warm–loving). There are other semantic dimensions contained within this set of words, but the antonymic and metaphorical dimensions are the most relevant. In this study, the control subjects used both the antonymic and metaphorical dimensions as bases for responding. The LHD aphasic patients relied mostly on metaphorical equivalence and showed less-than-normal use of the antonymic dimension. In contrast, the RHD patients relied mostly on antonymic links and showed less-than-normal use of metaphorical equivalence. Again, in this and other linguistic tasks (52), RHD patients showed a clear dissociation in which aspects of meaning they were most attuned to, that is, a decreased sensitivity to metaphorical meaning relative to control subjects and to LHD, aphasic patients.

When interpreting the excessive literalness of RHD patients, one should note that the tasks used to study metaphor interpretation all require deliberate semantic judgments by subjects; that is, a subject is asked to reflect consciously on the meanings of words or phrases, and, implicitly, to generate his or her own task strategy. These deliberative tasks do not reveal the precise nature of the impairment—whether the problem is really one of deliberation or one restricted to metaphoric extension of meaning. The Winner and Gardner (50) anecdote concerning the abilities of RHD patients to explain nonliteral meaning suggests a decrease in self-directed access to nonliteral knowledge rather than a total loss.

An alternative paradigm illustrates how task requirements can be altered to rely less on self-generated deliberative processing and more on unconscious processing. Tompkins (53) has used a lexical-decision task in which a subject sees a string of letters on each trial and decides as quickly as possible whether the string is an English word. The task itself does not require that the subject make any overt judgment about word meaning. On some trials, the target letter string is preceded by a "prime" word that may be related to the target. The usual result (for non-brain-damaged control subjects) is that a semantically related prime word facilitates a subject's lexical decision for the following target string. For example, the prime "bread" makes it possible for subjects to decide more quickly that "butter" is a word (54). When the proportion of trials containing a related prime is low overall, subjects do not consciously use primes to predict targets. Also, when a prime word is followed very quickly by a target, the subject has too little time to predict actively what exactly will appear as a target string.

Using this basic design, Tompkins (53) tested RHD patients' appreciation of metaphorical meaning when they were not explicitly required to reflect on that meaning. She used primes such as "loving" designed to facilitate access to the metaphorical meaning of letter strings (words) such as "warm." The general result was that RHD patients showed normal priming effects in this "automatic" processing condition, which suggests that, at least in some conditions, these patients' access to metaphorical meaning is intact. Also, in a different condition in the same study, RHD patients showed an impaired ability to apply response strategies in a deliberate, conscious manner. Preliminary results reported by Brownell and Molloy (55) corroborate the intact processing of metaphorical meaning by RHD patients. In the Brownell and Molloy priming task, RHD patients (as well as controls) showed facilitation when ambiguous, potentially metaphorical primes ("warm") preceded targets ("loving") that were related to the metaphorical meaning of the prime. Finally, Tompkins and her colleagues (56) extended the scope of preserved nonliteral comprehension to the automatic processing of idiomatic phrases.

In conclusion, several studies have demonstrated a clear deficit at the level of single words and familiar phrases that reflects specifically the effects of right-sided brain injury. The effect does not seem to reflect a loss of knowledge (since RHD patients can, under some conditions, process metaphorical and idiomatic meaning), but rather a limitation in processing: when patients are required to explore and choose on the basis of their own deliberations, they are more likely to show impaired understanding.

The processing deficit in metaphor/idiom interpretation can be viewed as an example of excessive literalness or as just one example of a broader inability to appreciate *any* different, alternative meanings for stimuli, including other ambiguous items such as homonyms (e.g., "cabinet") and indirect requests ("Can you tell me the time?") that can be interpreted literally or figuratively (52,57). As suggested by Chiarello (58), this more general characterization links the abnormalities on metaphor and idiom processing to others documented using words, phrases, and sentences with alternative interpretations, even if both of them are literal. (Representative studies will be discussed below.) The existence of a general problem apprehending the alternative meanings of linguistic elements is secure. Beyond this general impairment, though, there may still exist a separate impairment specific to metaphorical stimuli (52).

NARRATIVE-DISCOURSE-PROCESSING

Most communication is accomplished through the production and comprehension of sets of sentences that make up conversations, stories, or jokes. This suprasentential level of analysis treats individual utterances as pieces of a discourse that derive their meaning by virtue of their relation to the other utterances. Extracting what is often termed the "macrostructure" or main theme(s) of a discourse requires inferences that are based on the sentences themselves and also on prior context and world knowledge (59). Because of the ubiquity of discourse in human interaction, dysfunction at this level severely limits the social success of RHD patients. We discuss first *narrative* discourse (e.g., stories, instructions, coherent descriptions) and then *conversational* discourse.

The prime characteristic of coherent text is that a theme is maintained throughout such that the individual sentences fit together. In narrative comprehension, the task for the listener is to extract that main idea, gist, or macrostructure. Once the theme has been identified, a listener can then use it to evaluate subsequent utterances, which, by virtue of their common membership in a single discourse, ought to interrelate. The most salient feature of RHD patients' narrative performance is that they fail to perform all of the necessary inferences to understand how sentences all fit together. Without this conceptual anchor, their understanding falls prey to tangential associations and misinterpretation.

A series of studies by Hough and her colleagues (20,60) has examined LHD and RHD patients' use of main themes in narrative comprehension. One manipulation was whether a main theme for a paragraph-long story, e.g., receiving flowers from a fiance on Valentine's Day, was presented at the beginning or at the end of the story. After listening to the story, subjects answered comprehension questions and selected an appropriate main theme. Control subjects and also LHD, aphasic patients showed little effect of the manipulation of theme placement, suggesting that their inferential capacities were not overtaxed by the task. However, RHD patients performed significantly worse when presentation of the theme was delayed until near the end of the paragraph. One interpretation is that the RHD patients were impaired at providing their own thematic organization for even these brief stories. When left to their own devices, they were unable to extract a commonality from the disparate parts, and they were unable to use the theme to review the story and to put the component sentences together retrospectively. Similar dysfunction has been illustrated using other paradigms. Schneiderman, Murasugi, and Saddy (61) and Delis, Wapner, Gardner, and Moses (62) tested subjects' ability to rearrange jumbled sentences to form a coherent text. Beeman (63) examined how quickly subjects decided whether a string of letters formed an English word when the word was related to an inference that should have been made during comprehension. In all these studies, RHD patients exhibited difficulty performing the integration of information necessary for narrative comprehension.

Narrative productions of RHD patients reflect what appears to be the same basic deficit. In one recent study Myers and Brookshire (64) asked RHD patients to explain illustrations by Norman Rockwell. One painting used by these authors was that of a waiting room in a doctor's office or hospital in which two men (one with a bandaged head) and a boy are seated. In their narrations, the RHD patients often failed to mention the waiting room, the central feature of the painting. Myers and Brookshire refer to this deficit as a decrease in the informative content. The omission of a main theme in picture explanation is consistent with the Hough (20) comprehension results and also with other studies of narrative production in which patients were asked to narrate pictorially presented stories (65,66). Perhaps as a result of missing a main theme, RHD patients' narrations tend to be less selective than those of control subjects in that the patients mention a higher proportion of unimportant detail: they possess no overarching organization to determine which information is central to a story and which is peripheral. In addition to problems inferring what an organizing theme might be, RHD patients respond to their confusion in peculiar ways, i.e., by confabulating and by embellishing their narratives. Wapner et al. (66) and Myers (67) report that, in addition to an excessive attention to unimportant details, RHD patients mention stray elements and then make up some account to justify their inclusion in the story. These confabulations often make sense when viewed in isolation but do not fit with the central theme of the story at hand.

While previously cited studies have shown that RHD patients fail to extract a sense of gist, other work has addressed their problems using and revising a theme once they have it. One study examined patients' abilities to revise their understanding as a simple "story" unfolded. Brownell, Potter, Bihrle, and Gardner (68) presented subjects with two-sentence stimulus stories constructed to require a *revision* of an initial interpretation. From the initial sentence "Sally brought a pen and pencil with her to meet the movie star," most listeners infer that Sally is an autograph hound intent on collecting a new signature for her collection. This is a common, reasonable association to make based on knowledge of the world. In this study, the initial inference (based on a single sentence) was designed to be obvious and easy for subjects to make, and both control subjects and RHD patients were apparently able to make this initial inference. However, as often happens in natural conversation or stories, the next sentence ("The article would include famous people's opinions on nuclear power") did not fit with the established interpretation. To make the second and first sentence fit together under a single interpretation, listeners needed to revise their original model of the discourse to determine that Sally is more likely a journalist than an autograph collector: what used to be the main thrust of the story turns out to be tangential in the final analysis. As indicated by their performance on a series of true–false questions presented after each stimulus story, control subjects had no trouble performing the needed repair of their sense of gist, but RHD patients often got stuck on their first inference and failed to revise their initial interpretation. This failure to reinterpret provides one model for how a patient might develop a misguided understanding of a story. Whenever the surface flow of the narrative takes a detour due to the speaker's departure from standard narrative form, the RHD patient will be less able to infer or, in some cases, return to the main theme. A similar argument has been used to account for RHD patients' deficits in understanding jokes, in which the humor rests on the listener's revising his or her interpretation of how the punchline relates to the situation established in the body of the joke. (See Ref. 69 for a review and Ref. 63 for a more recent analysis of RHD patients' inference impairments.)

CONVERSATIONAL-DISCOURSE PROCESSING

Closely related to narrative deficits are the problems RHD patients exhibit understanding utterances, in conversations. Rehak, Kaplan, and Gardner (70) examined subjects' appreciation of the conventions governing cooperative discourse as outlined by Grice (71). For example, Grice's convention of *relevance* specifies that, all else being equal, an utterance in a conversation should maintain the topic being discussed. Rehak et al. (70) tested how subjects responded to a tangential comment that abruptly shifted the topic under discussion in a conversation. Relative to control subjects, RHD patients more often judged conversations containing a tangential insertion as normal, and they more often judged a tangential insert as a speaker's attempt to continue talking about the same topic. Control subjects typically interpreted the insertion as reflecting a speaker's attempt to change the topic. In sum, the patients failed to appreciate fully the coherence linking utterances in a conversation.

Discourse comprehension requires listeners to use a variety of contextual information to identify sarcasm, a form of nonliteral language canonically used to convey displeasure (72). Sarcastic utterances are often indicated by, for example, a characteristic tone of voice; thus, any receptive prosodic impairment exhibited by RHD patients will affect sarcasm comprehension. In addition, though, some studies have tried to eliminate speech prosody as an obvious cue and to examine the roles of other kinds of information relevant to conversations.

A recent study by Brownell, Carroll, Rehak, and Wingfield (73) tested subjects' use of three different kinds of information: the mood of a speaker, the plausibility of a response to a question, and the presence of a pronoun that links an utterance to the ongoing conversation by referring to a character mentioned previously. According to the analysis put forth above, as overlearned, rule-governed linguistic markers, pronouns are relatively easy for RHD patients to use. On the other hand, speaker mood and plausibility require attention to the overall context and, accordingly, will be harder for RHD patients. The following sample stimulus illustrates how these factors were manipulated in the study:

> Mrs. Moran is upset with her husband. He spilled grape juice on the living-room rug while giving a piggyback ride to their daughter Nancy. As he cleans up, Mr. Moran asks his wife, "Where did Nancy go?" Mrs. Moran replies . . .

A vignette could end with any of four types of utterances, which was always presented (via audiotape) to subjects in a neutral tone of voice that did not suggest sarcasm or jest. One type of concluding utterance ("She went to the kitchen to get some more grape juice") was a very straightforward answer to the preceding question, and it contained a pronoun that linked the utterance to the preceding question.

A second utterance ("There's more grape juice in the kitchen") was also a straightforward answer to the question but did not contain a linking pronoun. Here subjects had to perform more of an inference to ascertain the coherence of the response with the preceding conversation.

A third utterance ("She's buying a new carpet") contained a pronoun linking the response to the preceding question, but the content was simply not plausible: daughters young enough to play piggyback with their fathers do not visit carpet sales without their parents. This reply, produced by an angry respondent, reflects a violation of the expectations of normal polite discourse and thereby invites some nonstandard interpretation such as sarcasm.

The final utterance type ("There's a sale in the carpet store") also indicated an implausible activity for a young daughter, and there was no pronoun used to link it to the preceding conversation. There was, then, little basis for thinking this was an answer to the question asked by Mr. Moran.

After hearing a vignette, subjects were asked to choose one of the following four interpretations of the respondant's utterance at the end of the vignette:

What Mrs. Moran said was

(a) not a sensible answer to the question
(b) an attempt to answer the question as asked
(c) joking or in fun
(d) sarcastic and nasty

Results for the two affectively charged alternatives, (c) and (d), revealed that RHD patients showed *less than normal* use of mood information. For example, when the respondent was angry, RHD patients were less likely than controls to choose the sarcasm interpretation, and when the respondent was happy, the RHD patients were less likely than controls to choose the joking interpretation. These effects show that RHD patients underutilize context in the form of mood information, even when that information is explicit. In contrast, RHD patients showed *greater than normal* effects due to the presence/absence of pronouns: when a response contained a pronoun linking it to the person under discussion, RHD patients were often *more* likely than controls to think the response was an attempt to answer the question as asked, and *less* likely than controls to think the response was uninterpretable. This result highlights that RHD patients have preserved use of some discourse features, i.e., those that require application of overlearned rules of language structure, and at the same time reduced use of others. As a result, their perception of sarcasm and other forms of literal and nonliteral language rests on an abnormal use of the contextual cues that all listeners use in conversation. It follows that RHD patients' evaluation of the emotional tone and intent of an exchange will at times be inaccurate.

A different form of dysfunction reflects alteration in patients' use of social conventions and can be illustrated by requiring subjects to choose an appropriate degree of formality when referring to someone in conversation (74,75). The major question asked in this study was how well a speaker in a conversation takes into account a listener's knowledge. A speaker's sensitivity to a listener's knowledge has recently become a major topic in the developmental literature under the rubric of "theory of mind," i.e., the understanding of other people's knowledge and beliefs (76). To illustrate, imagine a conversation between two people meeting for the first time in the office where they work. If neither the speaker nor the listener is well-acquainted with a third person named Oliver Harding who is not present, then a formal "Mr. Harding" is often considered the appropriate term of reference. When the speaker is a personal friend of the referent but the listener is not, using the more formal "Mr. Harding" is still canonically considered more polite than using just the first name: the more formal reference avoids "name-dropping" by the speaker as a form of boasting. Only when both a speaker and a listener are personal friends of the referent is the informal use of just the first name "Oliver" appropriate. This example illustrates how a term of reference reflects norms of politeness and also a speaker's appreciation of what his or her listener knows. Brownell et al. (74) asked subjects to listen to a conversation and to select an informal or formal label for a third person, who was not present, as part of a concluding utterance. A sample stimulus follows:

> You have just met Fran Hill, who, like you, is about to start working as a reservations clerk for American Airlines. You are describing your hopes about the job, when she says to you: "I heard that the other clerk who works in the reservations office is getting a big prize for having broken the reservations record this month." It comes out in conversation that you are good friends with Oliver Harding, the other clerk she is referring to, but that she has never met him.
> Which of the following would you choose to respond to Fran Hill?
> (a) "Well, Oliver must be a really hard worker."
> (b) "Well, Mr. Harding must be a really hard worker."

In different vignettes, the speaker ("you" in the vignette) knew the referent very well or not at all, and the listener knew the referent very well or not at all. As expected, based on conventional rules of polite reference, the control subjects generally preferred formal terms *except* when *both* the speaker and listener knew the referent well. RHD patients did not consistently show this sophisticated use of speaker and listener knowledge together. They at times responded on the basis of how well the speaker knew the referent or how well the listener knew the reference, but they were worse than the controls at restricting their use of informal responses to the one case in which both the speaker and listener knew the referent well. It remains to be seen the extent to which this deficit observed in the RHD patients' performances reflects a problem in reflecting on others' knowledge states (i.e., a problem in their theory of other minds), a reduced sense of politeness, or both. Although preliminary, this finding shows how nuances of conversational exchange may be lost to patients in subtle ways that make their social life less successful.

RELATIONS AMONG DEFICITS

No one underlying impairment provides a completely successful account for the range of problems discussed above, but several offer useful perspectives for different subsets of problems. One issue is what portion of a deficit is due to patients' inability to perceive basic information needed to support interpretation. For example, perception of prosodic information is often impaired in RHD patients, as is their ability to perceive complex visual displays including faces (77). If RHD patients cannot accurately perceive a sneer on a speaker's lips and cannot easily perceive a sarcastic sentence intonation, then they must rely more than non-brain-damaged listeners on attentional and inferential abilities, which are also at risk.

A pervasive affective disorder may limit patients' ability to interpret whatever prosodic information is accurately perceived. Abnormal reasoning about affective content may also reduce or skew patients' use of even explicitly stated mood information, which would affect social interaction (73,78). It is also worth considering the reverse: the extent to which poor communication could contribute to an affective impairment. Poor understanding of the nuances of conversation, whatever the cause of the impairment, would render a patient less able to understand fully many situations and less able to behave appropriately.

Other candidate accounts do not include the aprosodias but do address many other examples of deficit in lexical semantics and narrative. One suggestion by Chiarello (58) is that RHD patients exhibit different manifestations of a single underlying deficit in making deliberate use of alternative meanings of any ambiguous linguistic element and that one function of the intact right hemisphere is the maintenance of alternative readings for possible consideration during language understanding. This account incorporates under one umbrella deficits in nonliteral language understanding, homonyms (e.g., "cabinet"), and some inference deficits, and also has received support from laterality studies performed with neurologically intact control subjects. In the same vein, Beeman and colleagues (63,79) have outlined different, although complementary, roles for the right and left hemispheres in normal language comprehension. The right hemisphere contributes significantly to broadly focused, coarse-grained semantic analysis that is sensitive to overlapping and multiple meanings and to links between distantly related linguistic elements. The left hemisphere, in contrast, mediates the more narrowly focused, fine-grained analysis needed, for example, to identify the single most relevant meaning in a particular context.

The ability to attend to and integrate information is a fundamental aspect of cognition and communication. Attentional impairments are strongly associated with right-sided lesions (80,81) and have been proposed as an account for lexical and narrative-level communication impairments (82). The character of these accounts depends on how the construct of attention is considered. Attention can be viewed in terms of a general function, such as arousal or capacity, which is reduced in RHD patients (82). Similarly, measures of left neglect correlate with many different cognitive abilities. [See Myers (67) for a brief review.] One research goal is to determine just how many of the lexical and discourse impairments reviewed above can be explained in terms of a general decline of arousal associated with right-sided brain injury or with the severity of neglect as a marker.

Alternatively, one can subdivide the construct of attention into components such as vigilance, alerting, and orienting and then test for associations between an attentional component and specific communication deficits. Posner and Peterson (81), for example, favor a componential approach to attention and consider the evidence strongest for a link between RHD and a deficit in maintaining a state of alertness. Prather, Jarmulowicz, Brownell, and Gardner (83) reported that RHD patients can detect features in complex visual displays requiring many different components of attention, but show an impaired ability to conjoin or integrate visual features. One strategy for future work is to take further advantage of the theoretical precision available in the attention literature and to tie selective deficits in attention to specific components of language ability.

The notion of an integration deficit that Prather et al. (83) discussed in the context of a circumscribed visual attention task has been proposed more generally to account for RHD patients' performances on many disparate tasks. One compelling demonstration of the generality of this account was provided by Benowitz and his colleagues (84,85). These authors reported correlations between the visospatial and constructional deficits of RHD patients and their problems integrating linguistic information in, for example, narratives. The description fits: RHD patients focus on details, whether single sentences or parts of a geometric design, and they fail at combining the parts to form well-organized wholes, either complete stories or accurate block designs. Whether the dominant deficit is one of maintaining or directing attention or one of integrating the information gleaned from attending, successful explanations for communication impairments will certainly include a general cognitive basis.

CONCLUSIONS

RHD patients exhibit dysfunction in a variety of domains within cognition including affect, visuospatial processing, attention, and integration. These problems contribute to, and may well help explain, RHD patients' disrupted communication abilities. Nonetheless, in light of their relevance for daily life, deficits in communication deserve separate and special status in patient description and management. Although documenting the prevalence of RHD patients' communication problems and the pattern(s) of dissociation among them are tasks that remain for future investigations, one clear sign of success already achieved is the widespread acknowledgment that the intact right hemisphere plays a large role in mediating normal communication.

ACKNOWLEDGMENTS

Preparation of this chapter was supported by the Research Service of the Department of Veterans Affairs; NIH grants 2 R01 NS27894, AG 10496, and 5P01 DC00102; and Harvard Project Zero.

REFERENCES

1. Caplan D. Neurolinguistics and linguistic aphasiology. Cambridge: Cambridge University Press, 1987.
2. Head H. Aphasia and kindred disorders of speech. Cambridge: Cambridge University Press, 1926.
3. Geschwind N. Disconnexion syndromes in animals and man. Brain 1965;88: 237-294, 585-644.
4. Blumstein S. A phonological investigation of aphasic speech. The Hague: Mouton, 1973.
5. Goodglass H, Baker E. Semantic field naming and auditory comprehension in aphasia. Brain Lang 1976;3:359-374.
6. Grodzinsky Y. Theoretical perspectives on language deficits. Cambridge, MA: MIT Press, 1990.
7. Brookshire RH, Nicholas LE. Comprehension of directly and indirectly stated main ideas and details in discourse by brain-damaged and non-brain-damaged listeners. Brain Lang 1984;21:21-36.
8. Eisenson J. Language and intellectual modifications associated with right cerebral damage. Lang Speech 1962;5:49-53.
9. Gardner H. The shattered mind. New York: Alfred A Knopf, 1975.
10. Wechsler A. The effect of organic brain disease on recall of emotionally charged versus neutral texts. Neurology 1973;23:130-135.
11. Joanette Y, Goulet P, Hannequin D. Right hemisphere and verbal communication. New York: Springer-Verlag, 1990.
12. Brownell HH, Joanette Y, eds. Narrative discourse in neurologically impaired and normal aging adults. San Diego: Singular Publishing Group, 1993.
13. Code C. Language, aphasia, and the right hemisphere. Chichester: Wiley, 1987.
14. Joanette Y, Brownell HH, eds. Discourse ability and brain damage: theoretical and empirical perspectives. New York: Springer-Verlag, 1990.
15. Pimental PA, Kingsbury NA. Neuropsychological aspects of right brain injury. Austin, TX: PRO-ED, 1989.
16. Weinstein EA, Kahn RC. Denial of illness, symbolic and physiological aspects. Springfield, IL: Charles C Thomas, 1955.
17. Prigatano GP, Schacter DL, eds. Awareness of deficit after brain injury: clinical and theoretical issues. New York: Oxford University Press, 1991.
18. Semmes J. Hemispheric specialization. Neuropsychologia 1968;6:11-26.
19. Bihrle AM, Brownell HH, Powelson JA, Gardner H. Comprehension of humorous and non-humorous materials by left and right brain damaged patients. Brain Cogn 1986;5:399-412.
20. Hough M. Narrative comprehension in adults with right and left hemisphere brain damage: theme organization. Brain Lang 1990;38:253-277.
21. Cancelliere AEB, Kertesz A. Lesion localization in acquired deficits of emotional expression and comprehension. Brain Lang 1990;13:133-147.
22. Heilman KM, Watson RT, Valenstein E. Neglect and related disorders In: Heilman KM, Valenstein E, eds. Clinical neuropsychology. 2nd ed. New York: Oxford University Press, 1985:243-294.
23. Brown P, Levinson SC. Politeness: some universals in language usage. Cambridge: Cambridge University Press, 1987.

24. Knapp ML, Hall JA. Nonverbal communication in human interaction. 3rd ed. Fort Worth, TX: Holt Rinehart and Winston, 1992.
25. Rosenthal R, Hall JA, DiMatteo MR, Rogers PL, Archer D. Sensitivity to nonverbal communication: the PONS test. Baltimore: Johns Hopkins University Press, 1979.
26. Mesquita B, Frijda NH. Cultural variations in emotions: a review. Psychol Bull 1992;112:179–204.
27. Monrad-Krohn H. The third element of speech: prosody and its disorders. In: Halpern L, ed. Problems of dynamic neurology. Jerusalem: Hebrew University Press, 1963:101–117.
28. Monrad-Krohn GH. Dysprosody or altered "melody of language." Brain 1947; 70:405–415.
29. Colsher PL, Cooper WE, Graff-Radford N. Intonational variability in the speech of right-hemisphere damaged patients. Brain Lang 1987;32:379–383.
30. Shapiro BE, Danly M. The role of the right hemisphere in the control of speech prosody in propositional and affective contexts. Brain Lang 1985; 25:19–36.
31. Handel S. Listening: an introduction to the perception of auditory events. Cambridge, MA: MIT Press, 1989.
32. Alpert M, Rush M. Comparison of affects in Parkinson's disease and schizophrenia. Psychopharmacol Bull 1983;19:118–120.
33. Gorelick PB, Ross ED. The aprosodias: further functional-anatomical evidence for the organization of affective language in the right hemisphere. J Neurol Neurosurg Psychiatry 1987;50:553–560.
34. Ross ED. The aprosodias: functional-anatomic organization of the affective components of language in the right hemisphere. Arch Neurol 1981;38:561–569.
35. Ross ED, Mesulam MM. Dominant language functions of the right hemisphere? Prosody and emotional gesturing. Arch Neurol 1979;36:144–147.
36. Ross ED, Rush J. Diagnosis and neuroanatomical correlates of depression in brain-damaged patients: implications for a neurology of depression. Arch Gen Psychiatry 1981;38:1344–1354.
37. Blonder LX, Gur RE, Gur RC. The effects of right and left hemiparkinsonism on prosody. Brain Lang 1989;36:193–207.
38. Heilman KM, Bowers D, Speedie L, Coslett HB. Comprehension of affective and nonaffective prosody. Neurology 1984;34:917–921.
39. Weintraub S, Mesulam MM, Kramer L. Disturbances in prosody: a right-hemisphere contribution to language. Arch Neurol 1981;38:742–744.
40. Brådvik B, Dravins C, Holtås S, Rosén I, Ryding E, Ingvar DH. Disturbances of speech prosody following right hemisphere infarcts. Acta Neurol Scand 1991;84:114–126.
41. Darkins AW, Fromkin VA, Benson DF. A characterization of the prosodic loss in Parkinson's disease. Brain Lang 1988;34:315–327.
42. Emmorey KD. The neurological substrates for prosodic aspects of speech. Brain Lang 1987;30:305–320.
43. Tucker DM, Frederick SL. Emotion and brain lateralization. In: Wagner H, Manstead T, eds. Social psychophysiology and emotion: theory and clinical application. New York: John Wiley, 1988:27–70.

44. Tucker DM, Watson RT, Heilman KM. Discrimination and evocation of affectively intoned speech in patients with right parietal disease. Neurology 1977;27: 947–950.
45. Heilman KM, Scholes R, Watson RT. Auditory affective agnosia: disturbed comprehension of affective speech. J Neurol Neurosurg Psychiatry 1975;38:69–72.
46. Gardner H, Denes G. Connotative judgments by aphasic patients on a pictorial adaptation of the semantic differential. Cortex 1973;9:183–196.
47. Lyons J. Introduction to theoretical linguistics. London: Cambridge University Press, 1968.
48. Myers PS, Linebaugh CW. Comprehension of idiomatic expressions by right-hemisphere-damaged adults. In: Brookshire RH, ed. Clinical aphasiology: conference proceedings. Minneapolis: BRK Publishers, 1981:254–261.
49. Van Lancker DR, Kempler D. Comprehension of familiar phrases by left but not by right hemisphere damaged patients. Brain Lang 1987;32:265–277.
50. Winner E, Gardner H. The comprehension of metaphor in brain-damaged patients. Brain 1977;100:717–729.
51. Brownell HH, Potter HH, Michelow D, Gardner H. Sensitivity to lexical denotation and connotation in brain damaged patients: a double dissociation? Brain Lang 1984;22:253–265.
52. Brownell HH, Simpson TL, Bihrle AM, Potter HH, Gardner H. Appreciation of metaphoric alternative word meaning by left and right brain-damaged patients. Neuropsychologia 1990;28:375–383.
53. Tomkins CA. Knowledge and strategies for processing lexical metaphor after right or left hemisphere brain damage. J Speech Hear Res 1990;33:307–316.
54. Meyer DM, Schvaneveldt RW. Facilitation in recognizing pairs of words: Evidence of a dependence between retrieval operations. J Exp Psychol 1971;90: 227–234.
55. Brownell HH, Molloy R. Lexical priming in right-hemisphere damaged patients. Conference presentation. Baltimore, MD: Academy of Aphasia, 1990.
56. Tompkins CA, Boada R, McGarry K. The access and processing of familiar idioms by brain-damaged and normally aging adults. J Speech Hear Res 1992; 35:626–637.
57. Weylman ST, Brownell HH, Roman M, Gardner H. Appreciation of indirect requests by left and right brain-damaged patients: the effects of verbal context and conventionality of wording. Brain Lang 1989;36:580–591.
58. Chiarello C. Semantic priming in the intact brain: separate roles for the right and left hemispheres? In: Chiarello C, ed. Right hemisphere contributions to lexical semantics. Heidelberg: Springer-Verlag, 1988:59–69.
59. van Dijk T, Kintsch W. Strategies of discourse comprehension. New York: Academic Press, 1983.
60. Hough MS, Pierce RS. Contextual and thematic influences on narrative comprehension of left and right hemisphere brain-damaged adults. In: Brownell HH, Joanette Y, eds. Narrative discourse in neurologically impaired and normal aging adults. San Diego: Singular Publishing Group, 1993:213–238.
61. Schneiderman EI, Murasugi KG, Saddy JD. Story arrangement ability in right brain-damaged patients. Brain Lang 1992;43:107–120.

62. Delis DC, Wapner W, Gardner H, Moses JA. The contribution of the right hemisphere to the organization of paragraphs. Cortex 1983;19:43–50.
63. Beeman M. Semantic processing in the right hemisphere may contribute to drawing inferences from discourse. Brain Lang 1993;44:80–120.
64. Myers PS, Brookshire RH. The effects of visual and inferential complexity on the picture descriptions of non-brain-damaged and right-hemisphere-damaged adults. In: Lemme M, ed. Clinical aphasiology. Vol 22. Austin, TX: PRO-ED. In press.
65. Joanette Y, Goulet P, Ska B, Nespoulous JL. Informative content of narrative discourse in right-brain-damaged right-handers. Brain Lang 1986;29:81–105.
66. Wapner W, Hamby S, Gardner H. The role of the right hemisphere in the apprehension of complex linguistic materials. Brain Lang 1981;14:15–33.
67. Myers PS. Narrative expressive deficits associated with right-hemisphere damage. In: Brownell HH, Joanette Y, eds. Narrative discourse in neurologically impaired and normal aging adults. San Diego: Singular Publishing Group, 1993:279–296.
68. Brownell HH, Potter HH, Bihrle AM, Gardner H. Inference deficits in right brain damaged patients. Brain Lang 1986;27:310–321.
69. Molloy R, Brownell HH, Gardner H. Discourse comprehension by right hemisphere stroke patients: deficits of prediction and revision. In: Joanette Y, Brownell HH, eds. Discourse ability and brain damage: theoretical and empirical perspectives. New York: Springer-Verlag, 1990:113–130.
70. Rehak A, Kaplan JA, Gardner H. Sensitivity to conversational deviance in right-hemisphere-damaged patients. Brain Lang 1992;42:203–217.
71. Grice HP. Logic and conversation. In: Cole P, Morgan JL, eds. Syntax and semantics. Vol 3. New York: Academic Press, 1975:41–58.
72. Sperber D, Wilson N. Relevance: foundations of pragmatic theory. Cambridge, MA: Harvard University Press, 1986.
73. Brownell HH, Carroll JJ, Rehak A, Wingfield A. The use of pronoun anaphora and speaker mood in the interpretation of conversational utterances by right hemisphere brain-damaged patients. Brain Lang 1992;43:121–147.
74. Brownell HH, Winner E, Pincus D. Theory of mind and politeness: the effects of brain damage on patients' use of terms of personal reference. Conference presentation. Toronto, Ontario: Academy of Aphasia, 1992.
75. Murphy GL. Personal reference in English. Lang Soc 1988;17:317–349.
76. Astington JW, Harris PL, Olson DR. Developing theories of mind. New York: Cambridge University Press, 1988.
77. Benton A. Visuoperceptual, visuospatial, and visuoconstructive disorders. In: Heilman KM, Valenstein E, eds. Clinical neuropsychology. 2nd ed. New York: Oxford University Press, 1985:151–185.
78. Cicone M, Wapner W, Gardner H. Sensitivity to emotional expressions and situations in organic patients. Cortex 1980;16:145–158.
79. Beeman M, Friedman RB, Grafman J, Perez E, Diamond S, Lindsay MB. Summation priming and coarse semantic coding in the right hemisphere. J Cogn Neurosci 1994;6:26–45.

80. Mesulam MM. Principles of behavioral neurology. Philadelphia: FA Davis, 1985.
81. Posner MI, Peterson SE. The attention system of the human brain. Annu Rev Neurosci 1990;13:25–42.
82. Coslett HB, Bowers D, Heilman KM. Reduction in cerebral activation after right hemisphere stroke. Neurology 1987;37:957–962.
83. Prather P, Jarmulowicz L, Brownell HH, Gardner H. Selective attention and the right hemisphere: a failure in integration not detection. Conference presentation. San Diego: International Neuropsychological Society Meeting, 1992.
84. Benowitz LI, Moya KL, Levine DN. Impaired verbal reasoning and constructional apraxia in subjects with right hemisphere damage. Neuropsychologia 1990; 23:231–141.
85. Moya KL, Benowitz LI, Levine DN, Finklestein S. Covariant deficits in visuospatial abilities and recall of verbal narrative after right hemisphere stroke. Cortex 1986;22:381–97.

13

Language in Aging and Dementia

Kathryn A. Bayles

National Center for Neurogenic Communication Disorders,
University of Arizona, Tucson, Arizona

To discuss the effects of normal aging and dementing diseases on language, it is appropriate to define the term *language*. For purposes of this chapter, language is defined as knowledge of phonology, syntax, semantics, and pragmatics, and the ability to process and produce meaningful linguistic expressions. Thus, language is both something we know and something we do, and it involves the processes of comprehension and production.

Clinicians need to consider the integrity of patients' knowledge of phonological, syntactic, semantic, and pragmatic rules and their ability to manipulate these rules if language is to be comprehensively evaluated. They also need to consider that the different types of linguistic knowledge are represented in different areas of the brain and can be differentially impaired. This fact is especially important in understanding the profile of language impairment of individuals with dementing diseases.

CAN A LANGUAGE PROBLEM BE DESCRIBED AS A MEMORY PROBLEM?

Consider the situation of an individual who encounters a familiar person in the grocery store but cannot think of the person's name. Is the failure to produce the linguistic representation of the name a loss of linguistic knowledge or a loss of the ability to use linguistic knowledge? Perhaps it is both.

Suppose that the failure is in the ability of the individual to retrieve the name; should that failure then be called a language problem? An argument could be made that it is a memory problem.

Now suppose that the reason the individual could not produce the name is that the mental representation of the name no longer exists. Is this a language problem or a memory problem? Clearly our linguistic representations are a form of memory. So also are the cognitive procedures by which linguistic representations are manipulated. The point of this example is that a loss of language knowledge or the ability to use linguistic knowledge can be described as a loss of memory substance and/or process. Thus, Alzheimer's dementia patients, with their severe memory problems, can be said to have difficulty with linguistic communication.

LANGUAGE TASKS TYPICALLY TEST MORE THAN LANGUAGE

Tasks that clinicians and researchers commonly refer to as language tasks typically require more than the integrity of linguistic knowledge; they also require perception, attention, memory, and association. For example, naming is commonly referred to as a language task, yet it requires attention to a stimulus, perception of its features, activation of the concept of the stimulus within semantic memory, retrieval of the linguistic representation of the concept, and planning and production of the articulated or written word. Dementia patients may fail a naming task not because of a language deficit but because the demands on attention or other cognitive processes are too great. Because language is nonorthogonal to other aspects of cognition, attempts to ferret out the effects of normal aging and dementing diseases on language is methodologically challenging. Both the normal elderly and dementia patients are known to suffer changes in perception, memory, and information processing. When the literature related to normal aging and language is interpreted, it is important to keep these points in mind.

If clinicians are to be able to distinguish mild dementia patients from the normal elderly, they must be knowledgeable of the effects of normal aging on language. In the first segment of this chapter, the effects of normal aging on language are summarized. In the second segment, a summary is given of the effects of dementing diseases on language.

NORMAL AGING AND LANGUAGE

Language was defined as both knowledge of rules and the ability to use these rules; in general, age has a greater effect on the latter. Capacities critical to the processes of linguistic communication are diminished by age, among them hearing (1) and vision (2). The presbycusis and presbyopia of the average elderly cause them to make more language performance errors. The aged are also slower in movement and information processing. Birren and Schaie (3) have emphasized that the most significant change with age is slowing. Thus, in aging studies, when the task is timed and highly dependent upon visual and auditory acuity, an age effect is generally reported. When, however, time constraints are not imposed and care is taken to make sure stimuli are audible and visible, age effects are less likely to be reported.

Effects of Aging on Language Knowledge

Semantic/Vocabulary

Most studied is the effect of normal aging on vocabulary. Many investigators (4–7) have reported that vocabulary is well maintained over the life span; indeed, some (8,9) have reported vocabulary growth. Others (10) have described a decrement in advanced age. The variability in these reports likely results from differences in the task and educational characteristics of the subjects (11). When subjects have to provide definitions for words (12–14) or retrieve a specific word (7), they perform more poorly (15,16) than when they are presented with a multiple-choice format (7). Also, subjects whose occupations have provided them with continued opportunity for exposure to new words—for example, teachers—tend to perform better (17–20).

Phonology

No reports exist of an age-related loss of knowledge of the sounds of language and the rules for their combination. Elders are able to pronounce words as well as they did when they were younger. The presbycusis they suffer may make it difficult to hear high-frequency sounds.

Syntax/Grammar

Grammatical knowledge comprises the individual's knowledge of how to combine words meaningfully. Although there are no reports that grammatical knowledge is lost as a result of normal aging, simpler grammatical constructions are more frequently used by elderly individuals (21). Certain elaborate syntactic constructions, such as embedding, place a heavier load on memory (21), which may explain why elders have a tendency to use them less frequency.

Pragmatics

Pragmatic knowledge comprises the rules people have internalized for using language in different ways, e.g., to greet, deny, declare, propose, object. As yet, standardized tests of pragmatic knowledge are unavailable, making measurement of the effects of normal aging on language use difficult. Nonetheless, anecdotal evidence of loss of pragmatic knowledge with age is virtually nonexistent. Healthy normal elders know how to use language for different purposes and can recognize the intentions of other speakers.

One type of pragmatic knowledge is knowing how to use language to greet and say good-bye. These overlearned and much-used phrases are preserved even in Alzheimer's dementia patients. If Alzheimer's disease is exaggerated aging as has been suggested (22), then the preservation of social phrases suggests their immunity to the effects of normal aging.

Effects of Aging on Linguistic Comprehension and Production

Comprehension

Studies of the effects of normal aging on the ability to comprehend language have produced conflicting results. Table 1 summarizes reports of studies of word and sentence comprehension. Consensus is lacking not only in whether an age effect is present but in regard to whether the effect takes the form of an across-the-decades decline.

What investigators do agree about is that comprehension is slower. Therefore, when reaction time is the dependent variable in comprehension studies, age effects are typically reported. If the dependent variable is the number correct, an age effect is not always observed.

Production

The ability to produce language takes many forms, from the production of a single word to the production of verbal or written discourse. When the task is to name on confrontation, many investigators (23,24) have reported an age effect. The findings of a study by Bowles, Obler, and Albert (25) are characteristic of studies of aging and language; that is, the performance of elder normals is not *dramatically* different from that of young normals. In the Bowles study, the mean for young adults was 59 of 63 whereas the mean for older adults was 55 of 63.

When the naming task requires enumeration of items in a category (generative naming), the effect of aging is more apparent (26–28). Animal generative naming was the task used by Borod and colleagues (28), who reported a gradual across-the-decades decline with age. Whereas adults younger than 40 provided an average of 27 names in 1 minute, adults in their 50s averaged 21 and adults in their 70s averaged 19.

Production of Discourse. Bayles et al. (29) recently completed a study of the effects of normal aging on discourse production in a sample of 207 subjects, using a picture stimulus. The samples were analyzed for total numbers of words and information units and conciseness of expression. Nonparame-

Table 1 Summary of Research on Comprehension and Aging

Task	Age difference
Story/prose retelling	
Ulatowska et al., 1986 (34)	Yes
Taub, 1979 (100)	Yes
Moenster, 1972 (101)	Yes
Gordon and Clark, 1974 (102)	Yes
Spilich, 1983 (103)	Yes
Kemper, 1986 (104)	Yes
Recall of main information	
Petros et al., 1983 (105)	Yes
Zelinski et al., 1984 (106)	Yes
Cohen, 1979 (35)	Yes
Dixon et al., 1982 (107)	Yes
Spilich, 1983 (103)	No
Byrd, 1981 (110)	No
Zelinski et al., 1980 (108)	No
Dixon et al., 1984 (109)	Mixed
Meyer and Rice, 1981 (111)	No
Recall of supplemental information	
Spilich, 1983 (103)	Yes
Petros et al., 1983 (105)	Yes
Zelinski et al., 1984 (106)	Yes
Byrd, 1981 (110)	Yes
Zelinski et al., 1980 (108)	Yes
Dixon et al., 1984 (109)	Yes
Cohen, 1979 (35)	No
Dixon et al., 1982 (107)	No
Meyer and Rice, 1981 (111)	No
Explicit or direct linguistic information	
Belmore, 1981 (112)	Yes
Ulatowska et al., 1986 (34)	No
Cohen, 1979 (35)	No
Till and Walsh, 1980 (113)	No
Camp, 1981 (114)	No
Implicit or inferred linguistic information	
Ulatowska et al., 1986 (34)	Yes
Cohen, 1979 (35)	Yes
Till and Walsh, 1980 (113)	Yes
Belmore, 1981 (112)	No
Camp, 1981 (114)	No
Walsh and Baldwin, 1977 (115)	No

tric and parametric analyses revealed a tendency for the elderly to produce fewer total words and information units and to be less concise. The effect was most pronounced for conciseness and became apparent in individuals in their late 70s. It is important to emphasize, however, that not all elders in their 70s were inferior to younger normals; considerable variability existed.

Shewan and Henderson (30) used a picture-description task to elicit discourse from subjects ranging in age from 45 to 74. No consistent relation was observed between the amount of information expressed and increasing age. However, the youngest individuals were significantly more efficient in communication when the dependent variable was the number of content units divided by time.

Cooper (31) administered a picture-description task to 80 subjects who ranged in age from 20 to 78. No association was observed between aging and speech production, elaborateness, complexity, dysfluency, conciseness, or amount of information. The elderly did tend to produce more prepositional phrases, indefinite words, and longer pauses.

When the discourse-production task was something other than picture description, elders produced fewer prepositions (32), fewer steps in procedural discourse (33), impairment of reference (34), errors in reference when retelling a story (35), and fewer words per clause and fewer clauses (36).

Using an object-description task to elicit discourse, Bayles and colleagues (7) evaluated the performance of 10 healthy individuals of normal intelligence from each decade of life from the third to the eighth. One point was awarded for each nonredundant, relevant piece of information provided by subjects in their descriptions. Although a possible age effect on subject performance was observed, it did not manifest as an across-the-decades decline. The best performance was given by subjects in their 30s and 40s. Although these individuals were significantly better than those in their 70s, subjects in their 50s and 60s did not perform differently from those in their 20s.

The object-description subtest of the Arizona Battery for Communication Disorders of Dementia (37) has been given to elders (mean age 71) and a group of young normals (mean age 20). The mean score of the elders was 9.2 while that of young normals was 10.9; the difference, although small, was statistically significant ($t = 3.47$, $p = 0.01$).

Discourse Production in Conversation. Studying age effects on naturally occurring conversation is complex. If the investigator controls the conversation, it becomes unnatural. There is thus a dearth of data on this topic. However, results of laboratory studies suggest how some age-related changes may affect conversation. Rabbitt (38) observed that keeping track of which speaker made a statement in a multispeaker interaction was difficult for individuals over the age of 70. Numerous investigators have reported difficulty in word retrieval in the elderly, a potential problem in conversation (39–42). Koriat and colleagues (43) observed that older adults were poorer in their ability to recall whether words had already been used and hence they repeated words. Kausler and Hakami (44) found that younger adults were better able than elders to recall topics discussed within a session.

Summary

In summary, convincing evidence does not exist of an age-related linear decline in linguistic knowledge and in the ability to use that knowledge. Language knowledge and use is not definitely diminished for 50-year-olds compared to 40-year-olds or for 60-year-olds compared to people in their 50s. When age effects are observed, they tend to occur on tests of language comprehension and production in the very elderly, especially when speed is a component of the task. The elderly show marked variability in performance; it is inappropriate for a clinician to assume inferior performances for individuals just because of their age.

WHY IS IT DIFFICULT TO CONCLUDE THAT AN AGE EFFECT EXISTS FOR LANGUAGE?

One of the reasons it is difficult to evaluate possible age effects is that the aged are heterogeneous; in fact, no segment of the population is more so. Consider, for example, a group of elders at age 65. Some individuals in the group are genetically destined to die in the next few years, whereas others will be centenarians. The future centenarians are more vigorous. When older humans are near death (45), their performance diminishes. This fact alone makes age-related research difficult. If a sufficient number of individuals in a sample of older subjects die shortly after their participation in the research project, the effects of impending death, and not normal aging, may affect performance. Nonetheless, age at death is almost never reported in studies of age effects.

Not only are the elderly heterogeneous in physical health and psychological function, but they also differ in education and social and economic history. Affluent and better educated and socially integrated individuals are likely to have a better self-image, which improves their performance (46).

Another variable that most investigators have failed to control is drug intake. The average elder is taking six drugs at any point in time (47) because of chronic diseases. The typical elder has 3.5 chronic conditions (48). Drugs affect mental status and motivation, and their effects may mistakenly be interpreted as age effects.

Yet another condition that can affect performance is depression. Most investigators have failed to control for the presence of depression in research subjects, even though the incidence of depression is greater among the elderly (3). As with drug-induced mental-status changes, the effects of depression can be mistaken for age effects.

Many researchers group together everyone over the age of 50 or 60, and the range of age in some samples is 50 to 90. This problem is exacerbated by the small sample sizes in many studies; although the extreme performance of an individual can skew the results, only group data are provided.

EFFECTS OF DEMENTIA ON LANGUAGE

Dementia is a syndrome associated with numerous diseases and conditions. Before the diagnosis of dementia can be given, evidence must be obtained of progressive intellectual decline sufficient to interfere with social and occupational functioning (49). The most distinguishing characteristic of dementia appears to be episodic memory failure, perhaps because it is the hallmark feature of early Alzheimer's disease (AD), the most prevalent of the dementing diseases. Because the meaningful use of language depends on the integrity of episodic memory, as well as other intellectual capacities, language will inevitably be affected when episodic memory and other intellectual functions are diminished. What is of interest is the nature of the effect on language.

To discuss the influences of dementia on language, it is necessary to specify the etiology of the dementia. Dementia takes different forms in different diseases because of variations in the type and distribution of morphological change in the brain. The following section considers the effects on language of Alzheimer's, Pick's, and Parkinson's diseases. The discussion is limited to the most common forms of cortical and subcortical dementing disease.

Dementia and Language in Alzheimer's Disease Patients

Effects on Language Knowledge

Phonology. No evidence exists that AD patients lose their knowledge of the sounds of their native language. Even the neologisms AD patients produce respect the rules of their native language, and severe AD patients spontaneously correct phonological errors in sentences they repeat (50,51). Whitaker (50) was the first to observe the phenomenon of spontaneous correction in a case study of an advanced AD patient. Subsequently, Bayles and Boone (51) demonstrated that spontaneous correction of phonological errors was not idiosyncratic with Whitaker's patient but common in severely demented AD patients.

Grammar/Syntax. The AD patients discussed by Bayles and Boone (51) and Whitaker (50) spontaneously corrected errors of phonology and grammar in sentences they repeated for the examiner. For example, to the stimulus sentence "The lady has two dress," patients responded, "The lady has two dresses."

Phonological and syntactic rules are complicated and cannot be recited by anyone but an informed linguist, yet these rules are applied automatically and unconsciously in routine linguistic communication. What phonological and syntactic rules have in common is that they are finite and predictable. The same sounds and structures are used over and over throughout life, enabling the brain to carry out this processing without our conscious thought. Such rules tend to be spared in the early and mid stages of AD.

Many investigators have observed the preservation of grammar in the language of AD patients (51–56), although some reports exist of simplification of grammar (57). If simplification does exist, it does not necessarily signify loss of knowledge of syntax and phonology but may reflect the need to use structure that is less demanding of memory. In a study by Bayles and Boone (51), AD patients retained their ability to judge the grammaticality of simple sentences and correct grammatical errors. The preservation of grammar contrasts dramatically with the loss of semantic well-formedness of language.

Semantic/Vocabulary. Semantic knowledge, the knowledge of the meaning and reference of words, progressively diminishes during the course of AD (53,58–60). AD subjects in the studies by Bayles and Boone (51) and Whitaker (50) never corrected semantic errors in sentences. Unlike phonology and syntax, meaning is unpredictable and requires conscious attention. Many factors contribute to progressively poorer performance on vocabulary tests: diminishing perception, deteriorating semantic memory, and lexical access difficulty.

Over the disease course, the utterances of AD patients become semantically more aberrant. Consider the following samples over a 5-year period from the same patient, describing the Normal Rockwell picture of a mother and children going to church on Easter Sunday without the father.

AD patient HM at year 1, Easter Morning Picture Description

Test time 1

Examiner: Now I'd like you to look at that picture there.
AD patient: Too many children.
Examiner: Yes. Describe what's happening in the picture.
AD patient: Well, here's a man reading something. It's happening but he's not looking at the reading. See he's looking someplace else and he's he's talking to these beautiful ladies here, and also reading his own paper beside. And here's his little boy. Isn't he cute?

Examiner: Tell me more.

AD patient: Well the father's gotten a little tired of reading all this, see, so he's just getting rid of that one at a time as they march past him going to their own reading or whatever else they do [laugh]. That's real good. And he has his own great big great big newspaper. And then he has a few down here like this. Two feet for all that. That's a cute thing right there [laughing].

Test time 3

Examiner: Describe what's going on in this picture.

AD patient: Well, they look like the pictures that uh don't want to be pick-picketed, or or made made up into an odd creature in in the meantime.

Examiner: Is there anything else that you want to say about that?

AD patient: Yes, they do. They they they they they actually look so actable that it makes you want to run away for some reason or other. But um, they have their their special *aqualelge* over. The way people take uh take uh an *actoba* that they don't even know anything about. But they just don't try to bother with these other people who have their.

Examiner: Okay, great, thank you.

Test time 5

Examiner: Tell me about this picture. Describe what is happening?

AD patient: Yes. Mmhm. It must be a ah, ah, somebody that really thought themselves really gone and close way.

Examiner: What's happening in this picture?

AD patient: No.

Examiner: What's happening in this picture?

AD patient: Well, there's, that's something that we'd be supplied with it, but usually goes away with a.

Examiner: OK. Good.

Notice that although meaningfulness deteriorates, nouns and other parts of speech are placed appropriately. The ability of the AD patient to position nouns and other parts of speech correctly, without regard for effects on meaning, demonstrates the dissociability of knowledge of word class, pronunciation, and even spelling from knowledge of word meaning. Further, these different types of word knowledge may be represented in different areas of the brain.

One of the principal debates among the scientists who study the neurobehavioral effects of AD is whether semantic, or conceptual, knowledge is lost, degraded, or inaccessible. Results of a study by Bayles et al. (61) suggest that accessibility is affected, primarily by the demands of the task the patient is asked to perform. Bayles and colleagues (61) used a paradigm in which AD subjects were administered 11 tasks with the same 13 conceptual stimuli, enabling the researchers to assess the effects of task demand on performance. If conceptual knowledge were lost, the concept should be missed on all 11 tasks, an event that almost never occurred in the 69 subjects studied. Instead, the task difficulty predicted whether a concept was missed. Moderately severe subjects typically missed a concept in harder tasks such as coordinate naming (naming examples of other things in the same category), superordinate naming (naming the larger category of things to which the stimulus concept belongs), and definition, but got the same concept correct in easier tasks such as auditory comprehension, oral reading, and reading comprehension (61). Although these data indicate that access to conceptual knowledge is affected, I suspect that conceptual knowledge ultimately is degraded and lost in late-stage AD when the neuropathology is severe and widespread.

Loss of Conceptual Knowledge: Bottom Up or Top Down? Another argument among behavioral scientists who believe conceptual knowledge is lost is whether it is lost from the "top down" or "bottom up." Several investigators have argued that it occurs from the bottom up (55,62–66); that is, the knowledge of specific attributes of an object is lost prior to the loss of categorical knowledge. Results of a study by Cox, Bayles, and Trosset (66), in which subjects were asked to demonstrate knowledge of attributes and categories both implicitly and explicitly, call into question the bottom-up theory and the methodology used to evaluate the theory. In this study no convincing pattern of decline in attribute knowledge was found relative to categorical knowledge. At the conclusion of the study, Cox and colleagues posed the intriguing question of whether categorical knowledge can be studied separately from attribute knowledge. To have categorical knowledge may require attribute knowledge; indeed, it is a particular collection of attributes that defines a category.

Pragmatic. Certain types of pragmatic knowledge are spared in AD, while others are prominently affected. The use of language for greeting people, saying good-bye, and other highly routinized automatisms are well preserved in most patients through the early and middle stages of the disease (67). Such forms of language use appear to be carried out without the attention of higher intellectual processes, as is true of the processing of phonology and syntax. Other uses of language, however, do require conscious attention and therefore are dramatically affected because they, like the content of language, are unpredictable and infinite. There is no way of knowing whether the speaker will use language to persuade, cajole, intimidate, explain, deny, incriminate, or entertain, to name a few possibilities. Speakers unpredictably shift from one use to another.

AD patients become progressively impaired in their ability to use language for these complex purposes, in part because of profound disease effects on episodic memory. To carry out a complex speech act, AD patients must be able to remember their intention to relate it to the context. Remembering one's linguistic intention and the context is extremely difficult when consciousness has become like a continuously fading dream.

Effects of AD on Linguistic Comprehension and Expression

Comprehension. Deterioration in episodic and semantic memory cause associated deficits in the comprehension of language (53). AD patients forget what they just heard or read, making it difficult to comprehend stimuli that do not remain in their perceptual field. In tests of word, sentence, or paragraph comprehension, AD patients have performed inferiorly to normal control subjects. Further, the degree of comprehension difficulty is proportional to the severity of the dementia.

To evaluate comprehension, some investigators have used disambiguation tasks (51,68,69) or verbal reasoning tasks (70,71), which have proven to be particularly sensitive to mild dementia. Such tasks are relatively challenging to normals and are most sensitive for identifying the mild dementia patient. If a task is very easy for normal elders, such that they perform at ceiling, it may be too easy to reveal a mild dementia.

Production. In most AD patients, language can be elicited even in the advanced stages of the disease. Advanced patients can recognize when it is their turn to talk. They retain the ability to process the intonation patterns and pausal phenomena that tell them they have been asked a question or indicate when another speaker is through talking.

During the course of dementia, verbal and written output fall off (53,72). Very early, before prominent intellectual changes are apparent, some patients may become more talkative or exhibit logorrhea (67). By the middle stages, however, the impoverishment of thought reduces the production of meaningful language in the typical AD patient. Eventually, many patients become mute.

Tomoeda and Bayles (72) analyzed the discourse produced by three AD patients who were followed for 5 years. The prominent finding was the consistency of change in the three patients in quantity, quality, and efficiency of language. There was a diminution of total output and decimation of semantic substance. In the first year they were tested, the three patients produced 288, 364, and 183 words, respectively, in a picture-description task. In year 5, they produced, 0, 30, and 20.

Another type of language-production task is confrontation naming; impairment of naming is the most frequently reported language problem of patients with AD (73–84). Although naming impairment is common in AD patients and generally proportional to severity of dementia, there are exceptions (83,84). Some severely demented patients name well, and some mildly demented patients are severely dysnomic. Bayles and Trosset (83) observed that dementia severity, as defined by Global Deterioration Scale ratings (85), Mini-Mental State Examination scores (86), and combinations of them, was found to account for only one-third of naming-performance variability. These findings demonstrate the inadequacy of dementia severity for predicting confrontation naming in AD patients.

When misnamings occur, they are likely to be semantically or perceptually related to the stimuli, typically an attribute, or the name of something that looks like the stimulus object (87). Kirshner and colleagues (87) reported that perceptual difficulty influenced naming in demented and right-hemisphere stroke patients but not in aphasics and control subjects. Demented and right CVA patients also provided more visually related error responses. However, demented and aphasic groups also made significantly more semantically related and circumlocution errors than control and right CVA groups. In an analysis of the misnaming of AD patients, Bayles, Tomoeda, and Trosset (88) found that it was rare for an AD patient to give the name of a superordinate. Over the course of the disease, misnamings become less related to stimuli, and ultimately the patient is unable to respond.

Generative naming, or production of a series of words sharing a requested characteristic, has also been well studied in AD patients. This capacity is recognized as being more sensitive to disease effects than confrontation naming (56,89–91). In a study by Bayles and associates (92), normal control subjects named a mean of 14 examplars from a category, whereas testable AD patients averaged six.

Longitudinal Decline of Language in AD Patients

In a recently completed 5-year longitudinal study of the effect of AD on language in 94 patients, Bayles, Tomoeda, and Trosset (92) observed inexorable decline. The order of deterioration across tasks was determined by task difficulty. On very simple tasks, like the reading aloud of single words, decline was not seen in the early and middle stages. Similarly, decline was not observed on very difficult tasks in severely demented patients, because deterioration was below the range of the test. In Table 2, the tasks used in the Arizona longitudinal study are listed in order of difficulty for AD patients. Performance on the easier tasks was maintained longer than on the harder. The longitudinal data suggest that the typical AD patient loses approximately one-half of his/her ability per year and takes 5 to 6 years to progress from normal to nonfunctional performance on language tasks.

Table 2 Order of Task Difficulty for 5-Year NIMH Study (Means and Standard Deviations)

Normals	Mild AD	Moderate AD
Oral reading 12.96 (0.20)	Oral reading 12.44 (1.93)	Oral reading 11.30 (3.07)
Reading comprehension 12.87 (0.71)	Auditory comprehension 11.58 (1.74)	Reading comprehension 8.98 (3.39)
Superordinate ID 12.66 (0.56)	Reading comprehension 11.52 (2.22)	Auditory comprehension 8.94 (2.88)
Auditory comprehension 12.62 (0.74)	Pantomime recognition 9.80 (2.26)	Pantomime recognition 6.11 (3.45)
Pantomime recognition 12.56 (1.01)	Superordinate ID 9.59 (2.97)	Confrontation naming 5.83 (3.56)
Confrontation naming 11.82 (1.35)	Pantomime expression 8.60 (3.34)	Superordinate ID 5.64 (4.29)
Superordinate naming 11.67 (2.11)	Dictation 8.57 (2.71)	Dictation 5.52 (3.76)
Pantomime expression 11.52 (1.43)	Confrontation naming 8.27 (3.14)	Pantomime expression 4.78 (3.25)
Dictation 11.45 (1.43)	Definition 7.60 (2.91)	Definition 4.71 (2.35)
Definition 10.29 (1.79)	Superordinate naming 5.67 (4.30)	Superordinate naming 1.45 (2.11)
Coordinate naming 7.44 (3.91)	Coordinate naming 3.56 (3.62)	Coordinate naming 1.36 (1.96)

Pick's Disease: How It Affects Language

Another cortical dementing disease is Pick's disease. Far more rare than AD, Pick's is distinguished by severe cell loss and atrophy primarily in the frontal lobes and anterior portions of the temporal lobes. Consequently, aberrant behavior and changes in personality are likely to be presenting symptoms. To the degree that the frontal lobes influence judgment about language use, the Pick's patient may be verbally inappropriate.

Few in-depth reports of the effect(s) of Pick's on language exist in the literature. A theme in the few available studies is the tendency for these patients to become less talkative and eventually mute (93). Gustafson and colleagues (94) described the combination of mutism and preserved receptive language as typifying Pick's patients. Cummings (95) described Pick's patients as having a transcortical sensory aphasia and noted their tendency to be repetitive. Feher, Inbody, Nolan, and Pirozzolo (96) observed that language impairment is likely to be greater in Pick's disease patients than in AD.

Holland and associates (93) noted the loss of the formal syntactic elements of language in their patients who retained access to the semantic store throughout the disease. Consideration of language disorders in Pick's disease is also provided in Chapter 14.

Parkinson's Disease: Effects on Language

A majority of Parkinson's disease (PD) patients suffer some type of intellectual deficit. Cummings has written that "neuropsychological testing indicates that mental status changes are ubiquitous" in PD patients (97, p. 15). Current estimates of the frequency of frank dementia in PD range from 15 to 40% (98). In the demented PD patient, language will necessarily be affected. Of interest is whether it is affected similarly to language in AD patients. Bayles and Kaszniak (53) conducted a 3-year longitudinal study in which disease effects of PD and AD were compared. The language of demented AD and PD patients was observed to be more similar than different. Take, for example, the following language samples in which the patients were describing the Norman Rockwell Easter Morning picture. See if you can tell which was produced by a demented PD patient and which was produced by an AD patient.

Subject 1: School. The father's sitting around doing nothing. A student. A student. A teacher of the student. Employed. He's wearing shoes, he's wearing those shoes. Pajamas on. School teacher. High school teacher I guess. She's wearing enough shoes. Calendar. Him. He looks like he's upset or something. And, that's all I can think of. She's wearing a suit with shoes on. Looks like she's wearing shoes, going to school. I talked about these before. Teacher, student.

Subject 2: Well, looks like a bunch of scholars goin' through there and the old man sittin' here in the chair. I don't know if he's the instructor or teacher or what, but he's got a big paper up. Looks like they're going to school. There's a girl, she's got a bible in her hand. There's four of them in the row, going' someplace, and I don't know if this is supposed to be the teacher, principal or what.

Bayles (99) reviewed disease effects on language in the nondemented PD patient. In this paper, when the effects of nonlanguage cognitive deficits were controlled, the language "effect" disappeared. No evidence exists to date of loss of language knowledge in the nondemented PD patient. Reports of deficit come mainly from poor performance on linguistically oriented tasks, which can be explained by more fundamental problems in memory or mental flexibility. The first sample was produced by a PD patient.

Summary

The memory deficits that define the syndrome of dementia devastate the patients' ability to communicate normally. Dementia patients have progressive difficulty accessing concepts and their linguistic representations, generating meaningful discourse, and comprehending the meaning of words and contexts, but they retain the essentials of grammar. Occasionally a clinician who has engaged the mild patient in simple conversation may conclude that language is spared. However, if a comprehensive evaluation of language is carried out and the patient is challenged to process semantic and pragmatic information, disease effects will become evident.

ACKNOWLEDGMENTS

I would like to acknowledge the support of NIM,H grants R01 MH40827 and R01 MH43872 and the National Center for Neurogenic Communication Disorders DC-01409.

REFERENCES

1. Hayes D, Jerger J. Neurology of aging: The auditory system. In: Albert ML, ed. Clinical neurology of aging. New York: Oxford University Press, 1984: 362–380.
2. Fozard JL, Wolf E, Bell B, McFarland RA, Podolsky S. Visual perception in communication. In: Birren JE, Schaie KW, eds. The handbook of the psychology of aging. New York: Van Nostrand Reinhold, 1977:497–528.
3. Birren JE, Schaie W. Handbook of the psychology of aging. San Diego: Academic Press, 1990.
4. Lewinsky RJ. Vocabulary and mental measurement: A qualitative investigation and review of research. J Genet Psychol 1948;72:247–281.
5. Shakow D, Goldman R. The effect of age on the Stanford-Binet vocabulary scores of adults. J Educ Psychol 1938;29:241–256.
6. Thorndike RL, Gallup GH. Verbal intelligence of the American adult. J Genet Psychol 1944;30:75–85.
7. Bayles KA, Tomoeda CK, Boone DR. A view of age-related changes in language function. Dev Neuropsychol 1985;1:231–264.
8. Owens NA. Age and mental abilities: A longitudinal study. Genet Psychol Monogr 1953;48:3–54.
9. Fox C. Vocabulary activity in later maturity. J Educ Psychol 1947;38:482–492.
10. Lubinski R, ed. Dementia and communication. Philadelphia: BC Decker, 1991: 86.
11. Salthouse TA. Effects of aging on verbal abilities: Examination of the psychometric literature. In: Light LL, Burke DM, eds. Language, memory and aging. Cambridge: Cambridge University Press, 1988:17–35.

12. Botwinick J, Storandt M. Vocabulary ability in later life. J Genet Psychol 1974; 125:303–308.
13. Botwinick J, West R, Storandt M. Qualitative vocabulary test responses and age. J Gerontol 1975;30:574–577.
14. Looft WR. Note on WAIS vocabulary performance by young and old adults. Psychol Rep 1970;26:943–946.
15. Feifel H. Qualitative differences in the vocabulary responses of normals and abnormals. Genet Psychol Monogr 1949;39:151–204.
16. Ricks JH Jr. Age and vocabulary test performance: A qualitative analysis of the responses of adults. Doctoral dissertation, Columbia University. Dissertation Abstracts International 1958;19:182.
17. Garfield SL, Blek L. Age, vocabulary level, and mental impairment. J Consult Psychol 1952;16:395–398.
18. Lachman R, Lachman JL, Taylor DW. Reallocation of mental resources over the productive life-span: Assumptions and task analyses. In: Craik FIM, Trehub S, eds. Aging and cognitive processes. New York: Plenum, 1982:279–308.
19. Sorenson H. Mental ability over a wide range of adult ages. J Appl Psychol 1933;17:729–741.
20. Sward K. Age and mental ability in superior men. Am J Psychol 1945;58:443–479.
21. Kynette D, Kemper S. Aging and the loss of grammatical forms: A cross-sectional study of language performance. Lang Commun 1986;6:65–72.
22. Jolles J. Cognitive, emotional and behavioral dysfunctions in aging and dementia. In: Swaab DF, Fliers E, Mirmiran M, Van Gool WA, Van Haaren F, eds. Aging of the brain and Alzheimer's disease. Prog Brain Res 1986;70:15–39.
23. Bowles NL, Poon LW. Aging and retrieval of words in semantic memory. J Gerontol 1985;40:71–77.
24. Nicholas M, Obler LK, Albert ML, Goodglass H. Lexical retrieval in healthy aging. Cortex 1985;21:595–606.
25. Bowles NL, Obler LK, Albert ML. Naming errors in healthy aging and dementia of the Alzheimer type. Cortex 1987;23:519–524.
26. Spreen O, Benton A. Neurosensory Center Comprehensive Examination for Aphasia. Victoria, British Columbia: Neuropsychology Laboratory, Department of Psychology, University of Victoria, 1969.
27. Kamin LJ. Differential changes in mental abilities in old age. J Gerontol 1957; 12:66–70.
28. Borod JC, Goodglass H, Kaplan E. Normative data on the Boston Diagnostic Aphasia Examination, Parietal Lobe Battery, and the Boston Naming Test. J Clin Neuropsychol 1980;2:209–215.
29. Bayles KB, Rao SM, Trosset MW, Tomoeda CK. Effects of normal aging on production of descriptive discourse. In press.
30. Shewan CM, Henderson VL. Analysis of spontaneous language in the older normal population. J Commun Disord 1988;21:139–154.
31. Cooper PV. Discourse production and normal aging: Performance on oral picture description tasks. Gerontolog Soc Am 1990;45:210–214.

32. Light LL, Burke DM, eds. Language, memory and aging. New York: Cambridge University Press, 1988:175-176.
33. North AJ, Ulatowska HK, Macaluso-Haynes S, Bell H. Discourse performance in older adults. Int J Aging Hum Devel 1986;23:267-283.
34. Ulatowska HK, Hayashi MM, Cannito MP, Fleming SG. Disruption of reference. Brain Lang 1986;28:24-41.
35. Cohen G. Language comprehension in old age. Cogn Psychol 1979;11:412-429.
36. Walker VG, Hardiman CK, Hedrick D, Holbrook A. Speech and language characteristics of an aging population. In: Lass NJ, ed. Speech and language: Advances in basic research and practice. New York: Academic Press, 1981;6:144-202.
37. Bayles KA, Tomoeda CK. Arizona Battery for Communication Disorders of Dementia. Tucson: Canyonlands Publishing, 1991.
38. Rabbitt P. Talking to the old. New Soc 1981;55:140-141.
39. McCrae RR, Arenberg D, Costa PT. Declines in divergent thinking with age: Cross-sectional, longitudinal, and cross-sequential analyses. Psychol Aging 1987;2:130-137.
40. Obler LK, Albert ML. Language skills across adulthood. In: Birren JE, Schaie KW, eds. Handbook of the psychology of aging. New York: Van Nostrand Reinhold, 1985:463-473.
41. Schaie KW, Parham IA. Short-sequential analyses of adult intellectual development. Dev Psychol 1977;13:649-653.
42. Burke DM, Harrold RM. Automatic and effortful semantic processes in old age: Experimental and naturalistic approaches. In: Light LL, Burke DM, eds. Language, memory, and aging. New York: Cambridge University Press, 1988:100-116.
43. Koriat A, Ben-Zur H, Sheffer D. Telling the same story twice: Output monitoring and age. J Mem Lang 1988;27:23-39.
44. Kausler DH, Hakami MK. Memory for topics of conversation: Adult age differences and intentionality. Exp Aging Res 1983;9:153-157.
45. Kleemier RW. Intellectual changes in the senium. Proceedings of the Socal Statistics Section of the American Statistical Association, 1962:290-295.
46. Ryan EB. Normal aging and language. In: Lubinski R, ed. Dementia and communication. Philadelphia: BC Decker, 1991:84-97.
47. Bressler R, Conrad KA. Clinical pharmacology. In: Steinbert FU, ed. Care of the geriatric patient. St Louis, MO: CV Mosby, 1983:256-274.
48. Williamson J, Stokoe IH, Gray S, Fisher M, Smith A, McGhee A, Stephenson E. Old people at home: Their unreported needs. Lancet 1964;x:1117-1126.
49. American Psychological Association. Diagnostic and statistical manual-III-Revised. Washington, DC.
50. Whitaker HA. A case of isolation of the language function. In: Whitaker H, Whitaker HA, eds. Studies in neurolinguistics. Vol 2. New York: Academic Press, 1976:1-58.
51. Bayles KA, Boone DR. The potential of language tasks for identifying senile dementia. J Speech Hear Dis 1982;47:210-217.

52. Irigaray L. Le langage des dements. The Hague: Mouton, 1973.
53. Bayles KA, Kaszniak A. Communication and cognition in normal aging and dementia. Boston: Little, Brown, 1987.
54. Kempler D, Curtiss S, Jackson C. Syntactic preservation in Alzheimer's disease. J Speech Hear Res 1987;30:343-350.
55. Schwartz MF, Marin OSM, Saffran EM. Dissociations of language function in dementia: A case study. Brain Lang 1979;7:277-306.
56. Appell J, Kertesz A, Fisman M. A study of language functioning in Alzheimer's disease. Brain Lang 1982;17:73-91.
57. Hier DB, Hagenlocker K, Shindler AG. Language disintegration in dementia: Effects of etiology and severity. Brain Lang 1985;25:117-133.
58. de Ajuriaguerra J, Tissot R. Some aspects of language in various forms of senile dementia: Some comparisons with language in childhood. In: Lenneberg EH, Lenneberg E, eds. Foundations of language development: A multidisciplinary approach. Vol 1. New York: Academic Press, 1975:323-339.
59. Ernst B, Dalby MA, Dalby A. Aphasic disturbances in presenile dementia. Acta Neurol Scand 1970;46(suppl 43):99-100.
60. Kaszniak AW, Wilson RS. Longitudinal deterioration of language and cognition in dementia of the Alzheimer's type. Presented at the International Neuropsychological Society meeting, San Diego, 1985.
61. Bayles KA, Tomoeda CK, Kaszniak AW, Trosset MW. Alzheimer's disease effects on semantic memory: Loss of structure or impaired processing? J Cogn Neurosci 1991;3:166-182.
62. Warrington EK. The selective impairment of semantic memory. Q J Exp Psychol 1975;27:635-657.
63. Martin A, Fedio P. Word production and comprehension in Alzheimer's disease: The breakdown of semantic knowledge. Brain Lang 1983;19:124-141.
64. Martin A. Representation of semantic and spatial knowledge in Alzheimer's patients: Implications for models of preserved learning in amnesia. J Clin Exp Neuropsychol 1987;9:191-224.
65. Flicker CC, Ferris S, Crook T, Bartus RT. Implications of memory and language dysfunction in the naming deficits of senile dementia. Brain Lang 1987;31:187-200.
66. Cox D, Bayles KA, Trosset MW. Category and attribute knowledge in Alzheimer's disease. 1993. Submitted.
67. Obler LK. Narrative discourse style in the elderly. In: Obler LK, Albert ML, eds. Language and communication in the elderly. Lexington, MA: DC Heath 1980:75-90.
68. Bayles KA. Language function in senile dementia. Brain Lang 1982;16:265-280.
69. Cushman LA, Caine ED. A controlled study of processing of semantic and syntactic information in Alzheimer's disease. Arch Clin Neuropsychol 1987;2:283-292.
70. Perez FI, Gay JR, Taylor RL. WAIS performance of neurologically impaired aged. Psychol Rep 1975;37:1043-1047.
71. Crookes TG. Indices of early dementia on WAIS. Psychol Rep 1974;34:734.

72. Tomoeda CK, Bayles KA. Longitudinal effects of Alzheimer's disease on discourse production. Alzheimer Dis Assoc Disord. In press.
73. Bayles KA, Boone DR, Tomoeda CK, Slauson TJ, Kaszniak AW. Differentiating Alzheimer's patients from the normal elderly and stroke patients with aphasia. J Speech Hear Dis 1989;54:74–87.
74. Barker M, Lawson J. Nominal aphasia in dementia. Br J Psychiatry 1968;114: 1351–1356.
75. Bayles KA, Tomoeda CK. Confrontation naming impairment in dementia. Brain Lang 1983;10:98–114.
76. Hart S. Language and dementia: A review. Psychol Med 1988;18:99–112.
77. Kirshner HS, Webb WG, Kelly MP. The naming disorder of dementia. Neuropsychologia 1984;22:23–30.
78. Lawson JS, Barker MG. The assessment of nominal dysphasia in dementia: The use of reaction-time measures. Br J Med Psychol 1968;41:411–414.
79. Margolin DI, Pate DS, Friedrich FJ, Elia E. Dysnomia in dementia and in stroke patients: Different underlying cognitive deficits. J Clin Exp Neuropsychol 1990; 12:597–612.
80. Rochford G. A study of naming errors in dysphasic and demented patients. Neuropsychologia 1971;9:437–443.
81. Schwartz MF, Saffran EM, Williamson S. The breakdown of lexicon in Alzheimer's dementia. Presented at the Linguistics Society of America meeting, New York, 1981.
82. Skelton-Robinson M, Jones S. Nominal dysphasia and the severity of senile dementia. Br J Psychiatry 1984;145:168–171.
83. Bayles KA, Trosset MW. Confrontation naming in Alzheimer's patients: Relation to disease severity. Psychol Aging 1992;7:192–203.
84. Emery OB, Breslau LD. The problem of naming in SDAT: A relative deficit. Exp Aging Res 1988;14(4):181–193.
85. Reisberg B, Ferris SH, Crook T. Signs, symptoms, and course of age-associated cognitive decline. In: Corkin S, Davis KL, Growdon JH, Usdin E, Wurtman RL, eds. Aging. Vol 19. Alzheimer's disease: A report of progress. New York: Raven Press, 1982:177–181.
86. Folstein MF, Folstein SE, McHugh PR. Mini Mental State: A practical method for grading the cognitive state of patients for the clinician. J Psychiatr Res 1975; 12:189–198.
87. Kirshner HS, Casey PF, Kelly MP, Webb WG. Anomia in cerebral diseases. Neuropsychologia 1987;25:701–705.
88. Bayles KA, Tomoeda CK, Trosset MW. Naming and categorical knowledge in Alzheimer's disease: The process of semantic memory deterioration. Brain Lang 1990;39:498–510.
89. Benson DF. Neurologic correlates of anomia. In: Whitaker H, Whitaker HA, eds. Studies in neurolinguistics. Vol 4. New York: Academic Press, 1979:293–328.
90. Corkin S. Growdon JH, Nissen MJ, Huff FJ, Freed DM, Sagar HJ. Recent advances in the neuropsychological study of Alzheimer's disease. In: Wurtman RJ, Corkin SH, Growdon JH, eds. Alzheimer's disease: Advances in basic research and therapies. Cambridge, MA, 1984:75–93.

91. Bayles KA, Tomoeda CK. Confrontation and generative naming abilities of dementia patients. In: Brookshire RH, ed. Proceedings of the clinical aphasiology conference. Minneapolis, MN: BRK Publishers, 1983:304–315.
92. Bayles KA, Tomoeda CK, Trosset MW. Alzheimer's disease: Effects on language. Submitted for review.
93. Holland AL, McBurney DH, Moossy J, Reinmuth OM. The dissolution of language in Pick's disease with neurofibrillary tangles: A case study. Brain Lang 1985;24:36–58.
94. Gustafson L, Brun A, Risberg J. Frontal lobe dementia of non-Alzheimer type. In: Wurtman RJ, Corkin S, Growdon JH, Ritter-Walker E, eds. Advances in neurology: Alzheimer's disease. Vol 51. New York: Raven Press, 1990:65–71.
95. Cummings JL. Dementia of the Alzheimer type: Challenges of definition and clinical diagnosis. In: Whitaker HA, ed. Neuropsychological studies of nonfocal brain damage. New York: Springer-Verlag, 1988:86–107.
96. Feher EP, Inbody SB, Nolan B, Pirozzolo FJ. Other neurologic diseases with dementia as a sequela. Clin Geriatr Med 1988;4(4):799–815.
97. Cummings JL. The dementias of Parkinson's disease: Prevalence, characteristics, neurobiology, and comparison with dementia of the Alzheimer type. Eur Neurol 1988;28(1):15–23.
98. Brown RG, Marsden CD. How common is dementia in Parkinson's disease? Lancet 1984;ii:1262–1265.
99. Bayles KA. Language and Parkinson Disease. Alzheimer Dis Assoc Dis 1990; 4(3):171–180.
100. Taub HA. Comprehension and memory of prose materials ;by young and old adults. Exp Aging Res 1979;5:3–13.
101. Moenster P. Learning and memory in relation to age. J Gerontol 1972;27: 361–363.
102. Gordon SK. Clark WC. Application of signal detection theory to prose recall and recognition in elderly and young adults. J Gerontol 1974;29:64–72.
103. Spilich GJ. Life-span components of text processing: Structural and procedural differences. J Verbal Learn Verbal Behav 1983;22:231–244.
104. Kemper S. Imitation of complex syntactic constructions by elderly adults. Appl Psycholing 1986;7:277–288.
105. Petros T, Tabor L, Cooney T, Chabot RJ. Adult age differences in sensitivity to semantic structure of prose. Dev Psychol 1983;19:907–914.
106. Zelinski EM, Light LL, Gilewski MJ. Adult age differences in memory for prose: The question of sensitivity to passage structure. Dev Psychol 1984;20: 1181–1192.
107. Dixon RA, Simon EW, Nowak CA, Hultsch DF. Text recall in adulthood as a function of level of information, input modality, and delay interval. J Gerontol 1982;37:358–364.
108. Zelinski EM, Gilewski MJ, Thompson LW. Do laboratory tests relate to selfassessment of memory ability in the young and old? In: Poon LW, Fozard JL, Cermak LS, Arenberg D, Thompson LW, eds. New directions in memory and aging: Proceedings of the George Talland Memorial Conference. Hillsdale, NJ: Erlbaum, 1980:519–544.

109. Dixon RA, Hultsch DF, Simon EW, von Eye A. Verbal ability and text structure effects on adult age differences in text recall. J Verbal Learn Verbal Behav 1984;23:569–578.
110. Byrd M. Age differences in memory for prose passages. Unpublished doctoral dissertation, Department of Psychology, University of Toronto, 1981.
111. Meyer B, Rice GE. Information recalled from prose by young, middle, and old adult readers. Exp Aging Res 1981;7:253–286.
112. Belmore SM. Age related changes in processing explicit and implicit language. J Gerontol 1981;36:316–322.
113. Till RE, Walsh DA. Encoding and retrieval factors in adult memory for implicational sentences. J Verbal Learn Verbal Behav 1980;19:1–16.
114. Camp CJ. The use of fact retrieval vs. inference in young and elderly adults. J Gerontol 1981;36:715–721.
115. Walsh DA, Baldwin M. Age differences in integrated semantic memory. Dev Psychol 1977;13:509–514.

14

Primary Progressive Aphasia Syndrome

Howard S. Kirshner

Vanderbilt University School of Medicine, Nashville, Tennessee

INTRODUCTION

Although language has not been emphasized as a major aspect of the early cognitive deficit of dementia, Alzheimer's seminal case report (1) contained a clear description of a fluent aphasia. Macdonald Critchley (2) also called attention to words from Ecclesiastes regarding changes in speech with aging: "And all the daughters of musick shall be brought low." In Chapter 13 of this volume, Dr. Bayles elegantly reviews the evidence that language is one of the cortical functions most typically affected by dementia.

One way of summarizing the extensive evidence on language and dementia is to epitomize the course of language involvement in a "typical dementia" such as Alzheimer's disease (AD). The earliest stage often begins with memory loss, including deficient memory for names (3–5). Aphasia testing in early demented subjects often shows anomic aphasia. As the disease progresses, articulation, repetition, and oral reading remain largely intact, but the speech becomes progressively impoverished in discourse elements and abstract content. Reading comprehension and writing tend to be affected more severely than auditory comprehension and speech, but auditory comprehension also declines. In linguistic terms, syntax and articulation are preserved long after semantics and discourse fail. In the middle stages of the disease, aphasia testing often results in a classification of transcortical sensory or Wernicke's aphasia. In the final phase of the disease, patients become almost mute, uttering only expressions of biological need (6–8).

In distinction to this "common" pattern of language involvement in dementia, a less common but increasingly recognized group of elderly patients shows progressive language impairment, resembling aphasia from focal lesions such as strokes. In such cases, language deterioration is the presenting feature, and other cognitive functions remain preserved. While progressive language syndromes do not have as long a history as Alzheimer's disease, suggestive cases have been reported in the past, including Alajouanine's 1948 description of the progressive, fluent aphasia and musical illiteracy of the composer Maurice Ravel (9,10). Mesulam (11) called attention to such cases under the name *slowly progressive aphasia without generalized dementia*, later shortened to *primary progressive aphasia* (PPA) (12). Six patients were described in whom aphasia progressed over a period of years, in the absence of any impairment of right-hemisphere functions, memory, social graces, or reasoning. CT scanning and electroencephalography yielded evidence of focal left-hemisphere dysfunction in some cases. A single patient underwent biopsy of the left superior temporal gyrus. The sections showed only lipofuscin staining in neurons, an age-related change, but no specific pathological features of Alzheimer's or Pick's disease. Mesulam (11) postulated that these cases represented a selective degenerative disease, with a predilection for specific neurons in the left perisylvian language cortex.

CLINICAL FEATURES OF PRIMARY PROGRESSIVE APHASIA

In the ensuing years, numerous reports have appeared documenting the clinical entity of primary progressive aphasia. The syndrome is defined as a progressive disorder with prominent language deficits, preservation of other mental functions, and intact activities of daily living. To qualify, patients must have met these criteria for at least a 2-year period. Most patients with progressive aphasia do not appear demented, often maintaining ability to function well in nonverbal areas, pursuing hobbies, and even continuing to work (13). This preservation of cognitive function is what separates patients with progressive aphasia from those with generalized dementias such as Alzheimer's disease.

The pattern of language deterioration also differs from that of AD, but there is considerable variability in language profile. Weintraub and colleagues (13) pointed out that, whereas patients with Alzheimer's disease tend to have fluent aphasias of the anomic, transcortical sensory, and Wernicke's type, patients with primary progressive aphasia tend to have nonfluent syndromes such as Broca's and transcortical motor aphasia. Literal (phonemic) rather than verbal (semantic) errors in naming characterize PPA as compared with AD. Linguistically, the syntactic, morphological, and phonological aspects of language, which are typically preserved in Alzheimer's disease, are often affected in progressive aphasia, whereas the lexical and semantic aspects are more typically affected in AD (13). Karbe, Kertesz, and Polk (14) recently reported results of language testing in 10 patients with PPA. Anomia, reduced fluency, and mild agrammatism were characteristically seen in these patients, although nine of the 10 cases were classified as anomic aphasics. Language comprehension tended to remain preserved.

Not all patients with PPA, however, follow the pattern of reduced fluency and agrammatism. For example, cases have been reported with fluent aphasia (11,15–20) and with selective auditory-comprehension difficulty resembling pure word deafness (15,21,22). Caselli and Jack (23) recently reported, under the new name *asymmetric cortical degeneration syndromes*, 12 cases of progressive aphasia, of which seven were dysfluent, five were fluent. Two groups (24,25) have applied the term *semantic dementia* to patients with progressive aphasia with a deficit profile including fluent aphasia, severe anomia, poor comprehension, and poor semantic memory, with preserved phonology, spoken syntax, and comprehension of syntactic commands. Reading in some of these patients showed surface dyslexia (see Chapter 10). Specific language features are thus variable in PPA, and a "typical language syndrome" cannot be specified.

LABORATORY TESTING AND BRAIN IMAGING IN PPA

Standard laboratory testing is generally unrevealing in PPA. CT and MRI scans reveal either focal left perisylvian or generalized atrophy, electroencephalography shows variable slowing, and tests of spinal fluid and blood are unremarkable. In comparison to the relative insensitivity of structural brain imaging techniques such as CT and MRI, functional brain imaging with positron emission tomographic (PET) scanning has been very illuminating in progressive aphasia. Areas of focal, left-hemisphere hypometabolism have been consistently described in patients with this syndrome (18, 26,27). Tyrrell et al. (27) found that early cases of PPA had isolated areas of reduced cerebral blood flow in the left temporal lobe, while more advanced cases had involvement of the frontal and parietal lobes as well. These findings suggest that the disease process begins in the dominant temporal lobe and then spreads to adjacent cortical areas. Hodges et al. (25), in their report of "semantic dementia," also found evidence of focal, left temporal hypometabolism by PET in one patient and by SPECT in five patients. SPECT also showed focal, left frontotemoral hypometabolism in patients with progressive aphasia studied by Caselli and Jack (23) and in the frontal lobes in the case of Kartsounis and colleagues (28).

Recently, Tyrell and colleagues (29) reported three patients with progressive dysarthria and orofacial dyspraxia, followed by other cognitive deficits, in whom the changes on PET were predominantly frontal. The PET changes in all these cases are distinct from those reported in Alzheimer's disease, in which bilateral temporoparietal areas of reduced blood flow and metabolism are characteristic (30,31). Foster et al. (32) reported PET studies of patients with presumed Alzheimer's disease in which either aphasic or visuospatial deficits predominated; focal or unilateral left-hemisphere hypometabolism was seen in aphasic patients, right-hemisphere hypometabolism was reported in patients with visuospatial deficits, and patients with predominantly memory loss had no consistent asymmetry of metabolism. These patients did not have pathological confirmation of the diagnosis of Alzheimer's disease, and it is possible that some of the "aphasic" patients had the PPA syndrome.

Figure 1 shows a PET scan from a recently studied case of progressive aphasia. There is marked bifrontal hypometabolism.

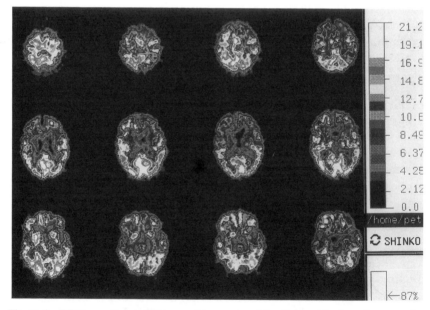

Figure 1 PET scan from a 70-year-old woman with a 2-year history of progressive nonfluent aphasia with severe anomia. Other cognitive functions appeared intact. The scan shows profoundly decreased metabolism (uptake of fluorodeoxyglucose) in both frontal lobes.

DISEASES CAUSING PROGRESSIVE APHASIA

A number of authors (15,34–37) have reported patients in whom aphasia was a presenting or disproportionate deficit, but in whom a generalized dementia could be diagnosed either at presentation or over time. These authors have questioned whether progressive aphasia is a true syndrome, or merely a point in the spectrum of typical dementing diseases in which the pathological changes happen to become evident first in relatively localized areas of the brain. Mesulam (11) has continued to define progressive aphasia as a separate entity from typical dementing illnesses such as Alzheimer's disease. Neuropathological studies in well-documented cases of progressive aphasia have been few, but the available studies support the concept that several different pathological substrates can produce the syndrome of progressive aphasia.

Pick's Disease

The first disease documented to cause progressive aphasia is Pick's disease. Pick's original case report (38) involved a patient in whom a prominent language deterioration accompanied a dementia. Pick anticipated contemporary studies in noting that the aphasia was similar to the syndrome of transcortical sensory aphasia, which had been described a few years earlier by Wernicke and Lichtheim in patients with focal brain lesions. Pick also addressed the issue of focal versus diffuse disease: "simple progressive brain atrophy can lead to symptoms of local disturbance through local accentuation of the diffuse process." The neuropathology of Pick's disease involves a focal, lobar atrophy affecting the frontal and temporal lobes of one or both hemispheres. Surviving cortical neurons may have large, silver-staining cytoplasmic inclusions called "Pick bodies."

Cases of pathologically proved Pick's disease have recently been reported in which aphasia was the presenting symptom. Wechsler (39) reported a single case of isolated, progressive, fluent aphasia; 2 years after onset, a generalized dementia had supervened. At postmortem examination, definite lobar atrophy and microscopic Pick inclusion bodies were found (40). Holland and colleagues (21) reported a patient with a 12-year history of progressive language deficits involving predominantly a pure word deafness. The patient was able to write notes to his family, keep his own financial records, and take public transportation to his appointments. Late in the course, behavioral disturbances developed. Graff-Radford and colleagues (19) reported an autopsy-proved case of Pick's disease in whom a profound anomia was the presenting symptom. These authors postulated that the localized degeneration of the left inferior and middle temporal gyri produced a relatively pure anomia, while later, more widespread degeneration of the left temporal lobe, bilateral frontal, and right temporal lobes produced the progressive aphasia and dementia. Karbe, Kertesz, and Polk (14) also reported, in their series of progressive aphasia cases, one with postmortem findings of left frontal and parietal atrophy and microscopic changes of Pick's disease.

Aphasia characteristics may be useful in separating patients with Pick's disease from patients with AD. In the series of Knopman et al. (41) and Gustafson and Nilsson (42), reduced speech fluency and echolalia were more prominent in Pick's disease. Mendez and colleagues (43) recently reported comparisons of behavioral deficits in pathologically confirmed cases of Pick's and Alzheimer's diseases. The most helpful features in diagnosing Pick's disease were presenile onset, initial personality change, hyperorality, disinhibition, and roaming behavior. Patients with Pick's disease often manifested reduced speech fluency, with echolalia and verbal stereotypies, while Alzheimer's disease patients tended to have fluent speech with paraphasic errors, but these language features did not reliably distinguish the two groups of patients. Late in Pick's disease, the Kluver-Bucy syndrome of hyperorality, hypersexuality, and visual agnosia may develop (42–44).

"Nonspecific" Neurodegenerative Diseases

Closely related to Pick's disease is the disorder reported by Morris and colleagues (45) termed *hereditary dysphasic dementia*. Ten cases were reported from three generations of a single family, four with autopsy confirmation, suggesting an autosomal dominant inheritance pattern. These patients presented with anomia and fluent aphasia, as well as generalized dementia. The pathology included frontal and temporal lobe atrophy. Microscopic changes were not characteristic of any one disease; the affected cortex contained senile plaques, gliosis, spongiform change, and loss of neurons, without Pick bodies. Neuronal loss was also present in the substantia nigra of the midbrain, the site of pathology in Parkinson's disease. This pathology seems most closely related to familial Pick's disease. A patient with progressive aphasia has been reported in whom autopsy showed focal left frontotemporal atrophy, neuronal loss, and gliosis, without Pick bodies; a diagnosis of atypical Pick's disease was made (46). Cases of familial (47) and nonfamilial (48) "atypical dementia" have had similar neuropathological changes, but without disproportionate or early language deterioration.

Two cases of progressive aphasia, reported previously in a clinical series of six patients (15), came to autopsy in our hospital (49). The first patient had a 10-year history of progressive word deafness and deterioration of expressive speech. His symptoms began with word deafness and a pattern of prefixing and suffixing extra syllables to words (*logoclonia*), which later gave way to complete jargon speech. Reading and writing, as well as deportment and memory, remained intact for more than 5 years into the illness. In late stages, he became mute, able to write only single words, and less able to read printed messages. He also began having temper outbursts with his family and ultimately required placement in a nursing home, where he became bedridden and died. The second patient had a mixed aphasia with anomia and paraphasic errors, more rapidly progressive than the first. This man later developed muscle atrophy and fasciculations suggesting motor neuron disease. At autopsy, both patients had focal atrophy of the left frontal and temporal lobes. Microscopically, both had a spongiform change, or vacuolation of the neuropil, present principally in the second cortical layer, along with neuronal loss and gliosis. Changes of Alzheimer's disease and Pick bodies were absent. While these pathological changes are nonspecific, the findings appear to confirm Mesulam's postulate of a focal degeneration of neurons in the left-hemisphere perisylvian language cortex. Recently, Green and colleagues (36) reported very similar changes at autopsy in a case of progressive aphasia.

Creutzfeldt-Jakob Disease

Another neurodegenerative disease recently reported to produce progressive aphasia is Creutzfeldt-Jakob disease (CJD). Usually, this disease is manifest by mood and personality changes, rapidly progressive dementia, and myoclonus, often with exaggerated or myoclonic responses to startle, and epileptic seizures. Most cases progress to death within several months (50). Mandell et al. (51) reported a patient with pathologically proved CJD in whom fluent aphasia was the sole presenting complaint and the only major deficit over an 8-month period. By 11 months after onset, however, progressive dementia had developed, and death from status epilepticus occurred at 13 months. In comparison to other cases of progressive aphasia, the progression to dementia in CJD tends to be much faster, and the patients typically have myoclonus, exaggerated startle responses, and a characteristically abnormal EEG. The pathology in CJD also differs from that of our two cases of progressive aphasia, in that the spongy change is seen through all six layers of the cortex and throughtout both hemispheres. The vacuoles are typically intracellular, while those in our cases were both intra- and extracellular (52).

Corticobasal Degeneration

Another rare neurodegenerative disease reported in association with progressive aphasia is corticobasal degeneration with neuronal achromasia. Lippa and colleagues (53) described a 69-year-old man with a 3-year history of progressive aphasia of transcortical motor type. Ultimately, his speech became limited to a few simple words, while he remained cognitively intact except for a short attention span. Right-arm posturing, decreased right-arm swing during walking, and a right upgoing toe were noted later in the course. At autopsy, focal cortical degeneration was found in the left frontal lobe, with remaining neurons showing swollen cytoplasm and loss of Nissl substance (*achromasia*), a pattern seen in patients with a combination of motor and cognitive deficits referred to as *corticobasal degeneration* (54).

Alzheimer's Disease

Alzheimer's disease is the most common disease producing dementia. Despite Alzheimer's description of aphasia as a prominent part of the dementia in his original patient (1), only a few cases of pathologically proved Alzheimer's disease have been reported in whom aphasia was an isolated presenting symptoms (14,18,36,55). Green and colleagues (36) reported eight cases of progressive aphasia ascertained from a large dementia study. Of two cases with autopsy data, one showed a spongiform change with neuronal loss, similar to the cases of Kirshner et al. (49), and the other had pathologically proved Alzheimer's disease. By the time of the autopsy, the changes of neuritic plaques and neurofibrillary tangles were widespread throughout the brain. Of the 10 cases reported by Karbe et al. (14), two came to postmortem examination; one had AD, the other Pick's disease. Both Green and colleagues (36) and Kempler et al. (18) predicted that most patients with progressive aphasia will prove to have Alzheimer's disease, since it is by such a large margin the most common cause of dementia. The pattern of progressive aphasia, however, with deficits restricted to the left-hemisphere language cortex over extended periods of time, appears to be uncommon in patients with Alzheimer's disease.

Other authors have considered whether Alzheimer's disease with prominent language degeneration differs clinically from the more typical cases of AD. One source of controversy has been the clinical dictum that early-onset cases of Alzheimer's disease are more likely to manifest "focal" deficits such as aphasia, apraxia, and agnosia than the senile cases (56–59). Recent studies by Selnes et al. (60) and Bayles (61) have not confirmed this association, finding only that language disorder correlates with severity of dementia. One recent study (62) did not find any significant differences between early- and late-onset cases of AD in terms of cognitive profile or rate of progression. It is not clear, therefore, that the presence of prominent language deficit can be used as a predictor of rapid progression. Prominent language disorder has also been found to be a predictor of familial Alzheimer's disease (63), but a more recent study found only that familial AD patients have a more rapid clinical course than nonfamilial cases (64).

FRONTAL LOBE DEMENTIA

Another "focal" variant of dementia, overlapping the primary progressive aphasia syndrome, is the progressive development of a frontal lobe syndrome, or *frontal lobe dementia*. Personality changes, rather than cognitive or memory loss, may predominante in the presenting clinical picture of these cases. Apathy, pathological unconcern, jocularity and disinhibition, obsessive traits, loss of social empathy and awareness, and distractability and poor attention characterize these patients (65). Many cases of Pick's disease present with personality changes rather than with cognitive or memory loss (66). As mentioned earlier, Tyrrell et al. (29) have reported three patients with frontal hypometabolism on PET who had a distinctive syndrome of dysarthria, orofacial apraxia, and later development of more widespread cognitive deficits. One patient had associated signs of motor neuron disease. No autopsy confirmation was available. These cases may be considered to represent a "frontal" variant of the progressive aphasia syndrome.

MOTOR NEURON DISEASE, PROGRESSIVE APHASIA, AND DEMENTIA

As mentioned earlier, a few cases of progressive aphasia have had associated changes of motor neuron disease (15,29). Motor neuron disease, or amyotrophic lateral sclerosis (ALS), is characterized by progressive weakness and muscle wasting, fasciculations or muscle twitches, and upper motor neuron signs such as spasticity and increased reflexes. Most cases of ALS have no associated mental or cognitive change. Wikstrom et al. (67) and Horoupian and colleagues (68) each described three patients with dementia and motor neuron disease. The neuropathology was that of an "atypical dementia" similar to that described by Kim et al. (47), Masse et al. (69), and Knopman et al. (41). The pathology in these cases involved neuronal loss and gliosis, with spongy change in the superficial cortical layers, without neurofibrillary tangles, senile plaques, or Pick bodies. Knopman et al. (41) found that these cases were as common as Pick's disease in their series.

Two recent studies (70,71) have likewise reported the association of "frontal dementia" and motor neuron disease, with postmortem confirmation of an atypical dementia with gliosis and spongiform change. These pathological changes are similar to those of some cases of progressive aphasia (49, 36), except for their more widespread distribution, and also to those of the "hereditary dysphasic dementia" syndrome (45). Similar spongy change of superficial cortical layers has also been described in dialysis encephalopathy (72), which involves speech and language abnormalities, and in the Parkinsonian-dementia complex of Guam (73), which features motor neuron degeneration. The range of histopathology underlying frontal dementia and dementia associated with motor neuron disease requires further study, as does the range of clinical phenomenology associated with the pathology of "atypical dementia."

SUMMARY AND CONCLUSIONS

This chapter has reviewed the clinical syndrome of primary progressive aphasia, in the absence of generalized dementia. These cases are distinct from the language deterioration that occurs in the course of generalized dementing diseases such as Alzheimer's disease, resembling more closely focal stroke syndromes with aphasia. In general, these patients do not suffer any generalized cognitive deterioration or any dysfunction in activities of daily living until late in the course, although subtle exceptions can be found in the musical abilities of a composer (9) or in the artistic productions of a commercial artist (74). The distinctions between "focal" and "generalized" disease are somewhat blurred, and there is still much to be learned about the spectrum of diseases that can produce progressive language impairment. Emerging brain imaging modalities such as positron emission tomography and continued clinical-pathological correlation should contribute to our knowledge of this interesting syndrome in the future.

REFERENCES

1. Alzheimer A. Uber eine eigenartige erkrankung der hirnrinde. Allg Zeitschrift für Psychiatrie und Psychisch-Gerichliche Med 1907;64:146–148. In: Rottenberg DA, Hochberg FH, eds. Neurological classics in modern translation. New York: Hafner Press, 1977:41–43.
2. Critchley M. And all the daughters of musick shall be brought low. Language function in the elderly. Arch Neurol 1984;41:1135–1139.
3. Bayles KA, Tomoeda CK. Confrontational naming impairment in dementia. Brain Lang 1983;19:98–114.
4. Kirshner HS, Webb WG, Kelly MP. The naming disorder of dementia. Neuropsychologia 1984;22:23–30.
5. Williams BW, Mack W, Henderson VW. Boston Naming Test in Alzheimer's disease. Neuropsychologia 1989;27:1073–1079.
6. Appell J, Kertesz A, Fisman M. A study of language functioning in Alzheimer patients. Brain Lang 1982;17:73–91.
7. Cummings JL, Benson DF, Hill MA, Read S. Aphasia in dementia of the Alzheimer type. Neurology 1985;35:394–397.
8. Faber-Langendoen K, Morris JC, Knesevich JW, LaBarge E, Miller JP, Berg L. Aphasia in senile dementia of the Alzheimer type. Ann Neurol 1988;23:365–370.
9. Alajouanine T. Aphasia and artistic realization. Brain 1948;74:229–241.
10. Sergent J. Music, the brain and Ravel. TINS 1993;16:168–172.
11. Mesulam M-M. Slowly progressive aphasia without generalized dementia. Ann Neurol 1982;11:592–598.

12. Mesulam M-M. Primary progressive aphasia – Differentiation from Alzheimer's disease. Ann Neurol 1987;22:533–534.
13. Weintraub S, Rubin NP, Mesulam M-M. Primary progressive aphasia: longitudinal course, neuropsychological profile, and language features. Arch Neurol 1990;47:1329–1335.
14. Karbe H, Kertesz A, Polk M. Profiles of language impairment in primary progressive aphasia. Arch Neurol 1993;50:193–201.
15. Kirshner HS, Webb WG, Kelly MP, Wells CE. Language disturbance. An initial symptom of cortical degenerations and dementia. Arch Neurol 1984;41: 491–496.
16. Sapin LR, Anderson FH, Pulaski PD. Progressive aphasia without dementia: further documentation. Ann Neurol 1989;25:411–413.
17. Mandell AM, Alexander MP, Carpenter S. Creutzfeldt-Jakob disease presenting as isolated aphasia. Neurology 1989;39:55–58.
18. Kempler D, Metter EJ, Riege WH, Jackson CA, Benson DF, Hanson WR. Slowly progressive aphasia: three cases with language, memory, CT and PET data. J Neurol Neurosurg Psychiatry 1990;53:987–993.
19. Graff-Radford NR, Damasio AR, Hyman BT, Hart MN, Tranel D, Damasio H, Van Hoesen GW, Rezai K. Progressive aphasia in a patient with Pick's disease: a neuropsychological, radiologic, and anatomic study. Neurology 1990;40: 620–626.
20. Benson DF, Zaias BW. Progressive aphasia: a case with postmortem correlation. Neuropsychiatry Neuropsychol Behav Neurol 1991;4:215–223.
21. Holland AL, McBurney DH, Moossy J, Reinmuth OM. The dissolution of language in Pick's disease with neurofibrillary tangles: a case study. Brain Lang 1985;24:36–58.
22. Croisile B, Laurent B, Michel D, LeBars D, Cinotti L, Mauguiere F. Differentes modalités cliniques des aphasies degeneratives. Rev Neurol (Paris) 1991; 147:192–199.
23. Caselli R, Jack CR. Asymmetric cortical degeneration syndromes. A proposed clinical classification. Arch Neurol 1992;49:770–780.
24. Snowden JS, Goulding PJ, Neary D. Semantic dementia: a form of circumscribed cerebral atrophy. Behav Neurol 1989;2:167–182.
25. Hodges JR, Patterson K, Oxbury S, Funnell E. Semantic dementia. Progressive fluent aphasia with temporal lobe atrophy. Brain 1992;115:1783–1806.
26. Chawluk JB, Mesulam M-M, Hurtig H, Kushner M, Weintraub S, Saykin A, Rubin N, Alavi A, Reivich M. Slowly progressive aphasia without generalized dementia: studies with positron emission tomography. Ann Neurol 1986;19: 68–84.
27. Tyrrell PJ, Warrington EK, Frackowiak RSJ, Rossor MN. Heterogeneity in progressive aphasia due to focal cortical atrophy. Brain 1990;113:1321–1336.
28. Kartsounis LD, Crellin RF, Crewes H, Toone BK. Primary progressive nonfluent aphasia: a case study. Cortex 1991;27:121–129.
29. Tyrrell PJ, Kartsounis LD, Frackowiak RSJ, Findley LJ, Rossor MN. Progressive loss of speech output and orofacial dyspraxia associated with frontal lobe hypometabolism. J Neurol Neurosurg Psychiatry 1991;54:351–357.

30. Frackowiak RSJ, Pozzilli C, Legg NJ, DuBoulay GH, Marshall J, Lenzi GL, Jones T. Regional cerebral oxygen supply and utilization in dementia: a clinical and physiological study with oxygen-15 and positron tomography. Brain 1981; 104:753–778.

31. Goto I, Takayuki T, Hosokawa S, Otsuka M, Ichiya Y, Ichimiya A. Positron emission tomographic (PET) studies in dementia. J Neurol Sci 1993;114:1–6.

32. Foster NL, Chase TN, Fedio P, Patronas NJ, Brooks RA, DiChiro G. Alzheimer's disease: focal cortical changes shown by positron emission tomography. Neurology 1983;33:961–965.

33. Foster NL, Chase TN. Diffuse involvement in progressive aphasia. Ann Neurol 1983;13:224–225.

34. Gordon B, Selnes O. Progressive aphasia "without dementia": evidence of more widespread involvement. Neurology 1984;34(suppl):102.

35. Poeck K. Luzzatti C. Slowly progressive aphasia in three patients. Brain 1988; 111:151–168.

36. Green J, Morris JC, Sandson J, McKeel DW, Miller JW. Progressive aphasia: a precursor of global dementia? Neurology 1990;40:423–429.

37. Mendez MF, Zander BA. Dementia presenting with aphasia: clinical characteristics. J Neurol Neurosurg Psychiatry 1991;54:542–545.

38. Pick A. 1892. Uber die beziehungen der senilen hirnatrophie zur aphasie. Prager Med Wochenschrift 1892;17:165–167. In: Rottenberg DA, Hochberg FH, eds. Neurological classics in modern translation. New York: Hafner Press, 1977: 35–40.

39. Wechsler AF. Presenile dementia presenting as aphasia. J Neurol Neurosurg Psychiatry 1977;40:303–305.

40. Wechsler AF, Verity A, Rosenschein S, Fried I, Scheibel AB. Pick's disease. A clinical, computed tomographic, and histologic study with Golgi impregnation observations. Arch Neurol 1982;39:287–290.

41. Knopman DS, Christensen KJ, Schut LJ, Harbaugh RE, Reeder T, Ngo T, Frey W. The spectrum of imaging and neuropsychological findings in Pick's disease. Neurology 1989;39:362–368.

42. Gustafson L, Nilsson L. Differential diagnosis of presenile dementia on clinical grounds. Acta Psych Scand 1982;65:194–209.

43. Mendez MF, Selwood A, Mastri A, Frey WH II. Pick's disease versus Alzheimer's disease: A comparison of clinical characteristics. Neurology 1993;43:289–292.

44. Cummings JL, Duchen LW. Kluver-Bucy syndrome in Pick disease: Clinical and pathological correlations. Neurology 1981;31:1415–1422.

45. Morris JC, Cole M, Banker BQ, Wright D. Hereditary dysphasic dementia and the Pick-Alzheimer spectrum. Ann Neurol 1984;16:455–466.

46. Caplan LR, Richardson EP. Case records of the Massachusetts General Hospital. N Engl J Med 1986;314:1101–1111.

47. Kim RC, Collins GH, Parisi JE, Wright AW, Chu YB. Familial dementia of adult onset with pathological findings of a "non-specific" nature. Brain 1981; 104:61–68.

48. Knopman DS, Mastri AR, Frey WH II, Sung JH, Rustan T. Dementia lacking distinctive histologic features: A common non-Alzheimer degenerative dementia. Neurology 1990;40:251-256.
49. Kirshner HS, Tanridag O, Thurman L, Whetsell WO Jr. Progressive aphasia without dementia: two cases with focal spongiform degeneration. Ann Neurol 1987;22:527-532.
50. Brown P, Cathala F, Castaigne P, Gajdusek DC. Creutzfeldt-Jakob disease: Clinical analysis of a consecutive series of 230 neuropathologically verified cases. Ann Neurol 1986;20:597-602.
51. Mandell AM, Alexander MP, Carpenter S. Creutzfeldt-Jakob disease presenting as isolated aphasia. Neurology 1989;39:55-58.
52. Masters CL, Richardson EP Jr. Subacute spongiform encephalopathy (Creutzfeldt-Jakob disease). The nature and progression of spongiform change. Brain 1978;101:333-344.
53. Lippa CF, Cohen R, Smith TW, Drachman DA. Primary progressive aphasia with focal neuronal achromasia. Neurology 1991;41:882-886.
54. Gibb WRG, Luthert PJ, Marsden CD. Corticobasal degeneration. Brain 1989; 112:1171-1192.
55. Pogacar S, Williams RS. Alzheimer's disease presenting as slowly progressive aphàsia. RI Med J 1984;67:181-185.
56. Seltzer B, Sherwin I. A comparison of clinical features in early and late-onset primary degenerative dementia: one entity or two? Arch Neurol 1983;40:143-146.
57. Chui HC, Tend EL, Henderson VW, Moy AC. Clinical subtypes of dementia of the Alzheimer type. Neurology 1985;35:1544-1550.
58. Berg L, Danzinger WL, Storandt M, Coben LA, Gado M, Hughes CP, Knesevich JW, Botwinick J. Predictive features in mild senile dementia of the Alzheimer type. Neurology 1984;34:563-569.
59. Filley CM, Kelly J, Heaton RK. Neuropsychologic features of early and late-onset Alzheimer's disease. Arch Neurol 1986;43:574-576.
60. Selnes OA, Carson K. Rovner B, Gordon B. Language dysfunction in early- and late-onset possible Alzheimer's disease. Neurology 1988;38:1053-1056.
61. Bayles KA. Age at onset of Alzheimer's disease. Relation to language dysfunction. Arch Neurol 1991;48:155-159.
62. Haupt M, Kurz A, Pollman S. Severity of symptoms and rate of progression in Alzheimer's disease: a comparison of cases with early and late onset. Dementia 1992;3:21-24.
63. Folstein MF, Breitner JCS. Language disorder predicts familial Alzheimer's disease. Johns Hopkins Med J 1981;149:145-147.
64. Luchins DJ, Cohen D. Hanrahan P, Eisdorfer C, Paveza G, Ashford JW, Gorelick P, Hirschman R, Freels S, Levy P, Semla T, Shaw H. Are there clinical differences between familial and nonfamilial Alzheimer's disease? Am J Psychiatry 1992;149:1023-1027.
65. Neary D, Snowden JS, Northen B, Goulding P. Dementia of frontal-lobe type. J Neurol Neurosurg Psychiatry 1988;51:353-361.

66. Munoz-Garcia D, Ludwin SK. Classic and generalized variants of Pick's disease: a clinicopathological, ultrastructural, and immunocytochemical comparative study. Ann Neurol 1984;16:467–480.
67. Wikstrom J, Paetau A, Palo J, Sulkava R, Haltia M. Classic amyotrophic lateral sclerosis with dementia. Arch Neurol 1982;39:681–6783.
68. Horoupian DS, Thal L, Katzman R, Terry RD, Davies P, Hirano A, DeTeresa R, Fuld PA, Petito C, Blass J, Ellis JM. Dementia and motor neuron disease: Morphometric, biochemical, and Golgi studies. Ann Neurol 1984;16:305–313.
69. Masse G, Mokol J, Brion S. Atypical presenile dementia. Report of an anatomo-clinical case and review of the literature. J Neurol Sci 1981;52:245–267.
70. Neary D, Snowden JS, Mann DMA, Northen B, Goulding PJ, Macdermott N. Frontal lobe dementia and motor neuron disease. J Neurol Neurosurg Psychiatry 1990;53:23–32.
71. Ferrer I, Roig C, Espino A, Peiro G, Matias Guiu X. Dementia of frontal lobe type and motor neuron disease. A Golgi study of the frontal cortex. J Neurol Neurosurg Psychiatry 1991;54:932–934.
72. Windelman MD, Ricanati ES. Dialysis encephalopathy: Neuropathological aspects. Hum Pathol 1986;17:823–833.
73. Tan NT, Kakulas BA, Masters CL, Chen K-M, Gibbs CJ Jr, Gajdusek DC. Clin Exp Neurol 1981;17:227–234.
74. Schwartz MF, Chawluk JB. Deterioration of language in progressive aphasia: A case study. In: Schwartz M, ed. Modular deficits in Alzheimer-type dementia. Cambridge, MA: MIT Press, 1990:245–296.

15

Language Impairment in Closed Head Injury

Sandra Bond Chapman

University of Texas at Dallas, Dallas, Texas

Harvey S. Levin

University of Maryland Medical System, Baltimore, Maryland

Kathleen A. Culhane

University of Houston, Houston, Texas

INTRODUCTION

One question frequently raised regarding the presence of language deficits in the closed-head-injured (CHI) population is whether aphasia occurs as a common neurobehavioral sequel. This question shows a bias toward defining language deficits within a narrow scope as observed in aphasia. As discussed in Chapter 1, aphasic patients represent a neurogenic population with primarily focal brain lesions typically of a vascular etiology as opposed to the diffuse injury following a closed head injury. While the conceptual framework of language–brain relationships established by classic aphasia theory has contributed to the understanding of potential language deficits following CHI, the framework has some limitations in explaining the nature of verbal deficits in this population. The limitations of restricting the language profile solely to aphasic characteristics arise from the distinctive and heterogeneous patterns of communication disorders found in CHI patients. The differences between CHI and aphasic populations are manifested in the pathophysiology, the subsequent neurobehavioral symptoms, and the underlying mechanisms. The neurological and cognitive sequelae of CHI interact with the language system in producing a different pattern of language deficits from that observed in classically defined aphasias.

This chapter focuses on the empirical evidence from recent investigations of language in CHI. The contents have theoretical and clinical significance in addressing how best to conceptualize the language abilities in this hetero-geneous, neurogenic population. From a theoretical perspective, there is growing evidence that the language disturbance in CHI should be viewed from a framework broader than that provided by classic aphasic theory. This more global framework suggests that the important issue is how one uses language to communicate, not simply how one performs on isolated linguistic measures. Such a broadened approach would explore which fac-tors, cognitive or linguistic, contribute to the breakdown of communica-tive competence. Nevertheless, aphasia theory has made important contribu-tions to the understanding of language deficits in CHI. As suggested below, certain language deficits may be explained in part by focal brain lesions that are commonly concomitant with the well-documented diffuse damage asso-ciated with CHI.

From a clinical perspective, the empirical findings relevant to language disturbances in CHI indicate that traditional language measures do not fully characterize the nature of linguistic sequelae. The language deficits are more readily discernible on tasks with greater cognitive demands than those in conventional measures. Recent neurolinguistic studies suggest that discourse measures may be a promising clinical tool for elucidating the interrelation-ship among linguistic and certain cognitive abilities.

The issues addressed in this chapter are:

1. The pathophysiological profile in CHI
2. Language abilities at early and late phases of recovery
3. The contributions and limitations of applying an aphasia model to CHI
4. The use of traditional language measures versus discourse measures in assessing language abilities in CHI
5. An integrated approach: the interdependency of language, cognition, and neurological profile
6. Critical issues related to recovery
7. A case for subgroups

DEFINITION AND PATHOPHYSIOLOGY

CHI, as used in this chapter, refers to a nonmissile head injury in which the primary traumatic force is a sudden acceleration or deceleration. The sud-den acceleration/deceleration imparted to a freely moving head, possibly combined with an external impact, produces a variety of neuropathological profiles, involving diffuse injury and focal brain lesions. Diffuse axonal injury (DAI) involves the tearing and stretching of nerve fibers due to the mechanical forces at the moment of impact. Severe DAI typically produces immediate coma and tends to occur more often in high-velocity injuries (e.g., motor vehicle crashes) than in lower-velocity injuries such as falls (1). Degeneration of the cerebral white matter, a common sequel of severe DAI, is reflected by lateral ventricular enlargement. Hypoxic-ischemic injury, a major cause of grey-matter insult, can result from hypoxia due to periods of apnea and increased intracranial pressure. Hypoxia seems to selectively affect the basal ganglia, hippocampus, and cerebral artery zones (2).

Focal brain lesions commonly identified in CHI patients include contusions and hematomas, which occur most frequently in the frontotemporal cortex. Contusions commonly result from transient in-bending of the skull or from penetration of a bone fragment subsequent to depressed skull fracture (3). The orbital surface of the frontal lobes and the anterior temporal lobes are particularly vulnerable to injury due to compression against the bony prominences of the sphenoid wing. Hematomas commonly occur in the same region of the frontotemporal cortex as contusions and may involve the extradural and/or intradural compartments. Intradural hematomas injure the brain by compression.

Impaired consciousness, which varies in depth and duration, is a characteristic feature of CHI and provides an index of severity of acute injury. The Glasgow Coma Scale (GCS), developed by Teasdale and Jennett (4), is the tool most commonly used to assess coma. As shown in Table 1, the GCS consists of three components: the minimal stimulus necessary to elicit eye opening, the best motor response to command or to painful stimulation, and the best verbal response. Determination of severity is derived by combining the component scores of the GCS (possible range 3 to 15). As defined by Jennett et al. (5), the acute CHI is considered severe if the patient's GCS is 8 or less (i.e., no eye opening, inability to obey commands, and vocalization limited to incomprehensible sounds) for a period of at least 6 hours. Recently, the 6-hour requirement for chronicity has been deleted. A moderate CHI is typically defined as a GCS of 9 to 12, indicating impaired consciousness without coma. A mild CHI is reflected by confusion and disorientation (a GCS score from 13 to 15).

Table 1 The Glasgow Coma Scale

Best eye opening		Best motor response		Best verbal response
4 Spontaneous	6	Obeys commands	5	Oriented
3 To speech	5	Localizes to pain	4	Confused
2 To pain	4	Flexion-withdrawal to pain	3	Inappropriate words
1 None	3	Abnormal flexion to pain	2	Incomprehensible
	2	Extension to pain	1	None
	1	None		

Conceptual Model

The mechanisms of brain injury commonly identified in CHI are depicted in Figure 1. As illustrated, the pathophysiology of the injury may include diffuse axonal injury, focal lesions, ischemia, and neurochemical changes. This mix of pathophysiological mechanisms interacts with the severity of the injury and the patient's premorbid status to produce diverse patterns of neurobehavioral deficits and islands of preserved function. Figure 1 identifies the most common areas of neurobehavioral impairment in CHI. These areas include general cognitive, visuospatial, language, memory, attention, and behavioral deficits. The purpose of this model is to illustrate the direct relationship between the pathophysiology and the neurobehavioral consequences of CHI that result in functional disability for an individual. Figure 1 does not represent a processing model in that it does not depict the complex interactions among the neurobehavioral sequelae.

Focal and Diffuse Lesions

The considerable heterogeneity in severity and type of injury after CHI reflects individual patterns of focal and diffuse insult. Adding to this variability are the premorbid characteristics (including comorbidities) of the patient. The lack of a predictable set of language consequences following CHI is hardly surprising, given this complex neurological pattern.

Acute onset of a language disorder after CHI often reflects the localization and size of contusions or hematomas, and recovery of linguistic skills typically parallels the resolution of these focal mass lesions. Subcortical lesions, involving regions such as the putaminal-capsular area, are associated

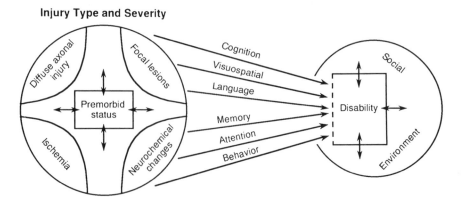

Figure 1 A conceptual model of neurobehavioral outcome of closed head injury.

with such speech disturbances as mutism (6). The long-term outcome of posttraumatic language disruption is determined by the residual focal lesions (e.g., gliosis) superimposed on diffuse insult. The considerable heterogeneity in severity and type of injury reflects the pattern of focal and diffuse insult.

Structural imaging using computed tomography (CT) and magnetic resonance imaging (MRI) has disclosed considerable heterogeneity in the type of brain lesions sustained as a result of CHI. The Traumatic Coma Data Bank has provided CT data on a large cohort of patients admitted to four neurotrauma centers (7). Analysis of the initial CT scan obtained for 753 patients sustaining severe CHI disclosed that 199 (27%) had potentially operable (15 cc or larger) focal mass lesions (either intracerebral or extracerebral), whereas 332 (55%) had bilateral diffuse brain swelling, defined as compressed or obliterated mesencephalic cisterns and/or small ventricles. CT findings were confined to minor abnormalities, such as small, focal lesions in 155 patients, or 21% of the cohort. Although the initial CT findings obtained in the Coma Data Bank indicated a relatively high percentage of focal brain lesions after CHI, more than half of these patients died. Extrapolating from this extensive study, it appears that about 15% of patients surviving severe CHI have focal brain lesions that could result in classic neurobehavioral deficits such as aphasia.

MRI studies (8) have disclosed focal regions of abnormal signal, often evident in areas with small or no lesions on CT. In mild to moderate CHI, areas of abnormal signal intensity have been found by MRI in about 80% of patients studied within the first week postinjury (8). In most cases, the MRI abnormalities after mild to moderate CHI partially or totally resolve within 3 months, whereas the residuals of severe CHI are found years after injury (8,9). Depth of lesion visualized by MRI is also related to the severity of impaired consciousness (9). Abnormal signal in the deep white matter and central gray matter is found in chronic survivors of severe CHI, whereas mild head trauma is associated with primarily cortical lesions. As with CT findings, on MRI areas of abnormal signal tend to be most widely represented in the frontotemporal region. MRI has been particularly informative in revealing white-matter abnormalities that may be the mechanism underlying hemispheric disconnection symptoms. Recent studies using functional imaging such as single-photon computed tomography have disclosed frequent instances of hypoperfusion in the frontal region despite minimal or no structural lesion on CT (10). The relationship of functional neuroimaging to posttraumatic language disorder, however, remains to be studied.

LANGUAGE IN CHI

Until recently, language received minimal attention in investigations of neurobehavioral sequelae in CHI relative to other cognitive abilities. The cursory attention given to language can be attributed to the evidence that CHI patients tend to score consistently lower on performance subtests of intelligence measures than on verbal subtests (11,12). Additionally, the course of language recovery appeared dramatic and complete in CHI, as manifested initially by a complete collapse of the language system, followed by gradual recovery until "normal speech" was attained for the majority of patients (13–15). Despite this impressive recovery, language investigations have shown that certain aspects of language remain impaired years after injury. Determining the presence of language deficits in CHI is influenced by the phase of recovery for the patient, by how one conceptualizes or defines a "language" disruption, by the nature of tasks used to assess language (i.e., traditional versus discourse measures), and by the severity of injury. The literature relevant to these issues is summarized below.

Early Phase of Recovery

For purposes of this chapter, the early phase of recovery is defined as the first 6 months of CHI, and the long-term phase of recovery is 6 months or more postinjury. Acutely, almost all CHI patients suffer linguistic impairment, although the profile of deficits is quite heterogeneous across individual cases (as a function of age at injury, injury severity, and other, probably as yet undefined, factors). The profile ranges from mutism to Sarno's subclinical aphasia (i.e., linguistic processing deficits) to no linguistic impairment in only the mildest injuries. The most common disruption during the early phase of recovery from CHI is anomia (16,17). Other deficits include reduced word fluency, impaired confrontation naming, impaired comprehension of complex oral commands, verbal paraphasic errors, and impairments of reading and writing (16,18–20). Whereas some studies reported relative preservation of comprehension and repetition in adult CHI (16), others have suggested that the comprehension of complex material (i.e., as measured by the Token Test and the Complex Ideational Material subtest from the Boston Diagnostic Aphasia Examination) and sentence repetition are impaired (21).

Language comprehension and production across all modalities show considerable improvement during the first month, with continued increments in performance over time. Groher (22) reported depressed communicative abilities, as measured by the Porch Index of Communicative Ability (PICA), in all modalities of expression—gestural, verbal, and graphic—in a group of severely impaired head-injured adults. Re-evaluations at 1-month intervals for 4 months revealed that the most dramatic improvements in language occurred during the first month after regaining consciousness. Continued improvement in language was measured across all modalities for the 3 subsequent months. A comparable pattern of recovery in memory performance was reported for these same patients. Groher concluded that receptive and expressive language abilities had recovered to a "grossly" functional level for conversational purposes within 4 months postinjury. Naming to confrontation was within normal limits for all the CHI patients at the final testing date, but persistent deficits were apparent in written language as evidenced by spelling errors, incomplete sentence construction, and syntax errors. Despite Groher's claim of a relatively good prognosis for language recovery, he commented that the conversation of many patients reflected confused thought content with irrelevant responses, even at the end of the 4-month recovery period.

A more recent study (23) evaluated 125 postcoma patients with the Neurosensory Center Comprehensive Examination for Aphasia. Consistent with earlier findings (20,24), Sarno et al. (23) found that all patients manifested some form of language disruption and/or dysarthria. The severity of the language disorder was related to the severity of the head injury. The reported linguistic deficits included impairments on measures of visual naming, word fluency, and comprehension of multistage commands.

Long-Term Phase of Recovery

The findings regarding the persistence of language deficits are equivocal. Thomsen (17) followed 12 severely injured CHI patients who initially showed marked language disturbances classified as aphasia from 1 to 4 years postinjury. At long-term follow-up, only one patient continued to show obvious language deficits. Seven of the 12 patients, however, continued to exhibit minor difficulties manifested by disruptions in the flow of language (slowed rate of speech, hesitations, and repetition of words or phrases), perseverative language, and verbal paraphasic errors. These difficulties were evident primarily on tasks that were linguistically and cognitively complex (e.g., picture-description task and use of antonyms, synonyms, and metaphors). While these findings supported the view that aphasia secondary to CHI has a good prognosis, the majority of the patients did show persistent residual linguistic deficits that were not necessarily characteristic of aphasia.

Subsequent investigations have extended Thomsen's (17) observations that minor language deficits may persist in CHI patients who manifest aphasia acutely. Levin, Grossman, Sarwar, and Meyers (18) identified three patterns of language and cognitive recovery in 21 CHI patients with acute aphasia, re-examined at least 6 months postinjury with the Multilingual Aphasia Examination (25). The three linguistic profiles included: (1) normal language (scores on all language tests were within normal limits), (2) specific linguistic disturbance (impairment of a single function, such as naming or repetition), and (3) a generalized disturbance (impairment in both receptive and expressive abilities). The CHI patients were equally distributed between the specific linguistic deficit category (n = 6) and the generalized linguistic impairment category (n = 6), with a few more in the normal language category (n = 9).

Levin and colleagues (18) pursued explanations for the three patterns of recovery in terms of initial severity of injury, neurological profile, and level of intellectual functioning. CHI patients who manifested generalized linguistic impairment at follow-up had longer coma duration than patients in the other two categories. In regard to neurological findings, some preliminary patterns were identified. For example, three of the six patients with a specific linguistic disturbance exhibited focal left-hemisphere injury on CT evaluation within a week of the injury. Patients with generalized linguistic deficits tended to show severe diffuse cerebral injury. As one might expect, comparison of intellectual and linguistic profiles revealed significantly lower scores on verbal and performance subtests of the Wechsler Adult Intelligence Scale for CHI patients with generalized language disturbances. Differences in intellectual level between the normal group and the specific linguistic deficit group were not significant.

In summary, linguistic function in CHI patients in the early phase of recovery, particularly within the first month postinjury, is frequently impaired on standardized aphasia measures. Fortunately, the prognosis for *improvement* in language ability is good following CHI. Approximately two-thirds of the CHI patients who manifest aphasia in the acute stage show overall improvement in linguistic abilities. Nonetheless, some residual language deficits (i.e., naming or word-finding problems) frequently remain in these patients. For severe CHI patients, the prognosis for linguistic recovery is less favorable. Generalized language deficits may persist in patients who sustain a severe CHI, as determined by coma duration and extent of neurological injury. Moreover, global cognitive impairment is likely to accompany generalized language deficits.

CONTRIBUTIONS AND LIMITATIONS OF THE APHASIA MODEL IN CHI

As indicated by the studies summarized above, specific language functions in CHI do not recover as completely as the early studies suggested. Indeed, many CHI patients exhibit persistent language deficits, as measured by aphasia batteries such as the Porch Index of Communicative Ability, the Neurosensory Center Comprehensive Examination for Aphasia, and the Multilingual Aphasia Examination. Renewed research has been directed at determining the presence and nature of the language dysfunction in CHI.

Traditional Language Measures

Many CHI patients exhibit difficulties in expressing their ideas, although their scores on traditional language measures are within normal limits. Moreover, clinical language measures do not consistently or reliably predict discourse ability (26). Consequently, the prevalence of language dysfunction in CHI may be underestimated when language disturbances are assessed solely with aphasia batteries. While aphasia batteries are useful in identifying certain linguistic deficits in CHI, these tests were not designed to evaluate the characteristic communicative deficits in CHI. Hagen (27) commented that CHI patients often appear to have minimal or no language impairment on the basis of available test instruments, yet manifest significant functional communication difficulties in real-life situations. Traditional tests, which measure language primarily at word and sentential levels, may be relatively insensitive to the language deficits that compromise communication following CHI.

Nonaphasic Language Disturbances

A number of terms appear in the literature to signal the distinction between language impairment in CHI and that in aphasia. For example, the language problems in CHI have been labeled as: a "subclinical" aphasic disorder (23), high-level language deficits (28), global disorganization of language (29), confused thought content (22,30), impaired language processing (27), and fragmented and tangential conversation (31).

These labels confirm that language is typically impaired following a head injury, but not in the classic aphasia sense, particularly for adult CHI patients. Levin, Benton, and Grossman (32) remarked that many CHI adults demonstrate an unspecified impairment in communicative skills despite the relative preservation of surface linguistic structure. For children with CHI, several researchers have argued that the resultant language disruption does not conform to any pattern characteristic of a developmental language disorder (28,33); that is, standardized developmental measures of language fail to detect the language sequelae in pediatric CHI populations. Traditional language measures have not been adequate to evaluate the nature of the language deficits in adults or children with CHI.

A number of researchers have argued that more sophisticated neurolinguistic measures are needed to characterize fully the language impairment following CHI (19,23,28,33). More specifically, better measures are needed to tap the consequences of cognitive impairment on the language system in CHI patients. Recent investigators have proposed that discourse studies may provide a way of elucidating the type of language and communication breakdown that occurs in head injury (26,34–36).

Discourse in CHI

Studies in Adults

Although evaluation of discourse in CHI populations has been undertaken only recently, higher-level discourse measures have proved useful in characterizing aspects of linguistic and communicative breakdown. Research in adult populations has focused on narrative, procedural, descriptive, and conversational discourse. Most investigations in adults have reported differences between normals and CHI patients.

The discourse in CHI adults has been characterized by reduction of information content, fewer cohesive ties, inefficient production, and increased use of repetitions and revisions (37,38). While Ehrlich (34) found a reduction in efficiency of production, he did not find a reduction in amount of information. The failure to find a reduction of information in CHI adults has varied with different tasks in different studies. Liles, Coelho, Duffy and Zalagens (39) reported that their CHI patients showed impairments of intersentential cohesion and episodic organization. This study demonstrated that not only was cohesion impaired but, at a more global level, story structure was disrupted as manifested in incomplete episodes.

Discourse measures have revealed differences not only in severely impaired CHI adults but also in CHI adults whose language has recovered to a high level (39). However, factors such as elicitation procedures and task complexity influence the sensitivity of the measures. For example, Liles and colleagues (39) found impairments in CHI patients as compared to normals for narratives elicited in a spontaneous-generation condition, but not for those elicited in a retell condition. While no differences were reported in amount of language (measured by number of sentences) or complexity of language (measured by clauses per sentence unit) between the two elicitation conditions, measures of intersentential cohesion and episodic structure revealed differences in the spontaneous-generation condition.

The study by Liles et al. (39) added to the emerging evidence that lower levels of language may recover, as shown by CHI group performance comparable to that of normals on measures of amount and complexity of language. However, linguistic abilities at the discourse level have a less favorable prognosis following CHI. The use of linguistic devices (e.g., cohesion) and the cognitive organization (e.g., episodic structures) of information in narrative discourse are typically impaired.

Discourse measures have also been utilized to describe the course of language recovery for individual CHI patients. Coelho, Liles, and Duffy (40) demonstrated different patterns of recovery in two CHI patients' discourse performance at early and long-term phase recovery periods. One patient produced appropriate but poorly organized narrative content. In contrast, the second patient's stories were reportedly well organized but with limited appropriate content. Over time, the former patient's narratives improved in organization, whereas the latter patient's narrative improved minimally. The researchers suggested that discourse evaluation at an early phase of recovery may have some prognostic value in determining which patients are likely to show improvement. Moreover, the pattern of discourse recovery matched the patient's functional recovery. The patient whose discourse improved returned to work successfully, while the second patient had problems returning to school.

Additional discourse deficits identified in CHI adults include impairment of both global and local coherence (41). The head-injured patients in the Glosser study were selected based on the presence of fluent language disorder. Global coherence was operationally defined as a relationship of a patient's response to the topic of conversation and was subjectively rated using a 5-point scale. Local coherence, also rated on a 5-point scale, was defined as the relationship between adjacent responses. Supporting previous findings of relative preservation of sentential-level language, the CHI patients in the Glosser and Deser study demonstrated normal syntactic complexity. Nonetheless, the CHI patients produced more syntactic errors than the normal control subjects. It is unclear whether the presence of syntactic errors represents a disturbance of the grammatical rules that define the well-formedness of sentences or whether the errors reflect formulation difficulties. The group's syntactic errors included omission of the subject, the main verb, required functors, and other grammatical morphemes. Other neurogenic populations have produced what appear to be paragrammatic responses but may be merely a reflection of formulation difficulties (42).

Investigations of conversational discourse in head-injured adults revealed deficits in the coherence and sequential organization (43,44). In both studies, the patients showed minimal language disturbances on standardized tests. Impairments included difficulties in topic management, in both appropriate selection and maintenance of conversational topic. Additional problems in topic management were noncoherent topic changes; ambiguous, unrelated, and incomplete ideational units; and unrelated responses. These responses led to a disruption of the overall coherence of the discourse. Moreover, the head-injured patients tended to be more passive conversational partners than the normal subjects, initiating fewer novel topics (43). CHI patients tended to use more pass-type turns as opposed to conversational turns that added new information. The head-injured patients relied more on the structure provided by the communication partner than did normal subjects.

Studies in Children

Compared to adult CHI studies of discourse, there is a paucity of research in head-injured children. Nonetheless, the preliminary findings also support the notion that discourse measures may provide a more complete way of characterizing the language deficits common to pediatric CHI populations. Language deficits at the discourse level reportedly persist despite marked improvement of performance on structured language measures (45).

Dennis and Barnes (26) documented discourse problems in a majority of their prediatric CHI subjects. The discourse deficits included problems in interpreting ambiguous sentences and metaphors, in drawing inferences from a stereotyped event sequence, and in generating sentences from key words.

Using conversational discourse, Campbell and Dollaghan (46) failed to find persistent deficits in a pediatric group of severely impaired CHI patients. However, these findings must be interpreted cautiously for two reasons. First, as noted by the authors, the group data may have obscured individual patterns of recovery. Of the nine patients evaluated, two showed early recovery and two exhibited recovery at 1 year. More importantly, however, five of the patients continued to show marked deficits after 1 year postinjury. Second, the selected variables did not include discourse-level measures; although Campbell and Dollaghan (46) obtained discourse samples, they evaluated the texts at lexical and sentential levels only. Nonetheless, this study provided important documentation that sentential-level language may not be immune to disruption following CHI in children. This finding emphasizes the importance of evaluating language function in CHI at multiple levels.

The findings regarding narrative discourse production in CHI children are somewhat equivocal. Jordan, Murdoch and Buttsworth (47) found no significant differences among mild CHI, severe CHI, or matched controls on measures of story grammar and use of intersentential cohesive devices. In contrast, Chapman and colleagues (36) reported significant differences on narrative-discourse measures for severely impaired CHI children as compared to mildly impaired CHI and normal control subjects. The differences included reduction in language and information and impairment of information organization. The differences across groups were not related to deficits on standardized measures of vocabulary or memory.

The incongruence between the two studies may be due, in part, to differences in the task, age differences, and/or selected measures. Jordan et al. (47) utilized a spontaneous story-generation task, whereas the study by Chapman et al. (36) involved an auditory story-retell task. Perhaps CHI patients are more proficient at self-generated narratives than retold discourse. From a different perspective, both the normal and CHI children in the study by Jordan et al. may have produced sparsely elaborated narratives on a spontaneous, self-generated task with minimal content support (e.g., producing a story when given a GI Joe toy soldier). Another possibility is that an auditory retell task (used in the study by Chapman et al.) may be more problematic for CHI populations because of concomitant memory problems. Although contribution of memory loss cannot be excluded, the impairment of discourse ability after severe head injury could not be accounted for entirely by a memory disturbance, as evaluated by a word-list recall measure in the Chapman study. With regard to age, Jordan's study was composed of younger patients than those in the Chapman study. Moreover, the measures of information organization differed across studies. Clearly, more studies of discourse in CHI children are needed to address the relevant issues.

In summary, a specific language disorder may or may not be present in CHI adult or pediatric populations, at least as measured by traditional language measures. Nonetheless, head-injured patients frequently demonstrate significant communicative difficulties. Recent evidence suggests that communication deficits in CHI may best be characterized by discourse measures. Discourse production in CHI is commonly impaired in one or more of the following domains: sequential organization of information, informativity (amount of accurate content), and semantic connectivity at either a global level of coherence (relevance of information to a unifying theme) or a local level (intersentential connectivity as marked by cohesive devices, e.g., reference, connectors, etc.). Impairment of sentential grammar is reported less frequently. While traditional naming ability is commonly disrupted in CHI patients, there does not appear to be a direct association between naming and discourse function (26,36). Therefore, a comprehensive assessment of language in CHI should include discourse measures (26,35, 36).

Are CHI Language Deficits Subtle?

The recent evidence of significant discourse impairment in CHI patients raises the question as to whether the term "subtle linguistic deficits" is appropriately applied to this population. It would be more accurate to say that traditional language measures are relatively insensitive to the language disturbances of CHI. However, one's perspective will depend on how one views the relationship between language and cognition. Some may argue that the discourse disturbances reflect an impairment of underlying cognitive processes and have little to do with the language system. Others might contend that language and cognition are interrelated processes and that the separation of the two is highly artificial. In the following section, a case for the latter perspective is developed. We believe that in order to understand the communication deficits in CHI, one must adopt an integrative approach that takes into account the interdependency of language and cognition.

INTEGRATIVE APPROACH

There is growing empirical and theoretical evidence that language and cognition are intricately related processes that do not function autonomously (42, 48,49). Consequently, the impact of cognitive and linguistic impairments are viewed as bidirectional; cognitive impairments affect language and communication, and language problems influence cognitive abilities.

The current trend in management of language problems in the head-injured population is not simply to ask whether the patients show deficits but rather to investigate how cognitive disturbances interact with the language system and vice versa. More importantly, the goal of the diagnostic process is directed toward examining how cognitive and linguistic disruptions hinder communicative competence. This approach is a broadened perspective on interpreting language disturbance within a classic aphasic framework.

Conceptualization of Discourse Processing

Figure 2 represents a conceptual schematic of discourse processing, depicting the interdependency of cognitive processes involved in manipulating information and the various levels of discourse representation. Aspects of discourse can be appreciated at multiple levels, some expressed through linguistic structures (e.g., word, clausal, sentential, intersentential cohesion) and some through information structures (e.g., propositions, superstructure, macrostructure, microstructure).

Discourse studies have recently provided a major contribution to the understanding of brain–language relationships and the effects of brain-injured populations. Joanette and Brownell (50) remarked that a full understanding of brain–language relationships and the effects of brain damage on communication requires a focus on discourse-level processes and the cognitive functions that become impaired subsequent to brain injury. One empirical fact that has evolved from aphasiology is that discourse deficits are not simply extensions of impairments at lower linguistic levels (i.e., sentential or lexical). Specifically, discourse production requires a mixture of linguistic and nonlinguistic knowledge as well as intactness of supporting cognitive abilities (memory, planning, and attention, to mention a few) (51). Thus, discourse studies may provide a promising methodology for understanding the nature and extent of language deficits in CHI patients with primary cognitive deficits.

The cognitive and neurological profile provides important background information necessary for understanding the nature of the language deficits in CHI. In the following discussion, the general profile of cognitive deficits

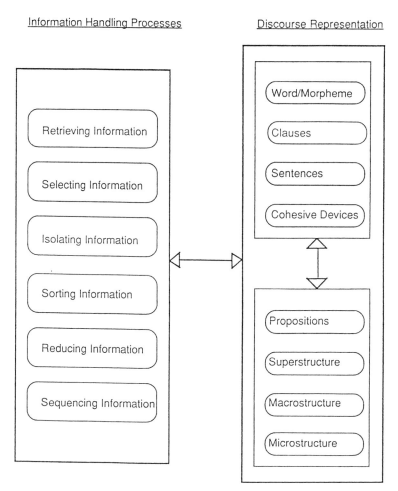

Information Handling Processes   Discourse Representation

Word/Morpheme

Clauses

Sentences

Cohesive Devices

Retrieving Information

Selecting Information

Isolating Information

Sorting Information

Reducing Information

Sequencing Information

Propositions

Superstructure

Macrostructure

Microstructure

Figure 2 A conceptual schema of discourse processes depicting the interdependency of cognitive information-handling processes and discourse representation at multiple levels in the linguistic and information structure domains. (From Ref. 36.)

is outlined, in terms of the common neurobehavioral sequelae in CHI. This information provides the foundation for building an integrative approach to assessing and managing the language problems in the CHI population, a population with primary cognitive deficits. In addition, focality of brain lesion is an important issue to consider in CHI. Whereas CHI was previously considered solely as a diffuse injury to the brain, recent MRI studies reveal persistent focal lesions in at least half the patients studied, in addition to the diffuse injuries. A deeper understanding of the language problems common to CHI may evolve from considerations of focal lesions.

General Profile of Cognitive Deficits

As discussed earlier, the various pathophysiological mechanisms involved in CHI produce a pattern of cognitive deficits that is quite heterogeneous across patients. Although no two patients are likely to have the same cognitive profile, certain areas appear to be particularly compromised in CHI. The most consistently reported cognitive deficits in this population are memory disturbances and decreased information-processing speed (32). Additionally, attentional abilities are often compromised. More recent studies have implicated higher-level executive functions such as planning and problem-solving. The general level of intellectual functioning is not necessarily affected in these patients, and visuoperceptual skills tend to be relatively well preserved. Language skills have also been thought to be relatively resistant to the effects of head injury. However, as argued previously, this sparing of language may be an artifact of the measurement of language by traditional aphasia tests, which are relatively insensitive to the deficits produced by CHI.

Relation Between Cognition and Language

In general, CHI patients exhibit impairments in memory, planning, problem-solving, self-monitoring, and impulse control. Although the impact of these deficits on language is not well understood, they undoubtedly contribute to the breakdown of communication. Dennis and Barnes (26), for example, found a correlation between subtests measuring discourse abilities and memory variables. Performance on a subtest measuring inferential abilities, an operation believed to be a prerequisite for discourse comprehension, was significantly correlated with performance on a working memory measure in children with CHI.

Nonetheless, the correspondence between cognitive and discourse deficits may not be straightforward. In regard to memory, it would seem reasonable to assume that memory capacity would be directly related to the ability to recall and reproduce a story presented through the auditory modality. However, Chapman and colleagues (36) found that performance on a story-retell task could not be accounted for entirely by a reduced working memory capacity, at least as measured by a word-recall task. According to discourse theory and the discourse processing model (Figure 2), it is not surprising that discourse recall is not completely explained by working memory. Empirical evidence suggests that text recall is better accounted for by hierarchical discourse theories (52,53), which conceptualize the retention of certain information and loss of other information. As depicted in the discourse model, retrieval of the information is only one aspect in the cognitive management of information handling. For example, the ability to select which story information to retrieve and make explicit may strongly influence story recall, as would the ability to sort the information according to importance. Moreover, Wyckoff (37) found that discourse performance was inconsistently correlated with performance on memory tests. In summary, discourse performance and measures of isolated cognitive functions may not be clearly related.

Global Processing Schemas

Recent evidence suggests that application of theoretical neuropsychological models of information processing may help elucidate the complex relationships between cognition and discourse (54,55). For example, a framework that incorporates a number of tasks to assess global processing strategies or global cognitive schemas across cognitive functions (including language, memory, and perception) may be more illuminating than simply quantifying performance on separate measures of cognitive and linguistic ability (29,55,56). Such an approach would provide a coherent explanation for the breakdown of cognitive processes that underlie a number of behaviors, including language. This framework has been applied with some success in explaining behavioral disruption in patients with frontal lobe lesions (55).

Deficits may appear across a variety of neurobehavioral measures because of problems in selecting information, solving problems, planning, initiating, monitoring, retrieving, or flexibility in thinking rather than impairments of the specific content. For example, a CHI patient who exhibits poor planning on specific cognitive tasks such as mazes or sequence of moves on a bead design (e.g., Tower of London) may manifest poor planning in discourse. Poor planning in discourse may be reflected in a variety of ways including poorly sequenced information (a failure to sequence information logically), false starts (restarting discourse), or revisions of information. A recent study by our group has demonstrated that both verbal and nonverbal measures of problem-solving and concept formation add significantly to the prediction of discourse organization in text recall. These measures provide information beyond that accounted for by measures of general verbal or nonverbal intellectual level (WISC-R Vocabulary and Block Design Scale scores) (56).

For CHI patients with memory problems, discourse may improve on tasks when the stimulus remains in front of the patient, reducing working memory demands, as compared to performance on tasks requiring recall of information. Moreover, differences in memory have been associated with specific lesion sites. For example, memory for unrelated word lists or numbers has been associated with temporal lobe function, whereas organized memory has been associated with frontal lobe function (e.g., recall of a list of food items). Parallel patterns in discourse may exist; that is, recall of isolated pieces of information from discourse may differ in localization from organization of discourse information.

To date, little evidence exists regarding the interrelationship between cognitive and language domains. The examination of this relationship, however, is the current trend in CHI studies. This approach has important implications for intervention, since manipulation of discourse information may be more important to everyday functioning than other cognitive contents.

Relation Between Neurological Profile and Discourse

Only a few investigations of discourse in CHI patients with focal lesions have been conducted. However, there is growing interest in the relationship between linguistic deficits in CHI patients and involvement of frontal brain regions. This interest is motivated by the empirical evidence that the frontal region is the most common site of focal lesions subsequent to CHI (as discussed above). Patients with frontal lobe lesions exhibit characteristic deficits on discourse measures (36,57–59).

Damage to the frontal region has been associated with diminished verbal output, initiation deficits, a tendency toward perseveration, confabulations, digressions, and problems in detecting the main idea of the text (36,57–59). Moreover, frontal patients displayed impairments in the organization of ideas. Kaczmarek posited that left frontal regions are involved in the organization and tracking of linguistic information, while right frontal areas are involved with global, nonlinguistic organization of information. In their review, Alexander et al. (57) summarized the discourse of patients with left prefrontal lesions as being unelaborated and sparsely detailed, whereas the discourse of right prefrontal patients tended to be tangential. In terms of the global organizing schemas discussed above, Chapman and colleagues (36) posited that frontal lesions may disrupt the organizational schema that guides discourse production.

CRITICAL ISSUES RELATED TO RECOVERY

Age of Injury and Cerebral Plasticity

Prior to the 1970s, the general viewpoint regarding the effects of age at injury was that the earlier the lesion, the more rapid and complete the language recovery (60). The better prognosis for recovery in younger children was attributed to the greater neuronal plasticity of the young brain. According to this view, localization of cerebral function (and language in particular) is poorly defined in very young children. As the brain matures, hemispheric specialization for language gradually becomes lateralized to the left hemisphere, perhaps at about the same time that handedness is established (61). Consequently, it was suggested that cognitive functions in young children may be assumed by brain regions not traditionally associated with language function or reserved for other cognitive abilities. Cotard (62) noted that very young children with severe left-hemispheric damage were indeed still able to acquire language. The implication from this observation was that either hemisphere could equally support language development. A number of reports seemed to substantiate this perspective, and this viewpoint persisted for nearly a century. Clarus (63) reported rapid recovery of acquired aphasia in children. Freud (64) commented that not only was language disturbance relatively transitory in children, but it also occurred with nearly equal frequency following lesions to either the left or right hemisphere.

In the 1970s, evidence emerged that recovery of language in children following brain insult was less complete than previously thought (65). Woods and Teuber (66) examined 64 cases of early-onset language disruption as well as 760 reported cases in the literature. They concluded that aphasia associated with unilateral right-hemisphere lesions was rare in children. More importantly, they found that language deficits persisted beyond age 2 years for many children. Dennis and Kohn (67) suggested that language could not develop normally in the absence of an intact left hemisphere.

Neurobiology of Recovery

Morphometric studies of the human frontal cortex (68) and positron emission tomography (PET) in infants and children have provided converging evidence that cerebral plasticity is present during early to middle childhood and subsequently declines. PET studies have shown that cerebral metabolic rate increases above adult levels during childhood, reaching a peak between 8 and 10 years and subsequently declining during adolescence to the adult level (69). Synaptic density in the human frontal cortex peaks above an adult level between 1 and 2 years (68) and later decreases, suggesting a "pruning" process that may be related to a reduced capacity for reorganization of function. An implication of this morphometric and imaging evidence is that the capacity for cerebral reorganization may be greatest during the period of peak metabolism and synaptic connectivity. In contrast, older children who sustain frontal lobe injury are less likely to compensate in their cognitive development.

The mechanisms underlying resolution of diffuse cerebral insult are not as well understood as those of focal brain lesions. However, reversibility of cerebral atrophy has been documented in children sustaining severe CHI (8,70). The relationship of diffuse cerebral insult to outcome 1 year after onset of posttraumatic aphasia has been studied using coma as the primary measure of CHI severity. Levin et al. (18) found that the overall severity of injury (as reflected by duration of coma) was a major determinant of recovery on measures of naming, verbal fluency, and language comprehension in adults who were aphasic during their initial hospitalization for CHI. In contrast, the presence of a focal brain lesion on the initial CT scan was related primarily to the persistence of specific language deficits such as problems in naming.

In summary, the notion of cerebral plasticity and recovery of function has been modified over recent years. While it is likely that age is an important factor in determining prognosis, age alone cannot predict recovery. There is growing evidence that language problems tend to persist even in children who sustained injuries to the brain at a very early age. The severity of diffuse cerebral insult is the major determinant of language competence 1 year after severe head injury. However, the mechanisms underlying recovery remain to be elucidated.

Recovery: Not an All-or-Nothing Phenomenon

Bates, Reilly, and Marchman (71) raised the question as to whether it is appropriate to talk about recovery in an absolute sense in a maturing organism. Recovery of function in children does not appear to be a once-and-for-all phenomenon that relates only to sparing and restoring of behaviors. Recovery in children is strongly influenced by how growth and development proceed in an injured brain (72). Bates and colleagues (71) suggest that children may have to recover from brain injury again and again at each subsequent stage of development.

The possibility of stage-by-stage recovery of language function may help explain the finding in head-injured children of deficits in later development of reading and writing abilities. Alajouanine and Lhermitte (73) found recovery to be the rule rather than the exception in a group including 32 neurologically impaired children, but none of the 32 subjects progressed normally in school. In particular, the children exhibited difficulty with classes that required more facility with language (i.e., reading and writing). Hagen (27) also found deficits in the written modality. More recent findings have confirmed the evidence that earlier injuries may disrupt writing to a greater extent than injuries in older children (28).

Ewing-Cobbs et al. (28) postulated that language functions in a rapid stage of development may be more affected by brain injury than well-established abilities. This perspective suggests that a brain insult has greater impact on the acquisition of new skills than recovery of previously learned functions. In contrast to earlier perspectives, Ewing-Cobbs and coworkers (28) suggested that the long-term linguistic sequelae of brain injury may be more devastating in younger children than in older children because language develops rapidly in the preschool years. At this point, it remains unclear whether the language impairment at later stages is reflected in slower *rate* of acquisition, lower *level* of performance, or different *sequence* of acquisition (72). The neurobiological mechanisms of recovery and development are important to consider.

A CASE FOR SUBGROUPS

The ability to sort out complex relations among linguistic deficits, cognitive deficits, biological parameters (e.g., plasticity), patient demographics (e.g., age at onset, sex, and socioeconomic factors), and patterns of neurophysiology will be dependent on establishing more homogeneous subgroups of CHI patients. Subgroups may be clustered according to shared behavioral profiles or to common neurological patterns. In the final analysis, the two domains will likely be related, as has been confirmed by the extensive literature on brain–behavior relations. The goal of establishing small, well-defined groups is to generate a description that is relatively broad, but not so broad that distinct patterns of impairment are obscured (74). On the other hand, the subclassification should not be so specific that the possibility of making any generalization is extremely limited.

Recent evidence suggests that it may be possible and advisable to classify CHI patients according to specific pathophysiological features. Such an approach may help to illuminate characteristic profiles of language disturbances following CHI. Peach (75) suggested that most studies fail to control for type of neurological damage in assessing language outcome in children and adults following head injury. To remedy this confound, Peach attempted to examine language performance in patients with a pattern of predominantly diffuse cerebral injury, excluding patients with focal aphasia-producing lesions. Chapman et al. (36) presented preliminary data on the potential effects on discourse of frontal lobe damage in individual children with focal frontal lesions following CHI. In addition, Chapman and colleagues included a patient with a traumatic aneurysm to evaluate the effects of well-defined frontal lesions without the contribution of diffuse cerebral insult. Hartley and Jensen (35) also suggested that characteristic language patterns may be identified in CHI patients with focal frontal lesions.

The importance of characterizing subgroups of CHI patients is exemplified using two cases from the Chapman study (36). Two CHI patients with frontal lobe damage — one primarily left frontal and one primarily right frontal as identified by MRI — were selected. Since there is growing evidence of a preponderance of frontal lobe injuries in CHI, studying patients with similar lesion foci may allow some degree of generalization to a larger number of patients.

The two patients' discourse performances were examined on a story-retell task involving a complex adventure story. The story consisted of four episodes and approximately 66 units of information (proposition). (See original story in the Appendix.) The patients' abilities to structure language and information on the narrative task were analyzed. The two patients' stories are as follows:

Patient 1: Three little boys were sailing in their boat. They fell asleep in the water. The boat crashed. The little boys were killed.

Patient 2: There were three boys camping in the woods . . . there were three boys camping in the woods. They got into a boat sail and sailed so they catch some fish. The boat started to flood, flooded the water. People started to fuss each other and say bad words and stuff. Also, they were trying to swim out the water, they were trying to swim out the water and swim to shore. After that they fished on the shore and on the grass. They got ropes and stuff. They brought all their supplies off the boat and jumped out and got a little boat. And they . . . a pet canary that talks.

Patient 1 experienced a severe head injury following a motor vehicle collision, and had an initial Glasgow Coma Score of 3. He was 7.14 years of age at time of injury and 9.29 years at time of testing. MRI examination at time of testing revealed a large lesion (2.0 cc) of the left inferior frontal gyrus and gyrus rectus. The most striking feature of patient 1's story is the sparse amount of information and marked reduction in language even as compared to other severe CHI children. Both sentential length and complexity are decreased. In regard to information, this patient's story shows disruption of story organization as measured by story components.

Patient 2, who had also sustained a severe head injury (GCS = 4), was 8 years old at time of injury and 11 years at time of evaluation. On MRI evaluation, he had parenchymal involvement (8.3 cc lesion) of the right superior and orbital frontal gyri. The most interesting aspect of this patient's story is the relative preservation in amount and complexity of language, unlike the reduction seen in patient 1. Patient 2 showed confabulation of story content and impaired sequence of information. However, like patient 1, he exhibited a severe disruption in story structure in that information about critical setting, action, and resolution was omitted.

What is of interest in these two case studies is that the discourse profile for these two CHI children with frontal lesions paralleled the pattern of frontal patients summarized by Alexander, Benson, and Stuss (57). The discourse of patients with left frontal lesions is reported as unelaborated and sparsely detailed, similar to that of our patient 1. In contrast, patients with right frontal lesions tend to produce tangential and irrelevant discourse, reminiscent of patient 2's story. While this association between frontal lesion and discourse profile remains speculative in children, the findings promise the establishment of more homogeneous subgroups of CHI patients based on lesion focus. Mcdonald (76) suggested that deficits in procedural discourse for two adult CHI patients may also be the consequence of frontal lobe involvement.

CONCLUSION

In summary, only a minority of closed-head-injury patients manifest classic aphasic syndromes. Basic sentential-level processes appear to show relatively good recovery for both children and adults who sustain severe head injury. Unfortunately, the apparent intactness of the surface-level aspects of language have led many to make inappropriate generalizations regarding a favorable prognosis for the entire language system following CHI.

Recent evidence indicates that there are major, long-term disturbances to the language system, particularly at a discourse level, following CHI. At present, these deficits are not adequately assessed by conventional language measures. While the language problems in CHI are likely associated with — and perhaps the consequence of — more generalized cognitive and memory deficits, the deficits to the language system are nonetheless real, requiring appropriate diagnostic and rehabilitative management. A conceptual approach that examines the complex interrelationships across cognitive behaviors including language will be the most promising in revealing the nature of language deficits in CHI.

As a final point, the likelihood of identifying a signature profile of language disturbance in CHI is remote, given the heterogeneity in pathopsysiological mechanisms, injury severity, and patients' premorbid characteristics. Nonetheless, the potential for identifying subgroups of CHI with common language disturbances will improve as measures of brain structure and function are improved, appropriate methodologies for assessing language especially discourse) are developed, and conceptual frameworks for examining the association across cognitive processes, including language, are established. The identification of prominent cognitive/linguistic deficits will then be more readily determined, and the rehabilitation program can be more effectively tailored to meet the individual needs of the CHI patient.

ACKNOWLEDGMENT
This investigation was supported by NIH grant NS-21889 and by The Greenery.

APPENDIX: "SHIPWRECKED"

Once there were three brothers who fished together in the ocean. They were good sailors and usually were gone from home for only a short time. One day, they all fell asleep on their boat. While they slept, the anchor broke loose and the boat drifted away in the dark night. It finally crashed against some rocks. The boys woke up frightened but then saw an island about a mile from the wreched boat. They swam for their lives and finally all reached the island. The boys were grateful to be alive, but they knew they were lost.

In the beginning, life on the island was very hard. The boys could not find fresh water or food. But they knew they could survive if they worked together. First they looked for coconuts. Then they caught birds with their bare hands and cooked them over an open fire. They always had enough to eat and drink and never felt hungry again.

The blazing sun was always hot on the island. But one day the rainy season began. The brothers knew they had to build a shelter. They searched the island and found parts of their wrecked boat. They tied the wood together and built a simple cabin and kept dry when the rain came.

The boys still dreamed every night of returning home to their family. One day, they spotted a ship. They became excited and set fire to some large bushes. The black smoke rose high in the sky and the ship's captain spotted it. He ordered his men to go ashore, where the sailors were welcomed by the three brothers. They shouted their thanks. After fifteen long months on the island, they were finally going home.

REFERENCES

1. Adams JH, Graham DI, Murray LS, Scott G. Diffuse axonal injury due to non-missile head injury in humans: An analysis of 45 cases. Ann Neurol 1982;12:557–563.
2. Namerow NS, Forney D. Traumatic brain injury: Post-acute management. J Neurolog Rehab 1990;4:193–201.
3. Gurdjian ES, Gurdjian ES. Cerebral contusions: Re-evaluation of the mechanism of their development. J Trauma 1976;16:35–51.
4. Teasdale G, Jennett B. Assessment of coma and impaired consciousness: A practical scale. Lancet 1974;ii:81–84.
5. Jennett B, Teasdale G, Galbraith, et al. Severe head injuries in three countries. J Neurol Neurosurg Psychiatry 1977;40:291–298.
6. Levin HS, Madison CF, Bailey CB, Meyers CA, Eisenberg HM, Guinto FC. Mutism after closed head injury. Arch Neurol (Chicago) 1983;40:601–606.
7. Eisenberg HM, Gary HE, Aldrich EF, et al. Initial CT findings in 753 patients with severe head injury. J Neurosurg 1990;73:688–698.
8. Levin HS, Mendelsohn D, Bruce D, et al. Reversibility of cerebral atrophy after head injury in children. Neurosurgery 1992;31:1117–1122.
9. Levin HS, Williams D, Crofford M, et al. Relationship of depth of brain lesions to consciousness and outcome after closed head injury. J Neurosurg 1988;69:861–866.

10. Newton MR, Greenwood RJ, Britton KE, et al. A study comparing SPECT with CT and MRI after closed head injury. J Neurol Psychiatry 1992;55:92–94.
11. Chadwick O, Rutter M, Brown G, Shaffer D, Traub M. A prospective study of children with head injuries. II. Cognitive sequelae. Psycholog Med 1981;11: 49–61.
12. Winogron HW, Knights RM, Bawden HN. Neuropsychological deficits following head injury in children. J Clin Neuropsychol 1984;6:269–286.
13. Caveness WF. Introduction to head injuries. In: Walker E, Caveness W, Cutchley M, eds. The late effects of head injury. Springfield, IL: Charles C Thomas, 1969.
14. Hooper R. Patterns of acute head injury. Baltimore: Williams & Wilkins, 1969.
15. Russell WR. Cerebral involvement in head injury. Brain 1932;55:549–603.
16. Heilman KM, Safran A, Geschwind N. Closed head trauma and aphasia. J Neurol Neurosurg Psychiatry 1971;34:265–269.
17. Thomsen IV. Evaluation and outcome of aphasia in patients with severe closed head trauma. J Neurol Neurosurg Psychiatry 1975;3:713–718.
18. Levin HS, Grossman RG, Sarwar M, Meyers CT. Linguistic recovery after closed head injury. Brain Lang 1981;12:360–374.
19. Levin HS, Grossman RG, Kelly PJ. Aphasic disorder in patients with closed head injury. J Neurol Neurosurg Psychiatry 1976;39:1062–1070.
20. Sarno MT. The nature of verbal impairment after closed head injury. J Nerv Ment Dis 1980;168(11):685–692.
21. Payne-Johnson JC. Evaluation of communication competence in patients with closed head injury. J Commun Disord 1986;19:237–249.
22. Groher M. Language and memory disorders following closed head trauma. J Speech Hear Res 1977;20:212–223.
23. Sarno MT, Buonaguro A, Levita E. Characteristics of verbal impairment in closed head injury. Arch Phys Med Rehab 1986;67:400–405.
24. Sarno MT. Verbal impairment after closed head injury: Report of a replication study. J Nerv Ment Dis 1984;172:475–479.
25. Benton AL. Problems of test construction in the field of aphasia. Cortex 1967; 3:32–58.
26. Dennis M, Barnes MA. Knowing the meaning, getting the point, bridging the gap, and carrying the message: Aspects of discourse following closed head injury in childhood and adolescence. Brain Lang 1990;39:428–446.
27. Hagen C. Language disorders in head trauma. In: Holland A, ed. Language disorders in adults. San Diego: College-Hill Press, 1984:247–281.
28. Ewing-Cobbs L, Levin HS, Eisenberg HM, Fletcher JM. Language functions following closed head injury in children and adolescents. J Clin Exp Neuropsychol 1987;9:575–592.
29. Wiig EH, Alexander EW, Secord W. Linguistic competence and level of cognitive functioning in adults with traumatic closed head injury. In: Whitaker HA, ed. Neuropsychological studies on non-focal brain damage: dementia and trauma. New York: Springer-Verlag, 1988:186–201.
30. Wertz RT. Language disorders in adults: State of the clifnical art. In: Holland AL, ed. Language disorders in adults. San Diego: College Hill Press, 1984:1–78.

31. Levin HS, Grossman RG, Rose JE, Teasdale G. Long-term neuropsychological outcome of closed head injury. Neurosurgery 1979;50:412–422.
32. Levin HS, Benton AL, Grossman RG. Neurobehavioral consequences of closed head injury. New York: Oxford University Press, 1982.
33. Jordan FM, Ozanne AE, Murdoch BE. Long-term speech and language disorders subsequent to closed head injury in children. Brain Injury 1988;2:179–185.
34. Ehrlich JS. Selective characteristics of narrative discourse in head-injured and normal adults. J Commun Disord 1988;21:1–9.
35. Hartley LL, Jensen PJ. Narrative and procedural discourse after closed head injury. Brain Injury 1991;5(3):267–285.
36. Chapman SB, Culhane KA, Levin HS, et al. Narrative discourse after closed head injury in children and adolescents. Brain Lang 1992;43:42–65.
37. Wyckoff LH. Narrative and procedural discourse following closed head injury. Doctoral dissertation, University of Florida, Gainesville, 1984.
38. Mentis M, Prutting CA. Cohesion in the discourse of normal and head-injured adults. J Speech Hear Res 1987;30:88–98.
39. Liles BZ, Coelho CA, Duffy RJ, Zalagens MR. Effects of elicitation procedures on the narratives of normal and closed head-injured adults. J Speech Hear Disord 1989;54:3:356–375.
40. Coelho CA, Liles BZ, Duffy RJ. Discourse analyses with closed head injured adults: Evidence for differing patterns of deficits. Arch Phys Med Rehab 1991;72:465–468.
41. Glosser G, Deser T. A comparison of changes in macrolinguistic aspects of discourse production in normal aging. J Gerontol 1990;47:266–272.
42. Ulatowska HK, Chapman SB. Discourse studies. In: Lubinski R, ed. Dementia and communication. Philadelphia: BC Decker, 1991.
43. Mentis M, Prutting CA. Analysis of topic as illustrated in a head-injured and a normal adult. J Speech Hear Res 1991;34:3:583–595.
44. Milton SB, Prutting CA, Binder GM. Appraisal of communicative competence in head injured adults. In: Brookshire RH, ed. Clinical aphasiology: Conference proceedings. Minneapolis: BRK Publishers, 1984:114–123.
45. Ylvisaker M. Language and communication disorders following pediatric head injury. J Head Trauma Rehab 1986;1:48–56.
46. Campbell TF, Dollaghan CA. Expressive language recovery in severely brain-injured children and adolescents. J Speech Hear Disord 1990;55:567–581.
47. Jordan FM, Murdoch BE, Buttsworth DL. Closed head-injured children's performance on narrative tasks. J Speech Hear Res 1991;34:572–582.
48. Bayles K, Boone D, Tomoeda C, Slauson T, Kaszniak A. Differentiating Alzheimer's patients from the normal elderly and stroke patients with aphasia. J Speech Hearing Disord 1989;54:74–87.
49. Ulatowska HK, Allard L, Donnell A, et al. Discourse performance in subjects with dementia of the Alzheimer type. In: Whitaker HA, ed. Neuropsychological studies in non-focal brain damage: trauma and dementia. New York: Springer-Verlag, 1988.
50. Joanette Y, Brownell H, eds. Discourse ability and brain damage. New York: Springer-Verlag, 1990.

51. Patry R, Nespoulous J. Discourse analysis in linguistics: Historical and theoretical background. In: Joanette Y, Brownell H, eds. Discourse ability and brain damage. New York: Springer-Verlag, 1990.
52. Kintsch W, VanDijk T. Toward a model of text comprehension and production. Psycholog Rev 1978;85:363-394.
53. Labov W. Language in the inner city: Studies in the black vernacular. Philadelphia: University of Pennsylvania Press, 1972.
54. Luria AR. Traumatic aphasia. The Hague: Mouton, 1970.
55. Shallice T, Burgess P. Higher-order cognitive impairments and frontal lobe lesions in man. In: Levin HS, Eisenberg HM, Benton AL, eds. Frontal lobe function and dysfunction. New York: Oxford University Press, 1991:125-138.
56. Culhane K, Chapman SB, Levin HS. The relationship of discourse and cognitive task performance following closed head injury. Paper presented at the meeting of the International Neuropsychology Society, Galveston, TX, 1993.
57. Alexander MR, Benson DF, Stuss DT. Frontal lobes and language. Brain Lang 1989;37:656-691.
58. Kaczmarek BL. Neurolinguistic analysis of verbal utterances in patients with focal lesions of frontal lobes. Brain Lang 1984;21:52-58.
59. Novoa OP, Ardila A. Linguistic abilities in patients with prefrontal damage. Brain Lang 1987;30:206-225.
60. Basser LS. Hemiplegia of early onset and the faculty of speech with special reference to the effects of hemispherectomy. Brain 1962;85:427-460.
61. Lenneberg E. Biological foundations of language. New York: John Wiley, 1967.
62. Cotard J. Études sur l'atrophie partielle du cerveau. Thèses de Paris, 1968.
63. Clarus A. Uber aphasie bei kindern. Jahresh Kinderheilkd 1874;7:369-400.
64. Freud S. Infantile cerebral paralysis, 1897. Rusin LA, trans. Coral Gables, FL: University of Miami, 1968.
65. Woods BT, Carey S. Language deficits after apparent clinical recovery from childhood aphasia. Ann Neurol 1979;6:405-409.
66. Woods BT, Teuber HL. Early onset of complementary specialization of cerebral hemispheres in man. Trans Amer Neurolog Assoc 1973;98:113-115.
67. Dennis M, Kohn B. Comprehension of syntax in infantile hemiplegia after cerebral decostication: Left hemisphere superiority. Brain Lang 1975;2:472-482.
68. Huttenlocher PR. Synaptic density in human frontal cortex—developmental changes and effects of aging. Brain Res 1979;163:195-205.
69. Chugani HT, Phelps ME, Mazziotta JC. Positron emission tomography study of human brain functional development. Ann Neurol 1987;22:487-497.
70. Bruce DA, Alavi A, Bilaniuk L, Dolinskas C, Obrist W, Uzzell B. Diffuse cerebral swelling following head injuries in children: The syndrome of malignant brain edema. J Neurosurg 1981;54:170-178.
71. Bates E, Reilly J, Marchman E. Discourse and grammar after early focal brain injury (abstr). Academy of Aphasia meeting, Toronto, Oct 25-27, 1992.
72. Fletcher JM, Miner M, Ewing-Cobbs L. Age and recovery from head injury in children: Developmental issues. In: Levin HS, Graufman J, Eisenberg HM,

eds. Neurobehavioral recovery from head injury. New York: Oxford University Press, 1987:279-292.

73. Alajouanine TH, Lhermitte F. Acquired aphasia in children. Brain 1965;88: 653-662.

74. Martin A. Neuropsychology of Alzheimer's disease: The case for subgroups. In: Schwartz MF, ed. Modular deficits in Alzheimer's-type dementia. Cambridge: MIT Press, 1990:143-176.

75. Peach RK. Factors underlying neuropsychological test performance in chronic severe traumatic brain injury. J Speech Hear Res 1992;35(4):810-818.

76. McDonald S. Pragmatic language skills after closed head injury: Ability to meet the informational needs of the listener. Brain Lang 1993;44(1):28-46.

16

Acquired Childhood Aphasia

Bryan T. Woods

Texas A&M University School of Medicine, Temple, Texas

INTRODUCTION

Of all the problems with language encountered in children, acquired aphasia is one of the least common. Thus, the strong interest it has held for neurologists, psychologists, and linguists has been based as much on its bearing on theories of language and the brain as on practical considerations. The history of the gradual refinement and changes in understanding of childhood aphasia since the mid-nineteenth century mirrors the major developments in behavioral neurology that have occurred since then. The localization of language functions in one hemisphere was and remains the premier example of hemispheric specialization in man, and childhood aphasia offers critical data on the how and when of that localization.

Earlier definitions of aphasia in children were very broad, and their refinement is part of the history reviewed below; in modern usage the term *acquired aphasia of childhood* is understood to mean a loss of previously acquired language functions. It is to be distinguished from a primary delay or failure in language acquisition, usually termed *developmental dysphasia.* It should also be distinguished from mutism, in which the child does not attempt to speak, and from mechanical difficulties in speech production, such as stuttering. Childhood aphasia usually implies age of onset from infancy through preadolescence, although the age boundaries themselves have been debated. The clinical characteristics of the aphasia depend in large part on the same variables of etiology and localization of lesion that are important in adults, but the picture is significantly modified by age at time of lesion.

HISTORICAL BACKGROUND

The earliest study of childhood aphasia, that of Cotard in 1868 (1), appeared as a thesis 7 years after Broca had localized speech function in the left third frontal convolution. Cotard examined the brains of a number of persons dying as adults who had been hemiplegic since childhood. He found that the brains of seven right-hemiplegic patients, who in life had normal development of speech and intelligence, showed destruction of either the left frontal lobe or the entire left hemisphere. He concluded that, if either hemisphere is destroyed in early infancy, the other can take over its functions, including language. He also concluded, incorrectly, that aphasia did not occur in childhood. This latter misconception was soon set right; by 1874 Clarus (2) had collected reports of 50 cases of childhood aphasia. Ten years later, Bernhardt (3) listed a number of principles of childhood aphasia, among which were the favorable prognosis and brief duration, the predominance of motoric (expressive) aphasias, and the ability of the right hemisphere to take over speech in the case of a left-hemisphere lesion.

In 1893 Sigmund Freud (4) published a monograph on cerebral palsy in which he reviewed the by then extensive literature on childhood aphasia. He clearly distinguished between acquired aphasia and a primary delay in speech development. He also pointed out that many authors had frequently encountered aphasia accompanying left hemiparesis (crossed aphasia) in children, in contrast to its infrequency in adults.

In 1925 Mingazzini (5) interpreted the high incidence of crossed aphasia and the rapid recovery of language in childhood as evidence that in early years both the right and left hemisphere play an active role in speech production. In 1962 Basser (6) provided further evidence in support of the proposition that the right hemisphere can take over speech after left-hemisphere damage. He described three children who had become aphasic after left-hemisphere lesions but recovered speech. The patients some time later underwent left hemispherectomy for the relief of intractable seizures. In two of the three cases, the hemispherectomy did not result in any recurrence of the aphasia, leading one to conclude that in these patients the remaining right hemisphere had completely taken over language functions.

In 1967 Lenneberg (7) summed up the conclusions about childhood aphasia that had emerged from the clinical experience. He laid stress on the frequent occurrence of crossed aphasia and the customarily rapid recovery of language function if the lesion had occurred prior to adolescence. He surmised that both the left and right hemispheres initially played an active role in speech, with the left gradually becoming more and more dominant, until by adolescence the right hemisphere had lost all of its active role. He concluded that complete recovery was still possible only as long as both hemispheres were active in speech.

This formulation received general acceptance for a time, but was graddually noted to be somewhat at variance with several types of evidence from other investigators that pointed to left-hemisphere dominance for language (at least in right-handers) from the outset of postnatal development and language acquisition.

First of all, neuroanatomical studies in adults (8), neonates (9,10), and fetuses (11) demonstrated that in most individuals the planum temporale of the left temporal lobe is larger in area and more convoluted than that on the right. Since this area is one of those critical for comprehension of spoken language, there appears to be an innate anatomical predisposition to lateralization of language in the left hemisphere.

Another line of research, using auditory evoked responses, showed infants to have a more prominent left-sided response to speech sounds but not to nonspeech sound (12). Still a third group of studies, utilizing the dichotic listening technique, appeared for the most part to demonstrate that right-ear preference is already present in most children even as early as age 3, the earliest practical age for testing in this manner (13,14).

As a consequence of these results, the clinical data, which had been interpreted as indicating initial bihemispheric involvement in language functions, appeared to be at variance with other neuropsychological findings. The concept of a progressive lateralization of language to the left hemisphere (LH), not complete until the onset of puberty, was partially revised by Krashen (15). He reinterpreted Lenneberg's data as to age threshold, concluding that the lateralization to LH was complete after age 5. This new model left unmodified the premise of initial bilaterality.

Woods and Teuber (16) offered a resolution of this apparent conflict by observing that the great predominance of crossed aphasias in children had occurred prior to 1942, and that in studies of approximately 300 children with aphasia acquired after 1942 the frequency of crossed aphasia was no greater than 5% when known left-handers were excluded. The authors further proposed that the difference between the earlier and the more recent clinical experience may have arisen because of a shift in the common etiologies of childhood aphasia away from bacterial infections, with their diffuse brain involvement, to more discrete focal vascular lesions.

This study and a further in-depth assessment of language function in children with acquired aphasia (17) also indicated that some modifications of other clinical teachings about this disorder might also be required. In particular, the view that there is a threshold age, before which complete recovery from an acquired aphasia will take place (7,15), appears to be an oversimplification. Woods and Carey (17) found that if the level of analysis of language function in children with acquired aphasia was strictly clinical, then observable aphasic language did not persist permanently in children who were below a certain age at time of lesion (age 8 was the critical age in their series). On the other hand, when analysis of language function was quantitative, then the group of children who had initially been aphasic, but had recovered clinically, showed significant persistent impairments of language function vis-à-vis children who had acquired right hemiparesis but no initial aphasia.

Another previously postulated feature of childhood aphasia that was called into question was the rapidity of recovery of language in the younger children; one child, age 5 at time of lesion, required more than 2 years for clinical language recovery (16). This same child served as a counterexample to the supposed absence of fluent or "jargon" aphasia with childhood lesions. As will be seen below, subsequent clinical studies appear to support all four of these "revisionist" positions: (1) scarcity of true crossed aphasia in children, (2) subtle language impairments even after early left-hemisphere speech area lesions, (3) marked variation in time required for clinical recovery, and (4) a small but noticeable occurrence of fluent aphasias even in early childhood.

CLINICAL FEATURES OF CHILDHOOD APHASIA

Table 1 lists the currently more important causes of acquired aphasia in children. In earlier times, systemic bacterial infection with encephalopathy and focal lesions (18) was an important cause of hemiplegia and aphasia, but such cases have been virtually eliminated in countries with modern medical care.

A few special syndromes that are seen in children should be noted. First of all, thrombotic strokes are not as rare in children as has been commonly believed (19,20). In a recent report on a 15-year experience with 3900 newborns who underwent brain imaging following admission to St. Louis Children's Hospital, it was noted that 46 had large artery territory infarctions (21).

The etiology of cerebral thrombotic infarcts is uncertain in most cases; certainly they are not due to atherosclerosis. Onset is accompanied by convulsions more frequently than is the case in adult vascular disease. The stroke may come on during, or soon after, an apparently mild upper respiratory infection. Except for patients with the moya-moya syndrome (20), progression or recurrence is rare.

Table 1 Causes of Acquired Aphasia in Children

 I. Generalized central nervous system lesions due to any cause
 II. Focal brain lesions
    A. Vascular
        1. Arterial occlusion
           a. Thrombosis of a major vessel; arteritis
           b. Embolism, usually of cardiac or pulmonary origin
        2. Arteriovenous malformation with hemorrhage
        3. Venous thrombosis, related to infection or dehydration
           a. With seizures and lesion extension
        4. Hemorrhage
           a. Aneurysmal
           b. Associated with hemophilia
    B. Trauma
        1. Blunt head injury
           a. With epidural hemorrhage
         2. Penetrating head injury
         3. Carotid artery trauma in neck
    C. Tumor
    D. Infectious process
        1. Abscess
        2. Herpes simplex encephalitis
        3. Tuberculous meningitis with large-vessel thrombosis
    E. Seizure disorder
        1. HHE syndrome (hemiconvulsions, hemiplegia, epilepsy)
        2. Sturge-Weber disease with convulsions
        3. Syndrome of acquired aphasia with convulsive disorder
    F. Migraine with aphasic aura
    G. Alternating hemiplegia

There is another syndrome of children that has sometimes been related to this stroke syndrome but should probably be kept separate: severe prolonged convulsions followed by hemiparesis and epilepsy (HHE syndrome) (22). In this disorder, if the hemiparesis is right-sided, aphasia is often present as well. In some of these patients the hemiparesis may develop only gradually. It has been suggested that there is a pre-existing focal lesion that sets up the seizures, but the seizures themselves then lead to focal hypoxia and tissue damage with extension of the deficit (23).

Loss of speech may be the only clinical manifestation of an underlying seizure disorder (24,25). The diagnosis may depend on the presence of paroxysmal discharges on the electroencephalogram. Prognosis is variable, and may correlate inversely with age of onset (26,27), but this has been disputed (28). Treatment with anticonvulsants is recommended (29). Steroids have also been advocated for treatment (30), but not all reports support their value (31).

PATTERNS OF DEFICIT

It was formerly held that one sees only nonfluent, expressive aphasia in children. While there is no doubt that this form of aphasia predominates, it is not the only one seen. Posterior lesions, such as temporal lobe abscesses (32), can present first with receptive aphasia. In young children this receptive aphasia may be followed by a gradual loss of all expressive speech. The initial report of jargon aphasia in a child by Woods and Teuber (16) has been followed by a number of other descriptions of fluent aphasia in children. In a recent case report and review Klein et al. (33) noted 30 such cases in the literature.

The predominance of expressive aphasia in children has been attributed to fundamental characteristics unique to the immature nervous system, but it is possible that the explanation may rather be found in a combination of several, more prosaic factors. First, prior to the advent of CT scanning, it is likely that there was a bias toward recognizing (and reporting) aphasia in a child more readily if it was accompanied by hemiplegia. Second, there are now many more specialists in the language pathologies of childhood, and accurate characterization of the precise nature of the language disturbance is more likely, especially given the ready accessibility of correlative imaging. Finally, the relative rarity of embolic strokes in children, as compared to adults, could be expected to diminish the likelihood of isolated Wernicke's-area lesions in children. Nonetheless, it now seems likely that the differences in prevalence of types of aphasia between children and adults are quantitative, not qualitative. For example, Aram et al. (34) described a capsular/striatal aphasia in a 7-year-old, and Martins et al. (35) a conduction aphasia in a 10-year-old.

Finally, as noted above, the older view that aphasia is common following right unilateral lesions in children is not supported by more recent observations (36,37). Martins et al. (35) reported only a single case of crossed aphasia in their series of 31 aphasic children.

EFFECTS OF PRE- OR PERINATAL
UNILATERAL LESIONS

If a cerebral lesion involving the language area of one hemisphere occurs before a child has begun to talk, then by convention one does not speak of the presence or absence of an acquired aphasia. Nevertheless, the subsequent language development of such patients is of great theoretical interest because it bears on the two major questions posed by childhood aphasia: hemispheric commitment and hemispheric plasticity. That children with early-life left-hemisphere language-area lesions develop apparently normal language functions has been known since Cotard (1), and the role of the right hemisphere in this development had already been suggested in the nineteenth century (3). However, only with the study of hemispherectomy cases by Dennis and Kohn (38) was it suggested that there was a limitation on the language capabilities of the remaining intact right hemisphere.

At present, the data about hemispheric differences in language capabilities following lesions of the contralateral hemisphere are equivocal. Dennis and Whittaker (39) described syntactic limitations in their left hemispherectomy patients vis-à-vis those with right hemispherectomies. Woods and Carey (17) found patients with early left-hemisphere lesions to have low verbal and performance IQ scores but no specific language deficits. Vargha-Khadem et al. (40) found that even perinatal left-hemisphere-lesion patients had specific language deficits, but that there was nevertheless an inverse relationship between age at lesion and deficit severity. Aram and colleagues (41,42), investigating the same issue, also found specific language defects after left perinatal lesions, but did not find any inverse relationship between deficits and age at time of lesion. Vargha-Khadem et al. (43) have also looked at left- and right-hemispherectomy cases in which both the age of lesion onset and the side of the lesion varied. They concluded that all the left-hemispherectomy cases and the early-lesion right-hemispherectomy case had specific language defects. Most recently, a longitudinal study by Feldman et al. (44) found that language onset was delayed after both left and right early lesions, but that levels of specific language function eventually attained were not different from those of normal controls.

RELATED COGNITIVE DEFICITS AND HANDEDNESS

It has long been suspected that recovery of specific cerebral functions after early unilateral brain lesions occurs only at a price (45). If so, then data about other cognitive functions in children with acquired aphasia should shed light on the nature and limitations of mechanisms of recovery of speech. Similarly, the strong correlation between handedness (hemispheric motor dominance) and hemispheric language dominance makes data about handedness shifts after early hemispheric lesions relevant to any discussion of childhood aphasia.

Satz (46) recently reviewed the results of several large data sets on handedness and speech lateralization after early lesions. His observations, based on 735 observed or reported left-hemisphere lesion patients (plus generally accepted normal percentages), have been retabulated as follows:

	Age at lesion onset		
	< 6 years	≥ 6 years	Controls
Left-hemisphere language dominance (LHLD)	44%	80%	96%
Left-hemisphere motor dominance (LHMD)	38%	69%	90%

Not all shifts in dominance were concordant, but 75% of concordant shifts occurred with early lesions.

Vargha-Khadem et al. (40) related handedness to time of left-hemisphere lesion using three groups: perinatal lesions, early lesions (before age 5), and later lesion (up to age 14). They found LHMD in approximately 15% of the perinatal-, 25% of the early-, and 60% of the later-lesion groups.

In addition to age at lesion, severity of motor deficit also influences motor dominance. Klein and Aram (47) studied eight children with prenatal and 18 with early and later childhood left-hemisphere lesions. None of the prenatal group retained LHMD, but five of 18 of the postnatal group did; on a variety of measures these latter five patients had superior (and often normal) right-hand motor function.

A number of studies have used Wechsler IQ test verbal and performance scores as indices of respective left- and right-hemisphere cognitive function. Lansdell (48) studied children who all had right-hemisphere language dominance (RHLD) after left-hemisphere lesions and found that the earlier-lesion group had higher VIQ scores and lower PIQ scores than the later-lesion group. In contrast, the left-hemisphere-lesion patients studied by Woods and Teuber (49) had similar VIQ and PIQ scores whether their lesion was early or late. Vargha-Khadem et al. (40) found that early left-hemisphere lesions lowered both VIQ and PIQ, but that later lesions had a more severe effect on VIQ than on PIQ. Ballantyne et al. (50) looked only at early-lesion patients and found that for left-sided-lesion patients mean VIQ and PIQ were both significantly lower than those of controls, while not significantly different from each other. Riva et al. (51) found neither early nor late left-lesion VIQ and PIQ scores to differ from each other, but they noted that both early-lesion scores were significantly lower than control scores. The early-lesion group of Riva et al. (51) were basically perinatal lesion patients, while their later-lesion group spanned the age range from 2½ to 12½ years. It is important to note that the differences between these series apply to the effects of later left-hemisphere lesions; all series indicate that early left-hemisphere lesions lower PIQ at least as much as VIQ, but only two of the five studies found VIQ to be lower than PIQ after later lesions.

PROGNOSIS

As has already been pointed out, the conclusions that early childhood aphasias due to unilateral lesions last only a short time and are followed by complete recovery of language function are in need of qualification. First, the presence of a receptive component to childhood aphasia appears to prolong recovery (52,53). Second, the recovery of language function is less complete than is apparent on the standard clinical neurological examination. Third, scholastic achievement may be more impaired than would be predicted from language function alone. Two-thirds of the patients of Alajouanine and Lhermitte (54), who were aged 5–15 years at the onset of their aphasias, appeared to recover, but as a group they tended to do poorly in their subsequent schoolwork. Rust and Volpe (21) noted that 21 of their 46 children with major cerebral artery infarcts observed with brain imaging had subsequent learning disabilities. Aram (55), looking separately at reading, writing, spelling, and math function, noted the following: the incidence of reading difficulties reported by various observers after early lesions range from 100% to a low of 25% in her own series; "written language generally is found to be the most severe and persistent area of academic difficulty . . . particularly when the left hemisphere is involved"; spelling deficits are also common; and mathematics deficits may be widespread as well, but are poorly characterized and not clearly related to side of lesion.

In reviewing the data from a number of studies, it is clear that prognosis is variable because it is importantly affected by at least four factors: etiology, location of lesion, age at time of lesion, and associated disturbances (particularly generalized seizures).

It is evident that progressive disorders have a poor prognosis, and the same is true of disorders producing diffuse bilateral cortical and subcortical involvement. The prognosis after a unilateral nonprogressive lesion is much better, but the data suggest that patients with anterior (Broca's area) lesions recover language more readily than those with posterior (Wernicke's area) lesions. The relatively few modern-era childhood crossed aphasias have as a rule recovered quickly.

It has proven difficult to demonstrate that size of lesion by itself has a major bearing on outcome. Thal et al. (56), looking at perinatal lesions, detected a ∪-shaped relationship, with the largest and smallest lesions associated with better outcomes than the mid-sized lesions. They suggested that the largest lesions were more likely to result in a shift in speech lateralization, leading to a more favorable outcome than that of the medium-sized lesions.

Age at the time of lesion remains an important prognostic variable, such that the earlier the lesion the better the prognosis. As noted above, however, even after quite early lesions there may be subtle deficits. This inverse relationship between age and prognosis may be true of young adults as well (57). Finally, the development of severe and persistent seizures in the aphasic child is associated with a less benign outcome, and such seizures are more common in children than in adults with comparable lesions.

MECHANISMS OF LANGUAGE RECOVERY IN CHILDREN

Theories about the neurology of language development in children and the basis for recovery of language after childhood aphasia have been very strongly influenced by the perceived clinical evidence. Because childhood aphasia was thought to lack the diversity of forms seen in adult aphasia, it was assumed that the neurological substrate of language was less differentiated in children than in adults. Because crossed aphasia was believed to be common in children, it was concluded that the ability of the right hemisphere to develop language after a left-sided lesion depended on the right hemisphere's playing an initially active role in language functions. The more recent clinical results described in this review lead to different conclusions. First, the distinctions among different components of overall language function (e.g., comprehension and production, semantic content, and syntactic form) that have anatomical correlates in adults are likely to have the same anatomical relevance for children. Second, hemispheric potential for language acquisition does not necessarily imply a prior active role in speech for that hemisphere.

The most fundamentally important mechanism of language recovery in childhood is the one first described in 1868: the complete takeover of language function by the uninjured right hemisphere. After 125 years, many questions remain about why, how, how often, and until when this shift may occur. Speech-lateralization data on patients undergoing cortical removal of seizure foci indicate that language does not shift to the right hemisphere unless the left-hemisphere lesions involve classical speech areas (58). The age range over which such a shift can take place is unknown; it has been suggested that it can still take place in adult life. Kinsbourne (59) reported three adults who had some recovery of language after left-hemisphere lesions and had subsequent Wada tests indicating language shift to the right side. Burklund and Smith (60) have reported partial recovery of language, especially comprehension, in two left-hemispherectomized, right-handed adults aged 41 and 47 years. Gott (61) reported a similar partial recovery after left hemispherectomy in a 12-year-old girl.

Although right-hemisphere potential for language does not initially depend on right-hemisphere activity for speech, it is likely that optimal right-hemisphere development of speech can take place only if control of language shifts from the damaged left to the undamaged right side. If so, then the failure of language to recover after later-life lesions via the mechanism of right-hemisphere takeover could arise in two ways: first, by a loss of the right hemisphere's potential for language development, in which case a shift of control to the right would do no good, or second, by a primary loss of the ability to shift language control, even though considerable right-hemisphere potential for language development was still present.

The latter mechanism is attractive because it holds out the hope that some treatment might be found that would permit speech to shift to the right hemisphere in adults, as it does in children, and thus improve the prognosis for adult aphasias. One tantalizing clue that potentially beneficial shifts of language control to the right hemisphere in aphasic adults are blocked by some inhibitory process is the complete and otherwise unexplained recovery of language occasionally seen in adults who have had a complete destruction of the speech areas of the dominant hemisphere (62). (A possible inhibitory effect of the damaged left hemisphere on the right hemisphere's ability to subserve reading is discussed in Chapter 10.) Nevertheless, a preponderance of data suggest that the more likely reason that the right hemisphere cannot take over language functions adequately in most adults after left-hemisphere speech areas have been destroyed is that the right hemisphere of the adult has largely lost its original potential for speech acquisition. The question, then, is why should this potential decrease with maturation? If the right hemisphere has never played an active role in language, then the answer cannot be that it gives up its active role to the left hemisphere. One plausible explanation is that the right hemisphere gradually becomes increasingly committed to its own proper functions and thus has less reserve capacity available for language acquisition, should destruction of the left hemisphere make this necessary. The corollary of the hypothesis of progressive commitment as an explanation for decreasing recovery of language function with age is the hypothesis that an *early* shift of language to the right hemisphere would be at the expense of the right-hemisphere functions.

A complete shift of language function to the other hemisphere is not the only mechanism by which language function might recover in children. The motor function of speech might shift to the right hemisphere while comprehension and overall control remained on the left. Such a reorganization has been invoked for adults in order to explain the rapid recovery sometimes seen after a Broca's aphasia (63). A partial shift of language functions may also take place after posterior lesions, as is demonstrated in a case described by Rasmussen and Milner (64). A recent study by Kurthen et al. (65) indicated that such shifts of only receptive or only expressive speech function do occur, albeit with a frequency of less than 3% in their 144 patients.

Alternatively, in patients with restricted left anterior lesions, contiguous areas may be able to take over expressive speech functions rather quickly (66), and this might be particularly true in children. It has been suggested that such ipsilateral shifts in localization are more characteristic for lesions acquired after age 6 (64).

Table 2 summarizes the relationships of six variables to age: left- and right-hemisphere language *function*, hemispheric *potentials* for language

Table 2 Relationship of Six Variables to Age

Age	Language function of		Language potential of		Ultimate consequences of damage localized to	
	LH	RH	LH	RH	LH	RH
Early prenatal	None	None	Full	Full	No specific language impairment; generalized functional impairment	Same as LH
Perinatal	Beginnings of activity	Little or none	Full	Slight reduction	Delayed development; subtle impairment of specific language functions	Generalized functional impairment only
1–5 yr	Essentially full development of spoken language	Little or none	Potential largely actualized	Mild reduction	Transient aphasia likely; only subtle permanent language deficits	Impairment limited to specific RH functions
5–8 yr	Development of reading and writing	None	Potential almost fully actualized	Marked loss of language potential	Clinically overt aphasia may persist; residual deficits present on formal testing	Specific impairment of RH functions
≥ 9 yr	Essentially adult-level function	None	Essentially full actualization	Minimal language potential	Similar to those in adults	Similar to those in adults

development, and the *consequences* for language of lesions of either hemisphere. It is speculative in indicating that the right hemisphere has full potential for language development in the early prenatal period, but this seems plausible given the occurrence of right-hemisphere language dominance in many normal left-handers and a few normal right-handers. It furthermore assumes that language *function* lateralization is an all-or-none process while loss of language acquisition *potential* by the nonspeaking hemisphere is gradual. Interestingly, new developments in functional brain imaging utilizing magnetic resonance (67) should make it possible to explore these issues much more definitively and further validate the importance of the study of the fortunately uncommon problem of childhood aphasia for understanding the unfortunately all too common developmental language disorders.

REFERENCES

1. Cotard J. Etude sur l'atrophie partielle du cerveau. Thesis, Paris, 1868.
2. Clarus A. Uber Aphasie bei Kindern. Jahresbuch für Kinderheilkunde 1874;7: 369–400.
3. Bernhardt M. Ueber die spastische Cerebralparalyse im Kindesalter (Hemiplegia spastica infantilis) nebst einem Excurse uber "Aphasie bei Kindern." Virchows Archiv fur Pathologische Anatomie und Physiologie und fur Klinische Medicin 1885;102:26–80.
4. Freud S. Infantile cerebral paralysis (Infantile Cerebrallahmung). 1893. Russin L, trans. Coral Gables, FL: University of Miami.
5. Mingazzini G. Uber den heutigen Stand der Aphasielehre. Klinische Wochenschrift 1925;4:1289–1294.
6. Basser L. Hemiplegia of early onset and the faculty of speech with special reference to the effects of hemispherectomy. Brain 1962;85:427–460.
7. Lenneberg E. Biological foundations of language. New York: John Wiley, 1967.
8. Geschwind N, Levitsky W. Human brain left-right asymmetries in the temporal speech region. Science 1968;161:186–187.
9. Witelson S, Pallie W. Left hemisphere specialization for language in the newborn: Neuroanatomical evidence of asymmetry. Brain 1973;96:641–646.
10. Wada J, Clarke R, Hamm A. Cerebral hemispheric asymmetry in humans. Cortical speech zones in 100 adult and 100 infant brains. Arch Neurol 1975;32:239–246.
11. Chi J, Dooling E, Gilles F. Left-right asymmetries of the temporal speech areas of the human fetus. Arch Neurol 1977;34:345–348.
12. Molfese D, Freeman R, Palermo D. The ontology of brain lateralization for speech and non-speech stimuli. Brain Lang 1975;3:356–368.
13. Kimura D. Speech lateralization in young children as determined by an auditory test. Compar Physiolog Psychol 1963;56:899–902.
14. Kinsbourne M, Hiscock M. Does cerebral dominance develop? In: Segalowitz S, Gruber F, eds. Language development and neurological theory. New York: Academic Press, 1977:171–191.

15. Krashen S. Lateralization, language learning, and the critical period. Lang Learn 1973;23:63–74.
16. Woods BT, Teuber HL. Changing patterns of childhood aphasia. Ann Neurol 1978;3:273–280.
17. Woods B, Carey S. Language deficits after apparent clinical recovery from childhood aphasia. Ann Neurol 1979;6:405–409.
18. Ford F, Schaffer A. Etiology of infantile acquired hemiplegia. Arch Neurol Psychiatry 1927;18:323–347.
19. Shillito J. Carotid arteritis: A cause of hemiplegia in childhood. J Neurosurg 1964;21:540–551.
20. Suzuki J, Takaku A. Cerebrovascular "moyamoya" disease. Arch Neurol 1969; 20:288–299.
21. Rust RS, Volpe J. Long-term sequelae of neonatal stroke. Ann Neurol 1991; 30:487.
22. Gastaut H, Poirier F, Payan H. HHE syndrome: hemiconvulsions, hemiplegia, epilepsy. Epilepsia 1960;1:418–447.
23. Norman R. Neuropathological finding in acute hemiplegia in childhood with special reference to epilepsy as a pathogenic factor. Little Club Clin Develop Med 1962;6:37–48.
24. Landau W, Kleffner F. Syndrome of acquired aphasia with convulsive disorder in children. Neurology 1957;7:523–530.
25. Worster-Drought C. An unusual form of acquired aphasia in children. Develop Med Child Neurol 1957;13:563–571.
26. Dulac O, Billard C, Arthuis M. Aspects electrocliniques et evolutifs de l'epilepsie dans le syndrome aphasie-epilepsie. Arch Franc Pediatr 1983;40:299–308.
27. Bishop DVM. Age of onset and outcome in "acquired aphasia with convulsive disorder" (Landau-Kleffner syndrome). Devel Med Child Neurol 1985;27:705–712.
28. Dugas M, Gerard CL, Franc S, Sagar D. Natural history, course and prognosis of the Landau and Kleffner syndrome. In: Martins IP, Castro-Caldas A, van Dongen HR, van Hout A, eds. Acquired aphasia in children. Boston: Kluwer Academic Publishers, 1991.
29. Mantovani JF, Landau WM. Acquired aphasia with convulsive disorder: Course and prognosis. Neurology 1980;30:524–529.
30. McKinney W, McGreal D. An aphasic syndrome in children. CMA J 1974;110: 637–639.
31. Van de Sandt-Koenderman WME, Smit IAC, van Dongen HR, van Hest JBC. A case of acquired aphasia and convulsive disorder: Some linguistic aspects of recovery and breakdown. Brain Lang 1984;21:174–183.
32. Brunner H, Stengel E. Zur Lehre von den Aphasien im Kindesalter. Zeitschrift fur die gesamte Neurologic and Psychiatrie 1932;142:430–450.
33. Klein SK, Masur D, Farber K, Shinnar S, Rapin I. Fluent aphasia in children: Definition and natural history. J Child Neurol 1992;7:50–59.
34. Aram DM, Rose DF, Rekate HL, Whitaker HA. Acquired capsular/striatal aphasia in childhood. Arch Neurol 1983;40:614–617.

35. Martins IP, Ferro JM. Acquired conduction aphasia in a child. Devel Med Child Neurol 1987;29:529–540.
36. Carter RL, Hohenegger MK, Satz P. Aphasia and speech organization in children. Science 1982;218:797–799.
37. Hecaen H. Acquired aphasia in children: Revisited. Neuropsychologia 1983; 21:581–587.
38. Dennis M, Kohn B. Comprehension of syntax in infantile hemiplegics after cerebral hemidecortication: Left hemisphere superiority. Brain Language 1975;2:472–482.
39. Dennis M, Whitaker H. Language acquisition following hemidecortication. Linguistic superiority of the left over the right hemisphere. Brain Lang 1976; 3:404–433.
40. Vargha-Khadem F, O'Gorman AM, Watters GV. Aphasia and handedness in relation to hemispheric side, age at injury and severity of cerebral lesion during childhood. Brain 1985;108:677–696.
41. Aram DM, Ekelman BL, Whittaker HA. Spoken syntax in children with acquired unilateral hemisphere lesions. Brain Lang 1986;27:75–100.
42. Aram DM. Language sequelae of unilateral brain lesions in children. In: Plum F, ed. Language, communication, and the brain. New York: Raven Press, 1988.
43. Vargha-Khadem F, Isaacs EB, Papaleoudi H, Polkey CE, Wilson J. Development of language in six hemispherectomized patients. Brain 1991;114:473–495.
44. Feldman HM, Holland AL, Kemp SS, Janosky JE. Language development after unilateral brain injury. Brain Lang 1992;42:89–102.
45. Woods BT, Teuber HL. Early onset of complimentary specialization of cerebral hemispheres in man. Trans Am Neurol Assoc 1973;98:59–63.
46. Satz P. Symptom pattern and recovery outcome in childhood aphasia: Amethodological and theoretical critique. In: Martins IP, Castro-Caldas A, von dongen HR, van Hout A, eds. Acquired aphasia in children. Boston: Kluwer Academic Publishers, 1991.
47. Klein SK, Aram DM. Recovery of hand function after hemispheric infarction in children. Ann Neurol 1991;30:475–476.
48. Lansdell H. Verbal and non-verbal factors in right-hemisphere speech: Relation to early neurological history. J Compar Physiolog Psychol 1969;69:734–738.
49. Woods BT. The restricted effects of right-hemisphere lesions after age one: Wechsler Test data. Neuropsychologia 1980;18:65–70.
50. Ballantyne AO, Scarvie KM, Trauner DA. Verbal and performance I.Q. patterns in children after perinatal stroke. Ann Neurol 1991;30:487–488.
51. Riva D, Pantaleoni C, Milani N, Devoti M. Late sequelae of right vs. left hemispheric lesions. In: Martins IP, Castro-Caldas A, van Dongen HR, van Hout A, eds. Acquired aphasia in children. Boston: Kluwer Academic Publishers, 1991.
52. Potzl O. Uber sensorische Aphasie im Kindersalter. Zeitschrift fur Ohrenheilkunde und fur die Krankheiten der Luftwege 1926;14:190–216.
53. Van Dongen H, Loonen M. Factors related to prognosis or acquired aphasia in children. Cortex 1977;13:131–136.

54. Alajouanine T, Lhermitte F. Acquired aphasia in children. Brain 1965;88:635–662.
55. Aram DM. Scholastic achievement after early brain lesions. In: Martins IP, Castro-Caldas A, von Dongen HR, van Hout A, eds. Acquired aphasia in children. Boston: Kluwer Academic Publishers, 1991.
56. Thal DJ, Marchman V, Stiles J, Aram D, Trauner D, Nass R, Bates E. Early lexical development in children with focal brain injury. Brain Lang 1991;40:491–527.
57. Kertesz A, McCabe P. Recovery patterns and prognosis in aphasia. Brain 1977;100:1–18.
58. Milner B. Hemispheric specialization: scope and limits. In: Schmitt F, Worden F, eds. The neurosciences: third study program. Cambridge, MA: MIT Press, 1974.
59. Kinsbourne M. The minor cerebral hemisphere as a source of aphasic speech. Arch Neurol 1971;22:1126–1132.
60. Burkland C, Smith A. Language and the cerebral hemispheres: Observations of verbal and non-verbal responses during 18 months following left ("dominant") hemispherectomy. Neurology 1977;27:627–633.
61. Gott P. Language after dominant hemispherectomy. J Neurol Neurosurg Psychiatry 1973;36:1082–1088.
62. Geschwind N. Late changes in the nervous system: An overview. In: Stein D, Rosen J, Butters N, eds. Plasticity and recovery of function in the central nervous system. New York: Academic Press, 1974:467–508.
63. Nielsen J. Agnosia, apraxia, aphasia. New York: Hafner Publishing, 1962.
64. Rasmussen T, Milner B. The role of early left-brain injury in determining lateralization of cerebral speech functions. Ann NY Acad Sci 1977;299:355–369.
65. Kurthen M, Helmstaedter C, Linke DB, Solymosi L, Elger EE, Schramm J. Interhemispheric dissociation of expressive and receptive language functions in patients with complex-partial seizures: An amobarbital study. Brain Lang 1992;43:694–712.
66. Mohr J. Rapid amelioration of motor aphasia. Arch Neurol 1973;28:77–82.
67. Connelly A, Jackson GD. Functional mapping of activated human primary cortex with a clinical MR imaging system. Radiology 1993;188:125–130.

17

Language Batteries in Aphasia

Wanda G. Webb

Vanderbilt University School of Medicine, Nashville, Tennessee

In an era of sophisticated neurodiagnostic assessment procedures such as CT scans, MRI, and PET, language remains one of the behavioral functions for which assessment must include human interaction with the patient. This interaction must be sophisticated in itself. It should be of adequate length, using valid and reliable measures of language comprehension and production. It should also include synthesis of information gathered from sources beyond the neuroradiological findings and the results of the language testing. If the purposes of assessment, as cited below, are to be achieved, this interaction must be interpreted utilizing informal observation data, information gathered from family and others, premorbid history, research data, and clinical judgment and experience.

THE PURPOSE OF ASSESSMENT

The purposes of language assessment may be varied in clinical practice depending on the setting. For acute care, rehabilitation, and outpatient settings, the primary purpose of assessment of aphasia patients will be one or several of the following:

1. To provide differential diagnosis, including presence or absence of aphasia as well as type and classification of aphasia, if appropriate

2. To make a prognosis regarding recovery
3. To establish a treatment plan and make recommendations concerning follow-up
4. To assess and document progress and change

In most of these clinical settings, the person most qualified to accomplish the language testing and make these critical decisions is the speech–language pathologist. Neuropsychologists and physicians in the practice of neurology and physical medicine and rehabilitation also often contribute information critical to the accurate assessment of the language functioning of these patients.

TYPES OF ASSESSMENT

This chapter concentrates primarily on comprehensive aphasia batteries and their use. There are other types of testing, however, that can and should be used in daily practice. The frequency and appropriateness of their use depends on the setting and the purpose of assessment. The three types of assessment that will be discussed in this chapter are screening tests, aphasia batteries, and supplementary testing with individual tests of various modalities.

Screening or Bedside Assessment

In an acute-care setting particularly, the purpose of testing may be to document the presence or absence of aphasia and make recommendations regarding follow-up assessment or treatment. The testing should allow some information to be gathered from the family about the patient's premorbid language. It also provides information for the clinician to give the family about the current level of language functioning and suggestions for ways to facilitate communication. Because of the usual briefness of stay, it may be possible to complete only screening tests of speech and language at bedside.

The following assessment instruments are well standardized and widely used for such purposes. As Davis (1) points out, a well-trained clinician could accomplish an accurate bedside assessment with only a few objects and some paper and a pen; the use of these types of instruments, however, provides consistency in and support for the diagnosis while facilitating convenience and consistency in measurement of progress or change.

Halstead-Wepman Aphasia Screening Test

The Halstead-Wepman Aphasia Screening Test (2) provides a quick survey of language skills, primarily to establish the presence or absence of aphasia. In its present modified form it is still being used by some neurologists as an adjunct to the clinical neurological exam (3).

Sklar Aphasia Scale

One of the older screening tests, the Sklar (4) tests each modality with five subtests of five items each. There is also a 5-point scoring system, with the higher scores indicating greater impairment.

Aphasia Language Performance Scales

The authors of the Aphasia Language Performance Scales (ALPS), Keenan and Brassell (5), have developed a highly useable standardized informal measure of aphasia that can be easily administered at bedside. A few objects that can be carried in the examiner's pocket are used to assess a hierarchy of skills in the four modalities tested: listening, speaking, reading, and writing.

Bedside Evaluation Screening Test

The Bedside Evaluation Screening Test (BEST), developed by Fitch-West and Sands (6) in 1987, takes a unique approach utilizing cartoons and other more conversational stimuli to test language. It thus includes assessment of conversational skill as well as the more typical naming, reading, and repetition. Unfortunately, the cartoon stimuli are difficult for some patients to see, making the test less useful for some populations than tests using objects or better picture stimuli.

Often clinicians have individual approaches to the screening of language function at bedside, or will use a protocol developed and utilized by the department or institution. Chapter 1 contains such a bedside examination. For experienced clinicians this approach works well and interpretation is accurate. It is vital, however, that consistency in measurement be a primary consideration. The use of standardized procedures facilitates such consistency.

Comprehensive Aphasia Batteries

Most of the popular aphasia batteries in use today were designed to diagnose aphasia, and their content is thus skewed primarily toward the defining features of the aphasia (1). Utility of an aphasia battery depends in theory on the inclusion of the following components as design features: (1) successful minimization of the effect of internal and external influences on language behavior (e.g., education, intelligence, socioeconomic status), (2) independent assessment of each language modality, (3) inclusion of a range of items to assess language along a continuum of complexity, and (4) adequate number of items or adequate scoring system to describe accurately a behavior as variable as language.

Discussed here are the major utilization and prominent strengths and weaknesses of the most widely used comprehensive aphasia batteries employed in the United States.

Minnesota Test for Differential Diagnosis of Aphasia

Hildred Schuell's (7) considerable skills as a clinician are evident in the principal objective of the Minnesota Test for Differential Diagnosis of Aphasia (MTDDA): to assess systematically a wide range of behavior in the principal language modalities and use the findings as a guide to effective treatment planning. Based on psychometric standardization that was very sophisticated for the time, the MTDDA's classification system yielded five major profiles of language impairment and two minor profiles. Major classifications include simple aphasia, aphasia with visual involvement, aphasia with sensorimotor involvement, aphasia with scattered findings compatible with generalized brain damage, and irreversible aphasic syndrome. The two minor profiles are mild aphasia with persisting dysfluency and aphasia with intermittent auditory imperception.

Although these classifications are not often used now, the "Minnesota" or "Schuell," as it is frequency called, has several strengths for use in clinical practice. It is the only aphasia battery that measures reading rate. It contains a much wider range of verbal tests than most assessments, including giving biographical information, retelling a paragraph, and defining words.

The extensive range of subtests within the MTDDA makes it time-consuming to administer and has raised the criticism that it goes beyond the measurement of speech and language and ventures into measurements traditionally used in intelligence testing (8). A "general" factor closely related to the g factor of intelligence tests was found on factor analysis, but Schuell and Jenkins (9) considered it a general *language* factor.

Many clinicians today use the MTDDA as a battery from which they select the subtests most useful to them in assessing the language of their patient. Since the subtests are independent and were developed by a master clinician, this is a very useful feature.

The Porch Index of Communicative Ability

The Porch Index of Communicative Ability (PICA) (10,11) is a highly standardized assessment tool designed to conform to a model of language involving several input modalities, a central processor, and a number of possible output modalities. The author's contribution to assessment is the design of a multidimensional scoring system that describes a range of behaviors in a manageable numerical scoring system. While this scoring system is to be applauded, it is one of the most criticized features of the test (12,13). The PICA does not cluster its 18 subtests according to modality of response. Rather, it utilizes 10 common objects throughout the subtests and clusters the most difficult subtest for each modality at the beginning of the tests of verbal, gestural, and auditory ability. Graphic subtests are the final section, also putting the most difficult subtests first.

The PICA has been used widely to chart progress of patients and to attempt to predict recovery using data obtained 1 month postonset. This has not been well validated and is not routinely utilized by many clinicians. Because of the difficulty with obtaining the formal training (40 hours) needed to learn to use the scoring system accurately and reliably, the PICA is not employed now as widely as in previous years. It remains a very useful tool for the well-trained clinician to chart recovery. Its lack of tests for the milder disorders in all modalities limits its use to certain groups of more involved patients.

Neurosensory Center Comprehensive Examination for Aphasia

Although not used in the United States as frequently as the other comprehensive batteries discussed here, the Neurosensory Center Comprehensive Examination for Aphasia (NCCEA) (14) is a highly respected, valuable tool for the assessment of aphasia. Its limitations are similar to those of the PICA in testing the milder aphasic deficits. There are 20 subtests, with four extra tests to be used when visual or tactile deficits are suspected as contributing to the performance. Four arrays of eight common objects are used in eight of the subtests. Administration time may be shortened by the provision of a set of items for initial testing in several subtests, allowing the examiner to screen those functions. Only if errors are made within the initial items does the examiner administer a second set of items for more detailed assessment of performance. The NCCEA contains tests of word-finding, immediate verbal memory, verbal production and fluency, decoding ability, reading and writing, and articulation.

Although the test was originally developed in 1969, normative data were not available until 1977. The NCCEA has also been shown to be useful in measuring the language development of children (15,16).

Boston Diagnostic Aphasia Examination

Because of its wide acceptance by research and clinical neurologists, neuropsychologists, and speech–language pathologists, the Boston Diagnostic Aphasia Examination (BDAE) (17) has become one of the most frequently utilized aphasia batteries. Kaplan (18) describes its design as following the clinical neuropsychological orientation that prefers description of apparently strategic behavior rather than depending simply on scores. This is a "process approach" to analyzing performance, according to Kaplan.

The BDAE has been used by researchers and clinicians alike to classify aphasic patients into the traditional Boston classifications of Broca's, Wernicke's, conduction, anomic, transcortical motor, transcortical sensory, and global aphasia syndromes (see Chapter 4). The test consists of 27 subtests assessing fluency, auditory comprehension, oral expression, repetition, reading, and writing. The manual also includes suggestions for supplementary testing of verbal and nonverbal functions divided into psycholinguistic explorations and spatial-quantitative testing. The presence of finger agnosia or constructional apraxia could be detected with the spatial-quantitative battery.

New normative data were gathered on the Boston exam between 1976 and 1982, and a revised version was published in 1983. Raw scores are related to percentiles in the 1983 version, replacing the z-scores originally used. Cutoff scores are given for persons over 60 and for individuals with fewer than 9 years of education. Profiles are provided for comparison purposes in classifying syndromes. Because of limited reliability data and lack of summary scores, the BDAE has not been typically used in the literature to document recovery. Data from patients has been used to document progress with certain treatment regimes (19,20).

Western Aphasia Battery

The author of the Western Aphasia Battery (WAB), Dr. Andrew Kertesz (21), hoped to minimize the subjective nature of syndrome classification with the BDAE by designing a test similar in content and purpose but with specific test scores assigned to the profiles and an additional advantage of access to summary scores. Although utilized by many for studies of aphasia taxonomy and recovery for several years prior, the complete test was not published until 1982.

Summary scores available after administering the test battery, which is very similar in content design to the BDAE, are as follows:

1. Aphasia quotient (AQ). The four sections of the auditory and spoken language tests yield the AQ as a summary of performance. Much of the score (40%) is derived from the scale for rating spontaneous speech.
2. Language quotient (LQ). This is a modification (22) to the original scoring of the test. It includes scores from the reading and writing tests as well as the AQ subtest scores.
3. Performance quotient (PQ). Reading, writing, apraxia, and construction tasks were originally folded into a performance score.
4. Cortical quotient (CQ). This score represents performance on all verbal and nonverbal tests. The WAB CQ includes performance on the Ravens Colored Progressive Matrices, which must be administered to obtain a cortical quotient.

The CQ and the AQ are the only two scores mentioned in the test manual.

As mentioned, the BDAE and the WAB are employed widely in the classification of aphasia into the traditional Boston aphasia syndromes. A study by Wertz et al. (23) found only 27% agreement in classifications between the WAB and the BDAE. A 1984 study (24) on the agreement in classification between the WAB and clinical impressions of those administering it showed only a 54% agreement, with the most disagreement occurring for fluent aphasias. It is suggested that clinical descriptions be used to supplement test batteries in assigning classifications.

Additional Batteries

Although the batteries discussed above are the primary tests used by most clinicians for comprehensive testing, other tests are available. A limited number of aphasia batteries have been translated to use in other languages, but only one test is available to aphasiologists that has equivalent versions in several languages. The Multilingual Aphasia Examination was developed by Benton and Hamsher (25) to meet the need for an aphasia test that not only would be translated into another language but would have equivalent content for each language, allowing real comparisons across cultures. The design of the test is similar to that of the NCCEA. It has been found to be a highly useful instrument for diagnostic and treatment decisions.

Other aphasia batteries do not quite qualify as comprehensive because the range of difficulty of the items is limited. However, they are aphasia batteries because they assess a number of modalities (listening, speaking, reading, writing, and gesture).

The Communicative Abilities in Daily Living (CADL) test was authored by Dr. Audrey Holland (26) to assist the clinician in assessing a patient's functional language skills, with the primary functions of language—understanding and conveying a message—as the main skills to be assessed. The CADL focuses much less on the adequacy of the linguistic components of the message than traditional aphasia tests, as long as the substance of the message is conveyed. Holland incorporated natural language activities and natural style to offset the usual formal, unnatural testing situation. She also incorporated humor, metaphor, social conventions, and role-playing into the testing situation. The CADL does not take the place of observation of the patient in actual communication situations, but it provides a useful adjunct to the more formalized testing, especially when assessing strengths of a patient's retained language abilities.

The Boston Assessment of Severe Aphasia (BASA) (27) is similar to the CADL in that it was developed by individuals immersed in clinical practice who wished to look for retained language abilities upon which to build or facilitate better communication. Most of the items on the BASA were selected because research had shown that many of the more severely impaired aphasic patients could naturally perform some language tasks that formal testing failed to identify. Tasks such as identifying famous people, repeating emotionally loaded words, or matching numbers to coins evoke residual skills in some patients. By noting mode of response and overall communicativeness (i.e., how much of the intended message could be understood?) rather than just scoring + / −, a more accurate assessment of a severely aphasic patient can be obtained than with the comprehensive batteries.

Recently published is a new assessment instrument called the Aphasia Diagnostic Profiles (ADP) (28). The ADP does not strictly meet the criteria for an aphasia battery in that reading and writing are only minimally assessed. The ADP serves a quite useful function for assessment in allowing the clinician to document not only the nature and severity of impairment but also the degree to which certain abilities are spared and the general social-emotional state of the patient. A classification profile is provided for analyzing whether the aphasia fits into any of the traditional fluent or nonfluent classifications of the Boston system. There is a "borderline fluent" classification in the profile that is not related to a certain aphasia classification. The ADP is an extremely utilitarian instrument because of its good standardization data and efficiency of administration in many different settings. It will assist the clinician in making decisions about further testing with a more in-depth battery or with supplementary tests listed in the next section. It also allows the clinician to begin treatment taking advantage of the information gathered about the spared language competencies of the patient.

Table 1 Tests that Assess Skill in Different Modalities Contributing to the Language Performance of Aphasia Patients (These tests may be used to supplement aphasia batteries or may be used instead of a comprehensive battery.)

Modality	Tests
Auditory comprehension	Revised Token Test (28)
	Auditory Comprehension Test for Sentences (29)
Gesture	Pantomime Recognition Test (30)
	Assessment of Nonverbal Communication (31)
Reading comprehension	Reading Comprehension Battery for Aphasia (32)
	Nelson-Denny Reading Test (33)
	Stanford Diagnostic Reading Battery (34)
	Test of Reading Comprehension (35)
Writing	Writing Process Test (36)
	Test of Written Language (37)
Limb apraxia	Limb Apraxia Test (38)
	Test of Oral and Limb Apraxia (39)
Verbal expression	Boston Naming Test (40)
	Word Fluency Measure (41)
	The Reporter's Test (42)
	Northwestern Syntax Screening Test (43)
	Shewan Spontaneous Language Analysis (44)
	Test of Adolescent/Adult Word-Finding (45)

Supplementary Testing

Although the information gathered from aphasia batteries is very useful to the physician and the speech–language pathologist, there is more often than not a need for further testing before a truly adequate treatment plan for an aphasic patient can be firmly established. An aphasia battery must be long enough to establish the presence of a disorder and to identify and compare the deficits in the various language modalities; however, it must also be short enough to explore language in a time- and cost-efficient manner. Therefore, once the primary characteristics of the aphasia are identified and a prognosis and treatment decision are made, the clinician often needs to expand the exploration of the territories that we call the language modalities: auditory comprehension, speaking, gesturing, reading, and writing. Table 1 lists various tests currently available for use in a more in-depth assessment of language performance in each of these areas.

TRAUMATIC BRAIN INJURY: SPECIAL CONSIDERATIONS

Due to the different mechanism of etiology in a closed head injury, more than one type of language disorder may be found upon assessment of patients. One may find a true aphasia similar to that caused by a vascular etiology. This results from focal damage to a particular area of the brain specialized for language. One may also find that the patient exhibits a *cognitive-communicative disorder* in combination with the aphasia or that there is no true aphasic component, in the traditional sense, to the language problem. Cognitive-communicative disorders result from the widespread, diffuse brain damage occurring after trauma and the consequent impaired attention, information processing, and cognition (46). Therefore, the clinician will go beyond the traditional language testing of the aphasia batteries and supplementary tests discussed previously. Diagnostic language testing for cognitive-communicative disorders includes examination of such areas as perception, discrimination, organization, recall, convergent thinking, deductive reasoning, inductive reasoning, divergent thinking, and problem-solving. Table 2 lists several assessment tools used by speech–language pathologists and neuropsychologists to examine cognitive processes involved in language. Speech–language pathologists also use some of these assessments with aphasic patients with a vascular etiology, especially if the therapy is going to be designed on a cognitive intervention model (47).

NEW DIRECTIONS IN THE ASSESSMENT OF APHASIA

Perusal of both the research and clinical literature on diagnosis and treatment of aphasia shows a move toward less dependence on the traditional

Table 2 Assessment Instruments Frequently Used in Evaluation of the Cognitive-Linguistic Status of Patients Who Have Had Traumatic Brain Injury (These may also be used in testing patients with mild aphasia and more subtle deficits.)

Woodcock-Johnson Test of Cognitive Abilities (48)
Brief Test of Head Injury (49)
Detroit Test of Learning Ability—Adult (50)
General Abilities Battery (51)
Rivermead Behavioral Memory Test (52)
Scales of Cognitive Ability for Traumatic Brain Injury (53)
Ross Information Processing Assessment (54)
Woodcock Language Battery (55)
Attention Processing Test (56)
The Word Test (57)
California Verbal Learning Test—Research Edition (58)
Prospective Memory Screening Test (59)
Test of Problem Solving (60)
Test of Nonverbal Intelligence (61)

aphasia batteries and greater use of supplementary testing utilizing standardized tests such as those listed above or experimental versions of other assessments. Beyond tests in the areas previously mentioned, there are two other directions into which aphasia assessment is branching.

Discourse Analysis

The traditional examination of discourse had been limited to a descriptive analysis such as that used in the MTDDA, BDAE, and WAB. The analysis was also limited to more of a description of the performance than an actual analysis of the content in terms of syntax, grammar, and/or semantics. In the past few years, the clinical research literature has frequently included studies of and recommendations for using a more expanded analysis of discourse with aphasic patients (62–65). Diagnosticians are cautioned to recognize that there are different types of discourse (1). One may design a task that requires descriptive, procedural, narrative, or conversational discourse. Different types of procedures are available to analyze the corpus of language depending on whether the primary interest is in the syntactical/grammatical performance, the semantic content, or the efficiency and communicativeness of the output.

Psycholinguistic Approach

Most clinicians and others interested in the assessment and remediation of the language disorder demonstrated by aphasic patients readily recognize the limitations of the aphasia batteries currently available. The syndrome-oriented approach to aphasia classification also has tremendous limitations. Most clinicians will try to specify the nature of the disturbance in the performance of the language tasks even if a classification has been assigned.

Dr. David Caplan (66) has provided a valuable tutorial in the speech-language pathology literature that discusses activation of major classes of linguistic representations by psycholinguistically defined language processors. In this article he describes a battery for psycholinguistic assessment of language disorders that he and his colleague Dr. Daniel Bub are developing and standardizing for clinical use. The availability of norms for psycholinguistic batteries would allow the well-trained clinician to administer such tests and accurately interpret performance. Caplan notes that the overall goal of such an assessment is a description of the language disorder that relates it to the major components of the language-processing system. Results of the analysis would indicate which types of linguistic representations (e.g., simple words, word formations, sentences, or discourse) are processed abnormally in each of the four major modalities usually assessed in aphasia. Further examined would be whether the disturbance affects linguistic forms, semantic meanings, or both. This would not necessarily preclude the traditional classification effort but would enhance the description and, perhaps, eventually lead to more finite classifications. Broader explorations of the language code may also contribute greatly to remediation efforts.

CONCLUSION

The assessment of the language disorder of aphasia has a rich history and a promising future. Through the collaboration of speech–language pathologists, neuropsychologists, neurologists, and others interested in aphasia, development of better assessment and treatment methods will add further promise to the future of individuals debilitated by the disorder.

REFERENCES

1. Davis GA. A survey of adult aphasia and related language disorders. 2nd ed. Englewood Cliffs, NJ: Prentice Hall, 1993.
2. Sall M, Wepman JM. A screening survey of organic impairment. J Speech Hear Disord 1945;10:283–286.
3. Love RJ. Aphasia rehabilitation: state of the art. Monographs in contemporary speech and language. Vol 1, No. 1. Upper Darby, PA: Instrumentation Associates, 1982.
4. Sklar M. Sklar aphasia scale. Revised ed. Los Angeles: Western Psychological Services, 1973.
5. Keenan JS, Brassell EG. Aphasia language performance scales. Murfreesboro, TN: Pinnacle Press, 1975.

6. Fitch-West J, Sands ES. Bedside evaluation screening test. Rockville, MD: Aspen, 1987.

7. Schuell H. Differential diagnosis of aphasia with the Minnesota test. Minneapolis: University of Minnesota Press, 1965.

8. Spreen O, Risser A. Assessment of aphasia. In: Sarno MT, ed. Acquired aphasia. New York: Academic Press, 1981.

9. Schuell HM, Jenkins JJ. The nature of language deficit in aphasia. Psycholog Rev 1959;66:45–67.

10. Porch BE. Porch index of communicative ability: theory and development. Vol 1. Palo Alto, CA: Consulting Psychologists Press, 1967.

11. Porch BE. Porch index of communicative ability: administration, scoring and interpretation. Vol 2. Palo Alto, CA: Consulting Psychologists Press, 1973.

12. Martin AD. Aphasia testing: a second look at the porch index of communicative ability. J Speech Hear Disord 1977;42:547–561.

13. McNeil MR. Porch index of communicative ability. In: Darley FL, ed. Evaluation of appraisal techniques in speech and language pathology. Reading, MA: Addison-Wesley, 1979.

14. Spreen O, Benton AL. Neurosensory center comprehensive examination for aphasia. Revised ed. Victoria, BC: University of Victoria Neuropsychology Laboratory, 1977.

15. Crockett DJ. Component analysis of within correlations of language-skill tests in normal children. J Spec Ed 1974;8:361–375.

16. Gaddes WH, Crockett DJ. The Spreen-Benton aphasia tests: normative data as a measure of normal language development. Brain Lang 1975;2:257–280.

17. Goodglass H, Kaplan E. The assessment of aphasia and related disorders. 2nd ed. Philadelphia: Lea & Febiger, 1983.

18. Kaplan E. The process approach to neuropsychological assessment. Aphasiology 1988;2:309–312.

19. Sparks RW, Helm NA, Albert ML. Aphasia rehabilitation resulting from melodic intonation therapy. Cortex 1974;10:303–316.

20. Helm NA, Barressi B. Voluntary control of involuntary utterances: a treatment approach for severe aphasia. In: Brookshire RH, ed. Clinical aphasiology conference proceedings. Minneapolis: BRK, 1980.

21. Kertesz A. Western Aphasia Battery. New York: Grune & Stratton, 1982.

22. Shewan CM, Kertesz A. Reliability and validity characteristics of the Western Aphasia Battery (WAB). J Speech Hear Disord 1980;45:308–324.

23. Wertz RT, Deal JL, Robinson AJ. Classifying the aphasias: a comparison of the Boston Diagnostic Aphasia Exam and the Western Aphasia Battery. In: Brookshire RH, ed. Clinical aphasiology conference proceedings. Minneapolis: BRK, 1984.

24. Swindell CS, Holland AL, Fromm D. Classification of aphasia: WAB type versus clinical impression. In: Brookshire RH, ed. Clinical aphasiology conference proceedings. Minneapolis: BRK, 1984.

25. Benton AL, Hamsher K. Multilingual aphasia examination. 2nd ed. Iowa City: AJA Associates, 1989.

26. Holland AL. Communicative abilities of daily living. Baltimore: University Park Press, 1980.

27. Helm-Estabrooks N, Ramsberger G, Morgan AR, Nicholas M. Boston assessment of severe aphasia (BASA). Chicago: Riverside, 1989.
28. McNeil M, Prescott TE. Revised token test. Baltimore: University Park Press, 1978.
29. Shewan CM. Auditory comprehension test for sentences. Chicago: Biolinguistics Clinical Institutes, 1979.
30. Varney NR, Benton AL. Pantomime recognition test. Iowa City: Benton Laboratory of Neuropsychology, 1978.
31. Duffy RJ, Duffy JR. Assessment of nonverbal communication. Austin, TX: PRO-ED, 1984.
32. LaPointe LL, Horner J. Reading comprehension battery for aphasia. Chicago: Riverside, 1979.
33. Brown JI, Fishco VV, Hanna G. Nelson-Denny reading test. Chicago: Riverside, 1993.
34. Karlsen B, Gardner E, Madden R. Stanford diagnostic reading test. 3rd ed. San Antonio: Harcourt Brace Jovanovich, 1986.
35. Brown VL, Hammill DD, Wiederholt JL. Test of reading comprehension. Austin, TX: PRO-ED, 1986.
36. Warden MR, Hutchinson TJ. The writing process test. Chicago: Riverside, 1993.
37. Hammill DD, Larsen SC. Test of written language. Austin, TX: PRO-ED, 1983.
38. Duffy JR, Duffy RJ. The limb apraxia test: an imitative measure of upper limb apraxia. In: Prescott TE, ed. Clinical aphasiology conference proceedings. Minneopolis: BRK, 1989.
39. Helm-Estabrooks N. Test of Oral and Limb Apraxia. Chicago: Riverside, 1991.
40. Goodglass H, Kaplan E. Boston naming test. Philadelphia: Lea & Febiger, 1983.
41. Borkowski JG, Benton AL, Spreen O. Word fluency and brain damage. Neuropsychologica 1967;5:135–140.
42. DeRenzi E, Ferrari C. The reporter's test: a sensitive test to detect expressive disturbances in aphasics. Cortex 1978;14:279–293.
43. Lee L. Northwestern syntax screening test. Evanston, IL: Northwestern University Press, 1971.
44. Shewan CM. The Shewan spontaneous language analysis (SSLA) system for aphasic adults: description, reliability, and validity. J Commun Disord 1988; 21:103–138.
45. German D. Test of adolescent/adult word-finding. Allen, TX: Developmental Learning Materials, 1990.
46. Adamovich LB, Henderson JA. Traumatic brain injury. In: LaPointe LL, ed. Aphasia and related neurogenic language disorders. New York: Thieme Medical Publishers, 1990.
47. Chapey R. Cognitive intervention: stimulation of cognition, memory, convergent thinking, divergent thinking and evaluative thinking. In: Chapey R, ed. Language intervention strategies in adult aphasia. 2nd ed. Baltimore: Williams & Wilkins, 1986.
48. Woodcock RW, Johnson MB. Woodcock-Johnson tests of cognitive ability. Allen, TX: Developmental Learning Materials, 1990.

49. Helm-Estabrooks N. Brief test of head injury. Chicago: Riverside, 1991.
50. Hammill D, Bryant B. Detroit test of learning ability—adult. Austin, TX: PRO-ED, 1991.
51. Schubert HJP. General abilities battery. East Aurora, NY: Slosson, 1986.
52. Wilson B, Cockburn J, Baddeley A. Rivermead behavioral memory test. 1986.
53. Adamovich LB, Henderson JA. Scales of cognitive ability for traumatic brain injury. Chicago: Riverside, 1992.
54. Ross DG. Ross information processing assessment. Austin, TX: PRO-ED, 1986.
55. Woodcock RW. Woodcock language proficiency battery—revised. Allen, TX: Developmental Learning Materials, 1991.
56. Mateer CA, Sohlberg MM, Barber J. Attention processing test. Puyallup, WA: Association for Neuropsychological Research and Development. No publication date.
57. Jorgensen C, Barrett M, Husingh R, Zachman L. The word test. Moline, IL: LinguiSystems, 1981.
58. Delis D, Kramer JH, Kaplan E, Ober BA. California verbal learning test—research edition. San Antonio: Psychological Corporation, 1987.
59. Sohlberg MM, Mateer CA. Prospective memory screening test. Puyallup, WA: Association for Neuropsychological Research and Development, 1992.
60. Zachman L, Jorgensen C, Huisingh R, Barrett M. Test of problem-solving. Moline, IL: LinguiSystems, 1984.
61. Brown L, Sherbenou RJ, Johnsen SK. Test of nonverbal intelligence. Austin, TX: PRO-ED, 1982.
62. Ulatowska HK, Cannito MP, Hayashi MM, Fleming SG. Language abilities in the elderly. In: Ulatowska HK, ed. The aging brain: communication in the elderly. San Diego: Singular, 1985.
63. Holland AL, et al. Rapid recovery from aphasia: a detailed language analysis. Brain Lang 1985;24:156–173.
64. Yorkston KM, Buekelman DR. An analysis of connected speech samples of aphasic and normal speakers. J Speech Hear Disord 1980;45:27–36.
65. Shewan CM. Expressive language recovery in aphasia using the Shewan spontaneous language analysis (SSLA) system. J Commun Disord 1988;21:155–169.
66. Caplan D. Toward a psycholinguistic approach to acquired neurogenic language disorders. Am J Speech Lang Pathol 1993;2:1:59–83.

18

Aphasia Therapy

Audrey L. Holland and Pelagie M. Beeson

*National Center for Neurogenic Communication Disorders,
University of Arizona, Tucson, Arizona*

INTRODUCTION

This chapter concerns treatment for aphasia, the disorder of symbol retrieval and formulation that can affect any or all language modalities. Thus, in its clinical sense, aphasia includes comprehension and formulation of spoken speech, reading, and writing, and comprehension and formulation of manual sign in deaf individuals. Aphasia is a "prototype disorder," possibly the most frequently occurring neurolinguistic communication impairment. For example, in 1979, the National Institutes of Health estimated that there were 1 million Americans with aphasia. Aphasia also is a prototype disorder in the sense that treatment for it has been the foundation and the model on which other intervention strategies for neurogenic disorders have been built.

It must be emphasized at the outset that professionals who treat neurogenic communication disorders actually work with a spectrum far broader than mere aphasia. Included are the language problems associated with strokes to the right hemisphere, such as disorganization of language, difficulty with its usage in social interaction, and problems in making linguistic judgments and inferences. Neurolinguistic problems associated with closed head injury that seemingly span left and right hemispheres are also the focus of therapy. Finally, there is a growing appreciation that intervention has some potential for maintaining functional performance in some individuals with progressive dementias.

In addition to these *language* disorders, it must also be noted that treatments for two related and often co-occurring *speech* disorders are also available. That is, speech–language pathologists work with individuals who experience dysarthria (more frequent following brainstem or cerebellar stroke than cortical or subcortical hemispheric stroke) or who have the cortically engendered disorder of motor programming called by most modern investigators *apraxia of speech.*

Despite this range of neurogenic speech and language disorders, for the sake of brevity this chapter discusses treatment only as it applies to the aphasia prototype. It begins with a discussion of the efficacy of treatment for aphasia. In succeeding sections, some examples of treatment are provided. Finally, some thoughts about the future of aphasia treatment are shared.

EFFICACY OF TREATMENT FOR APHASIA

The *general* question of efficacy of aphasia treatment, as opposed to efficacy studies designed to validate specific approaches, has been addressed in at least 14 moderate- to large-group studies. Of the eight studies detailed in Table 1, only two (1,2) constitute randomized controlled trials of treatment versus no treatment; an additional study (3) compares two forms of treatment in a randomized controlled trial. Although not a randomized controlled trial, the study by Poeck et al. (4) statistically partialed out improvements resulting from spontaneous recovery and used only the remaining differences for a subsequent comparison of treatment versus no treatment. The rest of the studies listed in Table 1 compare language and communication performance in the same subjects before and after treatment for their aphasia.

It should be noted that the large-group studies differ in both quality and results. Whereas both studies by Wertz et al. had positive results in favor of individual treatment for aphasic patients, Lincoln et al. found no effects of treatment. Concerning quality of studies, it is of interest to note that patients with a variety of disorders, including dementia, were included in the study by Lincoln et al. This study also failed to control amount and type of treatment. [For a complete critique of the Lincoln study, see Wertz et al. (5).] As can be seen in Table 1, six of the eight large-group studies reviewed, and almost all small-group and single-subject studies, support the general value of treatment for aphasia. Nevertheless, much controversy still exists in the minds of many who are in a position to refer aphasic patients for treatment. It is also the case that many legitimate questions remain concerning the efficacy of various types of treatment, as well as how and when treatment for aphasia should be delivered.

One particularly interesting question is which patients are good candidates and which are not good candidates for treatment of their aphasia. In this

Table 1a Treatment Outcome Studies

		Study subjects			Comparison groups			
Ref.	Purpose Study design Setting	Deficit	Time since onset	Inclusion/ exclusion criteria	Treatment group	Intensity/ duration	Sample size	Baseline comparability
Basso et al., 1979 (25)	To determine if lang. signif. improves specific lang. skills beyond improvement associated with spontaneous recovery. Nonrandomized control trial. Inpatient and outpatient Tx.	Aphasia	Recent: <2 mo Intermediate: 2–6 mo Long-standing: >6 mo	Fluent or nonfluent aphasia due to CVA, trauma, tumor. Excluded progressive cerebral disease	Classified as either fluent or nonfluent and moderate or severe.	≥ 3 sessions/wk, 5 mo, 1 session = 45–50 min	281 total: 162 Tx, 119 no Tx	Comparable distribution re: gender, education, nature of lesion. Mean age of no Tx group > Tx group by 5 yr.
Butfield and Zangwill, 1945 (27)	To review outcome of re-education in individuals with aphasia due to a variety of etiologies, early and late post-onset (i.e., during and after spontaneous recovery period). Descriptive study. Brain injuries unit.	Aphasia	Early: <6 mo Late: >6 mo	Excluded due to unfavorable prognosis, gross comprehension deficits, and psychiatric problems.	Most 20–45 yr; traumatic vascular, neoplastic etiologies.	2 sessions/day, 1 session = 30 min, 5–290 sessions.	65 total: 52 in early, 13 in late group	Varied re: aphasia severity, type. Differential group size precluded statistical analysis.

(continues)

447

Table 1a (Continued)

Ref.	Purpose Study design Setting	Deficit	Time since onset	Inclusion/ exclusion criteria	Treatment group	Intensity/ duration	Sample size	Baseline comparability
			Study subjects			Comparison groups		
Hartman and Landau, 1987 (26)	To compare effectiveness of traditional lang. therapy to supportive counseling therapy. Randomized assignment to group. Hospital setting.	Aphasia	1 mo	R-handed, with first LH vascular stroke, mostly thromboembolic. Native English speakers.	Randomly varied re: age, ed., aphasia type and severity, site of lesion, and other neurolog. def.	2 sessions/wk, 6 mo	60 total: 30 aphasia Tx, 30 counseling Tx (71 others rejected or died)	Equivalent re: age. No analysis re: severity comparability, but appeared equiv. NS diffs. −Ravens.
Lincoln et al., 1984 (1)	To determine whether speech Tx produces a better lang. outcome than natural recovery alone. Randomized control trial. Inpatient and home treatment.	Aphasia	10 wk	Single or multiple strokes. Excluded severe and mild aphasia and severe dysarthria.	Varied aphasia types. Additional disabilities.	2 hr/wk,[a] 24 wk	191 total: 104 Tx, 87 no Tx	No group diffs. re: age, gender distribution, aphasia type, or severity.
Poeck et al., 1989 (4)	To determine whether intensive lang. therapy leads to improvement that is > spontaneous recovery. Is therapy efficacious after 12 mo?	Aphasia	Early: 1-4 mo Late: 4-14 mo Chronic > 12 mo	LH vascular lesions. R-handed. Native German speakers. No group diffs. for age/ gender.	Early n = 23; late n = 23; chronic n = 19	9 hr/wk, 6-8 wk	68 Tx group, 92 control Ss for early (62 controls for late)	Early group and controls of comparable aphasia severity. Late group aphasia severity > than controls.

Study	Design / Purpose	Diagnosis	Time post-onset	Subjects		Treatment	N	Comparability
	Nonrandomized design with unselected control group from prior study. Inpatient Tx.							
Shewan and Kertesz, 1984 (6)	To determine if speech-lang. gains are greater for Rx vs. no Tx; to compare 2 Txs administered by SLPs and 1 Tx by non-SLPs. Randomized assignment to Tx group, self-selected control group. Hospital.	Aphasia	Within 7 wk	Unilateral (predom. LH) occlusive stroke or stable hemorrhage. Functional English speakers.	Global, Broca's, Wernicke's, anomic, and conduction aphasia. Mild to severe.	3 hr/wk, up to 1 yr	100 (25 per condition); lost 21 = 79	Similar age, ed., SES, etiology, gender dist. Tx groups stratified for aphasia type and severity. Control group less severe.
Wertz et al., 1981 (3)	To document lang. improvement associated with individual and group Tx; To determine the efficacy of Tx (after 6 mo postonset to eliminate effects of spontaneous recovery).	Aphasia	4 wk	Male, 40–80 yr, first thromboembolic stroke, premorbid English literacy, sensory screening. Overall PICA 15–75th %ile.	Selected from 1071; 4 cohorts: 11 wk, 22 wk, 33 wk, 44 wk	8 hr/wk, up to 44 wk	67 total: 35 individual Tx, 32 group Tx; 34 completed 44 wk	Age, ed, lang. severity at intake equivalent across groups and cohorts ($p > 0.05$).

(continues)

Table 1a (Continued)

Ref.	Study subjects			Comparison groups			
Purpose Study design Setting	Deficit	Time since onset	Inclusion/ exclusion criteria	Treatment group	Intensity/ duration	Sample size	Baseline comparability
Wertz et al., 1981 (3) (continued)	Random assignment to Tx group. VA centers.						
Wertz et al., 1986 (5)	To determine the effects of Tx vs. no Tx and of Tx administration by trained volunteers; to study the effect of delayed Tx. Random assignment to group. VA centers.	Aphasia	2–24 wk (X = 6–7 wk)	Male, ≤75 yr, single thrombo-embolic stroke. No existing major med. or psych. disorder. Overall PICA ≥ 10th %ile.	Traditional Tx: clinic w/SLP or home w/ volunteer; deferred Tx.	8–10 hr/wk, 12 wk	121	NS diffs. on PICA overall scores. NS diffs. BDAE lang. severity rating.

[a]Data reported regardless of actual number of hours of therapy.

Table 1b Treatment Outcome Studies

Ref.	Method	Follow-up Time	n	Outcome measures	Results	Conclusions/comments
Basso et al., 1979 (25)	Stimulation therapy (stimulus-response Tx), supplemented by group and homework.	≥ 6 mo	281: 162 Tx, 119 no Tx	Standard lang. exam: oral expression, aud. comp., reading, writing. Improvement defined as ≥ 2 points on composite score for modality (0–4 range).	Effects of Tx signif. overall ($p < 0.001$) and for each modality. Trend for comprehension (aud. and reading) to improve more than expression (spoken and writing). Increased time post-onset and aphasia severity negatively affected improvement. Type of aphasia (fluent vs. nonfluent) and effects of age NS.	Rehabilitation (≥3 sessions/wk) had a signif. positive effect on improvement in all lang. skills. Greatest improvement in Ss treated closer to onset of aphasia.
Butfield and Zangwill, 1945 (27)	Individual Tx directed toward deficit remediation.	Varied	65	Improvement rating based on clinical staff opinion, testing, and clinical records. Much improved/improved/unchanged.	78% of Ss improved with Tx. Speech was judged much improved in 1/2 of early Tx group and 1/3 of late Tx group. 10 of 13 Ss > 6 mo post-onset improved. Less improvement in reading, writing, and calculation. More improvement w/ lesser aphasia severity.	Majority of Ss improved with daily Tx, including Ss who were past spontaneous recovery period. Most favorable outcome with traumatic etiology, and with relatively mild, expressive aphasia type.
Hartman and Landau, 1987 (26)	Traditional task-oriented Tx by SLP vs. nondirective unstructured counseling by SLP.	7 and 10 mo post-stroke	60 at 7 mo, 50 at 10 mo	PICA change score (PICA at 1 mo compared to PICA at 7 and 10 mo).	No signif. differences between 2 groups at mo 7 and 10 (p set at 0.01). PICA change scores slightly favor traditional Tx at mo 10, and counseling Tx at mo 7.	Conventional therapy (2 sessions/wk) in acute stroke-induced aphasia was no more beneficial than support offered to family and patient through supportive counseling by SLP.

(continues)

451

Table 1b (Continued)

Ref.	Method	Follow-up Time	n	Outcome measures	Results	Conclusions/comments
Lincoln et al., 1984 (1)	Assessed Ss at 4 wk and randomly assigned to Tx and no Tx groups. Standard clinical Tx initiated at 10 wk post-stroke	22 and 34 wk post-stroke	47 Tx for ≥24 sessions, 47 controls	PICA overall severity, Functional Communication Profile.	No signif. differences between Tx and no-Tx groups (p value not reported). Did not report whether performance of either group improved signif. over 24-wk period. Did not indicate how many actual hr of therapy received by Tx group; however, 47 individuals received a minimum of 1 hr of therapy/wk. No signif. diffs. when comparing those Ss to 47 matched Ss in control group. Only 27 Ss received >36 sessions of Tx.	Concluded that Tx (avg 1/wk) did not improve lang. abilities more than achieved by spontaneous recovery.
Poeck et al., 1989 (4)	Lang.-oriented Tx directed at specific deficit. 5 individual and 4 group sessions.	> 18 mo	160	Aachen Aphasia Test; scores were corrected to control for effects of spontaneous recovery.	Early: Treated group improved more than untreated group (p = 0.033). 78% of Tx single cases improved significantly. Late: NS diff. b/t treated and untreated groups (p = 0.307). 46% of Tx single cases improved significantly. Chronic: 68% of Tx single cases improved significantly.	Greatest improvement during 1-4 mo. Signif. improvement with Tx beyond that explained by spontaneous recovery during late and chronic stage. Single cases showed improvement with Tx beyond 12 mo post-onset. Globals frequently failed to improve in late and chronic stages.

Study	Treatment	Duration	N	Measures	Results	Conclusions
Shewan and Kertesz, 1984 (6)	Lang.-oriented Tx; stimulation-facilitation Tx; unstructured stimulation by non-SLPS; no Tx.	Up to 1 yr	79	Western Aphasia Battery (Cortical and Lang. Quotient) and Aud. Comprehension Test for Sentences	Used ANCOVA to adjust for severity imbalances in Tx and no-Tx groups. Tx groups showed signif. greater improvement than no Tx ($p < 0.01$). Tx by non-SLPs was not signif. better than no Tx ($p = 0.09$), but was not signif. diff. from SLP Tx. LOT and ST Tx by SLP were NS different ($p = 0.98$).	Tx was signif. factor in greater recovery of Tx group for lang. and more general cortical index. Greatest gains made during first 3 mo.
Wertz et al., 1981 (3)	1 SLP at each site admin. both Tx's. Individual = 4 hr traditional stimulus-response Tx and 4 hr machine-assisted Tx. Group = 4 hr conversation group and 4 hr group recreation.	11, 22, 33, and 44 wk	67	PICA, Token Test, Word Fluency Test, Colored Progressive Matices, informant's rating, conversational rating.	Overall PICA improved for both groups in all cohorts ($p < 0.05$). Signif. diffs. b/t individual and group Tx existed for some PICA subtests in favor of individual Tx ($p > 0.05$). Few signif. diffs. on other outcome measures. Continued improvement noted with Tx after 6 mo post-onset ($p < 0.05$).	Signif. improvement associated with both individual and group Tx from 4–48 wk post-onset. Individual Tx > group Tx on standardized lang. test only. Signif. improvement in Ss treated beyond 6 mo post-onset (after traditional time for spontaneous recovery).
Wertz et al., 1986 (5)	Clinical and home Tx = traditional stimulus-response Tx 12 wk then no Tx 12 wk. Deferred Tx = 12 wk no Tx, then 12 wk clinic Tx.	12 and 24 wk	94 Clinic = 29 Home = 36 Deferred = 29	PICA overall %ile scores	After 12 wk: clinic Tx > no Tx ($p < 0.05$); home Tx vs. no Tx ($p > 0.05$); home Tx vs. clinic Tx NS ($p > 0.05$); after 24 wk; deferred Tx vs. clinic Tx and home Tx NS ($p > 0.05$).	Tx improved more than no Tx. Home Tx by trained volunteers resulted in gains intermediate to clinic Tx and no Tx. Delaying Tx was not detrimental to ultimate performance at 24 wk.

regard, the bulk of the research evidence supports the conclusion that most patients who have suffered a single, left-hemisphere thromboembolic stroke will profit from aphasia treatment. Nevertheless, initial severity of aphasia plays a major role in moderating effectiveness of treatment. Shewan and Kertesz (6) observed greatest improvement in individuals with moderate aphasia, followed next by the severe and then the mild group, wherein ceiling effects on criterion tests may have occurred. No studies directly address the issue of age and treatment, although Sarno (7) has suggested that when there are no complicating circumstances, elderly aphasic subjects appear to profit as much as their younger counterparts. However, Holland and Bartlett (8) noted that elderly aphasic patients seldom have a poststroke picture that is not medically compromised in some way, and their research also indicated that such patients do not make as full a recovery as younger cohorts. Other factors, concerning imprecise variables such as level of motivation, pretraumatic response to challenge, and other personality factors, probably also modulate the effects of treatment for aphasia. But, as with many other problems that intersect the behavioral and the medical, no clear answer is available as to precisely which patient characteristics are consistently associated with success in aphasia treatment and which are consistently associated with failure.

Extrapersonal variables that influence the efficacy of treatment include time post-onset of aphasia, and duration and intensity of treatment. Basso, Capitani, and Vignolo (9) and Vignolo (25) found that patients treated closer to onset of aphasia improved more than did patients who began treatment further from onset. Other investigators (2,3,6,10) observed greatest change in the first 6 months. However, change after the first 6 months, when the effects of spontaneous recovery are no longer thought to be significant, is documented as well (3,4,27). Sarno and Levita (11) noted that in globally aphasic patients, change started later post-onset than in less severely impaired patients. The bulk of single-case studies that show improvement were conducted on patients who were well beyond 6 months post-stroke. Wertz et al. (2) noted that delaying treatment for 3 months, at least during the first 6 months post ictus, did not influence ultimate outcome. In short, there is no clearcut evidence to guide the practitioner in terms of the duration or intensity of treatment, or of when it should begin. For example, our own experimental clinic treats only patients who have run out of third-party reimbursement and are a minimum of 6 months post-stroke. Yet many of our chronic patients continue to improve, as measured by increased scores on standard aphasia tests.

TREATMENTS FOR REHABILITATING APHASIC PATIENTS

The techniques that make up the portfolios of most speech–language pathologists are vast, ranging from didactic application of stimulus–response programs to pragmatic approaches that stress functional communication. There are approaches that teach compensatory and facilitative strategies, and others that focus on deficits that underlie the aphasic problem. There are approaches that attempt to modify aphasic persons' communicative environments as well as techniques for counseling aphasic persons and their families.

In addition to these varied foci of intervention, some clinical activities may be more appropriately applied in some phases of the postictal period than others. For example, there are treatment approaches specifically geared to newly aphasic patients in acute settings, others geared to in- and outpatient rehabilitation settings, and still others that specifically target chronic patients, often with the goal of maintaining previously taught skills.

Circumstances also dictate forms of therapy. For example, telephone and interactive video approaches for patients who live in settings remote from a hospital or rehabilitation setting are being developed, as are approaches that take advantage of the latest computer technology (12,13).

Last, but certainly not least, techniques respecting most of the above constraints are available that specifically address a particular aphasic patient's pattern of strengths and deficits. Perhaps the most interesting recent developments of this type are those that derive directly from cognitive neuropsychology and its detailed case analyses. These approaches attempt to pinpoint the precise nature of aphasic deficit, as postulated by explicit models of the cognitive processing of normal language.

Obviously, it is not possible to describe all aphasia treatment approaches in detail here. Therefore, in the following sections, an illustrative method is described for a number of the above treatment approaches. Because efficacy is a concern, only techniques that have been evaluated, at least by appropriate single-subject designs or by group pre- and posttreatment comparisons, will be presented.

Language-Oriented Treatment: An Example of a Stimulus–Response Approach

Stimulus–response approaches have long formed the centerpiece of aphasia treatment techniques, particularly in the United States. Most of the general efficacy studies have used variants of these approaches, in some cases with quite creative embellishments. In fact, Peach (14) devoted over half of a recent chapter summarizing aphasia treatment in the United States to the description of these so-called "traditional" techniques. They appear not only to be robust but to have retained their vigor since at least the end of World War II, when most authorities agree aphasia rehabilitation became well established in the United States.

Perhaps the most comprehensive approach to aphasia management arranged according to learning principles (in this case, operant conditioning and behavior modification) is the approach of Shewan and Bandur (15) called Language-Oriented Treatment (LOT). LOT's underlying assumptions are that aphasia represents not only a loss of access to language but a fundamental loss of language itself and a disturbance of language-processing mechanisms. LOT is a set of modality-specific guidelines for the treatment of aphasia, in which hierarchially arranged tasks are intended to train auditory processing and comprehension, visual processing and reading, oral expression, writing, and gestural communication. Language-based activities appropriate to an aphasic patient's presenting difficulties are the focus, and hierarchical progression follows only when a patient meets a given task's performance criterion. For example, the hierarchy for auditory processing has as its earliest levels the awareness and recognition of auditory stimuli; its highest level tasks concern comprehension of narratives and discourse. Each task level provides the clinician with suggestions for increasing difficulty in the 10 stimulus-item blocks that comprise a "step"; also included is information concerning how to provide cues, how to score responses, how to provide feedback to the patient regarding progress, and so on. Efficacy data demonstrate LOT's utility as measured by performance on a comprehensive aphasia test, the Western Aphasia Battery (16), and the Auditory Comprehension Test for Sentences (17). No data examining the extent to which effects on communication in everyday life or normal conversation have been provided.

Promoting Aphasic Communicative Effectiveness: An Example from Pragmatic Approaches

Peach (14) notes that in the United States the model for clinical intervention in aphasia has been evolving away from a symptom-based model toward a socially based one that includes concepts such as disability and handicap. This has meant a therapeutic reconsideration, emphasizing compensatory strategies and functional communication. The result is the development of a group of approaches that focus on the patient's communication, despite the limitations on language imposed by aphasia. These approaches attempt to capitalize on aphasic patients' remaining communicative strengths instead of attempting to overcome their linguistic deficits. Although the importance of verbal communication is not underestimated, these approaches also stress nonverbal and even augmentative communication, where appropriate. They also attempt to help the patient circumvent the effect of language loss on everyday communication.

Perhaps the best known of such pragmatic approaches is Promoting Aphasic Communicative Effectiveness (PACE) (18), a treatment context that does not focus on the structure and content of language per se, but shifts the emphasis to interpersonal communicative exchange. A typical PACE activity might have patient and clinician sitting across from each other, with a stack of drawings lying face down between them. The task is for each participant to communicate, for example, the name of the drawn picture. PACE has the four following principles, all of which approximate normal communication:

1. New information is exchanged, since neither patient nor clinician knows the name of the drawing.
2. Both participants act as senders and receivers of information.
3. All channels of communication are viewed as equally good, because sending and receiving information is the focus. The point is to get the message across.
4. Feedback is simply the consequent success or failure to communicate.

PACE therapy is in widespread use, and a number of elaborations of its simple theme have been forthcoming. For example, giving and following complex directions, using the technique in groups, and combining it with role-playing and other functionally meaningful activities have all been used. [An interesting example is furnished by Springer et al. (19).] Most PACE variants, as well as PACE as it is described above, have been evaluated for their clinical utility.

Treating Aphasic Perseveration: An Example of Therapy for a Deficit That Underlies Aphasic Performance

Aphasia is frequently accompanied by other behavioral deficits that negatively interact with the aphasia, and that frequently intensify or at least complicate the aphasia. Among such deficits are difficulty in general ability to represent the environment through use of symbols, buccofacial and limb apraxia, and perseveration. All have been the focus of treatment for the aphasic adult, and one of the most interesting of these approaches is Treatment of Aphasic Perseveration (TAP) (20). TAP teaches aphasic perseverators to be alert to perseverations and to understand the nature of their perseverative behaviors, as well as their effects on aspects of language such as word retrieval. Finally, TAP systematically teaches patients techniques, such as taking a brief time out, for modifying perseveration. The goal is to demonstrate for the aphasic patient the effects of such strategies in modifying perseveration during naming activities and to facilitate the patient's self-monitoring of perseverative behavior.

Mapping Therapy: An Example of Therapy Directed to Particular Deficits

Speech–language pathologists have long recognized the fact that effective "generic therapy" probably does not exist. In each of the above approaches, clinicians typically design treatment tasks and strategies geared to improving upon or compensating for a patient's particular pattern of deficits and strengths. For example, auditory comprehension tasks would constitute a major aspect of an appropriate therapy regimen for a patient with a significant Wernicke's aphasia, as would tasks designed to improve self-monitoring, and to reduce press of speech, if present. Or, for the patient with a severe anomia, tasks designed to facilitate word search or retrieval might be the focus of therapy, using techniques derived from any of the above approaches.

Recently, researchers have become interested in the application of cognitive processing models to various aspects of aphasia, directing their attention first to discovering where, in terms of such models of language processing, language in aphasic conditions appears to break down. Once extensive testing has been completed, and the stage of processing difficulty defined, therapy is specifically designed to modify behavior at the hypothesized level of breakdown. Clinical manipulation of aphasic performance by cognitive-processing experts is motivated by its potential to validate a given model of normal processing. Nevertheless, this fresh way of conceptualizing aphasia in terms of its specific processing breakdown has resulted in the development of a number of new, clinically relevant approaches to treatment. A recently well rationalized and designed example is mapping therapy, an approach to remediating sentence comprehension and production difficulties in agrammatic individuals (21). Agrammatic patients have demonstrable difficulty using syntactic structure in assigning thematic roles in sentences. In passive sentences, when they can rely on the semantics to help them figure out who is doing what to whom, they perform relatively well. (An example of a nonreversible passive is "The dinner is prepared by Julia".) However, sentences that lack such semantic guidance produce performances by agrammatic patients that are near chance level. (Such a passive sentence is "The man is kissed by Julia.") Saffran and her colleagues (21) have developed a training program consistent with their mapping-deficit hypothesis in agrammatism. This hypothesis holds that agrammatic patients, rather than having a general syntactic deficit, have a problem limited to understanding the syntactic relationships that exist between constituent structure and thematic role. Thus, they have elected to train agrammatic patients specifically on sentences that increase their understanding of the process of assignment of roles by the nature of the stimuli used, forcing the patient to an "explicit consideration of the relationship between the verb and its noun arguments" (21).

This training program is fairly traditional in format, although it has a number of interesting innovations, such as the required use of color-coding in an attempt to reinforce distinctions among a given sentence's thematic relationships. This type of cross-modal insight-building technique was first successfully used by Byng (22), in what is perhaps the germinal attempt to train deficit behaviors pinpointed by cognitive neuropsychological processing theories.

Such highly explicit therapies are still in their formative stages. Nevertheless, a number of active aphasia researchers are following cognitive processing models to develop remediation approaches with some success. One expects that much more of this work will appear in the future, and much of it will have immediate clinical application by speech–language pathologists.

Approaches Targeting a Specific Time Post-Ictus

The clinical approaches described to this point have all been developed for, and clinically evaluated with, individuals whose aphasia has stabilized. They are designed for patients beyond the stage of spontaneous recovery; that is to say, patients close to their end of their stays in acute hospitals, those in residency in rehabilitation centers and skilled nursing facilities, and those who are receiving outpatient speech-language pathology services. Many clinical researchers question the applicability of such approaches in the earliest stages of recovery from aphasia, in which spontaneous recovery is at its maximum acceleration and changes in a given patient's language profile may occur even daily. Nor are these techniques designed to meet the social needs of those quite chronic aphasic individuals who probably have gained much from traditional clinical activities but still can profit from clinical support. It should be noted, however, that far from being "unreachable" by techniques aimed at modifying aphasic performance directly, chronic patients have often been the experimental subjects for clinical treatment development, and many continue to profit from direct intervention. Nevertheless, for patients who are acutely aphasic, and many of those who are still experiencing its residual effects long post-stroke, still other techniques are probably appropriate. Two examples illustrate therapy at these widely separate points in the time course of aphasia.

An Example of an Approach to Patients in Acute-Care Settings

Holland (23) developed a conversationally oriented approach for use with patients who have recently incurred aphasia-producing strokes, and their families. This approach emphasizes remaining communicative strengths, which have a higher likelihood of surfacing during "normal" conversational activities than during more structured therapy tasks. Concurrently, the approach uses the subtle but reliable improvements in observed deficit behaviors to illustrate and explain to both patients and their families the nature of spontaneous recovery from aphasia. Counseling is provided to patients and families concerning the problem and what to expect in the future. By focusing on residual abilities in this acute stage, when behaviors change rapidly (often independently of the clinician), patients and families are prepared for the more language-centered activities of rehabilitation. It is also designed to provide both patients and families with an opportunity to deal with the emotions that inevitably accompany the fact of stroke and the onset of aphasia and, finally, to prevent the development of maladaptive behaviors and strategies.

A Therapeutic Approach for Chronic Patients:
The North York Aphasia Centre

At the other pole of the post-stroke aphasia time course, conversation again is highlighted. In this instance, the focus has shifted to real-world issues of maximizing re-entry of chronic aphasic individuals into the normal world of social interaction and its unique human currency, talking to other people. The North York Aphasia Centre is an appropriate example. Located in Ontario, the Centre has an ongoing 4-day weekly program serving well over 100 chronic aphasic patients and their families. Although the program is overseen by a small group of professionals, its board of directors includes both aphasic persons and the volunteers who vitalize and staff the program. This program is described in detail by Kagan and Gailey (24).

Rather than focus on the impairment of stroke or the disability that results from it, Kagan and Gailey point out that the focus of the North York Centre is on the social *handicap* brought about by aphasia. The Centre trains volunteers and families to serve as conversational partners for individuals with aphasia, who in turn function to foster the fullest possible involvement of aphasic individuals in the communicating world. The major medium of interaction at North York is conversation groups consisting of aphasic patients of complementary skill levels and nonaphasic, trained volunteers. These groups systematically learn to use nonverbal as well as verbal means for communicating. Other Centre initiatives include advocacy (by patients, staff, and volunteers) for aphasic persons, as well as an extensive program of public education. (One of the most fascinating of the Centre outreach programs, incidentally, is a short but extremely effective program that teaches interns, residents, and physicians how to communicate more effectively with their aphasic patients.)

The Centre's focus on the chronic social handicap of aphasia, its emphasis on conversation and group interaction, and its skillful use of volunteers to assist both aphasic individuals and their families is perhaps a portent of the future of aphasia treatment. As health-care reform and cost-containment issues influence service delivery to aphasic patients, upbeat and beneficial approaches such as this one may well become the model for chronic post-stroke intervention.

CONCLUSIONS

This chapter attempts to provide medical personnel with a guided tour of aphasia rehabilitation as it is practiced in North America at the close of the century. One expects that most of the illustrated rehabilitation approaches will remain viable for some time to come. But it is also quite likely that, as the knowledge base about aphasia continues to grow, the application of that knowledge base to aphasia treatment will continue to expand. New approaches to treatment will continue to be generated, and efficacy data shall continue to mount, and to become more specific.

Further, as progress is made in medical management of stroke, it is expected that changes will occur in aphasia treatment. For example, it appears that more individuals with severe strokes are likely to survive as a result of improved ability to manage the disorder. This should increase the number of surviving aphasic patients who have severe, or even global, aphasia. At the other end of the severity continuum, improved medical management should result in an increasing number of individuals who escape serious aphasia but have the mild and often extremely frustrating aphasias that impede their ability to return to work. These are the two problems in aphasia for which the fewest approaches to treatment are currently available. One expectation is that new techniques especially geared to these aphasic polar opposites will increase in the near future.

Finally, it should be noted that there has been an increasing understanding among medical practitioners of the significant role that speech–language pathologists can perform, not only in assessment, but in management of individuals with aphasia. This is a positive change that promises to benefit all concerned: the relevant professionals, of course, but, more importantly, aphasic patients and their families.

ACKNOWLEDGMENT

This chapter was supported in part by the National Center for Neurogenic Communication Disorders (grant DC-01409).

REFERENCES

1. Lincoln N, McGuirk E, Mulley G, Lendrem WI, Jones A, Mitchell J. Effectiveness of speech therapy for aphasic stroke patients: A randomised controlled trial. Lancet 1984:1197–1200.
2. Wertz RT, Weiss D, Aten J, Brookshire R, Garcia-Bunuel L, Holland A, Kurtzke J, LaPointe L, Milianti F, Brannegan R, Greenbaum H, Marshall R, Vogel D, Carter J, Barnes N, Goodman R. Comparison of clinic, home, and deferred lan-

guage treatment for aphasia: A Veterans Administration cooperative study. Arch Neurol 1986;43:653–658.

3. Wertz R, Collins M, Weiss D, Kurtzke J, Friden T, Brookshire R, Pierce J, Holtzapple P, Hubbard D, Porch B, West J, Davis L, Matovitch V, Morley G, Resurreccion E. Veterans Administration cooperative study on aphasia: A comparison of individual and group treatment. J Speech Hear Res 1981;24:580–594.

4. Poeck K, Huber W, Willmes K. Outcome of intensive language treatment in aphasia. J Speech Hear Disord 1989;54:471–479.

5. Wertz R, Deal J, Holland A, Kurtzke J, Weiss D. Comments on an uncontrolled aphasia no treatment trial. ASHA 1986;28:31.

6. Shewan C, Kertesz A. Effects of speech and language treatment on recovery from aphasia. Brain Lang 1984;23:272–299.

7. Sarno MT. Language rehabilitation outcome in the elderly aphasic patient. In: Obler L, Albert M, eds. Language and communication in the elderly. Lexington, MA: DC Heath, 1980.

8. Holland A, Bartlett C. Age and spontaneous recovery from aphasia. In: Ulatowska H, ed. The aging brain. San Diego: College Hill, 1985.

9. Basso A, Capitani E, Vignolo L. Influence of rehabilitation of language skills in aphasic patients: A controlled study. Arch Neurol 1979;36:190–196.

10. Hagan C. Communication abilities in hemiplegia: Effect of speech therapy. Arch Phys Med Rehab 1973;54:454–463.

11. Sarno M, Levita E. Natural course of recovery in severe aphasia. Arch Phys Med Rehab 1971;52:175–178.

12. Weinrich M, Steele R, Carlson G, Kleczewska M, Wertz R, Baker E. Processing of visual syntax by a globally aphasic patient. Brain Lang 1989;36:391–405.

13. Wertz R, Dronkers N, Sterling L, Bernstein-Ellis E, Lieber S. Utilizing technology to provide treatment for aphasia in remote settings. Presentation at the annual convention of the American Speech Language Hearing Association, San Antonio, 1992.

14. Peach R. Clinical intervention for aphasia in the United States of America. In: Holland A, Forbes M, eds. Treatment for aphasia: world perspectives. Vol 1. San Diego: Singular Press, 1993.

15. Shewan C, Bandur D. Treatment of aphasia: a language-oriented approach. San Diego: College-Hill, 1986.

16. Kertesz A. Western aphasia battery. New York: Grune & Stratton, 1982.

17. Shewan C. Auditory comprehension test for sentences (ACTS). Chicago: Biolinguistics Clinical Institutes, 1979.

18. Davis G, Wilcox J. Adult aphasia rehabilitation: applied pragmatics. San Diego: College Hill, 1985.

19. Springer L, Glindemann R, Huber W, Willmes K. How efficacious is PACE therapy when language systematic training is incorporated? Aphasiology 1991; 5:391–399.

20. Helm-Estabrooks N, Emery P, Albert M. Treatment of aphasic perseveration (TAP) program. Arch Neurol 1987;44:1253–1255.

21. Saffran E, Schwartz M, Fink R, Myers J, Martin N. Mapping Therapy: An approach to remediating agrammatic sentence comprehension and production.

In: Cooper J, ed. Aphasia treatment: current approaches and research opportunities. NIDCD monograph 2. Bethesda: National Institutes of Health, 1993.

22. Byng S. Sentence processing deficits: Theory and therapy. Cogn Neuropsychol 1988;5:629–676.

23. Holland A. A model treatment approach for acutely aphasic patients. In: Brookshire R, ed. Proceedings: clinical aphasiology conference. Minneapolis: BRK Publishers, 1984.

24. Kagan A, Gailey G. Functional is not enough: Training conversational partners for aphasic adults. In: Holland A, Forbes M, eds. Treatment for aphasia: world perspectives. Vol 1. San Diego: Singular Press, 1993.

25. Vignolo L. Evolution of aphasia and language rehabilitation: A retrospective exploratory study. Cortex 1964;1:344–367.

26. Hartman J, Landau W. Comparison of formal language therapy with supportive counseling for aphasia due to acute vascular accident. Arch Neurol 1987;24: 646–649.

27. Butfield E, Zangwill O. Re-education in aphasia: A review of 70 cases. J Neurol Neurosurg Psychiatry 1946;9:75–79.

19

Toward a Pharmacotherapy for Aphasia

Masaru Mimura

Boston University School of Medicine and Boston Veterans Affairs Medical Center, Boston, Massachusetts

Martin L. Albert

Boston University School of Medicine, Boston, Massachusetts, and Medical Research Service, Department of Veterans Affairs, Washington, D.C.

Patrick McNamara

State University of New York at Buffalo, Buffalo, New York

INTRODUCTION

Aphasia rehabilitation techniques should be designed to facilitate biologically possible recovery processes. Progress in neurobiology has provided two intersecting sets of data specifically important for understanding pharmacosystems and cognition. The first is the collection of detailed information concerning mechanisms of recovery following brain damage, such as "sprouting," "latent synapses," and "diaschisis" (1). For recovery of language function following brain damage, such neurobiological notions are no less critical than cognitive, psycholinguistic, or emotional issues. Modern techniques for aphasia treatment appear to be directed, to some extent, at stimulation of biological recovery. Melodic intonation therapy (2), visual action therapy (3), and visual communication therapy (4), for example, seem to facilitate the unblocking of latent synapses (5), bypassing damaged neurons in the zone of language. Luria et al. (6) have recommended the use of various chemical agents for "deinhibition" from diaschisis to restore higher cortical function. Pharmacotherapy for aphasia based on applied neurobiology may be one of the keys to successful treatment programs.

The second set of data relates to the emerging model of "neurocognitive networks" (7–10). According to this model, complex human cognition and behavior are processed through an integrated neural network that consists of (1) widely distributed, but interconnecting, sets of neural pathways that underlie anatomically localized operations and (2) chemically addressed pathways for modulating behavioral tone. Selected cognitive skills are organized in association with distinct neurotransmitter profiles. For example, dopaminergic pathways play a selective role in working memory (11,12). Even in the highly complicated realm of speech and language, specific neurobehavioral mechanisms, such as verbal fluency and verbal memory, can be postulated as being related to particular neurochemical systems.

The line of argument presented here leads directly to the suggestion that manipulation of neuropharmacosystems may ameliorate a deficit in aphasia. Specifically, we propose the following three-part hypothesis: (1) that clinical signs of aphasia are dependent on more basic deficits (processing deficits) in underlying neurobehavioral mechanisms, (2) that those underlying deficits are influenced by specific pharmacosystems, and (3) replacement or supplementation therapy with selected neurotransmitters targeted at the underlying processing deficit will relieve that deficit and thereby ameliorate the clinical aphasic signs and symptoms. In this chapter, we first review the concept of selective pharmacotherapy targeted at specific language symptoms, with special reference to dopaminergic and cholinergic systems. A considerable number of studies demonstrate that speech and language output is at least partially dependent on dopaminergic networks, and verbal memory on cholinergic networks. We then discuss briefly nonspecific pharmacotherapy that may ameliorate behavioral problems that could hinder conventional speech and language therapy.

LANGUAGE-TARGETED PHARMACOTHERAPY

Historical Background

The idea of treating aphasia with pharmacological agents has historical roots dating to ancient times. One of the earliest known treatments for aphasia is cashews (*Anacardium*) (13). In the middle of this century, Linn and colleagues (14,15) and others (16,17) demonstrated a beneficial effect of intravenous sodium amytal on aphasia. Linn and Stein (14) speculated that sodium amytal worked by reducing anxiety. Smith and Turton (18) demonstrated improvement in aphasic symptoms utilizing a vasodilating drug. Juria and colleagues (19) advocated the use of cholinergic agents (anticholinesterase) and drugs of other pharmacodynamic groups (caffeine, vitamin B_{12}, glutamic acid, gentian) in the treatment of aphasia.

Roumanian investigators systematically explored the value of drugs. Solomonovici et al. (20) and Voinescu and Gheorghita (21) reported that the antidepressant imipramine improved language function. More recently,

Gheorghita and colleagues (22,23) investigated other pharmacological agents in the treatment of aphasia. They showed a differential effect of drugs on different components of language. Among drugs administered, pyrithioxine (encephabol) had a significant and specific effect on aphasic symptoms. In decreasing order of effect, it benefited repetition and naming, reading and reception, and, finally, writing. Voinescu and Gheorghita (23) hypothesized that pyrithioxine exhibits its effect via enhanced cortical metabolic activity. In Germany, Willmes et al. (24) conducted a double-blind, placebo-controlled pilot study in which patients with aphasia treated with piracetam, a nootropic drug, showed greater improvement than the control group in certain subtests of the Aachen Aphasia Test.

Regardless of the mechanism by which a drug exerts its effect, these results suggest that pharmacological therapy may specifically influence language function in aphasic patients. In the United States, Benson (25) utilized dexedrine in the treatment of a small number of aphasic patients. Samuels (26) has routinely used L-dopa/carbidopa in the treatment of nonfluent aphasia. Thus, numerous investigators have demonstrated a beneficial effect on aphasia from a variety of pharmacological treatments, although no single agent stands out as clearly better than all others.

Dopaminergic Networks

Many of the drugs discussed above were considered to have their positive effect via the dopamine system. L-dopa/carbidopa specifically increases presynaptic dopamine synthesis and release within the central nervous system. Dexedrine increases activity within the catecholamine system, including dopamine and norepinephrine systems. The mechanism of pyrithioxine action is unknown, but some studies suggest that pyrithioxine may exert its effect by increasing dopaminergic activity within the central nervous system (27).

Dopaminergic activity may specifically mediate verbal fluency. This hypothesis results from both clinical and neurochemical findings. If this hypothesis is true, dopamine agonist therapy may be beneficial in the treatment of nonfluency in aphasia.

Clinical Observations

Parkinson's Disease. Strong evidence that dopamine mediates verbal fluency comes from clinical observations of speech and language in Parkinson's disease. Such deficits may include abnormalities of speech volume and timing, impaired verbal fluency, reduced phrasal and syntactic constructions, word-finding difficulties, paraphasias, and impaired verbal abstraction (28–30). Among these deficits, the most prominent features affected in Parkinson's disease seem to be reduced productivity, volume, phrase length, and prosody (31,32). Gotham et al. (33) found that verbal fluency in Parkinson's disease varies with dopaminergic therapy while other cognitive deficits do not. Their patients with Parkinson's disease were impaired on a measure of verbal fluency only when off levodopa. These findings suggest that Parkinson's disease is associated with verbal fluency deficits, which may be partially reversed with dopamine replacement therapy.

Akinetic Mutism. In 1981 Ross and Stewart (34) described a patient with akinetic mutism following removal of a tumor of the anterior hypothalamus who responded to bromocriptine, a postsynaptic dopaminergic agonist. They concluded that akinetic mutism may arise from loss of dopaminergic input to the anterior cingulate cortex or related structures, and direct dopamine agonists can successfully ameliorate the akinetic mutism. Other cases with akinetic mutism or milder abulia were subsequently reported with successful effect of bromocriptine (35,36). Crimson et al. (37) described specific improvement in speech and language, including intelligibility, spontaneity, and articulation of speech in three patients following bromocriptine. These reports suggest that dopaminergic agonists improve speech and language output, although this improvement may be the consequence of increased spontaneity.

Stuttering and Tourette's Syndrome. The success of haloperidol, a dopamine antagonist, in the treatment of Tourette's syndrome and stuttering provides another perspective (32,38). Several authors have suggested that stuttering may be linked to a central imbalance in dopaminergic activity (32,39).

Neuroanatomical and Neurochemical Correlates

Dopamine Network Projection. Midbrain dopaminergic systems project to medial frontal areas (mesocortical system), as well as to caudate and putamen (nigrostriatal system). Dopaminergic projections have predominance in the frontal cortex and also in the left hemisphere (40). From this preference of dopaminergic distribution one could anticipate that speech output, which seems to depend on left frontal regions, may be linked to dopamine.

Supplementary Motor Area. The supplementary motor area (SMA) plays a major role in mediating production of sequential, voluntary motor activity, of which speech is by far the most complex (41). As discussed in Chapter 4, lesions of the left medial frontal area, specifically SMA, can result in the syndrome of transcortical motor aphasia (42,43). The SMA is the principal cortical structure in the neural network that mediates the initiating mechanism of speech (44). Electrical stimulation within the SMA elicits vocalizations in both humans and monkeys (45). Regional cerebral blood flow studies demonstrate dramatic activation of SMA associated with silent counting and spoken recitation of overlearned items (46). SMA, together with anterior cingulate, forms a link with midbrain dopaminergic centers, receiving an important dopaminergic projection (40). Any site in this link, when lesioned, can produce transcortical motor aphasia. Naeser et al. (47) reported that severe nonfluency in aphasia was associated with combined lesions in the subcallosal fasciculus and periventricular white matter. The subcallosal fasciculus is a pathway of a dopaminergic system connecting SMA and anterior cingulate with striatal sites. Thus, SMA appears to regulate, through its network connections, both initiation of speech and its maintenance; dopamine is the facilitatory transmitter for this network. Impaired speech initiation and decreased verbal fluency may be due to interruption of the mesocortical dopaminergic projection.

Dopaminergic Therapy for Nonfluent Aphasia

Based on both clinical and anatomicochemical evidence that supports the hypothesis of dopaminergic mediation in verbal fluency, our research team undertook an open-label study of the effect of bromocriptine on nonfluent aphasia. Initially, we reported a patient with residual moderate transcortical motor aphasia following left frontal intracerebral hemorrhage who demonstrated dramatic improvement in speech and language during treatment with bromocriptine (48). His major fluency problems, including impaired initiation and hesitancies (long response latencies) of speech, responded well to pharmacotherapy. Both the number and proportion of pauses between and within utterances diminished significantly during free conversation. After cessation of drug therapy his language returned to baseline.

We also reported two additional cases (one with stable mixed anterior aphasia, the other with severe Broca's aphasia) who showed an increased use of novel words and an increased likelihood of conversation initiation at home, although they did not demonstrate obvious changes on formal testing (49). In addition to the mesocortical dopamine pathway discussed above, Bachman and Morgan (49) suggested an important role of the limbic system in influencing language function via dopaminergic pathways.

Subsequently, other studies described the beneficial effect of bromocriptine on fluency in aphasia. Gupta and Mlcoch (50) reported two nonfluent aphasia patients (one with Broca's aphasia, the other with transcortical motor aphasia) who showed considerable improvement in fluency after treatment with bromocriptine. Sabe et al. (51) noted that three patients with moderate nonfluent aphasia showed a significant improvement in language deficits after treatment with 30 to 60 mg per day of bromocriptine, while this improvement did not occur in four patients with severe nonfluent aphasia.

So far, all these clinical studies have methodological weaknesses, as noted in the original papers. The studies were uncontrolled; the subject samples were small; the drug trials were unblinded; and no placebo phases were included. MacLennan et al. (52) conducted a placebo-controlled study to verify the effect of bromocriptine on speech and language deficits. Although the number of words produced by their subjects increased during bromocriptine administration, the authors concluded that bromocriptine did not significantly affect any specific speech and language functions, and they cautioned against uncritical acceptance of bromocriptine treatment for improving communication capabilities of aphasic patients. We fully agree that a further placebo-controlled study with large numbers of subjects is warranted. In any future study, at least the following factors should be taken into account: aphasia type and severity, selection of dopaminergic agent, optimal dose, and side effects.

Aphasia Type and Severity. All patients who reportedly benefited from dopamine agonists had nonfluent aphasia. However, it is quite clear that not all patients with nonfluent aphasia improve with drug administration. Cases so far reported indicate that patients with transcortical motor aphasia respond more readily to dopaminergic agents than patients with other types of aphasia. This observation is consistent with the notion that transcortical motor aphasia may result from damage interrupting the mesocortical dopaminergic projection.

However, even patients with transcortical motor aphasia, who are theoretically most suited, may not always respond to treatment (52). In our laboratory, for example, one patient with transcortical motor aphasia did not show significant improvement with bromocriptine. This 70-year-old male who received bromocriptine 12 months after onset of aphasia did not respond to medication in any language-output measure, including average pause length, meaningful words per utterance, and meaningful words per total words. His aphasia-severity rating scale on the Boston Diagnostic Aphasia Examination (53) indicated severe dysfluency, and this severity may have been a reason for nonresponsiveness. Another possibility is that some subtype of transcortical motor aphasia could respond specifically well to bromocriptine, as transcortical motor aphasia may have variations according to lesion extension.

As far as severity is concerned, Sabe et al. (51) documented that patients with severe nonfluency did not respond well to bromocriptine treatment. Our experience also confirms this notion; none of our patients with very severe nonfluent or global aphasia has yet been successfully treated with bromocriptine. Of note, the case reported by Albert et al. in 1988 (48), who responded exceptionally well to bromocriptine, had an initial aphasia severity rating of 3.5 on the Boston Diagnostic Aphasia Examination, indicating only mild to moderate communication difficulty. Thus, at this early stage in our understanding of pharmacotherapy for aphasia, bromocriptine appears relatively less effective in situations in which dopaminergic postsynaptic receptors are severely damaged.

With a special interest in the correlation between lesion site and effect of pharmacotherapy, we reanalyzed the CT scan of our initial case (unpublished data) according to the method of Naeser et al. (47). This 62-year-old patient had a large left frontal lesion that partially included Broca's area. The lesion extended across to the lateral border of the left frontal horn. A large superior lesion extension was noted into the premotor and motor cortex areas, with patchy deep extension into the anterior one-third of the periventricular white matter (PVWM). The middle one-third PVWM (deep to motor and sensory cortex area for the mouth) was largely spared. There was a patchy lesion in the subcallosal fasciculus (ScF), but the supplementary motor area (cortical origin of the ScF pathway) was largely spared. We then analyzed the CT of another patient who showed overall improvement with bromocriptine treatment, a 55-year-old man who had a persistent Broca's aphasia 49 months post-onset. His CT scan showed no lesion in SMA, but a lesion rated half in the ScF and more than half in the middle one-third of the PVWM. Taking these two cases together, we conclude that for improvement to occur following bromocriptine therapy at least part of the supplementary motor area should remain intact, with some preservation also of its related subcortical pathways, the ScF and the PVWM.

Selection of Drug. Among dopaminergic agonists, bromocriptine is currently most widely used in pharmacotherapy for aphasia. This is an ergot derivative and a selective postsynaptic D2 receptor agonist. L-dopa increases presynaptic dopamine synthesis and release, and requires preserved presynaptic functions (54). The argument in favor of bromocriptine over L-dopa is that the former does not necessarily require presynaptic function. However, insufficient study has been done to confirm a preference of one drug over the other.

Liebson et al. (55) described a patient with multifocal head injury with residual severe dysarthria. Introduction of bromocriptine and carbidopa/L-dopa 2 and 3 years, respectively, after the injury resulted in extraordinary improvement in speech and motor functions. It was not until carbidopa/L-dopa was added to bromocriptine that dramatic improvements were seen. One explanation for this effect is that long-term low-dose bromocriptine primed the central nervous system, improving cell function sufficiently to facilitate response to carbidopa/L-dopa. Another is that the carbidopa/L-dopa by itself was the therapeutic agent, and that this drug combination effects a better delivery of dopaminergic activity to the central nervous system. We evaluated another patient who sustained a severe closed head injury as the result of a fall. This 20-year-old soldier also had a residual dysarthria, and his speech was unintelligible although he did not have other aphasic symptoms. We first administered L-dopa, then superimposed bromocriptine. Although L-dopa significantly improved his intelligibility, additional bromocriptine did not influence his speech functions.

Relation of Language to Other Cognitive Functions. Dopaminergic agents may affect not only speech and language functions but other cognitive functions as well. Indeed, the beneficial effect of dopamine on speech and language may be the fortunate, but nonspecific, consequence of the effect of dopamine on nonlinguistic functions. A considerable body of evidence supports the role of dopamine as a mediator of attention, memory, and motor function (12,56–58). No study has yet been published to determine if dopamine has a primary, direct effect on speech and language or a secondary effect working through its influence on other cognitive domains.

Optimal Dosage and Side Effects. Most of the open-label studies administered bromocriptine in both relatively low dose (10–20 mg) and relatively high dose (30–40 mg). Some cases demonstrated dose-dependent effect on fluency (50; case 1). However, the second patient of Gupta and Mlcoch (50) improved at 10 mg but got worse at 30 mg. They speculated that optimal dose might vary from person to person.

From the clinical point of view, a gradual increase in dose with careful observation is recommended. Maximum dosage so far reported for patients with chronic aphasia is 40 mg. Much higher doses (up to 110 mg per day) were administered in cases of akinetic mutism (34,36).

The most common side effects include dizziness, drowsiness, and faintness. Nausea, vomiting, and gastrointestinal discomfort are reported in some patients. All these symptoms are usually transient and frequently resolve if therapy is continued. Decrease in systolic blood pressure is reported in nearly 30% of patients upon initiation of therapy with bromocriptine (59). This decrease in blood pressure is often asymptomatic but requires regular blood-pressure examination. More serious side effects occur very rarely. These include exacerbation of a pre-existing psychosis, exacerbation of pre-existing movement disorder, confusion and disorientation, seizures, hypertension, and urinary dysfunction. Sabe et al. (51) reported severe dystonia in her four patients although this subsided after cessation of the treatment. We observed dose-related muscle cramps and spasms in the paretic leg of one aphasic patient. Caution is warranted in the use of dopaminergic drugs with brain-injured patients, as the long-term effects of these drugs in a nonparkinsonian brain are not yet well documented. It has been suggested that long-term use of dopaminergic agents may result in disturbances of visuospatial function (60).

Available data, thus, do not justify the routine administration of bromocriptine or other dopaminergic agents in the treatment of aphasia. However, there is little question that some patients with nonfluent aphasia improve with bromocriptine. Our current impression is that mild to moderate nonfluent aphasia may respond to bromocriptine, especially transcortical motor aphasia, and especially if the supplementary motor area is not completely destroyed. Further research studies are not only warranted but highly desirable.

Cholinergic Networks

Pharmacotherapy for fluent aphasia may also be feasible, utilizing cholinergic agents. Abundant data indicate that cholinergic pathways mediate verbal memory and spatial synthesis. Our hypothesis is that cholinergic agonists can improve selected aspects of naming deficit and comprehension dysfunction in aphasia to the extent that these aphasic disorders are influenced by verbal memory and spatial synthesis.

Neuroanatomical and Neurochemical Correlates

Acethylcholine is ubiquitous in the nervous system. Cerebral nuclei such as the nucleus basalis of Meynert and the substantia inominata have been demonstrated to be primary sources of cortical cholinergic innervation (61). In humans, cholinergic innervation may be asymmetrical, greater on the left than on the right, because choline acetyltransferase (ChAT) activity was found to be significantly higher in the left superior temporal gyrus than in the right (62). This study demonstrated that the ChAT activity in Brodmann area 22 had a greater left than right prevalence of enzymatic activity in cortical layers II and IV. From this dense and preferential cholinergic innervation in the left temporal lobe, it would be reasonable to suggest that cholinergic pathways might play a major role in verbal functions. Indeed, we already know that in dementia of Alzheimer's type, in which cholinergic activity is reduced (63), a significant verbal memory deficit is a characteristic feature (64).

Cholinergic System, Memory, and Language

Anticholinergic agents, such as scopolamine, impair verbal memory, with increased verbal intrusions/perseverations in healthy volunteers (65). The effect of anticholinergic agents on memory is consistent: they impair the ability to store new information in long-term memory, the ability to retrieve information from long-term memory, and the functioning of working memory systems (66,67). Deficits produced by anticholinergics (anticholinergic amnesia) have been considered as a model of memory deficits in elderly patients and in Alzheimer's disease (68,69), although the link between cognitive deficits and neurotransmitter deficiencies in Alzheimer's disease is clearly complex, and tied to multiple neuromodulators (70,71). Fuld et al. (72) demonstrated that patients with Alzheimer's disease frequently show verbal intrusions, correlated with verbal memory deficits, and that these verbal intrusions were also correlated with low levels of ChAT and high numbers of senile plaques.

Additional evidence of a cholinergic effect on verbal functions comes from a study of side effects of psychotropic agents. Five patients presented speech blockage after being treated with tricyclic antidepressants (73). The authors concluded that their patients' speech and language problems were the consequence of a tricyclic-exerted, central anticholinergic effect on higher cortical functions. They did not encounter the same language-related side effect when using desmethylimipramine, which causes fewer anticholinergic effects.

From these research results, and others not reported here, one can infer that cholinergic systems influence verbal memory processes. In contrast, dopamine pathways showed no significant effect on verbal memory (74,75).

Cholinergic System, Spatial Synthesis, and Grammatical Comprehension

Visuospatial deficits in normal aging and Alzheimer's disease have also been attributed to hypocholinergic function (76). Patients with Alzheimer's disease or progressive supranuclear palsy have been reported to show improvement on visuospatial, constructional, or spatial attentional abilities following treatment with the anticholinesterase agent physostigmine (77). Meador et al. (78) recently demonstrated that scopolamine impairs performance on visuospatial information processing, such as judgment of line orientation and complex figures, which require constructive skills. Zemishlany et al. (79) also noted that elderly subjects consistently showed impairment in constructional praxis following administration of scopolamine. Luria et al. (6) proposed that deficits in auditory comprehension of complex logicogrammatical constructions is a verbal manifestation of impaired spatial relationships. This deficit in comprehension of grammatical aspects of language, they argued, followed left parietal lesions, and frequently gave rise to a picture of semantic aphasia. Following Luria, we would speculate that comprehension of grammatical aspects of highly complex sentences and spatial synthesis may have a common neurochemical basis, mediated, in part, by cholinergic networks.

Cholinergic Therapy for Cognitive Disorders

Based on neurobiological findings that indicate that cholinergic pathways influence human memory and cognition, studies on pharmacological treatment of cognitive deficits began to appear in the 1970s and 1980s. Short-acting cholinergic agents such as physostigmine and arecoline have been demonstrated to enhance memory function transiently in various human conditions (76,80). Results of subsequent research focused on cholinergic therapy for memory difficulties in aging or primary degenerative dementia have been mixed. Some have reported positive results with physostigmine (81), physostigmine plus lecithin (82,83), and arecoline (84).

Thal et al. (82), for example, reported that six of eight patients with early Alzheimer's disease treated with oral physostigmine and supplemental lecithin demonstrated improvement in total recall and retrieval from long-term storage, with a decrease in verbal intrusions. The neuropsychological observations were highly correlated with inhibition of cholinesterase activity in cerebrospinal fluid, suggesting that the degree of improvement in memory function was related to the amount of physostigmine that reached the brain. Other neurotransmitters and metabolites in cerebrospinal fluid were unaffected by the physostigmine therapy, suggesting a specific effect of physostigmine on the cholinergic system. They concluded that small oral doses of physostigmine combined with lecithin ingestion have therapeutic benefit for some patients with Alzheimer's disease.

However, many others have reported negative results with long-term administration of cholinergic substances in different clinical conditions: elderly subjects (85), Alzheimer's disease (86,87), and progressive supranuclear palsy (88). Theoretical and methodological problems that remain to be resolved include the following: (1) cholinergic agents might not improve cholinergic function in patients with Alzheimer's disease who may not have sufficient cholinergic structures to respond; (2) improved memory with a single dose of physostigmine does not necessarily imply that long-term treatment would continue to produce such improvement; (3) cognitive deficits in brain disorders are undoubtedly due to dysfunction in several neuromodulator systems, and cannot be reduced to dysfunction in a single neurotransmitter system; and (4) dose-response relationships remain to be clarified. Similar methodological and theoretical problems must be addressed as we attempt to develop pharmacological approaches to therapy of aphasia.

Cholinergic Therapy for Fluent Aphasia

From the clinical and neurochemical evidence discussed above, we suggest that some aspects of language, specifically those based on anatomical networks regionalized to left posterior brain areas, may be mediated, in part, by the cholinergic system. Naming and comprehension in aphasia are partially dependent on verbal memory, and these language features may benefit from cholinergic supplementation.

Little research has looked directly at the effect of cholinergic agents on speech and language functions. Luria et al. (6) utilized "galanthamine," a powerful anticholinesterase agent, to obtain a "deinhibitory" effect on complex gnostic, praxic, and speech functions in brain damage. Galanthamine is said to have improved a wide range of cognitive dysfunctions. Electroencephalography (EEG) was used during treatment with galanthamine to obtain evidence of the changes in cortical neurodynamics. Activation of cortical function, as measured by EEG, following administration of galanthamine was found to take place only if the anatomical connections between the cortex and the mesencephalon remained intact. This observation suggested that galanthamine acted through cholinergic structures in the reticular formation of the mesencephalon, and that the activating effect of galanthamine might be nonspecific. However, they also noted a particularly strong effect on speech and language functions. Galanthamine improved motor speech problems including articulatory deficits, paraphasias, aphonia, and impaired fluency and tempo. In these studies, cholinergic medication was also effective in sensory disorders of speech; the range of acoustic perception of patients became wider, their understanding of speech was improved, the phenomena of alienation of word meaning were diminished, phonemic hearing was improved, and the time required for naming objects was shortened.

Interestingly, they observed no "deinhibitory" action by neostigmine therapy, while a drug of the same pharmacological group (galanthamine) clearly exhibited an effect. A possible explanation was that galanthamine, a tertiary amine, penetrates faster and to a greater degree into the central nervous system than neostigmine, a quaternary amine. Luria et al. (6) advocated that rehabilitation measures should include an attempt at pharmacological treatment with galanthamine (or other anticholinesterase drugs).

Moscowitch et al. (89) reported that a cholinergic agent (ameridin, an anticholinesterase agent) selectively improved language performance in semantic aphasia. Eight patients with semantic aphasia who were administered ameridin showed improvement after treatment compared with 13 control patients (age- and severity-matched) in comprehension of grammatical structures and in naming. Encouraged by this result, we have now performed an open-label trial of physostigmine in one patient with fluent aphasia. In this highly preliminary pilot study, the patient clinically improved in comprehension and naming following pharmacotherapy.

BEHAVIOR-TARGETED PHARMACOTHERAPY

More than 20 neurochemical substances have been identified as neurotransmitters in the human brain. Some of these substances appear promising as "cognitive enhancers," which may secondarily and nonspecifically have a beneficial effect on speech and language. These include noradrenaline, serotonin (5HT), peptides (e.g., substance P and opioid peptides), and amino acids (e.g., glutamic acid) (90). Adrenergic and serotonergic systems have shown much less evidence than dopaminergic and cholinergic systems of having direct effects on specific language functions. Both appear to be more implicated in mood and emotional aspects of behavior, although recent studies have demonstrated their influence on cognition (91,92). The possible effects of these drugs on speech and language remain intriguing challenges for future research and are not discussed here. Suffice it to say that we should open our minds to the possibility that drugs that influence limbic system function may have a nonspecific, beneficial effect on speech and language.

Patients who suffer from aphasia following brain damage may also display serious behavioral and psychiatric dysfunction. Although clinicians may not wish to consider treating these disorders pharmacologically as a first resort (93), medications occasionally ameliorate behavioral problems that could hinder language rehabilitation. Antidepressant agents, for example, may be useful adjuncts in aphasia therapy. Recently, beta-adrenergic antagonists (beta-blockers, such as propranolol) and serotonin agonists (selective serotonin reuptake inhibitors, such as fluoxetine, or 5HT A1 receptor agonists, such as buspirone or trazodone) have been reported to have a significant effect on aggressive and impulsive behavior (94,95). Administration of these medications may, in some cases, facilitate conventional speech and language therapy.

CONCLUSIONS

Cognitive functions cannot be explained by a reductionist approach to a single neurotransmitter system. Nevertheless, selected linguistic capacities, including verbal fluency and verbal memory, appear to be influenced by specific neurotransmitter systems. In light of this recognized chemicocognitive influence, it would be a mistake, we believe, to ignore the possibility that selected aphasic signs and symptoms may be ameliorated by targeted therapy with specific pharmacological agents. At this moment, we are aware of no neurochemical agent that has yet been rigorously proven to ameliorate specific language signs or symptoms, and it would be inappropriate to offer false hope to aphasic patients and their families.

The purpose of pharmacotherapy for aphasia would not be to replace traditional language therapy. Rather, when confronted with the devastating effects of loss of language on the person with aphasia and his or her family, one should employ all therapeutic possibilities based on each patient's condition. Both nonspecific (behavior-targeted) and specific (language-targeted) pharmacotherapy should be kept in mind as a potential adjunctive program. Clinicians and researchers should continue to seek any measure that can promote biological and functional recovery following brain damage. In this sense, pharmacotherapy for aphasia may be an important new avenue for discovery.

ACKNOWLEDGMENTS

We thank Dr. Lena Moscowitch for valuable comments based on her vast experience with pharmacotherapy for aphasia and Ms. Marjorie Nicholas for providing speech and language data.

REFERENCES

1. Albert ML. Neurobiological aspects of aphasia therapy. Aphasiology 1988; 2:215–218.
2. Albert ML, Sparks R, Helm N. Melodic intonation therapy for aphasia. Arch Neurol 1973;29:130–131.
3. Helm-Estabrooks N, Fitzpatrick P, Barresi B. Visual action therapy for global aphasia. J Speech Hear Disord 1982;47:385–389.
4. Gardner H, Zurif E, Berry T, Baker E. Visual communication in aphasia. Neuropsychologia 1976;14:275–292.
5. Wall P, Egger M. Formation of new connections in adult rat brains after partial deafferentation. Nature 1971;232:542–545.
6. Luria AR, Naydin VL, Tsvetkova LS, Vinarskaya EN. Restoration of higher cortical function following local brain damage. In: Vinken PJ, Bruyn GW, eds. Handbook of clinical neurology. Vol 3. Disorders of higher nervous activity. Amsterdam: North Holland Publishing, 1969:368–433.
7. Goldman-Rakic PS, Friedman HR. The circuity of working memory revealed by anatomy and metabolic imaging. In: Levin HS, Eisenberg HM, Benton AL, eds. Frontal lobe function and dysfunction. New York: Oxford University Press, 1991:72–91.
8. Goldman-Rakic PS. Topography of cognition: Parallel distributed networks in primate association cortex. Annu Rev Neurosci 1988;11:137–156.
9. Mesulam MM. Large-scale neurocognitive networks and distributed processing for attention, language, and memory. Ann Neurol 1990;28:597–613.
10. Posner MI, Peterson SE, Fox PT, Raichle ME. Localization of cognitive operations in the human brain. Science 1988;240:1627–1631.
11. Luciana M, Depue RA, Arbisi P, Leon A. Facilitation of working memory in humans by a D2 dopamine receptor agonist. J Cogn Neurosci 1992;4:58–68.
12. Sawaguchi T, Goldman-Rakic PS. D1 dopamine receptors in prefrontal cortex: Involvement in working memory. Science 1991;251:947–950.
13. Mettler CC. History of medicine. Philadelphia: Blackiston, 1947.
14. Linn L, Stein MH. Sodium amytal in treatment of aphasia. Preliminary report. Bull US Army Med Dept 1946;5:705–708.
15. Linn L. Sodium amytal in treatment of aphasia. Arch Neurol Psychol 1947;58:357–358.
16. Bergman PS, Green M. Aphasia: effect of intravenous sodium amytal. Neurology 1951;1:471–475.
17. Billow BW. Observation on the use of sodium amytal in the treatment of aphasia. Med Rec 1949;162:12–13.
18. Smith S, Turton EC. Restoration of speech in severe aphasia by intravenous and oral priscol. Br Med J 1951;2:891–892.
19. Luria AR. Traumatic aphasia. The Hague: Mouton, 1970.
20. Solomonovici A, Fradis A, Mihallescu L, Sevastopol M. Tratamental cu imipramina in afazille de origine vasculara. Stud Cerc Neurol 1962;7:257–263.
21. Voinescu I, Gheorghita N. Tratamentul afaziel cu imipramina. Neurol Psihiat Neurochir (Bucharest) 1973;18:423–430.

22. Gheorghita N. Immediate effects of neurodynamic substances on verbal performance in the treatment of aphasia. Rev Roum Med — Neurol Psychiat 1977; 15:95-101.
23. Voinescu I, Gheorghita N. Adjuvant drug therapy with psychologopedic rehabilitation of aphasic patients. Rev Roum Med — Neurol Psychiat 1978;16: 155-161.
24. Willmes K. Huber W, Poeck K, Poersch M. Die Wirkung von Piracetam bei der logopädischen Intensivtherapie von chronisch aphasischen Patienten. In: Von Helmchen H, ed. Sonderd ruck ans Wirkumgen und Wirksamkeit von Nootropika. Berlin: Springer-Verlag, 1988:177-187.
25. Benson DF. Presentation 10. In: Benton AL, ed. Behavioral changes in cerebrovascular disease. New York Harper & Row, 1970:77.
26. Samuels J. Personal communication, 1986.
27. Stoica E, Stefanescu E, Gheorghiu M. The restoration of the reactivity of higher autonomic centers by pyrithioxine administration in cerebral infarct patients. Europ Neurol 1972;7:348-363.
28. Critchley EMR. Speech disorders of Parkinsonism: a review. J Neurol Neurosurg Psychiatry 1981;44:751-758.
29. Illes J, Metter EJ, Hanson WR, Iritani S. Language production in Parkinson's disease: Acoustic and linguistic considerations. Brain Lang 1988;33:146-160.
30. Ruberg M, Agid Y. Dementia in Parkinson's disease. In: Iversen LI, Iversen SD, Snyder SH, eds. Handbook of psychopharmacology. Vol 20. New York: Plenum Press, 1988.
31. Cummings JL, Darkins A, Mendez M, Hill MA, Benson DF. Alzheimer's disease and Parkinson's disease: comparisons of speech and language alterations. Neurology 1988;38:680-684.
32. Rosenberger PB. Dopaminergic systems and speech fluency. J Fluency Disord 1980;5:255-267.
33. Gotham AM, Brown RG, Marsden CD. Frontal cognitive function in patients with Parkinson's disease "on" and "off" levodopa. Brain 1988;111:299-321.
34. Ross ED, Stewart RM. Akinetic mutism from hypothalamic damage: Successful treatment with dopamine agonists. Neurology 1981;31:1435-1439.
35. Eschiveri HC, Tattum WO, Merens TA, Coker SB. Akinetic mutism: pharmacologic probe of the dopaminergic mesencephalo frontal activating system. Pediatr Neurol 1988;4:228-230.
36. Barett K. Treating organic abulia with bromocriptine and lisuride: four case studies. J Neurol Neurosurg Psychiatry 1991;54:718-721.
37. Crimson MC, Childs A, Wilcox RE, Barrow N. The effect of bromocriptine on speech dysfunction in patients with diffuse brain injury (Akinetic mutism). Clin Neuropharmacol 1988;11:462-466.
38. Fisher W, Kerbeshian J, Burd L. A treatable language disorder: pharmacological treatment of pervasive developmental disorder. J Dev Behav Pediat 1986; 7:73-76.
39. Rastatter MP, Harr R. Measurements of plasma levels of adrenergic neurotransmitters and primary amino acids in five stuttering subjects: a preliminary report (biochemical aspects of stuttering). J Fluency Disord 1988;13:127-139.

40. Moore RY. Catecholamine neuron systems in brain. Ann Neurol 1982;12:321–327.
41. Rubens AB, Kertesz A. The localization of lesions in transcortical aphasias. In: Kertesz A, ed. Localization in neuropsychology. New York: Academic Press, 1983:245–268.
42. Albert ML, Goodglass H, Helm NA, Rubens AB, Alexander MP. Clinical aspects of dysphasia. New York: Springer-Verlag, 1981.
43. Freedman M, Alexander MP, Naeser MA. Anatomic bases of transcortical motor aphasia. Neurology 1984;34:409–417.
44. Botez MI, Barbeau A. A role of subcortical structures and particularly the thalamaus in the mechanisms of speech and language. Int J Neurol 1971;8:300–320.
45. Goldberg G. Supplementary motor area structure and function: Review and hypothesis. Behav Brain Sci 1985;8:567–615.
46. Larsen B, Skinhoj E, Lassen NA. Variations in regional cortical blood flow in the right and left hemispheres during automatic speech. Brain 1978;101:193–209.
47. Naeser MA, Palumbo CL, Helm-Estabrooks N, Stiassny-Eder D, Albert ML. Severe non-fluency in aphasia: Role of the medial subcallosal fasciculus plus other white matter pathways in recovery of spontaneous speech. Brain 1989;112:1–38.
48. Albert ML, Bachman DL, Morgan A, Helm-Estabrooks N. Pharmacotherapy for aphasia. Neurology 1988;38:877–879.
49. Bachman DL, Morgan A. The role of pharmacotherapy in the treatment of aphasia: Preliminary results. Aphasiology 1988;2:225–228.
50. Gupta S, Mlcoch A. Bromocriptine treatment of nonfluent aphasia. Arch Phys Med Rehabil 1992;73:373–376.
51. Sabe L, Leiguarda R, Starkstein SE. An open-label trial of bromocriptine in nonfluent aphasia. Neurology 1992;42:1637–1638.
52. MacLennan DL, Nicholas LE, Morley GK, Brookshire RH. The effects of bromocriptine on speech and language function in a man with transcortical motor aphasia. In: Prescott TE, ed. Clinical aphasiology. Santa Fe, 1990:145–155.
53. Goodglass H, Kaplan E. Assessment of aphasia and related disorders. Philadelphia: Lea & Febiger, 1984.
54. Riederer P, Sofic E, Konradi C, et al. The role of dopamine in the control of neurobiological functions. In: Flückiger E, Müller EE, Thorner MO, eds. The role of brain dopamine. Berlin: Springer-Verlag, 1989:1–17.
55. Liebson E, Walsh MJ, Jankowiak J, Albert ML. J Neuropsychiatry Neuropsychol Behav Neurol. In press.
56. Clark CR, Geffen GM, Geffen LB. Catecholamines and attention. I. Animal and clinical studies. Neurosci Biobehav Rev 1987;11:341–352.
57. Newman RP, Weingartner H, Smallberg SA, Calne DB. Effortful and automatic memory: Effects of dopamine. Neurology 1984;34:805–807.
58. Alexander GE, Crutcher MD. Functional architecture of basal ganglia circuits: neural substrates of parallel processing. Trends Neurosci 1990;13:266–271.
59. Physician's Desk Reference. 46th ed. Oradell, NJ: Medical Economics, 1992:2020–2023.

60. Moskowitch L. Personal communication, 1993.
61. Mesulam MM. Central cholinergic pathways: neuroanatomy and some behavioral implications. In: Anoli M, Reader TA, Dykes RW, Gloor P, eds. Neurotransmitters and cortical function. New York: Plenum Press, 1988:237–260.
62. Amaducci L, Sorbi S, Albanese A, Gainotti G. Choline acetyltransferase (ChAT) activity differs in right and left human temporal lobes. Neurology 1981;31:799–805.
63. McGeer PL, McGeer EG, Suzuki J, Dolman CE, Nagai T. Aging, Alzheimer's disease, and the cholinergic system of the basal forebrain. Neurology 1984; 34:741–745.
64. Liebson E, Albert ML. Cognitive changes in dementia of the Alzheimer's type. In: Calne DB, ed. Neurodegenerative diseases. Pennsylvania: WB Saunders, 1994:615–629.
65. Drachman DA, Leavitt J. Human memory and the cholinergic system. Arch Neurol 1974;30:113–121.
66. Drachman DA. Memory and cognitive function in man: Does the cholinergic system have a specific role? Neurology 1977;27:783–790.
67. Rusted JM, Warburton DM. Cognitive models and cholinergic drugs. Neuropsychobiology 1989;21:31–36.
68. Mohs RC, Davis KL, Darley C. Cholinergic drug effects on memory and cognition in humans. In: Poon LW, ed. Aging in the 1980s. Washington, DC: American Psychological Association, 1980:181–190.
69. Christensen H, Maltby N, Jorm AF, Creasey H, Broc GA. Cholinergic blockade as a model of the cognitive deficits in Alzheimer's disease. Brain 1992;115: 1681–1699.
70. Beatty WW, Butters N, Janowsky DS. Patterns of memory failure after scopolamine treatment: Implications for cholinergic hypotheses of dementia. Behav Neurolog Biol 1986;45:196–211.
71. Kopelman MD, Corn TH. Cholinergic "blockade" as a model for cholinergic depletion. Brain 1988;111:1079–1110.
72. Fuld P, Katzman R, Davies P. Intrusions as a sign of Alzheimer dementia: Chemical and pathological verification. Ann Neurol 1982;11:155–159.
73. Schatzberg AF, Jonathan OC, Blumer DP. Speech blockage: a tricyclic side effect. Am J Psychiatry 1978;135:600–601.
74. Cooper JA, Sagar HJ, Jordan N, Harvey NS, Sullivan EV. Cognitive impairment in early, untreated parkinson's disease and its relationship to motor disability. Brain 1991;114:2095–2122.
75. Litvan I, Grafman J, Gomez C, Chase TN. Memory impairment in patients with progressive supranuclear palsy. Arch Neurol 1989;46:765–767.
76. Bartus RT, Dean RL, Flicker C. Cholinergic psychopharmacology: An integration of human and animal research on memory. In: Meltzer HY, ed. Psychopharmacology: the third generation of progress. New York: Raven Press, 1987: 219–232.
77. Kertzman C, Robinson DL, Litvan I. Effects of physostigmine on spatial attention in patients with progressive supranuclear palsy. Arch Neurol 1990;47:1346–1350.

78. Meador KJ, Moore EE, Nicholas ME, et al. The role of cholinergic systems in visuospatial processing and memory. J Clin Exp Neuropsychol 1993;15:832–342.
79. Zemishlany Z, Thorne AE. Anticholinergic challenge and cognitive functions: a comparison between young and elderly normal subjects. Isr J Psychiatry Relat Sci 1991;28:32–41.
80. Davis KL, Mohs RC, Tinklenberg JR. Physostigmine: improvement of long-term memory processes in normal humans. Science 1978;201:272–274.
81. Drachman DA, Sahakian BJ. Memory and cognitive function in the elderly. A preliminary trial of physostigmine. Arch Neurol 1980;37:674–675.
82. Thal LJ, Fuld PA, Masur DM, Sharpless NS. Oral physostigmine and lecithin improve memory in Alzheimer disease. Ann Neurol 1983;13:491–496.
83. Peters BH, Levin HS. Effects of physostigmine and lecithin on memory in Alzheimer disease. Ann Neurol 1979;6:219–221.
84. Raffaele KC, Berardi A, Asthana S, Morris P, Haxby JV, Soncrant TT. Effects of long-term continuous infusion of the muscarinic cholinergic agonist arecoline on verbal memory in dementia of the Alzheimer type. Psychopharmacol Bull 1991;27:315–319.
85. Ferris SH, Sathananthan G, Reisberg B, Gershon S. Long-term choline treatment of memory-impaired elderly patients. Science 1979;205:1039–1040.
86. Christie JE, Shering A, Ferguson J. Physostigmine and arecoline: effects of intravenous infusions in Alzheimer presenile dementia. Br J Psychiatry 1981; 138:46–50.
87. Stern Y, Sano M, Mayeux R. Effects of oral physostigmine in Alzheimer's disease. Ann Neurol 1987;22:306–310.
88. Foster NL, Aldrich MS, Bluemlein L, White RF, Berent S. Failure of cholinergic agonist RS-86 to improve cognition and movement in PSP despite effects on sleep. Neurology 1989;39:257–261.
89. Moscowitch L, McNamara P, Albert ML. Neurochemical correlates of aphasia. Neurology 1991;41(suppl 1):410.
90. Gilman S, Newman SW. Chemical neuroanatomy. In: Manter and Gratz's essentials of clinical neuroanatomy and neurophysiology. 7th ed. Philadelphia: FA Davis, 1989:222–231.
91. Cuccaro ML, Wright HH, Abramson RK, Marsteller FA, Valentine J. Whole-blood serotonin and cognitive functioning in autistic individuals and their first-degree relatives. J Neuropsychiatry Clin Neurosci 1993;5:94–101.
92. Costall B, Barnes JM, Hamon M, Muller WE, Briley M. Biochemical models for cognition enhancers. Pharmacopsychiatry 1990;23(suppl 2):85–88.
93. Helm-Estabrooks N, Albert ML. Manual of aphasia therapy. Austin: PRO-ED, 1991.
94. Gedye A. Buspirone alone or with serotonergic diet reduced aggression in a developmentally disable adult. Biol Psychiatry 1991;30:88–91.
95. Ratey JJ, Sorgi P, O'Driscoll GA, et al. Naldol to treat agression and psychiatric symptomatology in chronic psychiatric inpatients: A double-blind, placebo-controlled study. J Clin Psychiatry 1992;53:41–46.

20

Neuropsychiatric Aspects of Aphasia

Ann H. Craig

UCLA School of Medicine, Los Angeles, California

Jeffrey L. Cummings

UCLA School of Medicine and West Los Angeles Veterans Affairs Medical Center, Los Angeles, California

INTRODUCTION

Neuropsychiatric disturbances are common among individuals with aphasic syndromes, but this area of neuropsychiatry has received relatively little investigation. The lack of studies of neuropsychiatric morbidity in aphasia may stem, in part, from the fundamental difficulty of assessing conditions with primarily verbal manifestations in individuals whose ability to communicate is compromised. Potentially treatable neuropsychiatric disorders may be overlooked because of impaired communication or because they are viewed as an appropriate psychological reaction to loss.

Aphasia is an acquired disturbance of linguistic communication produced by brain dysfunction. Etiologies of aphasia include stroke, head injury, neoplasms, central nervous system infections, and primary degenerative dementias. Focal brain injuries of the left hemisphere are associated with signature clinical syndromes: fluent aphasias occur with lesions of the posterior regions; nonfluent aphasia are associated with lesions of the anterior areas. More recently, regional affiliations of neuropsychiatric syndromes have also been studied. Although lacking the obligatory anatomical relationships observed with many neurobehavioral syndromes, neuropsychiatric disturbances exhibit anatomically contingent relationships manifested by an association between specific lesion sites and an increased vulnerability to neuropsychiatric disturbances. Depression has been associated with anteriorly located left brain lesions and psychosis with more posterior lesions and injuries involving the limbic system (1). In this chapter, the neuropsychiatric disorders associated with specific aphasia syndromes are reviewed. The anatomy, pathophysiology, and treatment of these disorders are presented.

CLASSIFICATION OF APHASIA-RELATED NEUROPSYCHIATRIC SYNDROMES

Aphasia-associated neurobehavioral and neuropsychiatric disorders may be divided into two broad categories (Table 1). First are the mood disorders, which include the syndromes of major and minor (or dysthymic) depression (2), the relatively brief dysphoric affective disturbance labeled the catastrophic reaction (3), and elevated mood states. Depression and catastrophic reaction occur with greater frequency in patients with nonfluent aphasia and anteriorly located left-hemisphere lesions (4,5). The second major category of aphasia-related neuropsychiatric disorders is psychosis, a disturbance associated with fluent aphasia and posteriorly located left-hemisphere lesions (6).

DEMOGRAPHY OF APHASIA-RELATED NEUROPSYCHIATRIC SYNDROMES

The incidence and prevalence of neuropsychiatric disorders among aphasics is unknown. About 100,000 new cases of aphasia are caused annually by stroke, and head injury is responsible for at least twice this number (7). In a recent study of patients with acute strokes (8), 53% of aphasic patients and 44% of patients without aphasia were found to be depressed. Extrapolation gives a figure of more than 150,000 potentially treatable cases of depression occurring annually in patients rendered aphasic from these causes

Table 1 Classification of the Principal Neuropsychiatric Syndromes Occurring in Patients with Aphasia

Neuropsychiatric syndrome	Associated aphasia	Hemispheric lesion site
Mood disorders		
Depression		
Major	Nonfluent	Anterior
Minor	Nonfluent > fluent	Anterior > posterior
Catastrophic reaction	Nonfluent	Anterior
Elevated mood	Fluent	Posterior
Psychosis	Fluent	Posterior

alone. The prevalence of aphasia-associated catastrophic reactions, elevated mood, and psychosis is unknown but these disorders are not uncommon among aphasic patients. The total frequency of neuropsychiatric morbidity among aphasia patients is substantial, and these behavioral disorders adversely influence the recovery and rehabilitation of aphasic patients.

DEPRESSION

Depression is the most commonly observed mood disorder following brain injury and the most extensively studied. Until recent years, depression following brain damage was considered solely a psychological reaction to the stress of severe disability. However, current research supports an important role for neurophysiological changes in the pathogenesis of the mood disorder. The study of depressive disorders in patients with aphasic syndromes has pointed to neuroanatomical factors important in the development of depression. Current evidence suggests that aphasia and depression are not causally related, but rather separate outcomes of anterior left frontal lobe lesions (8).

Frequency of Depression and Relationship to Disability

Robinson and coworkers (9) have studied post-stroke depression extensively, and are responsible for much of our current knowledge regarding post-stroke depressive disorders. They and others have found clinically significant depression in up to 50% of patients after acute stroke. Depression has also been found in approximately 30% of outpatient stroke populations (10–15). Folstein and colleagues (10) compared patients hospitalized for stroke rehabilitation with a group matched for degree of physical disability hospitalized for orthopedic injuries. They found a significantly higher frequency of depression among those with strokes (45% versus 10%). The finding of increased depression in stroke patients has been confirmed by a study comparing stroke patients with a randomly selected comparison group of physically impaired nonstroke patients in a rehabilitation facility (48% versus 0%) (11).

Several investigators (8,13,14,16–18) have found only weak or no correlations between degree of impairment and severity of depression in the acute poststroke period. The correlation between physical and cognitive impairment and depression increases over the first 6 months post-stroke (18,19). One study (20) found significant improvement in functional ability 1 year post-stroke only among nondepressed patients. These observations indicate that functional disability does not cause poststroke depression, but depressed patients have poorer recovery from stroke than nondepressed patients.

Characteristics of Stroke-Associated Depression

Robinson and colleagues (2,9) have phenomenologically separated post-stroke depression into major and minor (dysthymic) categories using the symptom criteria of the third edition of the *Diagnostic and Statistical Manual of Mental Disorders* (21) modified by omitting the duration requirements. Major poststroke depression was characterized by dysphoric mood or loss of pleasure or interest in usual activities with four or more of the following symptoms: anorexia or significant weight loss, insomnia, psychomotor retardation, loss of energy, loss of pleasure or interest in usual activities, impaired concentration, feelings of worthlessness, and suicidal ideation. Minor, or dysthymic, depression was diagnosed when there was prominent depressed mood that did not meet the severity criteria for major depression but included at least three of the following symptoms: sleep disturbance, fatigue, feelings of inadequacy, decreased productivity, social withdrawal, difficulty concentrating or thinking clearly, loss of interest in pleasurable activities, decreased activity or talkativeness, brooding, irritability, tearfulness, pessimism about the future, thoughts of death or suicide.

Important differences in lesion location, course, prognosis, and biological markers between stroke-associated major depression and poststroke dysthymia have been found. Major, but not minor, depression is strongly associated with anterior left cortical or subcortical brain injury and lesion proximity to the frontal pole (22). Major depression has a natural course similar to that of idiopathic major depression, with spontaneous remission 1 to 2 years after onset; whereas minor depression is not significantly improved after 2 years in most patients (23). Major, but not minor, depression is significantly associated with failure to suppress serum cortisol normally in a dexamethasone-suppression test, although false-positive tests are not uncommon (11,24).

Phenomenologically, idiopathic and poststroke major depression are similar, although psychomotor slowing was found to be more common following stroke, and impairment of interest and concentration was observed more often in idiopathic depression. There was also a significant difference in the frequency of familial psychiatric disorders in idiopathic depression compared to poststroke major depression (63% versus 13%) (25). Cognitive impairment similar to the dementia syndrome of depression has been observed in poststroke major depression. The occurrence of this disorder is independent of lesion size (26).

Anatomical Correlations

Robinson and coworkers have consistently found a strong correlation between lesion location and poststroke major depression. Major depression was significantly more frequent with left anterior hemispheric lesions (anterior lesion border proximal to 40% of the anterior-posterior distance on computerized tomography scan) than with any other lesion location (14,16, 18,22). This held for left-handed patients as well as those who were right-handed (27). Physical and cognitive impairment in one study of the acute poststroke period were found to account for only 10% of the variance in depression scores, whereas lesion proximity to the left frontal pole explained 50% (18). Patients with bilateral brain injury (28) and patients with closed head injuries (16) also exhibited the association between left anterior lesion and depression.

Not all investigators have found the marked predominance of left-sided compared to right-sided lesions in patients with poststroke depression (10, 13,29). Robinson and colleagues have suggested that such variables as length of time following stroke, diagnostic criteria for depression, existence of prior brain injury, history of psychiatric illness, and intrahemispheric lesion location might account for variable findings among investigators (2).

In studies comparing the effects of cortical and subcortical lesions, patients with left frontal cortex or left basal ganglia lesions had higher frequencies of poststroke major depression than those with left posterior cortical or thalamic lesions. In both cortical and subcortical lesion sites, proximity to the frontal pole was significantly correlated with severity of depression scores (22). There was an 88% frequency of major depression in patients with left basal ganglia lesions (including six of six with lesions involving the head of the caudate nucleus), compared to 0% of patients with thalamic lesions (30). Starkstein and colleagues (31) also found that cortical lesions produced depression combined with anxiety disorders, whereas left basal ganglia lesions produced depression without notable anxiety symptoms.

Patients with and without poststroke depression were matched for CT size and location of lesion in an effort to determine why some patients with left anterior lesions developed depression while others did not. A greater degree of subcortical atrophy was found in the depressed group, suggesting that this may be a predisposing factor in the development of poststroke depression (32).

Relationship Between Aphasia and Depression

Few empirical studies specifically address the relationship between aphasia and mood disturbances. Several investigators have failed to find a significant correlation between the occurrence of aphasia and poststroke depression (2,12,18,22). Starkstein and Robinson (8) studied a group of 113 patients consecutively admitted with acute stroke. They excluded those in whom it was not possible to verbally assess psychiatric symptoms due to moderate to severe comprehension deficits and those with impaired consciousness that precluded testing. In the remaining 103 patients, no significant difference in depression frequency was found between the 17% with aphasia and the remainder without language impairment (53% in aphasics versus 44% in nonaphasics). Likewise, the frequency of major and minor depression was not significantly different between the two groups (29% major versus 24% minor in aphasics).

Robinson and Benson (17) studied hospitalized patients with aphasia several months after brain injury. Nonfluent aphasics, all with frontal lobe lesions on CT, had significantly higher depression scale scores than did fluent or global aphasics, who scored similarly to one another. Depression scores did not correlate with cognitive impairment or physical dysfunction.

Signer, Cummings, and Benson (6) retrospectively reviewed information regarding chronic aphasics hospitalized for behavioral disturbances. On average, brain injury antedated first psychiatric hospitalization by 6.5 years. They found nonfluent aphasics to be 8.8 times more likely to be depressed than those with fluent or nonlocalizing aphasic syndromes.

Starkstein and Robinson (8) found no association between mood changes and language disturbance in 25 aphasic patients in the acute poststroke period. Nine were diagnosed with major depression, six with minor depression, and 10 were not depressed. Lesion location, however, was significantly associated with major depression. All patients with an identifiable lesion on CT and major depression had a lesion localized to the left anterior hemisphere. Only one of the nondepressed patients had a frontal lobe lesion on CT. They concluded that lesion location, rather than presence or type of aphasia, is the most relevant variable associated with major poststroke depression.

Caveats Regarding the Study of Mood in Aphasia

Exclusion of aphasic patients with severe comprehension deficits associated with posterior lesions may have resulted in the factitial association of depression with anterior lesions in studies of poststroke depression (8). However, this seems unlikely, since a low rate of depression has been found among patients with fluent aphasia who have the most severe comprehension deficits (17). It would also be inconsistent with the clinical observation of unconcern, and at times euphoria, in patients with fluent aphasia (4). In addition, patients with subcortical aphasias, who seldom have severe comprehension deficits, show the same significant association between proximity to the frontal pole and severity of depression as seen with cortical lesions (22).

Thus, current evidence suggests that depression is more common in patients with nonfluent aphasia, that this observation is not artifactual based on exclusion of patients with comprehension deficits, and that the anterior hemispheric location of the lesion is the principal determinant of the mood alterations.

Pathophysiology

Although psychological reaction to disability may contribute importantly to the development of poststroke depression, several lines of evidence support the etiological importance of neuropsychological or neurochemical processes initiated by structural brain injury. These include the lack of a strong association between depressive illness and degree of physical disability or presence of aphasia; the strong correlation between major depression and left anterior lesion location; the association of major poststroke depression with biological markers such as the dexamethasone suppression test; and the similarity of the natural course, phenomenology, and response to treatment of poststroke depression and idiopathic major depression.

Disturbances of catecholaminergic systems have been implicated in the etiology of idiopathic depression. Robinson and colleagues (2,22) postulate that there is damage to the asymmetric ascending biogenic amine pathways, resulting in differing emotional and behavioral responses dependent on the side of anterior cortical or subcortical hemispheric injury. Noradrenergic pathways arise in brainstem nuclei, project anteriorly through the median forebrain bundle, and disperse into the deep nuclei or pass into the frontal cortex, where widespread terminal projections ramify from anterior to posterior in the cortex. In animal studies, anterior cortical lesions disrupt these noradrenergic axons to a greater degree than do posterior lesions (33,34). There are lateralized differences in the behavioral responses to norepinephrine and dopamine depletion (35), and there is also preliminary evidence of neurotransmitter asymmetry in postmortem studies of human brains (36). Robinson and colleagues (2,22) hypothesize that anterior cortical and subcortical lesions cause greater interruption of terminal fibers, resulting in more severe biogenic amine depletion and thus more severe depression. They suggest that interhemispheric biochemical asymmetries may account for the production of depression after left, but not right, anterior hemisphere lesions. These asymmetries may be in biogenic amine content, receptor density, or structural integrity of biogenic amine pathways.

Alterations in dopamine function may also contribute to poststroke depression. Prefrontal and mesocortical dopaminergic systems play an important role in the behavioral functions of anticipation and expectancy, in reward, and in the mediation of stress responses. Disruption of hedonic, motivational, and stress-alleviating neurobiological mechanisms in conjunction with frontal lobe lesions could result in the psychological experience of worthlessness, helplessness, hopelessness, and dysphoria that categorize depression (37).

Limited functional imaging studies in patients with depression and brain injury have been pursued. These provide additional insight into the possible mechanisms of depression associated with focal brain injuries. Evidence of a lateralized biochemical response in humans after hemispheric stroke has recently been found. Increased serotonin S2 receptor binding in the temporal and parietal cortex was shown by positron emission tomography studies following right-, but not left-, hemisphere strokes. Decreased serotonin binding in the left temporal cortex correlated with depression severity (38). Starkstein and Robinson (2) propose that there may be less profound serotonin or norepinephrine depletion in left- than in right-hemisphere stroke, resulting in stimulation of compensatory serotonin receptor upregulation only on the right. The uncompensated biogenic amine depletion with left-hemisphere lesions would lead to the clinical manifestations of depression.

Treatment

Many investigators have noted that patients seldom receive therapy for depression after stroke. Many factors may contribute to this treatment reticence, including failure to diagnose depression and to recognize it as a potentially treatable condition, as well as concern over use of antidepressant medications in stroke patients, who are often elderly and often have multiple medical illnesses (11–13,39,40). Preliminary studies have shown, however, that antidepressants, psychostimulants, and electroconvulsive therapy can be effective in poststroke depression (39,41–44). Lipsey and colleagues (45) found significantly greater improvement in poststroke depression in patients treated with nortriptyline than in a similar group of patients receiving placebo in a double-blinded study. Treatment response correlated with nortriptyline serum concentrations (above 100 ng/ml) and duration of treatment (6 weeks in the treatment-responsive group). Patients with recent myocardial infarction, cardiac conduction abnormalities, urinary-outlet obstruction, and narrow-angle glaucoma were excluded from the study. Delirium was the most common side effect and was reversible. Other investigators have shown successful treatment of depression in stroke patients with trazodone (41) and psychostimulants (dextroamphetamine or methylphenidate) (42). Electroconvulsive therapy was also found to be safe and effective in a small retrospective study of stroke patients. Improvement was shown both in depression and in cognitive function (44).

CATASTROPHIC REACTION

Catastrophic reaction is a term first used by Goldstein (3) to describe a dysphoric emotional outburst observed in brain-damaged individuals. Catastrophic reaction, characterized by anxiety, crying, aggressive and hostile behavior, swearing, and withdrawal from testing was first systematically studied by Gainotti (46). He found a significantly higher frequency of catastrophic reactions (swearing, bursts of tears, anxiety, and renouncements and refusals of testing) in left than in right unilaterally brain-injured patients. Duration of catastrophic reaction was seconds to minutes. Those with Broca's aphasia had the highest frequency of such reactions. Their emotional outbursts were dramatic and occurred with minimal stimulus. Among aphasics, patients with Wernicke's aphasia had the lowest frequency of catastrophic reaction. The high frequency of catastrophic responses in left brain-injuried patients was in contrast to right brain-injured patients, who demonstrated more frequent indifference reactions, characterized by unconcern, joking, anosognosia, and minimization.

Terzian (47) observed "depressive/catastrophic" emotional reactions during left carotid sodium amytal injections in right-handed patients. Left carotid perfusion results in temporary anesthesia of the left hemisphere. Patients expressed feelings of guilt, nothingness, indignity, and worry about the future in association with anosognosia. They showed little concern over language or motor impairment. In contrast, euphoric reactions occurred exclusively with right-hemisphere injections. Lee and coworkers (48) also found changes in emotional expression after unilateral carotid amytal injections performed in candidates for epilepsy surgery. About 40% of patients had emotional reactions after right-sided injections and 30% after left carotid injections. Crying occurred only with left carotid injections. Laughter and elated mood were seen three times more often after right than after left injections. These findings were independent of general cognitive status, lateralization of seizure onset, crossflow to the contralateral hemisphere, or dose of amobarbital.

The association between catastrophic reaction and poststroke depression is not clear, nor has the anatomical basis of catastrophic reaction been studied beyond its association with nonfluent aphasia referable to the left frontal cortex. It is the only neurobehavioral disturbance noted to occur more commonly in aphasic than in nonaphasic patients (8). Its temporal relationship to the course of aphasia has not been investigated.

Theories of Pathogenesis

The etiology of catastrophic reactions is uncertain. Benson (4) attributed these outbursts to a psychological reaction to severe frustration and preserved awareness of deficit, and suggested that these reactions could be avoided by refraining from testing strategies likely to result in repeated failure. However, the studies of Terzian (47) and Lee et al. (48) of intracarotid amytal injection suggest that catastrophic reactions are independent of aphasia or psychological response to language impairment, as emotional reactions tended to occur as aphasia was resolving and the patients expressed no concern regarding linguistic disability.

It has been proposed that there is a hemispheric asymmetry for the expression of affect. Hypotheses derive from methodologically diverse investigations. Selective barbiturate injection studies suggest that ipsilateral subcortical structures influence the type and development of emotional reaction either through release of subcortical limbic structures from normal cortical control or through disruption of the normal balance between the two sides of the limbic system (48). Sackheim and colleagues (49) suggested that emotional outbursts associated with destructive lesions were due to disinhibition of contralateral centers subserving emotion, whereas outbursts associated with irritative lesions are due to excitation of ipsilateral centers. They proposed that there is affective hemispheric lateralization, perhaps resulting from neurotransmitter asymmetries between the two hemispheres. Silberman and Weingartner (50) concluded that the present level of knowledge suggests that emotional control may be based on an interactive inhibition between a right negatively biased and a left positively biased hemisphere.

However, Robinson and colleagues (2,51) postulate a more complex mechanism of affective symptom production after brain injury. Lipsey, Robinson and colleagues (28) studied 15 patients with bilateral hemispheric brain injury. They found the previously observed strong association between proximity of left brain lesion to the frontal pole and depression severity to be the principal determinant of post-brain-injury psychiatric disturbance. This was independent of lesion age, temporal sequence of lateralized brain injury, location of right brain injury, and degree of cognitive or physical impairment. They argue that if left anterior brain injury simply released inhibition of a negative right-hemisphere emotional bias, coexistent right-brain injury might be expected to modify depressive symptomatology. Such an influence was not observed in their study.

ELEVATED MOOD

Elation as a chronic personality alteration has been observed in patients with chronic fluent aphasic syndromes. It was noted in 29% of fluent aphasics hospitalized for management of behavioral disturbance (6). The patients seemed unaware of their language impairment and were elated without other features of hypomania such as pressured speech, grandiosity, flight of ideas, or insomnia. This mood disturbance was not observed in nonfluent aphasics.

PSYCHOSIS

The relationship between aphasic language disturbance and psychosis has received little attention. Several investigators have noted a striking association between fluent aphasias with lesions localized to the left posterior temporoparietal hemisphere and paranoid states, delusions, and psychosis. Fisher (52) reviewed 20 patients with Wernicke's aphasia and moderate to severe comprehension disturbance. He observed transient (days) behavioral manifestations of extreme anger with verbal and physical violence and "suspected" paranoia and delusional disturbances. He did not find similar behavior in nonfluent aphasics, nor did he observe any relation to premorbid personality or any predominant mood disturbances. Benson (4) also observed paranoid reactions, at times with violent behavior, in fluent aphasics with left temporoparietal cortical brain injury. He associated paranoid states with temporal auditory association area lesions and more severe impairment of language comprehension. Signer and colleagues (6) reviewed the records of chronic aphasics hospitalized for behavioral abnormalities, observing a preponderance of posterior/fluent aphasics among them. A strong association was found between the occurrence of delusions and posterior/fluent aphasic syndromes. Delusions were present in 58% of fluent aphasics and were primarily of a persecutory nature. This was compared to a frequency of 27% with nonlocalizing aphasic syndromes, and 25% among patients with anterior/nonfluent aphasias. The presence of delusions was independent of the occurrence of epilepsy or depressed mood.

Theories Regarding Pathogenesis

The pathogenesis of psychosis associated with aphasia is unknown. However, the occurrence of neuropsychiatric disturbances specific to aphasia type suggests a role for proximity of lesion sites, distant effects of structural lesions (diaschisis), or structural causes such as neurotransmitter system dysfunction. Fisher (52) first proposed that the behavioral abnormalities he noted in patients with Wernicke's aphasia might be related to limbic system dysfunction. Lateral temporal structures mediating language function are adjacent to medial temporal limbic structures often implicated in organic psychoses. Concurrent medial and lateral temporal dysfunction might be expected in the situation of traumatic, neoplastic, or vascular brain injury resulting on occasion in simultaneous aphasia and delusional syndromes (1). Cummings (53) observed that no single anatomical site can account for the occurrence of delusions, but has proposed a pathophysiological mechanism wherein limbic dysfunction results in paranoid delusions and psychosis. Nearly all structural lesions and diseases associated with organic psychosis involve dopaminergic projections, especially in the limbic system. Sustained dysfunction in these structures or their connections could result in abnormal valuation of experience with consequent inappropriate fear resulting in paranoia, the most commonly observed theme in organic psychosis.

Observations in epilepsy and trauma also support the association of psychosis and fluent aphasia. Kanemoto and Janz (54) reported that ictal aphasia characterized by impaired comprehension and paraphasia was associated with thought disorder in patients with complex partial seizures. Left temporal lobe seizure foci predominated in those with ictal aphasia and ictal thought disorder. In trauma patients, correlations have been observed between prevalence of organic psychosis after head trauma and left lateralization and temporal lobe localization of lesion (53).

The development of paranoia because of impaired language comprehension and lack of awareness of deficit resulting in misinterpretation of reality might play a role in the strong association between delusional disturbance and posterior hemispheric aphasic disturbances (4). However, the presence of delusions in three of four patients with chronic conduction aphasia and relatively preserved comprehension in the study of Signer and colleagues (6) supports the importance of factors other than linguistic misinterpretation in the etiology of psychosis. Reactive psychosis in response to severe disability is also made doubtful by observations that patients with more severe functional impairment (aphasia and hemiparesis) were less likely to be delusional than those with aphasia alone. The relationship between posterior hemispheric localization and delusions has also been found to be independent of the existence of epilepsy or presence of mood disturbance.

Psychosis is often of late onset relative to brain injury. Usually several years have elapsed between the onset of language disturbance and the emergence of the delusional disorder (6). A similar temporal relationship has been noted in epilepsy, especially with left temporal lobe seizure foci, for which an average of 14 years was reported between onset of seizures and recognition of psychosis (53). These findings suggest that long-term biochemical or neurophysiological alterations are important in the development of psychotic disturbances.

Other factors possibly contributing to the relationship of posterior brain injury and psychosis include genetic constitution, pre-existing personality characteristics, and exact location and size of the associated structural lesions. These may also explain why psychosis is not a constant feature of fluent aphasia syndromes (1).

Treatment

Patients with persecutory organic delusional beliefs not uncommonly act on them. Resultant refusal of medication or food for fear of poisoning, adoption of unnecessary security measures, increased domestic discord, and even murder or suicide attempts have been observed (1). Early recognition and treatment of psychotic disturbances are critical in the clinical management of aphasic patients. Organic psychoses are treated with the same neuroleptic agents used in idiopathic psychosis (53). More elementary and loosely held delusions respond better to medication than complex, rigidly structured delusional systems (1). The elderly, in whom organic psychoses are more common, require lower drug dosages and are more susceptible to the adverse consequences of therapy.

RESEARCH DIRECTIONS IN APHASIA-RELATED NEUROPSYCHIATRIC SYNDROMES

Investigation of depressive and delusional disorders associated with aphasic syndromes has relied on lesion localization by clinical aphasic syndrome and by computed tomography, when possible. More sensitive nuclear magnetic resonance imaging and functional imaging studies (positron emission tomography) have yet to be used extensively in the study of neuropsychiatric disturbances in brain-injured and aphasic patients. Positron emission tomographic imaging has previously been applied to the study of idiopathic psychiatric disturbances, and comparisons of functional imaging in patients with phenomenologically similar psychiatric disturbances with and without demonstrable structural lesions will likely be a fruitful source of insights into the as yet poorly understood etiology and pathogenesis of these neuropsychiatric disorders.

The precise roles of neurotransmitters in the regulation of mood also await further study. Combined positron emission tomography and neuropsychological studies in patients with structural cortical and subcortical lesions, subcortical degenerative syndromes, and idiopathic mood disorders are needed to extend our understanding of the relationship between frontal lobe and basal ganglia metabolism, laterality, and mood changes. Further positron emission tomography studies with specific neurotransmitter ligands as well as postmortem investigations are needed to elucidate the relationship of cellular, neurotransmitter, and receptor changes to mood alterations. The scope of neuropsychiatric disorders investigated in aphasic syndromes should be broadened. Changes in personality and the possible occurrence of anxiety have received virtually no study. The diversity of neuropsychiatric syndromes present in aphasic patients is probably underestimated. Much work remains in the development of a comprehensive understanding of the neurobiological basis of neuropsychiatric syndromes associated with local brain injury.

ACKNOWLEDGMENTS

This project was supported by the Department of Veterans Affairs and by a grant from the National Institute on Aging Alzheimer's Disease Core Center.

REFERENCES

1. Cummings JL. Organic delusions: phenomenology, anatomical correlations, and review. Br J Psychiatry 1985;146:184–197.

2. Starkstein SE, Robinson RG. Affective disorders and cerebrovascular disease. Br J Psychiatry 1989;154:170-182.

3. Goldstein K. Language and language disturbances. New York: Grune & Stratton, 1948.

4. Benson DF. Psychiatric aspects of aphasia. Br J Psychiatry 1973;123:555-566.

5. Gainotti G. Emotional behavior and hemispheric side of the lesion. Cortex 1972;8:41-55.

6. Signer S, Cummings JL, Benson DF. Delusions and mood disorders in patients with chronic aphasia. J Neuropsychiatry 1989;1:40-45.

7. Damasio AR. Aphasia. New England Journal of Medicine 1992;326:531-539.

8. Starkstein SE, Robinson RG. Aphasia and depression. Aphasiology 1988;2: 1-20.

9. Robinson RG, Starkstein SE. Current research in affective disorders following stroke. J Neuropsychiatry 1990;2:1-14.

10. Folstein F, Maiberger R, McHugh PR. Mood disorder as a specific complication of stroke. J Neurol Neurosurg Psychiatry 1977;40:1018-1020.

11. Finkelstein S, Benowitz CI, Baldessarini RJ. Mood, vegetative disturbance and dexamethasone supression test after stroke. Ann Neurol 1982;12:463-468.

12. Robinson RG, Price TR. Post stroke depression disorders: a follow-up study of 103 outpatients. Stroke 1982;13:635-641.

13. Sinyor D, Jacques P, Kaloupek DG, Becker R, Goldenberg M, Coopersmith H. Poststroke depression and lesion location: an attempted replication. Brain 1986; 109:537-546.

14. Robinson RG, Starr CB, Kubos KL, Price TR. A two year longitudinal study of post stroke mood disorder: findings during initial evaluation. Stroke 1983; 14:736-741.

15. Wade DT, Legh-Smith J, Hewer RA. Depressed mood after stroke: a community study of its frequency. Br J Psychiatry 1987;151:200-205.

16. Robinson RG, Szetela B. Mood change following left hemispheric brain injury. Ann Neurol 1981;9:447-455.

17. Robinson RG, Benson DF. Depression in aphasic patients: frequency, severity and clinicopathological correlations. Brain Lang 1981;14:282-291.

18. Robinson RG, Kubos KL, Starr LB, Rao K, Price TR. Mood disorders in stroke patients: importance of lesion location. Brain 1984;107:81-93.

19. Robinson RG, Starr LB, Lipsey JR, Rao K, Price TR. Two year longitudinal study of post stroke mood disorders: dynamic changes in associated variables over the first six months of followup. Stroke 1984;15:510-517.

20. Parikh RM, Lipsey JR, Robinson RG, Price TR. Two year longitudinal study of post stroke mood disorders: dynamic changes in correlates of depression at one and two years. Stroke 1987;18:579-584.

21. American Psychiatric Association Committee on Nomenclature and Statistics. Diagnostic and statistical manual of mental disorders. 3rd ed. Washington, DC: American Psychiatric Association, 1980.

22. Starkstein SE, Robinson RG, Price TR. Comparison of cortical and subcortical lesions in the production of post stroke mood disorders. Brain 1987;110:1045-1059.

23. Robinson RG, Bolduc PC, Price TR. Two year longitudinal study of post stroke mood disorders: diagnosis and outcome at one and two years. Stroke 1987;18: 837–843.
24. Lipsey JR, Robinson RG, Pearlson GD, Rao K, Price TR. The dexamethasone suppression test and mood following stroke. Am J Psychiatry 1986;142:318–323.
25. Lipsey JR, Spencer WC, Rabins PV, Robinson RG. Phenomenological comparison of poststroke depression and functional depression. Am J Psychiatry 1986;143:527–529.
26. Bolla-Wilson K, Robinson RG, Starkstein SE, Boston J, Price TR. Lateralization of dementia of depression in stroke patients. Am J Psychiatry 1989;146: 627–634.
27. Robinson RG, Lipsey JR, Bolla-Wilson K. Mood disorders in left-handed stroke patients. Am J Psychiatry 1985;142:1424–1429.
28. Lipsey JR, Robinson RG, Pearlson GD, Rao K, Price TR. Mood changes following bilateral hemispheric injury. Br J Psychiatry 1983;143:266–273.
29. Ebrahim S, Barer D, Nouri F. Affective illness after stroke. Br J Psychiatry 1987;151:52–56.
30. Starkstein SE, Robinson RG, Berthier ML, Parikh RM, Price TR. Differential mood changes following basal ganglia vs thalamic lesions. Arch Neurol 1988; 45:725–730.
31. Starkstein SE, Cohen BS, Federoff JP, Parikh RM, Price TR, Robinson RG. Relationship between anxiety disorders and depressive disorders in patients with cerebrovascular injury. Arch Gen Psychiatry 1990;47:246–251.
32. Starkstein SE, Robinson RG, Price TR. Comparison of patients with and without poststroke major depression matched for size and location of lesion. Arch Gen Psychiatry 1988;45:247–252.
33. Pickel VM, Segal M, Bloom FE. A radioautographic study of the efferent pathways of the nucleus locus ceruleus. J Comp Neurol 1974;155:15–42.
34. Morrison JH, Molliver ME, Grzanna R. Noradrenergic innervation of the cerebral cortex: widespread effects of local cortical lesions. Science 1979;205:313–316.
35. Robinson RG. Differential behavioral and biochemical effects of right and left hemispheric cerebral infarction in the rat. Science 1979;205:707–710.
36. Glick SD, Ross DA, Hough LB. Lateral asymmetry of neurotransmitters in human brain. Brain Res 1982;234:53–63.
37. Cummings JL. Depression and Parkinson's disease: a review. Am J Psychiatry 1992;149:443–454.
38. Mayberg HS, Robinson RG, Wong DF, et al. PET imaging of cortical S2 serotonin receptors after stroke: lateralized changes and relationship to depression. Am J Psychiatry 1988;145:937–943.
39. Finklestein SP, Weintraub RJ, Karmouz N, Askinazi C, Davar G, Baldessarini RJ. Antidepressant drug therapy for poststroke depression: retrospective study. Arch Phys Med Rehab 1987;68:772–776.
40. Rosse RB, Ciolino CP. Effects of cortical lesion location on psychiatric consultation referral of depressed stroke patients. Int J Psychiatry Med 1985-6:15: 311–318.

41. Reding MJ, Orto LA, Winter SW, Fortuna IM, Di Ponte P, McDowell FH. Antidepressant therapy after stroke: a double blind trial. Arch Neurol 1986;43: 763–765.
42. Masand P, Murray GB, Pickett P. Psychostimulants in post-stroke depression. J Neuropsychiatry 1991;3:23–27.
43. Federoff JP, Robinson RG. Tricyclic antidepressants in the treatment of post-stroke depression. J Clin Psychiatry 1989;50(7 suppl):18–23.
44. Murray GB, Shea V, Conn DK. Electroconvulsive therapy for post-stroke depression. J Clin Psychiatry 1986;47:258–260.
45. Lipsey JR, Robinson RG, Pearlson GD, Rao K, Price TR. Nortriptyline treatment of post-stroke depression: a double-blind study. Lancet 1984;1:297–300.
46. Gainotti G. Emotional behavior and hemispheric side of the lesion. Cortex 1972; 8:41–55.
47. Terzian H. Behavioral and EEG effects of intracarotid sodium amytal injection. Acta Neurochirurgica 1964;12:230–239.
48. Lee GP, Loring DW, Meader KJ. Hemispheric specialization for emotional expression: a reexamination of results from intracarotid administration of sodium amobarbital. Brain Cogn 1990;12:267–280.
49. Sackheim HA, Greenberg MS, Weiman AL, Gur RC, Hungerbuhler JP, Geschwind N. Hemispheric assymetry in the expression of positive and negative emotions. Arch Neurol 1982;39:210–218.
50. Silberman EK, Weingartner H. Hemispheric lateralization of functions related to emotion. Brain Cogn 1986;5:322–355.
51. Robinson RG, Boston JD, Starkstein SE, Price TR. Comparison of mania and depression after brain injury: causal factors. Am J Psychiatry 1988;145:172–178.
52. Fisher CM. Anger associated with dysphasia. Trans Am Neurolog Assoc 1970; 95:240–242.
53. Cummings JL. Organic psychosis. Psychomatics 1988;29:16–26.
54. Kanemoto K. Janz D. The temporal sequence of aura-sensations in patients with complex focal seizures with particular attention to ictal aphasia. J Neurol Neurosurg Psychiatry 1989;52:52–56.

21

Neurobehavioral Deficits Associated with Aphasia

Howard S. Kirshner

Vanderbilt University School of Medicine, Nashville, Tennessee

The goal of this chapter is to present information on a few of the major neurobehavioral syndromes related to aphasia. The emphasis is on the relationship of these deficits to language and communication disorders, rather than on a comprehensive discussion of each disorder, which would be a topic for a monograph in its own right. The reader is also referred to general neuropsychology textbooks such as those by Hecaen and Albert (1) and Heilman and Valenstein (2).

GERSTMANN'S SYNDROME

Gerstmann, a German physician, published an article in 1930 (3) establishing the association of four deficits — finger agnosia, right–left confusion, agraphia, and acalculia — with lesions of the dominant parietal lobe, specifically the "transitional area" between the angular and middle occipital gyri. By *finger agnosia*, Gerstmann meant the "inability to recognize, name, and select individual fingers of both hands." This difficulty may apply to both the patient's and the examiner's fingers. Gerstmann described a "lack of facility of individual movements and difficulty with coordinated movements," implying that the finger agnosia might be a causative factor in the writing and calculation deficits, via a disturbance of body schema. He also pointed to the central role of the fingers in writing and calculating. Gerstmann's patients lacked major deficits of aphasia, apraxia, agnosia, memory loss, or general intellectual compromise. Other associated deficits, such as alexia, hemianopia, color-recognition deficits, and apraxia, were inconsistently present. Gerstmann cited an autopsied case of Potzl and Hermann, involving a tumor of the area between the angular and middle occipital gyri, in the right hemisphere of an ambidextrous patient. He also cited two of his own cases, one a glioma, the other a "several month old cortical lesion." He stated that the syndrome could also result from a larger lesion, such as a stroke, in which an initially severe "sensory" aphasia gradually resolved, leaving the syndrome as a permanent residual deficit.

In the years since Gerstmann, there has been considerable controversy about the existence of Gerstmann's tetrad as a true syndrome. Both Benton (4) and Critchley (5) rejected its syndrome status, based on the absence of all four deficits in all patients and the frequent co-occurrence of combinations of these deficits with others such as alexia, aphasia, and memory loss. Nonetheless, more recent case reports (6–8) have documented that the four Gerstmann's deficits can occur as an isolated disorder. Benton (9), an early critic, has concluded on the basis of these reports that the combination of deficits is clinically meaningful in pointing to a lesion of the dominant angular gyrus. The four deficits can occur in any combination, or in groups of two or three in association with alexia, constructional apraxia, aphasia, or memory loss; the tetrad of deficits may be no more consistent as a syndrome than other combinations.

Morris and colleagues (10) have recently described the results of electrical stimulation of the angular and supramarginal gyri in a 17-year-old boy with epilepsy. Stimulation of discrete areas produced acalculia, agraphia, and finger agnosia in one site and right–left disorientation in another, although other nearby electrode locations produced alexia, anomia, and constructional apraxia in addition. Electrical stimulation thus confirms the evidence from destructive brain lesions that the left inferior parietal region is a localized site for the four functions that are disturbed in Gerstmann's syndrome, as well as for other cortical processes.

ANGULAR GYRUS SYNDROME

Benson and colleagues (11) described the *angular gyrus syndrome* as a variant of Gerstmann's syndrome and a mimicker of dementia. A patient with a single lesion in the left angular gyrus—documented by PET scan only, with no localized lesion by CT scan—had combined deficits of anomia and fluent aphasia, alexia, agraphia, acalculia, right–left disorientation, finger agnosia, and constructional apraxia. The sheer multiplicity of these deficits resembled a dementing illness. The angular gyrus has long been known to be important to reading, a role discussed in Chapter 10. Geschwind (12) pointed out the importance of the angular gyrus to the transfer of information between sensory modalities, a function important to reading but also to calculations and other higher functions.

ACALCULIA

The acalculia element of Gerstmann's syndrome points to the close relationship of deficits in calculation to the aphasias. Calculation disorders have long been associated with disease of the posterior portion of the left hemisphere (13). Hécaen and Angelergues (14) distinguished three types of acalculia: (1) inability to read and write numbers, (2) spatial acalculia, with inability to align numbers correctly in columns or order them properly, and (3) anarithmetia, or inability to perform mental arithmetic, unexplained by difficulty with writing or spatial functions. As expected, the first and third types correlated closely with posterior left-hemisphere lesions, while the spatial type was more associated with right-hemisphere lesions. It is important to analyze calculation difficulty in terms of these contributing factors.

A study by Jackson and Warrington (15) has confirmed that deficits in oral addition and subtraction were highly correlated with left-hemisphere lesions. Benson and Denckla (16) have pointed out that some aphasic patients may be unable to supply correct numbers orally, yet on multiple-choice tests they may show considerable ability to perform a silent calculation and choose the correct answer. Such dissociation of verbal versus silent calculation ability is also seen in aphasic patients who are able to continue to play card games such as bridge. Dahmen and colleagues (17), however, have pointed out that, even among aphasics, patients with posterior lesions and Wernicke's aphasia have more difficulty with spatial aspects of calculation than those with anterior lesions and Broca's aphasia. Other patients with posterior left-hemisphere lesions may have anarithmia without significant aphasia, suggesting that calculations may be impaired in the absence of aphasia (18). In general, calculation disturbances other than those clearly related to spatial dysfunction are an indicator of left parietal lobe dysfunction, and as such they can add localizing information in patients with language dysfunction.

APRAXIAS

Apraxia refers to a complex family of disorders having in common a loss of ability to carry out skilled or learned movements, as a result of brain disease. The German physician Liepmann (19) described the phenomena of apraxia and considered the deficit a *motor asymbolia*, or loss of the symbolism for learned movements. Norman Geschwind (20) more explicitly defined the apraxias as "disorders of the execution of learned movement which cannot be accounted for either by weakness, incoordination, or sensory loss, or by incomprehension of or inattention to commands." In other words, the apraxic patient cannot perform a motor act to command, yet he can understand the command and perform the same act in another context. Apraxia, thus defined, has a strong correlation with aphasia.

Liepmann described three principal varieties: ideomotor apraxia, ideational apraxia, and limb-kinetic apraxia. We shall briefly consider each. A number of other motor or behavioral dysfunctions have been labeled apraxias. *Apraxia of speech*, or verbal apraxia, is discussed in Chapter 3, with the conclusion that speech apraxia is a valid syndrome but only arguably an apraxia in the traditional sense. *Oral apraxia*, also alluded to in Chapter 3, is a form of ideomotor apraxia involving the oral and facial muscles, although considerable dissociation may occur between oral and limb apraxia in individual patients. *Constructional apraxia* and *dressing apraxia* are seen in patients with right-hemisphere lesions, reflecting disordered visual-spatial perception and faulty body image rather than primary motor dysfunction. *Oculomotor apraxia* refers to an inability to direct voluntary gaze; this disorder may be congenital, as in the syndrome of ataxia-telangiectasia, or it may be related to acquired, bilateral brain lesions (see the discussion of Balint's syndrome, under visual agnosias, later in this chapter). *Apraxia of eyelid opening* is seen in some movement disorders. *Gait apraxia* refers to an inability to walk, or an awkward gait, in the absence of muscular weakness or ataxia, as is seen in bilateral frontal lobe disease and hydrocephalus. Some patients have difficulty initiating gait but perform better as they continue to walk. Normal gait involves a complex sequence of muscle contractions, easily deranged by the motor planning deficits seen in frontal lobe syndromes.

Ideomotor Apraxia

Ideomotor apraxia is the principal apraxia described by Liepmann, a separation of the idea of a movement from its execution. The diagnosis of ideomotor apraxia requires that: (1) the patient cannot carry out a motor command, (2) he can be shown to understand the command, and (3) he can perform the same motor act in a different context. For example, an apraxic patient cannot demonstrate the use of a hammer, but he shows his understanding by describing verbally the act of hammering or by selecting the correct action from multiple choices demonstrated by the examiner. In addition, he performs the identical action by either manipulating a real hammer or imitating the examiner's pantomime. In general, patients with ideomotor apraxia perform poorly to command, better but still clumsily to imitation, and best in using the actual object. This apraxia is thus evident more in the testing situation than in real life. The diagnosis of ideomotor apraxia is important, however, in avoiding the misdiagnosis of a comprehension disorder.

The phenomena of ideomotor apraxia are closely tied to the concept of cerebral dominance for skilled movement. According to this concept, the left premotor cortex of a right-handed person programs not only the more adept right limbs in learned motor patterns, but also the less adept left limbs. Dominance for skilled movement does not always correlate with language dominance, and not even always with handedness. Heilman and colleagues (21) reported a left-handed patient with left hemiparesis secondary to a right-hemisphere stroke. The patient was not aphasic, but he showed apraxia for commands involving the nonparalyzed right limbs. The patient thus appeared to have "crossed" dominance, or left-hemisphere dominance for language, but right-hemisphere motor dominance. Studies on patients with surgical section of the corpus callosum also support left-hemisphere dominance for skilled movement. For example, patients with corpus callosotomy had more difficulty in programming movement of the right hand from visual displays of hand postures flashed to the right hemisphere (or left visual field) than in programming movement of the left hand from similar inputs to the left hemisphere (22).

Ideomotor apraxia is one of the classic disconnection syndromes, in which the behavioral disturbance can be explained not by direct damage to a cortical center, but by disconnection between two centers. Geschwind (20) provided a simple neuroanatomical model for understanding apraxia, similar to the model for conduction aphasia presented in Chapter 6. When a patient carries out a spoken command, the command must first be heard; then decoded into language in Wernicke's area; then transmitted, via the arcuate fasciculus, to the left prefrontal cortex, which is dominant for skilled movement. If the command requires use of the right extremities, the left premotor area activates the appropriate motor neurons in the left motor cortex; if the act requires the left extremities, the information is transmitted across the corpus callosum to the right premotor area, which in turn activates the right motor cortex. Heilman, Rothi, and Valenstein (23) have suggested an additional way-station in the left parietal lobe, a center for "visuokinesthetic engrams" of skilled movements. The Geschwind model, however, does not require this parietal center. The phenomena of ideomotor apraxia can be accounted for by lesions along the pathway from Wernicke's area to motor cortex.

A lesion in the left temporal lobe, or Wernicke's area, renders the patient aphasic, unable to follow commands because he cannot understand them. Such patients may have apraxia in addition to aphasia, however, in that they fail not only to follow commands, but also to imitate movements demonstrated by the examiner (24,25). This failure of imitation can be considered ideomotor apraxia, resulting from a disconnection of the perceived action from its execution in the left prefontal area. The apraxia involves movement of both sides of the body, as neither motor cortex can be properly activated, and also movement of the face and lips, or oral apraxia. Since most patients with Wernicke's aphasia have no hemiparesis, the apraxia is uncomplicated by weakness.

A lesion involving the arcuate fasciculus, between the temporal lobe and the prefrontal cortex, classically causes conduction aphasia. Benson and colleagues (26) pointed out that cases of conduction aphasia with parietal lesions also manifest ideomotor apraxia, while those with temporal lesions do not (see also Chapter 6). While this apraxia should involve both the right and left extremities and the face, some patients have an associated right hemiparesis, and the apraxia is then evident only in the nonparalyzed, left extremities.

A lesion of the left premotor cortex itself usually results in Broca's aphasia and right hemiparesis. Many Broca's aphasics have intact comprehension, yet they perform commands clumsily with their nonparalyzed left limbs. This abnormal motor performance may be mistaken for poor comprehension or dismissed as normal for the nondominant extremities. Normal people who are forced to use their left hand to write because of broken arms or similar injuries, however, rapidly become skillful in use of the nondominant hand. Geschwind (20) pointed out that this clumsy use of the left limbs in patients with left frontal lesions is the most common example of ideomotor apraxia and results from the lack of proper programming of learned movements by the damaged left prefrontal cortex.

The final lesion associated with ideomotor apraxia involves the anterior part of the corpus callosum, or the deep frontal white matter of either hemisphere, disconnecting the left from right premotor cortex. This *callosal apraxia* is a selective apraxia of the left limbs; since the pathway is intact for comprehension of commands, transmission to the left prefrontal cortex, and activation of the left motor cortex, the patient can move the right limbs normally to command. Callosal apraxia is important to our understanding of the function of the corpus callosum in connecting the two cerebral hemispheres.

Liepmann and Maas (27) described a patient with a right hemiplegia and apraxia and agraphia of the nonparalyzed left limbs. At autopsy, the patient had an infarction in the left pons, accounting for the right hemiplegia, and a second lesion in the territory of the left anterior cerebral artery, including parts of the left frontal lobe and anterior corpus callosum, disconnecting the intact right premotor area from input from the left hemisphere.

Geschwind and Kaplan (28) reported a patient with a left-hemisphere glioblastoma and postoperative infarction of the anterior portion of the corpus callosum in whom there was profound apraxia of the left limbs. This was the first modern description of the callosal syndrome. Other cases have been described involving either spontaneous lesions (29–31) or surgical section of the corpus callosum, performed for treatment of intractable epilepsy. These surgical cases have shown a more variable degree of apraxia, often milder than the syndromes described by Liepmann and Maas (27) and Geschwind and Kaplan (28). For example, some patients could not indicate with the fingers of the left hand the corresponding areas touched on the right hand by the examiner. These patients also showed apraxia in imitating pictures of hand postures flashed tachistoscopically to the ipsilateral visual field, suggesting that both of the separated hemispheres had difficulty in programming fine movements of the ipsilateral hand. Later research involving patients with corpus callosum surgery has also confirmed the presence of a mild apraxia of the left hand, especially involving fine finger movements in response to verbal commands (32,33).

Recent studies on ideomotor apraxia have generally verified the lesion localizations predicted by the anatomical model of Liepmann and Geschwind, and also the close correlation between apraxia and aphasia. DeRenzi and colleagues (24) reported a series of 180 patients with unilateral brain lesions, examined for apraxia with a test involving only the imitation of the examiner's skilled movements, thus permitting the diagnosis of apraxia even in patients with aphasia. Of the patients with aphasia, 80% also had apraxia, compared with only 5% of nonaphasic patients with left-hemisphere lesions and 20% of patients with right-hemisphere lesions. The three most common aphasia types—global, Broca's, and Wernicke's—were all closely associated with apraxia; there were too few conduction aphasics for meaningful correlation. The patients with right-hemisphere lesions tended to have milder degrees of apraxia. DeRenzi et al. (24), Kertesz, Ferro, and Shewan (34), and Goodglass and Kaplan (35) all found that the presence of aphasia and apraxia correlated closely, but the severity of the two deficits did not. Some patients had mild aphasia and severe apraxia; others had severe aphasia and mild apraxia. It is likely that the correlation between aphasia and apraxia relates to the anatomical proximity of the structures involved in language and praxis rather than to the shared symbolic nature of language and praxic behavior.

Investigations of oral or buccofacial apraxia have suggested that oral apraxia is not always correlated with limb apraxia (36,37). Left frontal lesions are most closely associated with oral apraxia, while both frontal and parietal lesions cause limb apraxia (37,38).

Apraxia in patients with right-hemisphere lesions is not easily explained by the disconnection model. Right-hemisphere lesions could cause apraxia by three possible mechanisms: (1) involvement of the deep frontal connections to the right premotor area, (2) right-hemisphere dominance for skilled movement, or (3) faulty spatial perception and direction of movement. The right hemisphere might contribute especially to clumsy movements on tests of imitation, in which the subject must watch a movement and then reproduce the same movement pattern, as in the study of DeRenzi and colleagues (24). More recently, Barbieri and DeRenzi (39) have attempted to distinguish the "executive" aspect of motor performance, in an imitation test, from the "ideational" aspect, as tested by asking the patient to gesture the use of an object. Of 56 subjects with left brain damage, 57% scored in the apraxic range on the imitation test, 50% on the use-of-objects test. Of 38 patients with right brain damage, 34% scored in the apraxic range on the imitation test, while only 13% were apraxic on the use-of-objects test. Imitation testing is thus more sensitive to right-hemisphere damage than apraxia testing to command.

Ideomotor apraxia has been reported not only with cortical lesions but also with lesions of the basal ganglia (40,41). There has been little investigation into the frequency of occurrence of apraxia in subcortical lesions. Ideomotor apraxia can also develop in dementing illnesses (42,43). Rapcsak and colleagues (43) found apraxic deficits in patients with Alzheimer's disease, involving the pantomiming of transitive limb movements more than intransitive limb movements or movements of the trunk. As in patients with focal lesions of the left hemisphere, the presence of apraxia correlated with language deficits, especially auditory comprehension.

Ideational Apraxia

Ideational apraxia, the second of Liepmann's three varieties, involves the loss of the "idea" or concept of a movement. In practice, ideational apraxia has been defined in two major ways. Liepmann's (19) original definition was the failure to carry out a sequential motor activity, when each component step could be performed separately. For example, the patient may be unable to use a coffeepot, coffee, and water to brew and pour a cup of coffee. The performance of a sequential act, of course, is more complex than a single action. Sequential acts require not only skilled movement but also memory storage and sequential motor planning, which requires the normal functioning of the frontal lobes. For these reasons, apraxia for sequential actions is very sensitive to frontal lobe disease and is also commonly seen in dementing diseases (43).

Another definition of ideational apraxia, that of DeRenzi and colleagues (44), is a loss of ability to manipulate actual objects. Apraxia for real-object use is a very different disorder from ideomotor apraxia, in that this apraxia interferes with everyday activities. Patients thus afflicted may be unable to care for themselves.

DeRenzi and Luchelli (45) investigated ideational apraxia in 20 right-handed patients with left-hemisphere lesions. The testing involved sequential actions involving real objects. Most of the errors involved omission, misuse, or incorrect location of the part of the object to be acted upon, while only a small minority of errors involved faulty sequencing of steps. Thus, ideational apraxia may be the same, whether defined as an inability to carry out a sequential action or a single action requiring use of a real object. In DeRenzi and Luchelli's patients (45), ideational apraxia correlated poorly with ideomotor apraxia, suggesting a true separation between these two types of apraxia. Most of the patients with ideational apraxia had lesions of the posterior left temporoparietal junction.

Ochipa, Rothi, and Heilman (46) have also studied ideational apraxia in a left-handed patient with a large left-hemisphere stroke. This patient spontaneously misused objects, for example, attempted to eat with a toothbrush or brush his teeth with a spoon. While he was initially aphasic, his language skills improved such that he could name objects, thus excluding an agnosic deficit, and he could point to the objects on command, excluding a language-comprehension deficit. In contrast, he was unable to identify objects by their function, to describe verbally the use of the objects, or to pantomime the use of the objects, and he could not demonstrate use of the actual objects. This patient thus appeared to have a loss of the "how" knowledge of the object's identity. This case is unusual because of the apparent crossed dominance for these two aspects of object knowledge. In the typical right-handed patient with a left-hemisphere stroke, both aspects are impaired, and the patient's loss of object knowledge is masked by aphasia (inability to name objects or comprehend commands regarding their use). Patients with large left-hemisphere strokes often misuse objects, but the nature of this misuse is unclear and is often referred to as "confusion" rather than ideational apraxia.

Limb-Kinetic Apraxia

Limb-kinetic apraxia, the third of Liepmann's apraxia types, involves a motor disability of one limb, in the absence of gross weakness or ataxia. Often the patient has difficulty with fine finger movements and manipulation of small objects, although gross strength in the hand and arm is normal. Many stroke patients recover muscle strength but remain clumsy in fine movements and rapid manipulations with the affected limbs. Contemporary neurologists generally regard this deficit as a mild pyramidal-tract dysfunction, or elementary motor disorder, and not a true apraxia.

AGNOSIAS

Agnosias are disorders of recognition. Freud (47) first used the term in describing disturbances in the recognition of objects. Milner and Teuber (48) later defined agnosia as a "normal percept . . . stripped of its meaning." In order to meet diagnostic criteria for agnosia, the patient must: (1) fail to recognize an object, (2) perceive the object normally, with no elementary disorder of the sensory modality tested, and (3) name the object once it is recognized, ruling out anomia as the cause of the patient's inability to identify the object. The patient must also not suffer from generalized dementia sufficient to explain the errors in recognition. In practice, the patient usually recognizes the object through presentation in a different sensory modality; e.g., the visual agnosic cannot identify a key ring until he feels the keys or hears them jingle. Agnosias are usually defined in terms of a specific sensory modality, such as visual, auditory, and tactile agnosia. Agnosias may be selective for one class of items within a sensory modality, such as agnosia for colors, agnosia for visual objects, or agnosia for faces (*prosopagnosia*). In each case, it is necessary to establish that the agnosia is separable from primary sensory disorders and from other cognitive dysfunctions such as aphasia or dementia. Naming deficits in aphasia or dementia should not be restricted to one sensory modality (see exceptions below), but rather should occur with all sensory stimuli.

Visual Agnosias

Cortical Visual Disturbances

Patients with bilateral occipital lobe damage may have complete blindness (*cortical blindness*), which is considered a primary sensory disorder rather than an agnosia (49). Cortical visual deficits, however, blend almost indistinguishably into the visual agnosias. Some patients with cortical blindness are unaware that they cannot see and confabulate seeing objects, a phenomenon called *Anton's syndrome* (50). Other patients with bilateral occipital damage claim blindness yet show evidence of residual vision of which they are not aware. This residual vision has been termed *blindsight* or *inverse Anton's syndrome* (51–53). Some patients describe visual hallucinations in blind fields (*Bonnet's syndrome*) (54). In both unilateral and bilateral visual-field defects, distortions of vision can occur, including *metamorphopsia* (distortion of shape) (55,56), macropsia and micropsia (apparent enlargement or reduction of visual images) (57), and peculiar perversions of shape and size known as the "Alice in Wonderland" syndrome, especially in association with migraine (58). Other cortical visual disturbances include *achromatopsia* (loss of color vision) (59–61), cerebral akinetopsia (loss of perception of motion) (62,63), and palinopsia (perseveration of visual images) (64,65). All these deficits are considered disturbances of higher visual perception rather than agnosias.

Balint's Syndrome and Simultanagnosia

A disorder more closely related to the agnosias is *Balint's syndrome*, which is usually associated with bilateral occipital lobe lesions (66). Patients with Balint's syndrome often act totally blind, even bumping into walls as they walk, yet they can describe fine details of objects in their central vision. The syndrome involves a triad of deficits: (1) psychic paralysis of gaze (difficulty directing the eyes away from central fixation, also called *ocular motor apraxia*) (67), (2) optic ataxia (incoordination of extremity movement under visual control, in the presence of accurate movement under proprioceptive control), and (3) impaired visual attention. These deficits result in the perception of only small details of a visual scene, with no ability to scan and perceive the "big picture"; patients literally cannot see the forest for the trees. Some patients have visual-field deficits, while others, with more anterior lesions, have full fields (68). Partial deficits related to Balint's syndrome have also been described. For example, cases of isolated optic ataxia of one (69,70) or both (71,72) upper limbs have been seen with unilateral or bilateral parietal lesions. The visual-attention part of Balint's syndrome is closely related to *simultanagnosia*, an inability to perceive simultaneously two visual items (73,74).

Visual Object Agnosia

Visual object agnosia refers to the inability to recognize objects visually, despite normal primary vision. Lissauer (75) distinguished two types of visual object agnosia: (1) apperceptive visual agnosia, in which subjects can see simple visual stimuli such as lines but cannot identify shapes, and (2) associative visual agnosia, in which subjects fail to recognize pictures or drawings but can copy them or match drawings with the appropriate objects. This classification implies a two-stage process of visual recognition: an apperceptive stage, in which the components of a visual image are synthesized into a whole object, and an associative stage, in which the meaning of the object is interpreted by association with previous visual and other sensory experiences.

Apperceptive Visual Agnosia. The first type, apperceptive visual agnosia, is difficult to separate from impaired perception or partial cortical blindness. Patients with apperceptive visual agnosia can pick out features of an object correctly, such as lines or angles, but fail to appreciate the whole object (76,77). For example, Luria's patient misnamed eyeglasses as a bicycle, pointing to the two circles and a crossbar (77). Posner (78) has suggested that an impaired "spotlight" of visual attention may be the key to the deficit. Thaiss and DeBleser (79) distinguished two separable functions of visual attention: a "wide-angle attentional lens," takes in the figure generally but perceives only gross features, and a narrow-angle "spotlight," which focuses on the finer visual details of one small area. The patient of Thaiss and DeBleser appeared to have a faulty wide-angle attentional beam, such that she could identify small objects within drawings but often missed the overall context. This ability to perceive fine details but not the whole picture is closely related to Balint's syndrome and simultanagnosia, discussed above.

As with all the cortical visual syndromes, apperceptive visual agnosia is usually seen in patients with bilateral occipital lesions. Warrington and James (80), however, have studied faulty visual object recognition in patients with unilateral, posterior right-hemisphere lesions. These deficits were especially apparent with recognition of degraded images such as drawings or silhouettes rather than actual objects.

Associative Visual Agnosia. Associative visual agnosia, Lissauer's second type, is more closely related to the aphasias than to primary disorders of vision. Some of these patients can copy or match drawings of objects that they cannot name, thus excluding a primary defect of visual perception. The failure to name the object is not considered an aphasic deficit, since the patients can identify the same object presented in the tactile or auditory modality (81). Patients with associative visual object agnosia often have other, related recognition deficits such as color agnosia, prosopagnosia (inability to recognize faces), and alexia, although visual agnosia can be present without alexia (82,83). With all these deficits, bilateral posterior hemisphere lesions are usually found (84,85), often involving the fusiform or occipitotemporal gyri, sometimes the lingual gyri, and adjacent white matter.

A recent, extremely well-documented case study of associative visual agnosia was presented by Jankowiak and colleagues (86). This patient, after bilateral parieto-occipital craniotomies for gunshot injuries, had nearly normal visual acuity and bilateral superior-half (*altitudinal*) visual-field defects. He had mild anomia and reading difficulty but normal performance on other language functions. Visual recognition was partially impaired for colors and severely deficient for faces, objects, and pictures. He not only could copy drawings that he could not recognize but could also produce accurate drawings from memory after they were flashed via tachistoscope for 100 ms, indicating preserved ability to perceive, extract, and reproduce the key features of a visual pattern during even a brief presentation. Other surprising abilities were the drawing of typical objects from memory, despite inability to identify these same objects, and accurate performance on categorization of drawings as real or unreal objects and as members of a specific class such as animals. The crux of this patient's deficit appeared to be a loss of ability to "match the internal visual percept 'in his mind's eye' with his representations of real visual stimuli" (86). The problem was not in the perception itself but in assigning meaning to the item perceived.

Geschwind (12) interpreted associative visual agnosia as a disconnection between the intact visual cortex and the more anterior centers where visual percepts are associated with past experiences, anatomically between the visual cortex and the language area. The syndrome thus bears similarity to the unilateral, left-hemisphere syndrome of alexia without agraphia (see Chapter 10), in which words and letters can be perceived by the right occipital cortex but are disconnected from the left-hemisphere language centers. Color agnosia, also called color anomia, has been postulated by Geschwind (87) to have a similar disconnection mechanism, as discussed in Chapter 10. One case of associative visual agnosia has been described with a unilateral lesion of the left temporo-occipital region, in the territory of the left posterior cerebral artery (88). This lesion did not involve the splenium of the corpus callosum or the right hemisphere by MRI scan, leading the authors to reject a disconnection explanation for the syndrome.

The subject of visual agnosia has long been controversial. The evidence just summarized indicates that patients do exist who are not aphasic, demented, or impaired in primary visual perception, yet who cannot recognize objects. Visual agnosia cannot be explained by a combination of primary visual perceptual deficits and dementia, as earlier asserted (89,90). Precise classification of individual cases in terms of the type of agnosia and the complete intactness of visual perception, however, is often difficult. Riddoch and Humphreys (91), for example, described a patient who appeared to have some visual perceptual difficulty as shown by improved performance with greater stimulus duration, yet he could copy objects that he could not recognize, an ability usually diagnostic of associative visual agnosia. The deficit could not be completely categorized as apperceptive or associative; the authors proposed a specific deficiency in "integration" of visual form information.

Optic Aphasia

The syndrome of *optic aphasia* or *optic anomia* is intermediate between the agnosias and the aphasias. In this syndrome, patients fail to name objects presented in the visual modality, yet they can demonstrate recognition of the objects by pantomiming or describing their use (92–94). This preserved recognition of the objects is what distinguishes optic aphasia from associative visual agnosia. Like visual agnosics, patients with optic aphasia can name objects presented in the auditory or tactile modalities, distinguishing them from anomic aphasics. In this syndrome, information about the object must reach the semantic system, such that the object is recognized, but the information is not sufficiently accessible to the language cortex to permit naming (94). Patients with optic aphasia may confabulate incorrect names when asked to name an object they clearly recognize. They often have alexia without agraphia and color-naming difficulty, suggesting a left occipital lesion.

By Geschwind's disconnection model (12), the optic aphasia syndrome, like pure alexia without agraphia (Chapter 10), is a disconnection between the occipital cortex and the left-hemisphere language cortex. One theory is that the right hemisphere recognizes the object but cannot transmit the information to the left hemisphere for naming (94,95); Plaut and Shallice (96) reviewed other disconnection explanations for optic aphasia, all involving a breakdown between visual perception and semantics or between semantics and naming.

The deficit of optic aphasia and that of pure alexia without agraphia, discussed in Chapter 10, are closely related. Just as the optic aphasic may recognize objects he cannot name, the pure alexic may show recognition of words he cannot read (91). In both cases, objects and words may be recognized in the right hemisphere. Most patients with pure alexia do not have difficulty recognizing and naming objects; their deficits are restricted to naming of words and colors. Subtle deficits in visual object naming have been described, however, such as greater difficulty with two-dimensional than with three-dimensional drawings of objects (97).

Prosopagnosia

Prosopagnosia refers to the inability to recognize faces. Patients fail to recognize close friends and relatives or pictures of famous people, unless they memorize details of size, hair style or color, and clothing. Prosopagnosia is restricted not only to the visual modality but to the class of faces; patients can recognize familiar people by voice, mannerisms, and unusual postures or gaits (98,99).

Facial recognition is often tested by matching of pictures of unfamiliar faces, taken from different angles. DeRenzi and colleagues (100) pointed out, however, that matching of unfamiliar faces is a different function from recognition of familiar faces. These authors suggested that failure to match new faces reflects an apperceptive facial recognition deficit (*apperceptive prosopagnosia*), while failure to recognize familiar faces is an *associative prosopagnosia*. The two functions are dissociated in some patients with prosopagnosia (100–102). Others have examined the recognition of emotional facial expressions, a function that appears localized to the right hemisphere (103). It is important to specify exactly which type of facial recognition is meant when describing deficits in prosopagnosia.

In clinical studies, prosopagnosia may be either an isolated deficit or a part of a more general visual agnosia for objects and colors. Even pure prosopagnosia may not be truly restricted to faces, in that deficits have been discovered in the recognition of other complex but familiar visual stimuli such as architectural landmarks or pets (104–106). Faces may thus not be a truly unique class of items that these patients cannot recognize, but they are surely the most individualized of visual displays. The syndrome of prosopagnosia usually involves bilateral parieto-occipital lesions (107,108), but cases with unilateral, posterior right-hemisphere lesions have been described (109,110).

Kluver-Bucy Syndrome

Another form of visual agnosia is the "psychic blindness" seen in Kluver-Bucy syndrome (111). This syndrome has been described in both animals and humans with bilateral temporal lobe lesions. An animal with bitemporal lesions may inappropriately try to eat or mate with objects or fail to show customary fear or hostility when faced with a natural enemy. Human patients manifest visual agnosia and often prosopagnosia, together with marked memory loss, variable aphasic deficits, and changes in behavior such as placidity, altered sexual orientation, and excessive eating (112). Human cases of Kluver-Bucy syndrome have been reported with bitemporal damage from surgical ablation (113), herpes simplex encephalitis (112,114), and dementing conditions such as Pick's disease (112,115). Patients with Kluver-Bucy syndrome appear to have no major deficits of primary visual perception, but connections appear to be disrupted between vision and memory and limbic structures, so that visual percepts do not arouse their ordinary associations.

Auditory Agnosias

Like cortical visual syndromes, cortical auditory disorders are complex conditions, ranging from complete cortical deafness to partial deficits of recognition of specific types of sound. As with the visual agnosias, most cortical auditory deficits require bilateral cerebral lesions, in this case of both temporal lobes, especially Heschl's gyri. Only rare patients with cortical deafness have no hearing at all; some have nearly normal pure tone hearing but have deficits in temporal sequencing or sound localization (116). As in visual agnosia, the distinction between cortical auditory deficits and auditory agnosia is difficult.

A patient with auditory agnosia can hear noises but not appreciate their meanings, as in identifying animal cries or sounds associated with specific objects, such as the ringing of a bell. Most such patients also cannot understand speech or appreciate music. Auditory agnosias can be divided into pure word deafness, pure nonverbal auditory agnosia, pure amusia, and mixtures of the other three deficits.

Pure Word Deafness

The syndrome of pure word deafness, as discussed in Chapter 4, refers to a failure of comprehension of spoken words, with preserved ability to hear and recognize nonverbal sounds. Patients with bilateral temporal lobe lesions and pure word deafness often manifest more general auditory deficits early in their course (117) and have abnormalities of other auditory parameters such as temporal sequencing (118), loudness discrimination and auditory threshold duration (119), or auditory reaction time (120). Such deficits link pure word deafness to primary auditory disorders and to an apperceptive rather than associative form of agnosia, by Lissauer's dichotomy for visual agnosia (75).

As stated in Chapter 4, pure word deafness has generally been explained as a disconnection of both primary auditory cortices from the left-hemisphere Wernicke's area. Coslett and colleagues (121), however, suggested that pure word deafness is caused by bilateral lesions of the auditory cortex, while nonverbal auditory sound recognition may be mediated by other parts of the auditory system, perhaps auditory association areas. Unilateral left-hemisphere lesions have also been associated with pure word deafness; Geschwind (122) postulated that such lesions are strategically placed so as to disconnect both primary auditory cortices from Wernicke's area. A recent case of pure word deafness with such a lesion has been reported (123). As discussed in Chapter 4, some patients with Wernicke's aphasia have more severe involvement of auditory comprehension than of reading, also resembling pure word deafness (124). In a review of pure word deafness, Goldstein (125) found that most cases have had paraphasic speech, further linking the syndrome to Wernicke's aphasia.

Auditory Nonverbal Agnosia

Auditory nonverbal agnosia refers to patients who have lost the ability to identify meaningful nonverbal sounds but who have preserved pure tone hearing and preserved language comprehension. Such cases are rare but well documented (126–128), usually involving bihemispheral lesions. Vignolo (124) distinguished a "semantic-associative" type, with loss of ability to recognize familiar sounds, from a "discriminative" type, involving failure to match two meaningless sounds. This distinction is closely related to the apperceptive-associative dichotomy of Lissauer (75) for visual agnosia. Vignolo tested each function in patients with unilateral lesions and found that the semantic-associative type correlated with aphasia and left-hemisphere damage, while the discriminative type correlated with right-hemisphere damage.

Amusias

The loss of musical abilities after focal brain lesions is complex, reflecting the complexity of musical appreciation and analysis. Evidence has been presented that recognition of melodies and musical tones may be a right temporal function, whereas analysis of pitch, rhythm, and tempo involves the left temporal lobe (129). Mapping of brain electrical activity, an EEG technique, showed relative right-hemisphere activation with melody, left temporal activation for scales (130). The left hemisphere may be called on more when a trained musician listens to a musical piece, as compared with an untrained listener (129), although a recent study using dichotic listening found only minimal differences between normal trained versus untrained subjects (131). A recent study (132) examined cortical activation by PET scanning during musical performance in 10 professional pianists. Sight reading of music activated both visual association cortices and the superior parietal lobes, areas distinct from those utilized in reading words. Listening to music activated both secondary auditory cortices, while playing of music activated frontal and cerebellar areas. The authors commented that, widespread as these areas were, the study did not examine the whole of musical experience, let alone the pleasure afforded by music.

The case studies of musical abilities in patients with focal brain lesions are surprisingly limited. Patients with bitemporal lesions and the syndromes of cortical deafness, auditory agnosia, and pure word deafness often have disturbance of musical abilities (116,124). Selective loss of ability to appreciate and produce music, recognize familiar tunes, and even make simple judgments about musical pitch or rhythm has been associated with right-hemisphere damage, especially right temporoparietal (133) but also right frontal (134) lesions. Right temporal lobectomy for epilepsy impairs perception of melody (135). Injection of barbiturates into the right carotid artery during the Wada test impairs singing (136). Kinsella and colleagues (137), however, found impaired singing with both left- and right-hemisphere lesions. Aphasic patients with left-hemisphere damage may seem normally able to appreciate music and sing tones, but the reading and writing of music may be disturbed by left-hemisphere lesions (138). As stated in Chapter 14, the composer Maurice Ravel suffered an illness of progressive fluent aphasia, in association with which he lost the ability to read or write music although he could still listen to and appreciate music (139,140). Polk and Kertesz (141) have also reported progressive musical dysfunction in two professional musicians with dementing illness.

While musical functions do not appear to be localized to specific or even unilateral brain foci, the evidence from patients with focal lesions does suggest a relative dominance of the right hemisphere for perception of auditory tones as music and of the left hemisphere for learned aspects of reading and writing music. Singing may be affected by lesions of either hemisphere. Considerable further research is needed on the complex relationships of music and the brain.

The preservation of unlearned musical abilities in patients with aphasia has been utilized in a form of speech therapy called melodic intonation therapy (142). Many aphasic patients can hum melodies and sing familiar songs. They can be trained to intune words, even when they cannot say the words without music. With repetition, subjects gradually become able to say the words without singing. Presumably, right-hemisphere musical abilities serve a facilitating role in the production of words.

Tactile Agnosias

As with the syndromes of cortical loss of auditory and visual perception, a range of sensory deficits is seen with cortical lesions. Patients with lesions of the parietal cortex may have preserved ability to feel pinprick, temperature, vibration, and proprioception, yet they fail to identify objects palpated by the contralateral hand or recognize numbers or letters written on the opposite side of the body (143,144). These deficits, called *astereognosis* and *agraphesthesia*, respectively, are considered to represent cortical sensory loss rather than a true agnosia. Alternatively, they could be considered apperceptive tactile agnosias. Rare cases have been described of patients who can describe the shape and features of a palpated object yet cannot identify the object (143). The patient can readily identify the object by sound or sight, thereby fulfilling the criteria for a true associative tactile agnosia.

Caselli (145) investigated 84 patients with unilateral hemisphere lesions for deficits in tactile perception. Seven patients were found with tactile agnosia for objects palpated by the contralateral hand. These deficits occurred in the absence of primary somatosensory loss. Some patients had severe hemiparesis or hemianopia yet performed well in tactile object recognition, but patients with neglect secondary to right-hemisphere lesions tended to have more severe deficits. In a second study (146), Caselli reported that only patients with neglect had bilateral tactile object-recognition deficits, while patients with left parietal lesions had tactile agnosia only for items in the contralateral hand. Caselli did not study patients with bilateral lesions, however, and agnosia in the visual and auditory modalities is clearly more profound when bilateral lesions are present.

The mechanisms of tactile agnosia may vary. First, appreciation of shape and perception of a tactile figure or ideogram may be properties of the sensory cortex itself. Second, the right parietal cortex is also involved in spatial and topographical functions, and spatial disorders may account for some of the tactile recognition deficits of patients with right parietal lesions. Third, attentional deficits and neglect seen with right-hemisphere lesions may increase the lack of tactile recognition (146). Fourth, disconnection syndromes may be involved in tactile agnosia. The famous patient of Geschwind and Kaplan (147) with a lesion of the corpus callosum could not identify objects with the left hand but could point to the correct object in a group. Patients with surgical section of the corpus callosum have similar deficits (148). Such patients clearly feel the characteristics of the object but cannot name it, presumably because the right parietal cortex is disconnected by the callosal lesion from left-hemisphere language centers.

Tactile Aphasia

Tactile aphasia is an inability to name a palpated object, despite intact recognition of the object and intact naming when the object is presented in another sensory modality (149). This syndrome is closely analogous to optic aphasia, discussed above.

REFERENCES

1. Hécaen H, Albert ML. Human neuropsychology. New York: John Wiley & Sons, 1978.
2. Heilman KM, Valenstein E. Clinical neuropsychology, 3rd ed. New York: Oxford University Press, 1993.
3. Gerstmann J. Zur symptomatologie der Hirnlasionen im Ubergangsgebiet der unteren Parietal- und mittleren Occipitalwindung (Das Syndrom: Fingeragnosie, Rechts-Links-Storung, Agraphie, Akalkulie). Nervenartzt 1930;691–695. Translated in: Rittenberg DA, Hochberg FH, eds. Neurological classics in modern translation. New York: Hafner Press, 1977:150–154.
4. Benton AL. The fiction of the Gerstmann syndrome. J Neurol Neurosurg Psychiatry 1961;24:176–181.
5. Critchley M. The enigma of Gerstmann's syndrome. Brain 1966;89:183–198.
6. Roeltgen DP, Sevush S, Heilman KM. Pure Gerstmann's syndrome from a focal lesion. Arch Neurol 1983;40:46–47.
7. Varney NR. Gerstmann syndrome without aphasia: a longitudinal study. Brain Cogn 1984;3:1–9.
8. Mazzoni M, Pardoni L, Giorgetti V, Arena R. Gerstmann's syndrome: a case report. Cortex 1990;26:459–467.
9. Benton AL. Gerstmann's syndrome. Arch Neurol 1992;49:445–447.
10. Morris HH, Luders H, Lesser RP, Dinner DS, Hahn J. Transient neuropsychological abnormalities (including Gerstmann's syndrome) during cortical stimulation. Neurology 1984;34:877–883.
11. Benson DF, Cummings JC, Tsai SI. Angular gyrus syndrome simulating Alzheimer's disease. Arch Neurol 1982;39:616–620.
12. Geschwind N. Disconnection syndromes in animals and man. Brain 1965;88: 237–294, 585–644.
13. Boller F, Grafman J. Acalculia: historical development and current significance. Brain Cogn 1983;2:205–223.
14. Hécaen H, Angelergues R. Étude anatomo-clinique de 280 cas de lesions retro-rolandiques unilaterales des hemispheres cerebraux. Encephale 1961;6:533–562.

15. Jackson M, Warrington EK. Arithmetic skills in patients with unilateral cerebral lesions. Cortex 1986;22:611–620.
16. Benson DF, Denckla MB. Verbal paraphasia as a cause of calculation disturbances. Arch Neurol 1969;21:96–102.
17. Dahmen W, Hartje W, Bussing A, Sturm W. Disorders of calculation in aphasic patients — spatial and verbal components. Neuropsychologia 1982;20:145–153.
18. Grafman J, Passafiume D, Faglioni P, Boller F. Calculation disturbances in adults with focal hemispheric damage. Cortex 1982;18:37–50.
19. Liepmann H. Das Krankheitsbild der apraxie ("motorischen asymbolie"). Monatschr Psychiatr Neurol 1990;8:15–44, 102–132, 182–197. Translated in part in: Rottenberg DA, Hochberg FA, eds. Neurological classics in modern translation. New York: Hafner Press, 1977:155–181.
20. Geschwind N. The apraxias: neural mechanisms of disorders of learned movement. Am Sci 1975;63:188–195.
21. Heilman KM, Coyle JM, Gonyea EF, Geschwind N. Apraxia and agraphia in a left-hander. Brain 1973;96:21–28.
22. Gazzaniga MS, Bogen JE, Sperry RW. Dyspraxia following division of the cerebral commissures. Arch Neurol 1967;16:606–612.
23. Heilman KM, Rothi LJ, Valenstein E. Two forms of ideomotor apraxia. Neurology 1982;32:342–346.
24. DeRenzi E, Motti F, Nichelli P. Imitating gestures: a quantitative approach to ideomotor apraxia. Arch Neurol 1980;37:6–10.
25. Kertesz A, Hooper E. Praxis and language: the extent and variety of apraxia in aphasia. Neuropsychologia 1982;20:276–286.
26. Benson DF, Sheremata WA, Bouchard R, Segarra J, Price D, Geschwind N. Conduction aphasia. Arch Neurol 1973;18:339–346.
27. Liepmann H, Maas O. Fall von linksseitiger Agraphie und Apraxie bei rechtsseitiger Lahmung. Zeitschrift für Psychologie und Neurol 1907;10:214–227.
28. Geschwind N, Kaplan E. A human cerebral deconnection syndrome. Neurology 1962;12:675–685.
29. Watson RT, Heilman KM. Callosal apraxia. Brain 1983;391–403.
30. Goldenberg G, Wimmer A, Holzner F, Wessely P. Apraxia of the left limbs in a case of callosal disconnection: the contribution of medial frontal lobe damage. Cortex 1985;21:135–148.
31. Graff-Radford NR, Welsh K, Goderski J. Callosal apraxia. Neurology 1987;37:100–105.
32. Zaidel E, Sperry RW. Some long term effects of cerebral commisurotomy in man. Neuropsychologia 1977;15:193–203.
33. Volpe BT, Sidtis JJ, Holtzman JD, Wilson DH, Gazzaniga MS. Cortical mechanisms involved in praxis and observation following partial and complete section of the corpus callosum in man. Neurology 1982;32:645–650.
34. Kertesz A, Ferro JM, Shewan CM. Apraxia and aphasia: the functional-anatomical basis for their dissociation. Neurology 1984;34:40–47.
35. Goodglass H, Kaplan E. Disturbance of gesture and pantomime in aphasia. Brain 1963;86:703–720.

36. Basso A, Capitani E, Della Sala S, Laiacona M, Spinnler H. Recovery from ideomotor apraxia: a study on acute stroke patients. Brain 1987;110:747–760.
37. Raade AS, Gonzalez-Rothi LJ, Heilman KM. The relationship between bucco-facial and limb apraxia. Brain Cogn 1991;16:130–146.
38. Tognola G, Vignolo LA. Brain lesions associated with oral apraxia in stroke patients: a clinico-neuroradiological investigation with the CT scan. Neuropsychologia 1980;18:257–272.
39. Barbieri C, DeRenzi E. The executive and ideational components of apraxia. Cortex 1988;24:535–543.
40. Agostoni E, Coletti A, Orlando G, Tredici G. Apraxia in deep cerebral lesions. J Neurol Neurosurg Psychiatry 1983;46:801–808.
41. DeRenzi E, Faglioni P, Scarpa M, Crisi G. Limb apraxia in patients with damage confined to the left basal ganglia and thalamus. J Neurol Neurosurg Psychiatry 1986;49:1030–1038.
42. Foster NL, Chase TN, Patronas NJ, Gillespie MM, Fedio P. Cerebral mapping of apraxia in Alzheimer's disease by positron emission tomography. Ann Neurol 1986;19:139–143.
43. Rapcsak SZ, Croswell SC, Rubens AB. Apraxia in Alzheimer's disease. Neurology 1989;39:664–668.
44. DeRenzi E, Pieczuro A, Vignolo LA. Ideational apraxia: a quantitative study. Neuropsychologia 1968;6:41–52.
45. DeRenzi E, Luchelli F. Ideational apraxia. Brain 1988;111:1173–1185.
46. Ochipa C, Rothi LJG, Heilman KM. Ideational apraxia: a deficit in tool selection and use. Ann Neurol 1989;25:190–193.
47. Freud S. On aphasia. 1891. Stengel E, trans. London: Imago, 1953.
48. Milner B, Teuber HL. Alteration of perception and memory in man. In: Weiskrantz L, ed. Analysis of behavioral change. New York: Harper & Row, 1968.
49. Aldrich MS, Alessi AG, Beck RW, Gilman S. Cortical blindness: etiology, diagnosis, and prognosis. Ann Neurol 1987;21:149–158.
50. Anton G. Ueber die Selbstwahrnehmungen der Herderkrankungen des Gehirns-durch den Kranken bei Reihdenblindheit und Rindentaubheit. Arch Psychiatry 1899;32:86–127.
51. Poppel E, Held R, Frost D. Residual visual function after brain wounds involving the central visual pathways in man. Nature 1973;243:295–296.
52. Perenin MT, Ruel J, Hécaen H. Residual visual capacities in a case of cortical blindness. Cortex 1980;605–612.
53. Hartmann JA, Wolz WA, Roeltgen DP, Loverso FL. Denial of visual perception. Brain Cogn 1991;16:29–40.
54. McNamara ME, Heros R, Boller F. Visual hallucinations in blindness: the Charles Bonnet syndrome. Int J Neurosci 1982;17:13–15.
55. Bender MB, Kanzer MG. Metamorphopsia and other psychovisual disturbances in a patient with a tumor of the brain. Arch Neurol Psychiatry 1941;45:481–485.
56. Brau RH, Lameiro J, Llaguno AV, Rifkinson. Metamorphopsia and permanent cortical blindness after a posterior fossa tumor. Neurosurgery 1986;19:263–266.

57. Hachinski VC, Porchawka J, Steele JC. Visual symptoms in the migraine syndrome. Neurology 1973;23:570-579.

58. Golden GS. The Alice in Wonderland syndrome in juvenile migraine. Pediatrics 1979;63:517-519.

59. Pearlman AL, Burch J, Meadows JC. Cerebral color blindness: an acquired defect in hue discrimination. Ann Neurol 1979;5:253-261.

60. Damasio A, Yamada T, Damasio H, Corbett J, McKee J. Central achromatopsia: behavioral, anatomic, and physiologic aspects. Neurology 1980;30:1064-1071.

61. Zeki S. A century of cerebral achromatopsia. Brain 1990;113:1721-1777.

62. Zihl J, von Cramon D, Mai N. Selective disturbance of movement vision after bilateral brain damage. Brain 1983;106:313-340.

63. Zeki S. Cerebral akinetopsia (visual motion blindness). A review. Brain 1991; 114:811-824.

64. Meadows JC, Munro SSF. Palinopsia. J Neurol Neurosurg Psychiatry 1977; 40:5-8.

65. Michel EM, Troost BT. Palinopsia: cerebral localization with computed tomography. Neurology 1980;30:887-889.

66. Balint R. Die seelenlahmung des "Schauens": Optische ataxia, Raumliche Storung des Aufmerksamkeit. Monatschr Psychiatr Neurol 1909;1:51-81.

67. Cogan DG, Adams RD. A type of paralysis of conjugate gaze (ocular motor apraxia). Arch Ophthalmol 1953;50:434-442.

68. Hécaen H, Ajuriaguerra J. Balint's syndrome (psychic paralysis of visual fixation) and its minor forms. Brain 1954;77:373-400.

69. Levine DN, Kaufman KJ, Mohr JP. Inaccurate reaching associated with a superior parietal lobe tumor. Neurology 1978;28:556-561.

70. Rizzo M, Rotella D, Darling W. Troubled reaching after right occipito-temporal damage. Neuropsychologia 1992;30:711-722.

71. Damasio AR, Benton AL. Impairment of hand movements under visual guidance. Neurology 1979;29:170-178.

72. Boller F, Cole M, Kim Y, Mack J, Patawaran C. Optic ataxia: clinico-radiological correlations with the EMI scan. J Neurol Neurosurg Psychiatry 1975; 38:954-958.

73. Wolpert I. Die Simultanagnosie—Storung der Gesamtauffasung. Zeitschrift für die gesamte Neurologie und Psychiatrie 1924;93:397-415.

74. Kinsbourne M, Warrington EK. A disorder of simultaneous form perception. Brain 1962;85:461-486.

75. Lissauer H. Ein Fall von Seelenblindheit nebst einem Beitrag zur Theorie derselben. Archiv für Psychiatrie und Nervenkrankenheit 1890;21:222-270.

76. Benson DF, Greenberg JP. Visual form agnosia: a specific defect in visual recognition. Arch Neurol 1969;20:82-89.

77. Luria AR. Higher cortical functions in man. London: Tavistock, 1966.

78. Posner MI. Orientation of attention. Quart J Exp Psychol 1987;32:3-25.

79. Thaiss L, DeBleser R. Visual agnosia: a case of reduced attentional "spotlight"? Cortex 1992;28:601-621.

80. Warrington EK, James M. Visual apperceptive agnosia: a clinico-anatomical study of three cases. Cortex 1988;24:13-32.

81. Rubens AB, Benson DF. Associative visual agnosia. Arch Neurol 1971;24: 305–316.
82. Levine DN. Prosopagnosia and visual object agnosia: a behavioral study. Brain Lang 1978;5:341–365.
83. Albert M, Reches A, Silverberg R. Associative visual agnosia without alexia. Neurology 1975;25:322–326.
84. Benson DF, Segarra J, Albert M. Visual agnosia-prosopagnosia: a clinicopathologic correlation. Arch Neurol 1974;30:307–310.
85. Albert ML, Soffer D, Silverberg R, Reches A. The anatomic basis of visual agnosia. Neurology 1979;29:876–879.
86. Jankowiak J, Kinsbourne M, Shalev RS, Bachman DL. Preserved visual imagery and categorization in a case of associative visual agnosia. J Cogn Neurosci 1992;4:119–131.
87. Geschwind N, Fusillo M. Color-naming deficits in association with alexia. Arch Neurol 1966;15:137–146.
88. McCarthy RA, Warrington EK. Visual associative agnosia: a clinico-anatomical study of a single case. J Neurol Neurosurg Psychiatry 1986;49:1233–1240.
89. Bay E. Disturbances of visual perception and their examination. Brain 1953; 76:515–551.
90. Bender MB, Feldman M. The so-called "visual agnosias". Brain 1972;95:173–186.
91. Riddoch MJ, Humphreys GW. A case of integrative visual agnosia. Brain 1987;110:1431–1462.
92. McCormick GF, Levine DA. Visual anomia: a unilateral disconnection. Neurology 1983;33:664–666.
93. Lhermitte F, Beauvois MF. A visual-speech disconnexion syndrome. Brain 1973;96:695–714.
94. Coslett HB, Saffran EM. Preserved object recognition and reading comprehension in optic aphasia. Brain 1989;112:1091–1110.
95. Coslett HB, Saffran EM. Preserved reading in pure alexia. Brain 1989;112: 327–359.
96. Plaut DC, Shallice T. Perseverative and semantic influences on visual object naming errors in optic aphasia: a connectionist account. J Cogn Neurosci 1993;5:89–117.
97. Damasio AR, McKee J, Damasio H. Determinants of performance in color anomia. Brain Lang 1979;7:74–85.
98. Bodamer J. Die Prosop-Agnosie (die Agnosie des Physiognomieerkennens). Archiv für Psychiatrie und Nervenkrankheiten 1947;179:6–53.
99. Hécaen H, Angelergues R. Agnosia for faces (prosopagnosia). Arch Neurol 1962;7:92–100.
100. DeRenzi E, Faglioni P, Grossi D, Nichelli P. Apperceptive and associative forms of prosopagnosia. Cortex 1991;27:213–221.
101. Benton AL, Van Allen MW. Prosopagnosia and facial discrimination. J Neurol Sci 1972;15:167–172.
102. Malone DR, Morris HH, Kay MC, Levin HS. Prosopagnosia: a double dissociation between the recognition of familiar and unfamiliar faces. J Neurol Neurosurg Psychiatry 1982;45:820–822.

103. Rapcsak SZ, Kaszniak AW, Rubens AB. Anomia for facial expressions: evidence for a category specific visual-verbal disconnection syndrome. Neurospychologia 1989;27:1031–1041.
104. Beyn ES, Knyazeva GR. The problem of prosopagnosia. J Neurol Neurosurg Psychiatry 1962;25:154–158.
105. Whiteley AM, Warrington EK. Prosopagnosia: a clinical, psychological, and anatomical study of three patients. J Neurol Neurosurg Psychiatry 1977;40: 395–403.
106. Damasio AR, Damasio H, Van Hoesen GW. Prosopagnosia: anatomic basis and behavioral mechanisms. Neurology 1982;32:331–341.
107. Meadows JC. The anatomical basis of prosopagnosia. J Neurol Neurosurg Psychiatry 1974;37:489–501.
108. Levine D, Calvanio R, Wolf E. Disorders of visual behavior following bilateral posterior cerebral lesions. Psycholog Res 1980;41:217–234.
109. Landis T, Regard M, Bliestle A, Kleihues P. Prosopagnosia and agnosia for noncanonical views. Brain 1988;111:1287–1297.
110. Michel F, Perenin MT, Sieroff E. Prosopagnosie sans hemianopsie après lesion unilaterale occipito-temporale droite. Rev Neurol 1986;142:545–549.
111. Kluver H, Bucy PC. Preliminary analysis of functions of the temporal lobes in monkeys. Arch Neurol Psychiatry 1939;42:979–1000.
112. Lilly R, Cummings JL, Benson DF, Frankel M. The human Kluver-Bucy syndrome. Neurology 1983;33:1141–1145.
113. Terzian H, Dalle Ore G. Syndrome of Kluver and Bucy reproduced in man by bilateral removal of the temporal lobes. Neurology 1955;5:373–380.
114. Marlowe WB, Mancall EL, Thomas TJ. Complete Kluver-Bucy syndrome in man. Cortex 1975;11:53–59.
115. Cummings JL, Duchen LW. Kluver-Bucy syndrome in Pick's disease: clinical and pathological correlations. Neurology 1981;31:1415–1422.
116. Jerger J, Weiker NJ, Sharbrough FW, Jerger S. Bilateral lesions of the temporal lobe: a case study. Acta Otolaryngol 1969;258(suppl):1–51.
117. Mendez M, Geehan GR. Cortical auditory disorder: clinical and psychoacoustic features. J Neurol Neurosurg Psychiatry 1988;51:1–9.
118. Tanake Y, Yamadori A, Mori E. Pure word deafness following bilateral lesions. A psychophysical analysis. Brain 1987;110:381–403.
119. Kanshepolsky J, Kelley JJ, Waggener JD. A cortical auditory disorder. Clinical, audiological and pathologic aspects. Neurology 1973;23:699–705.
120. Buchtel HA, Stewart JD. Auditory agnosia: apperceptive or associative disorder? Brain Lang 1989;37:12–25.
121. Coslett HB, Brashear HR, Heilman KM. Pure word deafness after bilateral primary auditory cortex infarcts. Neurology 1984;34:347–352.
122. Geschwind N. The organization of language and the brain. Science 1970;170: 940–944.
123. Takahashi N, Kawamura M, Shinotou H, Hirayama K, Kaga K. Shindo M. Pure word deafness due to left hemisphere damage. Cortex 1992;28:295–303.
124. Kirshner HS, Casey PF, Henson J, Heinrich JJ. Behavioural features and lesion localization in Wernicke's aphasia. Aphasiology 1989;3:169–176.

125. Goldstein MN. Auditory agnosia for speech ("pure word-deafness"). A historical review with current implications. Brain Lang 1974;1:195–204.
126. Spreen O, Benton AL, Rincham RW. Auditory agnosia without aphasia. Arch Neurol 1965;13:84–92.
127. Albert ML, Sparks R, von Stockert T, Sax D. A case study of auditory agnoszzia: linguistic and non-linguistic processing. Cortex 1972;8:427–443.
128. Motomura N, Yamadori A, Mori E, Tamaru F. Auditory agnosia. Analysis of a case with bilateral subcortical lesions. Brain 1986;109:379–391.
129. Bever TG, Chiarello RJ. Cerebral dominance in musicians and non-musicians. Science 1974;185:537–539.
130. Breitling D, Guenther W, Rondot P. Auditory perception of music measured by brain electrical activity mapping. Neuropsychologia 1987;25:765–774.
131. Prior M, Troup GA. Processing of timbre and rhythm in musicians and non-musicians. Cortex 1988;24:451–456.
132. Sergent J, Zuck E, Terriah S, MacDonald B. Distributed neural network underlying musical sight-reading and keyboard performance. Science 1992;257:106–109.
133. McFarland HR, Fortin D. Amusia due to a right temporoparietal infarct. Arch Neurol 1982;39:725–727.
134. Botez MI, Wertheim N. Expressive aphasia and amusia following right frontal lesion in a right-handed man. Brain 1959;82:186–202.
135. Shankweiler D. Effects of temporal lobe damage on perception of dichotically presented melodies. J Comp Physiol Psychol 1966;62:115–119.
136. Gordon HW, Bogen JE. Hemispheric lateralization of singing after intracarotid sodium amylobarbitone. J Neurol Neurosurg Psychiatry 1974;37:727–738.
137. Kinsella G, Prior M, Murray G. Singing ability after right and left sided brain damage. A research note. Cortex 1988;24:165–169.
138. Brust JCM. Music and language: musical alexia and agraphia. Brain 1980; 103:367–392.
139. Alajouanine T. Aphasia and artistic realization. Brain 1948;74:229–241.
140. Sergent J. Music, the brain and Ravel. TINS 1993;16:168–172.
141. Polk M, Kertesz A. Music and language in degenerative disease of the brain. Brain Cogn 1993;22:98–117.
142. Sparks R, Helm N, Albert M. Aphasia rehabilitation resulting from melodic intonation therapy. Cortex 1974;10:303–316.
143. Hécaen H, David M. Syndrome parietale traumatique: asymbolie tactile et hemisomatognosie paroxystique et douloureuse. Rev Neurol (Paris) 1945;77:113–123.
144. Semmes J. A non-tactual factor in astereognosis. Neuropsychologia 1965;3: 295–315.
145. Caselli RJ. Rediscovering tactile agnosia. Mayo Clin Proc 1991;66:129–142.
146. Caselli RJ. Bilateral impairment of somesthetically mediated object recognition in humans. Mayo Clin Proc 1991;66:357–364.
147. Geschwind N, Kaplan E. A human deconnection syndrome. Neurology 1962; 12:675–685.
148. Sperry RW. Mental unity following surgical disconnection of the cerebral hemispheres. Harvey Lect 1966-67;62:293–323.
149. Beauvois MF, Saillant B, Meininger V, Lhermitte F. Bilateral tactile aphasia: a tacto-verbal dysfunction. Brain 1978;101:381–401.

Index

About the Editor

HOWARD S. KIRSHNER is Vice Chair of, and a Professor in, the Department of Neurology at Vanderbilt University School of Medicine, Nashville, Tennessee, and Director of Neurology at Vanderbilt Stallworth Rehabilitation Hospital, Nashville, Tennessee. The author, coauthor, or coeditor of several books and numerous book chapters and professional publications, Dr. Kirshner is a Fellow of the American Neurological Association and the American Academy of Neurology. He is also a member of the American Society of Neurorehabilitation, the Academy of Aphasia, the World Federation of Neurology Research Group on Aphasia and Cognitive Disorders, and the American Heart Association Stroke Council, among others. He is also a member of the medical and scientific advisory board, National Aphasia Association. Dr. Kirshner received the B.A. degree (1968) in biology from Williams College, Williamstown, Massachusetts, and the M.D. degree (1972) from the Harvard Medical School, Boston, Massachusetts.